Orthopaedic Knowledge Update®

OKU® 2
Musculoskeletal Infection

Orthopaedic Knowledge Update®

OKU® 2

Musculoskeletal Infection

EDITOR

M. Daniel Wongworawat, MD, FAAOS

Professor, Department of Orthopaedic Surgery
Loma Linda University Health
Loma Linda, California

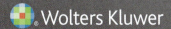

Philadelphia • Baltimore • New York • London
Buenos Aires • Hong Kong • Sydney • Tokyo

AAOS
American Academy of
Orthopaedic Surgeons

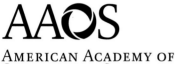

Board of Directors, 2023-2024

Kevin J. Bozic, MD, MBA, FAAOS
President

Paul Tornetta III, MD, PhD, FAAOS
First Vice President

Annunziato Amendola, MD, FAAOS
Second Vice President

Michael L. Parks, MD, FAAOS
Treasurer

Felix H. Savoie III, MD, FAAOS
Past President

Alfonso Mejia, MD, MPH, FAAOS
Chair, Board of Councilors

Joel L. Mayerson, MD, FAAOS
Chair-Elect, Board of Councilors

Michael J. Leddy III, MD, FAAOS
Secretary, Board of Councilors

Armando F. Vidal, MD, FAAOS
Chair, Board of Specialty Societies

Adolph J. Yates Jr, MD, FAAOS
Chair-Elect, Board of Specialty Societies

Michael P. Bolognesi, MD, FAAOS
Secretary, Board of Specialty Societies

Lisa N. Masters
Lay Member

Evalina L. Burger, MD, FAAOS
Member at Large

Chad A. Krueger, MD, FAAOS
Member at Large

Toni M. McLaurin, MD, FAAOS
Member at Large

Monica M. Payares, MD, FAAOS
Member at Large

Thomas E. Arend Jr, Esq, CAE
Chief Executive Officer (ex-officio)

Staff

American Academy of Orthopaedic Surgeons

Anna Salt Troise, MBA, *Chief Commercial Office*

Hans Koelsch, PhD, *Director, Publishing*

Lisa Claxton Moore, *Senior Manager, Editorial*

Steven Kellert, *Senior Editor*

Wolters Kluwer Health

Brian Brown, *Director, Medical Practice*

Tulie McKay, *Senior Content Editor, Acquisitions*

Stacey Sebring, *Senior Development Editor*

Janet Jayne, *Editorial Coordinator*

Erin Cantino, *Portfolio Marketing Manager*

Alicia Jackson, *Senior Production Project Manager*

Stephen Druding, *Manager, Graphic Arts & Design*

Margie Orzech-Zeranko, *Manufacturing Coordinator*

TNQ Technologies, *Prepress Vendor*

The material presented in the *Orthopaedic Knowledge Update®: Musculoskeletal Infection 2* has been made available by the American Academy of Orthopaedic Surgeons (AAOS) for educational purposes only. This material is not intended to present the only, or necessarily best, methods or procedures for the medical situations discussed, but rather is intended to represent an approach, view, statement, or opinion of the author(s) or producer(s), which may be helpful to others who face similar situations. Medical providers should use their own, independent medical judgment, in addition to open discussion with patients, when developing patient care recommendations and treatment plans. Medical care should always be based on a medical provider's expertise that is individually tailored to a patient's circumstances, preferences and rights. Some drugs or medical devices demonstrated in AAOS courses or described in AAOS print or electronic publications have not been cleared by the Food and Drug Administration (FDA) or have been cleared for specific uses only. The FDA has stated that it is the responsibility of the physician to determine the FDA clearance status of each drug or device he or she wishes to use in clinical practice and to use the products with appropriate patient consent and in compliance with applicable law. Furthermore, any statements about commercial products are solely the opinion(s) of the author(s) and do not represent an Academy endorsement or evaluation of these products. These statements may not be used in advertising or for any commercial purpose.

All rights reserved. No part of this publication may be reproduced, stored in a retrieval system, or transmitted, in any form, or by any means, electronic, mechanical, photocopying, recording, or otherwise, without prior written permission from the publisher. AAOS does not grant permission for AAOS-owned content to be ingested into any AI chatbot, unless approved.

ISBN 978-1-9752-0242-2

Library of Congress Control Number: Cataloging in Publication data available on request from publisher.

Printed in Mexico

Published 2025 by the American Academy of Orthopaedic Surgeons
9400 West Higgins Road
Rosemont, Illinois 60018

Copyright 2025 by the American Academy of Orthopaedic Surgeons

Acknowledgments

Editorial Board, Orthopaedic Knowledge Update®: Musculoskeletal Infection 2

Editor

M. Daniel Wongworawat, MD, FAAOS
Professor, Department of Orthopaedic Surgery
Loma Linda University Health
Loma Linda, California

Section Editors

Barry D. Brause, MD, FACP, FIDSA
Chief Emeritus
Division of Infectious Diseases
Department of Medicine
Hospital for Special Surgery
Attending Physician
New York Presbyterian Hospital
Professor of Clinical Medicine
Weill Medical College of Cornell University
New York, New York

Elie S. Ghanem, MD, FAAOS
Associate Professor
Department of Orthopedic Surgery
University of Missouri at Columbia
Columbia, Missouri

Brian A. Klatt, MD, FAAOS
Associate Professor
Chief, Division of Adult Reconstruction
Department of Orthopaedic Surgery
University of Pittsburgh
Pittsburgh, Pennsylvania

Sandra B. Nelson, MD
Associate Clinical Director
Division of Infectious Diseases
Massachusetts General Hospital
Assistant Professor
Harvard Medical School
Boston, Massachusetts

Aaron J. Tande, MD, FIDSA
Associate Professor of Medicine
Consultant, Division of Public Health, Infectious
  Diseases, and Occupational Medicine
Chair, Orthopedic Infectious Diseases Focus Group
Rochester, Minnesota

Charalampos G. Zalavras, MD, PhD, FAAOS, FACS
Professor, Department of Orthopaedic Surgery
University of Southern California
Los Angeles, California

Contributors

Serkan Akçay, MD
Attending, Orthopaedic Surgery and Traumatology
Department of Orthopaedic Surgery
Reyap Hospitals
Istanbul, Turkey

Keenan D. Atwood, MD
Department of Orthopaedics
West Virginia University School of Medicine
Morgantown, West Virginia

Maja Babic, MD
Assistant Professor
Department of Infectious Diseases
Cleveland Clinic Lerner College of Medicine
Cleveland Clinic
Cleveland, Ohio

Larry M. Baddour, MD, FIDSA, FAHA
Professor Emeritus
Division of Public Health, Infectious Diseases, and Occupational Medicine
Departments of Medicine and Cardiovascular Medicine
Mayo Clinic College of Medicine and Science
Rochester, Minnesota

Catalina Baez, MD
Postdoctoral Research Fellow
Department of Orthopaedic Surgery
University of Florida
Gainesville, Florida

Olivier Borens, MD
Professor, Bone and Motion Center
Clinic Bois-Cerf, Hirslanden
Lausanne, Switzerland

Victor R. Carlson, MD
Hip and Knee Fellow
OrthoCarolina
Charlotte, North Carolina

Laura Certain, MD, PhD
Clinical Associate Professor
Department of Medicine
University of Utah
Salt Lake City, Utah

Antonia F. Chen, MD, MBA, FAAOS
Associate Professor
Department of Orthopaedic Surgery
Harvard University
Brigham and Women's Hospital
Boston, Massachusetts

Niall Cochrane, MD
Department of Orthopaedics
Duke University
Durham, North Carolina

Lawson A. Copley, MD, MBA, FAAOS
Professor of Orthopaedic Surgery and Pediatrics
University of Texas Southwestern
Dallas, Texas

P. Maxwell Courtney, MD, FAAOS
Associate Professor
Department of Orthopaedic Surgery
Rothman Orthopaedics at Thomas Jefferson University
Philadelphia, Pennsylvania

Carl Deirmengian, MD, FAAOS
Professor, Rothman Orthopaedic Institute
Thomas Jefferson University
Philadelphia, Pennsylvania

Matthew J. Dietz, MD, FAAOS
Chair and Associate Professor
Department of Orthopaedics
West Virginia University School of Medicine
Morgantown, West Virginia

Bülent M. Ertuğrul, MD
Professor of Infectious Diseases and Clinical Microbiology
Department of Infectious Diseases
Reyap Hospitals
Istanbul, Turkey

Yale A. Fillingham, MD, FAAOS
Assistant Professor
Rothman Orthopaedic Institute
Thomas Jefferson University
Philadelphia, Pennsylvania

Contributors

Jonathon M. Florance, MD
Department of Orthopaedics
Duke University
Durham, North Carolina

Elie S. Ghanem, MD, FAAOS
Associate Professor
Department of Orthopedic Surgery
University of Missouri at Columbia
Columbia, Missouri

Jeremy M. Gililland, MD, FAAOS
Associate Professor
Department of Orthopaedic Surgery
University of Utah
Salt Lake City, Utah

Graham S. Goh, MD
Department of Orthopaedic Surgery
Boston University
Boston, Massachusetts

Sara F. Haddad, MD
Research Collaborator
Division of Public Health, Infectious Diseases, and Occupational Medicine
Department of Medicine
Mayo Clinic College of Medicine and Science
Rochester, Minnesota

Mark A. Haimes, MD, MS
Assistant Professor
Department of Orthopedic Surgery and Rehabilitation
University of Vermont
Burlington, Vermont

Michael W. Henry, MD
Associate Attending Physican
Department of Medicine
Hospital for Special Surgery
New York, New York

Noreen J. Hickok, PhD
Professor, Department of Orthopaedic Surgery
Thomas Jefferson University
Philadelphia, Pennsylvania

Carlos A. Higuera, MD
Chairman, Levitetz Department of Orthopaedic Surgery
Cleveland Clinic Florida
Weston, Florida

Joya-Rita Hindy, MD
Research Collaborator
Division of Public Health, Infectious Diseases, and Occupational Medicine
Department of Medicine
Mayo Clinic College of Medicine and Science
Rochester, Minnesota

Paul D. Holtom, MD
Adjunct Professor
Department of Medicine and Orthopaedics
Keck School of Medicine
University of Southern California
Los Angeles, California

Cole Howie, MD
Department of Internal Medicine
University of Iowa
Iowa City, Iowa

Jason E. Hsu, MD, FAAOS
Associate Professor
Department of Orthopaedics and Sports Medicine
University of Washington Medical Center
Seattle, Washington

Patrick Kelly, MD
Department of Orthopaedic Surgery
Duke University
Durham, North Carolina

Patrick J. Kellam, MD
Assistant Professor
Department of Orthopaedics
McGovern Medical School at The University of Texas Health Science Center at Houston
Houston, Texas

Jihye Kim, PharmD
Clinical Assistant Professor
Department of Pharmacy
Virginia Commonwealth University
Richmond, Virginia

Randall Marcus, MD, FAAOS
Professor, Department of Orthopaedic Surgery
Case Western Reserve University School of Medicine
Cleveland, Ohio

Willem-Jan Metsemakers, MD, PhD
Professor, Department of Trauma Surgery
University Hospitals Leuven
Leuven, Belgium

Andy O. Miller, MD
Associate Attending Physician
Department of Medicine
Hospital for Special Surgery
New York, New York

Sandra B. Nelson, MD
Associate Clinical Director
Division of Infectious Diseases
Assistant Professor
Harvard Medical School
Massachusetts General Hospital
Boston, Massachusetts

William T. Obremskey, MD, MPH, MMHC, FAAOS
Professor, Department of Orthopaedic Surgery
Vanderbilt University Medical Center
Nashville, Tennessee

Michael J. O'Malley, MD, FAAOS
Assistant Professor, University of Pittsburgh
Director of Education, UPMC Adult Reconstruction Fellowship
Department of Orthopaedic Surgery, UPMC
Pittsburgh, Pennsylvania

Tejbir S. Pannu, MD, MS
Orthopaedic Surgery Research Fellow
Levitetz Department of Orthopaedic Surgery
Cleveland Clinic Florida
Weston, Florida

Javad Parvizi, MD, FAAOS, FRCS
Professor of Orthopaedic Surgery
Department of Orthopaedic Surgery
Rothman Orthopaedic Institute
Philadelphia, Pennsylvania

Michael J. Patzakis, MD, FAAOS
Professor Emeritus
Department of Orthopaedic Surgery
University of Southern California
Los Angeles, California

Luis Pulido, MD
Orthopaedic Surgeon
North Central Florida Division of Florida Orthopaedic Institute
Gainesville, Florida

Jakrapun Pupaibool, MD, MS
Clinical Associate Professor
Department of Medicine
University of Utah
Salt Lake City, Utah

Noah J. Quinlan, MD
Department of Orthopaedic Surgery and Sports Medicine
Bassett Healthcare
Cooperstown, New York

James P. Reynolds, MD
Spine Fellow
OrthoCarolina
Charlotte, North Carolina

Julie E. Reznicek, DO
Associate Professor
Division of Infectious Diseases
Virginia Commonwealth University
Richmond, Virginia

William J. Rubenstein, MD
Orthopaedic Surgeon
Orthopaedic Arthroplasty Attending
Sports Medicine North
Peabody, Massachusetts

Jessica L. Seidelman, MD, MPH
Assistant Professor
Department of Medicine
Duke University
Durham, North Carolina

Parham Sendi, MD
Professor, Department of Infectious Diseases
Institute for Infectious Diseases
University of Bern
Bern, Switzerland

Thorsten M. Seyler, MD, PhD, FAAOS
Associate Professor
Department of Orthopaedics
Duke University
Durham, North Carolina

Claus S. Simpfendorfer, MD
Assistant Professor
Department of Diagnostic Radiology
Cleveland Clinic Lerner College of Medicine
Cleveland Clinic
Cleveland, Ohio

Contributors

John Sontich, MD, FAAOS
Associate Professor
Department of Orthopaedic Surgery
Case Western Reserve University School of Medicine
Cleveland, Ohio

Alex Soriano, MD
Department of Infectious Diseases
Clinic Hospital
Barcelona, Spain

Taylor Stauffer, BS
Medical Student
Duke University School of Medicine
Durham, North Carolina

Milan Stevanovic, MD, PhD, FAAM
Professor, Department of Orthopaedics
Keck School of Medicine of USC
Los Angeles, California

Paul Stoodley, PhD, FAAM
Professor, Departments of Microbial Infection and Immunity
The Ohio State University
Columbus, Ohio

Don Bambino Geno Tai, MD, MBA
Assistant Professor
Division of Infectious Diseases and International Medicine
University of Minnesota
Minneapolis, Minnesota

Saad Tarabichi, MD
Postdoctoral Research Fellow
Department of Orthopaedic Surgery
Rothman Orthopaedic Institute
Philadelphia, Pennsylvania

Alexander M. Tatara, MD, PhD
Clinical Staff
Division of Infectious Diseases
Massachusetts General Hospital
Boston, Massachusetts

Isaac P. Thomsen, MD, MSCI
Associate Professor
Pediatric Infectious Diseases
Vanderbilt University Medical Center
Monroe Carell, Jr. Children's Hospital at Vanderbilt
Nashville, Tennessee

Ilker Uçkay, MD
Titular Professor
Head of Infectious Diseases, Head of Clinical Research
Service of Infectious Diseases and Infection Control
Department of Orthopedic Surgery
Balgrist University Hospital
University of Zurich
Zurich, Switzerland

Kenneth L. Urish, MD, PhD, FAAOS, FAOA
Associate Professor
Department of Orthopaedic Surgery and Bioengineering
University of Pittsburgh
Pittsburgh, Pennsylvania

M. Daniel Wongworawat, MD, FAAOS
Professor, Department of Orthopaedic Surgery
Loma Linda University
Loma Linda, California

Marjan Wouthuyzen-Bakker, MD, PhD
Internist-Infectiologist
Department of Medical Microbiology and Infection Prevention
University Medical Center Groningen
University of Groningen
Groningen, The Netherlands

Charalampos G. Zalavras, MD, PhD, FAAOS, FACS
Professor, Department of Orthopaedic Surgery
University of Southern California
Los Angeles, California

Preface

Orthopaedic Knowledge Update®: Musculoskeletal Infection 2 is a comprehensive and updated guide to the diagnosis, prevention, and management of musculoskeletal infection, a complex and challenging problem that affects millions of people around the world. Musculoskeletal infection can cause severe complications for patients, their families, and the healthcare system, and it requires a multidisciplinary approach involving surgeons, infectious disease specialists, and basic scientists.

This book aims to provide a comprehensive and up-to-date overview of the current knowledge and best practices in the diagnosis, prevention, and treatment of musculoskeletal infection. Because the first edition of this book was published by AAOS in 2009, all chapters in this second edition have been newly written to reflect the recent advances in the field.

The first section discusses general aspects of musculoskeletal infection, such as epidemiology, risk factors, and risk reduction strategies. It also explores the basic science of infection, including diagnostic biomarkers and methods, microbiology of pathogens, biofilm biology, and irrigation solutions and techniques.

With recent advances in antibiotic therapy, an entire section is devoted to this topic. An in-depth review of antibiotic therapy is presented, covering general principles, local and systemic delivery, and specific considerations for different types of bone and joint infections. It also discusses the role of long-term antibiotic suppression in some cases.

The second half of the book addresses clinical scenarios of musculoskeletal infection—prosthetic joint infections, fracture-related infections, and other bone and joint and soft-tissue infections, including pediatric infections, hand and foot infections, spine infections, and necrotizing fasciitis. Chapters discuss the latest advances in diagnosis, surgical treatment, and antibiotic therapy for these conditions.

The editors and authors hope that this book will be a useful resource for residents, fellows, and practitioners who aim to provide optimal professional care to patients with musculoskeletal infection.

M. Daniel Wongworawat, MD, FAAOS
Editor

Contents

Section 1: General Considerations

SECTION EDITOR
Elie S. Ghanem, MD, FAAOS

Chapter 1
The Epidemiology of Musculoskeletal Infections 3
Cole Howie, MD
Elie S. Ghanem, MD, FAAOS

Chapter 2
Local Patient Risk Factors 11
Matthew J. Dietz, MD, FAAOS
Keenan D. Atwood, MD

Chapter 3
Systemic Patient Risk Factors 21
Tejbir S. Pannu, MD, MS
Carlos A. Higuera, MD

Chapter 4
Operating Room Environmental Risk Factors 31
Graham S. Goh, MD
Yale A. Fillingham, MD, FAAOS

Chapter 5
Perioperative Strategies to Reduce Surgical Site Infection 41
Jeremy M. Gililland, MD, FAAOS
Victor R. Carlson, MD
Patrick J. Kellam, MD
James P. Reynolds, MD

Chapter 6
Patient Optimization for Infection Prevention 47
Catalina Baez, MD
Luis Pulido, MD

Section 2: Basic Science

SECTION EDITOR
Barry D. Brause, MD, FACP, FIDSA

Chapter 7
General Diagnostics 61
Carl Deirmengian, MD, FAAOS
Yale A. Fillingham, MD, FAAOS
P. Maxwell Courtney, MD, FAAOS

Chapter 8
Microbiology of Musculoskeletal Infections 69
Michael W. Henry, MD
Andy O. Miller, MD

Chapter 9
Biofilm 81
Noreen J. Hickok, PhD
Kenneth L. Urish, MD, PhD, FAAOS, FAOA
Paul Stoodley, PhD, FAAM

Chapter 10
Irrigants and Irrigation 91
Antonia F. Chen, MD, MBA, FAAOS
William J. Rubenstein, MD

Section 3: Antibiotics

SECTION EDITOR
Sandra B. Nelson, MD

Chapter 11
Antibiotics: General Principles of Use in Orthopaedic Infections........105
Julie E. Reznicek, DO
Jihye Kim, PharmD

Chapter 12
Local Antibiotic Delivery Methods........................115
Niall Cochrane, MD
Taylor Stauffer, BS
Jonathon M. Florance, MD
Patrick Kelly, MD
Thorsten M. Seyler, MD, PhD, FAAOS

Chapter 13
Systemic Antibiotic Therapy.........129
Jessica L. Seidelman, MD, MPH
Marjan Wouthuyzen-Bakker, MD, PhD
Alex Soriano, MD

Chapter 14
Long-Term Antibiotic Suppression ...143
Alexander M. Tatara, MD, PhD
Sandra B. Nelson, MD

Section 4: Prosthetic Joint Infections

SECTION EDITOR
Brian A. Klatt, MD, FAAOS

Chapter 15
Diagnosis of Prosthetic Joint Infection..........................155
Saad Tarabichi, MD
Javad Parvizi, MD, FAAOS, FRCS

Chapter 16
Surgical Treatment of Hip and Knee Prosthetic Joint Infections.....165
Mark A. Haimes, MD, MS
Michael J. O'Malley, MD, FAAOS

Chapter 17
Surgical Management of Prosthetic Joint Infection of the Shoulder.......181
Noah J. Quinlan, MD
Jason E. Hsu, MD, FAAOS

Chapter 18
Antibiotic Treatment of Prosthetic Joint Infections....................195
Laura Certain, MD, PhD
Jakrapun Pupaibool, MD, MS

Section 5: Fracture-Related Infections

SECTION EDITOR
Charalampos G. Zalavras, MD, PhD, FAAOS, FACS

Chapter 19
Definition, Diagnosis, and Socioeconomic Effect of Fracture-Related Infections........ 209
Willem-Jan Metsemakers, MD, PhD
William T. Obremskey, MD, MPH, MMHC, FAAOS

Chapter 20
Prevention of Infection in Open Fractures........................ 221
Michael J. Patzakis, MD, FAAOS
Charalampos G. Zalavras, MD, PhD, FAAOS, FACS

Chapter 21
Management of Fracture-Related Infections 229
Charalampos G. Zalavras, MD, PhD, FAAOS, FACS
Paul D. Holtom, MD
John Sontich, MD, FAAOS
Randall Marcus, MD, FAAOS

Section 6: Bone, Joint, and Soft-Tissue Infections

SECTION EDITOR
Aaron J. Tande, MD, FIDSA

Chapter 22
Pediatric Musculoskeletal Infections   243
Isaac P. Thomsen, MD, MSCI
Lawson A. Copley, MD, MBA, FAAOS

Chapter 23
Septic Arthritis in Adults.   253
Don Bambino Geno Tai, MD, MBA
Olivier Borens, MD
Parham Sendi, MD

Chapter 24
Diabetic Foot Infections   263
Bülent M. Ertuğrul, MD
Serkan Akçay, MD
İlker Uçkay, MD

Chapter 25
Hand Infections   273
M. Daniel Wongworawat, MD, FAAOS
Milan Stevanovic, MD, PhD

Chapter 26
Infections of the Spine 281
Maja Babic, MD
Claus S. Simpfendorfer, MD

Chapter 27
Necrotizing Fasciitis and Other Complicated Skin and Soft-Tissue Infections 293
Joya-Rita Hindy, MD
Sara F. Haddad, MD
Larry M. Baddour, MD, FIDSA, FAHA

Index 307

SECTION 1

General Considerations

Section Editor:
Elie S. Ghanem, MD, FAAOS

CHAPTER 1

The Epidemiology of Musculoskeletal Infections

COLE HOWIE, MD • ELIE S. GHANEM, MD, FAAOS

ABSTRACT

As people live longer, in combination with increased morbidity and medical complexity, the projected trends suggest an increasing demand for elective and nonelective orthopaedic procedures with associated complications, including surgical site infection. The rate of surgical site infection after surgery, organism profile, and the organisms' evolving antibiotic resistance patterns can differ according to patient demographics, anatomic location, procedure performed, and several other confounding variables, creating a difficult scenario for all specialists involved in treating the infection. The patient faces high risk of treatment failure irrespective of treatment type, with burdensome and life-changing economic and social effects that can directly affect quality of life.

Keywords: economics; organism profile; prevalence; quality of life; surgical site infection

INTRODUCTION

Surgical site infections (SSIs) are devastating complications that may occur following elective orthopaedic surgery or a traumatic event. Rates of SSI vary across procedures and anatomic locations, which include primary joint arthroplasty (0.5% to 2%),[1] revision arthroplasty (3% to 9%),[2,3] fracture open reduction and internal fixation (ORIF) (1% to 5%),[4] and spine surgery (3.1%).[5] Treatment options across all specialties generally range from débridement, antibiotics, and implant retention[6] to staged revision surgery,[7] fusions, or even amputations for recalcitrant cases.[8] The natural history of SSI and subsequent treatment with a prolonged antibiotic course and recovery with extensive rehabilitation can be debilitating and costly for the patient, leading to disabilities and restricted activities, direct financial costs for treatment, indirect costs due to missed work or potential unemployment, and mental health burdens.[9] The hospital and health care workers also incur financial burdens consequent to repeated treatment strategies for recurrent infections with consequent readmissions and complications.[10] The patient's quality of life (QoL) can be greatly challenged by a musculoskeletal infection, affecting both the patient's physical and mental health with potential for irreversible disability compared with their initial functional state after the index procedure.[11,12]

PREVALENCE

The number of total hip arthroplasty (THA) and total knee arthroplasty (TKA) procedures performed each year is expected to increase by 2030, with a subsequent rise in incidence of prosthetic joint infections (PJI) thereafter.[13] The annual rate of PJI in the literature ranges anywhere from 0.5% to 2%[1] after primary total joint arthroplasty (TJA) and up to 7.0% after revision surgery.[14] The American Joint Replacement Registry 2020 Annual Report showed a steady increase in the rate of TKA revisions performed because of PJI since 2013 before peaking at 29.9% and subsequently dropping to 27.2% between 2019 and 2020 with similar findings reported for revision THA.[15]

Although total shoulder arthroplasty is performed less frequently than THA and TKA, their infection rates are

---

Dr. Ghanem or an immediate family member serves as a paid consultant to or is an employee of Symcel and has stock or stock options held in PSI. Neither Dr. Howie nor any immediate family member has received anything of value from or has stock or stock options held in a commercial company or institution related directly or indirectly to the subject of this chapter.

comparable and can reach up to 3%.[16] Similarly, the Mayo Clinic's Total Joint Registry found hemiarthroplasties to have a 1% infection rate[17] with approximately 98% infection-free survival rates at 5-, 10-, and 20-year follow-up. In contrast, reverse total shoulder arthroplasty performed on more complex cases showed a higher incidence of PJI, reportedly 3% to 4% in a 2020 study.[18] Another 2020 study reported that, of arthroplasty surgeries, total elbow arthroplasty (TEA) is the least commonly performed but has one of the highest postoperative infection rates of 3% to 8%; PJI comprised 43.5% of their primary TEA failures.[19]

A 2020 meta-analysis of spine surgeries found the prevalence of SSIs to be 3.1%, with superficial and deep SSI rates estimated at 1.4% and 1.7%, respectively.[5] This analysis concluded that the highest incidence of SSI was present in patients with neuromuscular scoliosis undergoing corrective deformity surgery (13%).[5] SSI rates for spinal deformity correction have been estimated at an overall rate of 1.2%, with kyphosis corrections reaching up to 2.4% compared with scoliosis and spondylolisthesis deformities (both 1.1%, $P < 0.0001$).[20] Similarly, SSI rates differ with the surgical approach used; a posterior-based approach (5.0%) has higher infection risk than an anterior-based approach (2.3%), and infection is less likely to develop after noninstrumented surgeries compared with instrumented surgeries (1.4% versus 4.4%).[5]

Infection rates are relatively higher for skeletal trauma surgeries, ranging from 1% to 4%, which is attributed to the injury mechanism disrupting the soft-tissue envelope, leading to potential contamination.[4] The anatomic location of the fracture plays a significant role in the incidence of fracture-related infection (FRI), with fractures of the elbow (6.6%), tibial plateau (7.6%), and tibial shaft (8.7%) occurring most often.[21] Open fractures are known to have an increased risk of FRI compared with closed fractures, with increasing frequency according to the Gustilo-Anderson classification, where type I, II, and III open fractures have zero to 2%, 2% to 12%, and 10% to 50% risk, respectively.[22]

ORGANISM PROFILE

Successfully treating a postoperative infection is heavily reliant on isolating the offending microbe at the surgical site and determining its antibiotic susceptibility, especially with the emergence of evolving drug-resistant organisms. The organism profile has been extensively described in TJA infection[23,24] (**Figure 1**). The most common culprit of TJA PJI is *Staphylococcus* species, with the incidence of *Staphylococcus epidermidis* (coagulase-negative staphylococci, CoNS) ranging between 20% and 35% and *Staphylococcus aureus* (including methicillin-sensitive *S aureus* and methicillin-resistant *S aureus* [MRSA]) from 8.5% to 21% for early-onset and late-onset infections.[24,25]

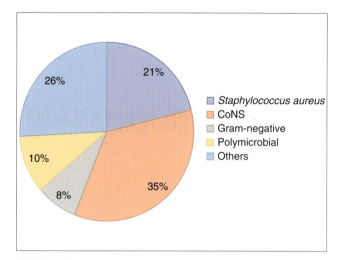

FIGURE 1 Graph showing the organism profile of bacteria commonly isolated from total hip arthroplasty and total knee arthroplasty prosthetic joint infection. CoNS = coagulase-negative staphylococci

CoNS and *Enterococcus faecalis* were found to be paired most frequently as copathogens in polymicrobial PJIs.[24] However, gram-negative and anaerobic pathogens are three times more likely to be in the mix of polymicrobial PJIs compared with gram-positive pathogens.[23] Anaerobic bacteria have been isolated in 3% to 6% of PJIs,[26] including *Cutibacterium* species, that are isolated more commonly in late infections.[27] Fungal organisms, although rare, have been reported in 1% of PJIs, with *Candida* being the most frequently identified pathogen.[28] Culture-negative infections occur in cases of high clinical suspicion of PJI with no culprit organism isolated and constitute 11% of infections but have no correlation with infection chronicity (acute versus chronic), implant type used, or antibiotic administration.[25] Culture-negative cases could be attributed to organisms that are challenging to culture in the laboratory or are rare pathogens not commonly isolated using routine culture methods, including *Coxiella burnetii*, *Brucella*, *Bartonella*, *Mycoplasma*, and mycobacterial and/or some fungal pathogens.[28]

The organisms causing PJI and their distinct profile, however, differ according to the anatomic location (**Figure 2**). A systematic review of shoulder PJI concluded that *Cutibacterium acnes* was the most frequent isolate, appearing in 38.9% of shoulder PJIs, followed by CoNS and *S aureus* in 14.8% and 14.5% of cases, respectively.[29] Other organisms that have been isolated in shoulder PJIs included *Enterobacter* (5.9%), *Finegoldia magna* (5.9%), and *Escherichia coli* (6.3%).[30] Polymicrobial infections occur in 11% of shoulder PJIs, whereas culture-negative cases are also relatively common, occurring in 5% to 15% of cases.[30] The literature on TEA microbiologic profile is scarce but shows a similar pattern of high CoNS prevalence (49%) followed by *S aureus* (12%).[31]

Chapter 1: The Epidemiology of Musculoskeletal Infections

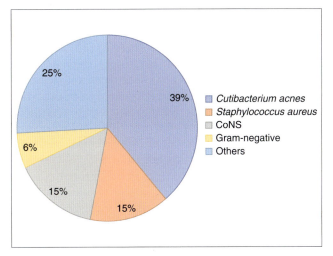

FIGURE 2 Graph showing the organism profile of bacteria commonly isolated from shoulder arthroplasty prosthetic joint infection. CoNS = coagulase-negative staphylococci

A 2020 meta-analysis also studied the prevalence of isolated organisms in spine surgery and found that the organism profile in the spine is similar to that of TJA, with most SSIs attributed to *S aureus* (37.9%) and CoNS (22.7%)[5] (**Figure 3**). Less-frequent organisms identified were *Escherichia* (13%), *Acinetobacter* (10%), *Klebsiella* (8.3%), *Enterococcus* (8.2%), and *Streptococcus* species (6.9%). Interestingly, one study found that approximately 18% of patients undergoing elective anterior cervical diskectomy and fusion had a subclinical infection in the cervical intervertebral disk, with *C acnes* constituting most bacteria.[32] Another study reported that *C acnes* was found to be the most common pathogen in patients who underwent spinal fusion, with late infections manifesting more than 1 year after surgery.[33]

FRIs are complex because of the nature of the trauma mechanism and environment, which creates variability in the microbiologic profile according to the anatomic location or severity of injury (**Figure 4**). *Staphylococcus* organisms are the most common offending organism isolated in FRIs (33.7% to 53.5%),[4,34] with *S aureus* present in 29% to 48%[34,35] and CoNS in 20% to 39%[36] of these patients. Other gram-positive pathogens present in FRI cases include *Streptococcus* and *Enterococcus* species.[35,36] *Enterobacter* species are the most common pathogens isolated from gram-negative monomicrobial FRIs (14% to 27%), whereas anaerobes and culture-negative FRIs make up 16% and 11% of infections, respectively.[36,37] Polymicrobial FRI rates have been reported to range from 14.3% to 57%,[34,38] with higher rates typically found in open fractures; pairings of *Enterobacter/Enterococci*, CoNS/*Enterobacter*, *Enterobacter/Serratia*, and CoNS/*Enterococci* were found to be most prevalent in these cases.[34] A 2018 study revealed that *S aureus* infections were more commonly isolated from FRIs after ORIF of closed fractures compared with open fractures (59% versus 41%, $P = 0.01$), whereas gram-negative organisms were more prevalent in FRIs that developed after treatment of open fractures (54% versus 46%, $P < 0.01$).[35]

RESISTANCE

The widespread use of antibiotics, especially in prophylactic settings, has introduced the emergence of antibiotic-resistant and multidrug-resistant bacterial species, with deaths related to treatment-resistant infection currently estimated to be 700,000 per year and projections estimated to spike to 10 million per year by 2050.[39] The incidence of treatment-resistant bacterial infections including MRSA and vancomycin-resistant *Enterococci*

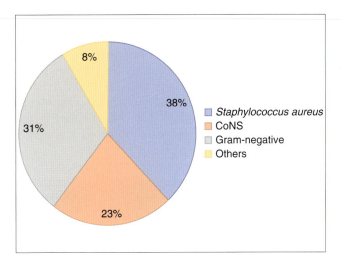

FIGURE 3 Graph showing the organism profile of bacteria commonly isolated from spine surgical site infection. CoNS = coagulase-negative staphylococci

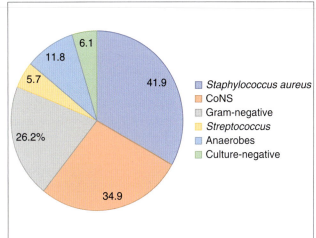

FIGURE 4 Graph showing the organism profile of bacteria commonly isolated from fracture-related infection. CoNS = coagulase-negative staphylococci

in PJI is increasing.[40] A 2018 review of TJA PJI reported that patients initially infected with a multidrug-resistant bacteria may subsequently acquire another treatment-resistant organism with further treatment strategies.[41]

Similarly, resistance to antibiotics used in preoperative prophylaxis is frequently encountered among patients undergoing spine surgery (up to 50% of cases).[42] The inciting resistant organism differs according to the location of surgery in which cefazolin-resistant enteric organisms (58.4% of SSIs) mostly affect the lower thoracic and lumbosacral spine, whereas methicillin-resistant gram-positive organisms (38.9% of SSIs) affect the cervical and upper thoracic spine.[42] Trauma patients are more likely to be in a catabolic state and therefore require longer stays in the intensive care unit and have higher exposure to treatment-resistant organisms. An FRI study found that speciation of at least one treatment-resistant organism occurred in 36% of infected patients, with 32% of the infections caused by MRSA and a smaller number caused by vancomycin-resistant *Enterococci* and multidrug-resistant organisms.[43] MRSA infections are isolated from 25% of open fractures, with a notable upward trend in incidence over time.[44]

ECONOMICS OF SSI

The cost of treating an increasing number of SSIs across all orthopaedic subspecialties places a major financial burden on both the patients and the healthcare industry. In the current healthcare setting, orthopaedic surgeons must recognize the financial burden SSIs impart and focus on delivering high-value surgical outcomes without compromising patient care. Alternative payment models such as the Bundled Payments for Care Improvement from the Centers for Medicare & Medicaid Services have been increasingly used to limit postoperative complications, including SSI, and generate greater value to the system, where the risk of patient complications and/or readmissions are shared with the hospital and clinician, during the entire care episode extending from the patient's admission through a 90-day postdischarge period for a certain diagnosis episode.[10]

For both THA and TKA PJI, costs can increase threefold to fourfold and take approximately twice as long to treat compared with matched patients without postoperative hip or knee PJI. The higher treatment costs of PJI are rooted in longer hospital stays, readmissions, longer course of antibiotic treatment, and extended rehabilitations postoperatively.[45] Treatment costs for TJA infections also vary according to the inciting organism: MRSA PJIs cost substantially more ($100,000) than methicillin-sensitive *S aureus* PJIs ($70,000) ($P < 0.001$).[46] Recent regression models project a national total cost of treatment for THA PJIs of $753.4 million and TKA PJIs to cost approximately $1.1 billion annually by 2030.[47]

Based on the limited data available, the average hospitalization cost to related to postoperative FRI is approximately $20,000, with potential to reach up to $100,000.[9,48] In addition, patients sustain an average income loss of $3,160 during the first year of treatment and accrue a loss of $6,080 per year starting 6 years posttreatment.[9] Taking inflation and FRI rates into account, lost earnings for all patients with FRI would exceed $1 billion per year. However, the window of opportunity to medically optimize trauma patients at higher risks for postoperative complications is nonexistent as in elective procedures. For example, patients undergoing nonelective joint arthroplasty because of trauma had a mean bundle payment loss of $23,122 with 91% of cases exceeding the target price, compared with bundled elective THA cases that generated an average $1,648 net profit per bundle ($P < 0.001$) and only 20% of cases going over target pricing ($P < 0.001$).[49]

Spine surgery also is negatively affected by the exuberant costs for treating SSI that can vary widely, dependent mostly on the procedure, with costs ranging from $16,000 to more than $300,000.[50,51] Treatment expenditures can reach up to 2.36 and 3.78 times higher for cervical and lumbar SSIs, respectively, compared with performing spine surgery for noninfectious etiologies.[51] The costs of treating shoulder arthroplasty PJI are staggering, with higher expenditures attributed to longer length of hospital stay, implant costs, medications, and various clinical tests required.[52] The average cost of treating a TEA PJI with two-stage exchange revision surgery has been reported to be on average twice as much as a primary TEA and 87% higher compared with the cost of revising a TEA for aseptic etiologies.[53]

QUALITY OF LIFE

Little is known about the effect of SSIs on a patient's long-term QoL. One study found that PJI after THA has a negative effect on QoL, including lower EuroQol-5 Dimension-5 Level index score and increased requirements for assisted living and walking aids compared with matched control patients with minimum 10-year follow-up.[54] A systematic review found similar findings in patients who underwent two-stage revision for hip PJI who had substantially lower physical QoL scores but mental health scores comparable with those of the general population after treatment.[55] Recurrence of PJI after treatment predisposes reinfected patients to lower health-related QoL scores compared with patients with successful treatment and no reinfections.[56] However, PJI successfully managed with débridement, antibiotics, and implant retention was not a significant risk factor for poor QoL, but patients sustained similar improvements in 12-Item Short Form scores from prearthroplasty to 12 months postarthroplasty compared with patients in whom PJI did not develop.[11]

Trauma patients who undergo ORIF of a tibial plateau fracture and in whom SSI develops are at higher risk for significantly poorer overall Knee Injury and Osteoarthritis Outcome Score and subscores for pain, activities of daily living, and QoL compared with patients without SSI.[57] Although vertebral osteomyelitis has a high mortality rate and leads to functional disability, surgical treatment leads to significantly improved QoL that remains well below the QoL levels of the general population.[58]

SUMMARY

SSIs are devastating complications that may occur following elective and nonelective orthopaedic surgery. Revision TJA and ORIF for open fractures have one of the highest rates of infection. Most orthopaedic infections are caused by *S aureus* and CoNS organisms except for shoulder arthroplasty infections, which are mostly attributed to *C acnes*. Polymicrobial infection with gram-negative organisms such as *Enterobacter* is isolated frequently from FRI cases after index ORIF of open fractures. Antibiotic-resistant SSIs, including MRSA and vancomycin-resistant enterococci, are becoming increasingly prevalent across different orthopaedic procedures. The cost to treat orthopaedic SSIs is at least double the cost of the index surgery across all subspecialties, with the major cost drivers including readmissions and extended length of hospital stay. Overall, orthopaedic infections even after treatment have a lifelong negative effect on patients' QoL and can diminish functionality with associated long-term disability.

KEY STUDY POINTS

- Prosthetic joint infections range from 0.5% to 3% of cases, with rates reaching up to 8% in elbow arthroplasty.
- The rate of FRIs is 1% to 4%, with much higher rates in open fractures.
- Most orthopaedic infections are caused by *Staphylococcus* species (*S aureus* and CoNS).
- Open fractures have higher rates of gram-negative and polymicrobial infections with *Enterobacter* species most prevalent in these cases.
- Antibiotic-resistant organisms are becoming increasingly prevalent in postoperative SSI.
- The cost of treating postoperative orthopaedic infections is more than double the cost of the primary index surgery, with the main drivers of cost including readmission, extended length of hospital stay, and prolonged antibiotic courses.
- Patients with postoperative infections can sustain loss of income and functionality, along with diminished QoL outcome scores.

ANNOTATED REFERENCES

1. Frank RM, Cross MB, della Valle CJ: Periprosthetic joint infection: Modern aspects of prevention, diagnosis, and treatment. *J Knee Surg* 2015;28(2):105-112.

2. Wickman JR, Goltz DE, Levin JM, Lassiter T, Anakwenze OA, Klifto CS: Early aseptic reoperation after shoulder arthroplasty increases risk of subsequent prosthetic joint infection. *JSES Int* 2021;5(6):1067-1071.

    This article analyzes the risk factors of infection after total shoulder arthroplasty procedures. The authors primarily look at infections that follow an aseptic revision of the shoulder prosthesis. Level of evidence: III.

3. Mortazavi SM, Schwartzenberger J, Austin MS, Purtill JJ, Parvizi J: Revision total knee arthroplasty infection: Incidence and predictors. *Clin Orthop Relat Res* 2010;468(8):2052-2059.

4. Motififard M, Teimouri M, Shirani K, Hatami S, Yadegari M: Prevalence of Bacterial surgical site infection in traumatic patients undergoing orthopedic surgeries: A cross-sectional study. *Int J Burns Trauma* 2021;11(3):191-196.

    This study assesses the rates of postoperative infection in orthopaedic patients. The authors also assess what specific organisms cause these postoperative infections.

5. Zhou J, Wang R, Huo X, Xiong W, Kang L, Xue Y: Incidence of surgical site infection after spine surgery: A systematic review and meta-analysis. *Spine (Phila Pa 1976)* 2020;45(3):208-216.

    This meta-analysis of postoperative spine infections analyzed 27 different studies. The article delves into specific causative organisms and infection rates for specific spine procedures. Level of evidence: III.

6. Morgenstern M, Kuehl R, Zalavras CG, et al: The influence of duration of infection on outcome of debridement and implant retention in fracture-related infection a systematic review and critical appraisal. *Bone Joint J* 2021;103-B(2):213-221.

    The purpose of this systematic review was to assess whether the timing of débridement had any effect on infection clearance in postoperative infections. Good success rates were noted when débridement was performed within 10 weeks and there was less success after 10 weeks.

7. Kunutsor SK, Wylde V, Beswick AD, Whitehouse MR, Blom AW: One- and two-stage surgical revision of infected shoulder prostheses following arthroplasty surgery: A systematic review and meta-analysis. *Sci Rep* 2019;9(1):232.

    This meta-analysis made comparisons on success rates between one-stage and two-stage revisions of shoulder prosthetic joint infections. The authors found that one-stage revisions were at least equally as successful as the traditional two-stage revisions.

8. Hungerer S, Kiechle M, von Rüden C, Militz M, Beitzel K, Morgenstern M: Knee arthrodesis versus above-the-knee amputation after septic failure of revision total knee arthroplasty: Comparison of functional outcome and complication rates. *BMC Musculoskelet Disord* 2017;18(1):443.

9. O'Hara NN, Mullins CD, Slobogean GP, Harris AD, Kringos DS, Klazinga NS: Association of postoperative infections after fractures with long-term income among adults. *JAMA Netw Open* 2021;4(4):e216673.

    This article sought to shed light on the indirect consequences of postoperative infections on patients. The authors found that patients experience significant income losses when dealing with postoperative infections.

10. Preston JS, Caccavale D, Smith A, Stull LE, Harwood DA, Kayiaros S: Bundled payments for care improvement in the private sector: A win for everyone. *J Arthroplasty* 2018;33(8):2362-2367.

    This study reported the benefits of bundle payment programs implemented at a joint arthroplasty practice. The driving factors of cost containment for total joint care episodes are outlined.

11. Aboltins C, Dowsey M, Peel T, Lim WK, Choong P: Good quality of life outcomes after treatment of prosthetic joint infection with debridement and prosthesis retention. *J Orthop Res* 2016;34(5):898-902.

12. Yagdiran A, Otto-Lambertz C, Lingscheid KM, et al: Quality of life and mortality after surgical treatment for vertebral osteomyelitis (VO): A prospective study. *Eur Spine J* 2021;30(6):1721-1731.

    This article looks into how patient QoL is affected during treatment for vertebral osteomyelitis. Although this condition is associated with high mortality rates, surgical treatment significantly improves the patient's QoL.

13. Sloan M, Premkumar A, Sheth NP: Projected volume of primary total joint arthroplasty in the U.S., 2014 to 2030. *J Bone Joint Surg Am* 2018;100(17):1455-1460.

    This study uses the National Inpatient Sample to project the future anticipated volume of TJA, and seeks to provide a better understanding of more predictive models to guide future practice needs.

14. Illingworth KD, Mihalko WM, Parvizi J, et al: How to minimize infection and thereby maximize patient outcomes in total joint arthroplasty: A multicenter approach – AAOS exhibit selection. *J Bone Joint Surg Am* 2013;95(8):e50.

15. Springer BD, Levine BR, Golladay GJ: Highlights of the 2020 American Joint Replacement Registry Annual Report. *Arthroplasty Today* 2021;9:141-142.

    This report by the American Joint Replacement Registry discusses the recent trends in how many surgeries are performed and for what purposes by joint replacement surgeons. The report outlines how many revision surgeries are performed because of PJIs on an annual basis as well.

16. Nezwek TA, Dutcher L, Mascarenhas L, et al: Prior shoulder surgery and rheumatoid arthritis increase early risk of infection after primary reverse total shoulder arthroplasty. *JSES Int* 2021;5(6):1062-1066.

    This 2021 study looks into infections rates after reverse shoulder arthroplasty and the relevant risk factors that can place patients at a higher risk for subsequent infections. Level of evidence: III.

17. Singh JA, Sperling JW, Schleck C, Harmsen W, Cofield RH: Periprosthetic infections after shoulder hemiarthroplasty. *J Shoulder Elbow Surg* 2012;21(10):1304-1309.

18. Contreras ES, Frantz TL, Bishop JY, Cvetanovich GL: Periprosthetic infection after reverse shoulder arthroplasty: A review. *Curr Rev Musculoskelet Med* 2020;13(6):757-768.

    This systematic review looks at the current literature on periprosthetic infections after reverse shoulder arthroplasty and updated literature on the treatment and management of these infections.

19. DeBernardis DA, Horneff JG, Davis DE, Ramsey ML, Pontes MC, Austin LS: Revision total elbow arthroplasty failure rates: The impact of primary arthroplasty failure etiology on subsequent revisions. *J Shoulder Elbow Surg* 2020;29(2):321-328.

    This study seeks to understand the indications for revision elbow arthroplasty in light of the high rates of revision failures. The most common revision etiologies in this patient cohort were infections and aseptic loosening. Level of evidence: IV.

20. Shillingford JN, Laratta JL, Reddy H, et al: Postoperative surgical site infection after spine surgery: An update from the Scoliosis Research Society (SRS) morbidity and mortality database. *Spine Deform* 2018;6(6):634-643.

    This is a retrospective review of infection rates after spinal deformity correction surgeries and the organism profiles of these infections. Level of evidence: III.

21. Bachoura A, Guitton TG, Smith RM, Vrahas MS, Zurakowski D, Ring D: Infirmity and injury complexity are risk factors for surgical-site infection after operative fracture care. *Clin Orthop Relat Res* 2011;469(9):2621-2630.

22. O'Brien CL, Menon M, Jomha NM: Controversies in the management of open fractures. *Open Orthop J* 2014;8(1):178-184.

23. Tai DBG, Patel R, Abdel MP, Berbari EF, Tande AJ: Microbiology of hip and knee periprosthetic joint infections: A database study. *Clin Microbiol Infect* 2022;28(2):255-259.

    The authors of this article look at the organism profiles of prosthetic joint infections within a single institution. Organism prevalence rates were also categorized by procedure and by certain risk factors.

24. Flurin L, Greenwood-Quaintance KE, Patel R: Microbiology of polymicrobial prosthetic joint infection. *Diagn Microbiol Infect Dis* 2019;94(3):255-259.

    This article looks specifically into the causes of polymicrobial prosthetic joint infections, a much less common finding compared with monomicrobial infections in joint replacements. The authors analyze the components of polymicrobial infections and the organisms most commonly cultured.

25. Watanabe S, Kobayashi N, Tomoyama A, Choe H, Yamazaki E, Inaba Y: Clinical characteristics and risk factors for culture-negative periprosthetic joint infections. *J Orthop Surg Res* 2021;16(1):292.

    This study looks into cases of culture-negative prosthetic joint infections and what the diagnosis of an infection should look like in the setting of negative cultures. Risk factors of infection without positive cultures are also assessed, as is the rate of culture-negative infections.

26. Tande AJ, Patel R: Prosthetic joint infection. *Clin Microbiol Rev* 2014;27(2):302-345.

27. Renz N, Mudrovcic S, Perka C, Trampuz A: Orthopedic implant-associated infections caused by Cutibacterium spp. – A remaining diagnostic challenge. *PLoS One* 2018;13(8):e0202639.

    This article discusses *Cutibacterium* species causing prosthetic joint infections, especially in shoulder joint, along with how these organisms are cultured properly to best detect and diagnose infection.

28. Beam E, Osmon D: Prosthetic joint infection update. *Infect Dis Clin North Am* 2018;32(4):843-859.

    This review article provides a vital update on recent trends seen in prosthetic joint infections. Proper treatment and management of these infections is discussed.

29. Nelson GN, Davis DE, Namdari S: Outcomes in the treatment of periprosthetic joint infection after shoulder arthroplasty: A systematic review. *J Shoulder Elbow Surg* 2016;25(8):1337-1345.

30. Richards J, Inacio MC, Beckett M, et al: Patient and procedure-specific risk factors for deep infection after primary shoulder arthroplasty. *Clin Orthop Relat Res* 2014;472(9):2809-2815.

31. Flurin L, Greenwood-Quaintance KE, Esper RN, Sanchez-Sotelo J, Patel R: Sonication improves microbiologic diagnosis of periprosthetic elbow infection. *J Shoulder Elbow Surg* 2021;30(8):1741-1749.

    This article looks at the rates of prosthetic elbow infections and the common pathogens isolated. The primary purpose of the article is to assess the effectiveness of implant sonication cultures in the diagnosis of infections.

32. Bivona LJ, Camacho JE, Usmani F, et al: The prevalence of bacterial infection in patients undergoing elective ACDF for degenerative cervical spine conditions: A prospective cohort study with contaminant control. *Global Spine J* 2021;11(1):13-20.

    The purpose of this study was to determine the true rate of postoperative infections following anterior cervical diskectomy and fusion procedures. The study looked at the most common bacteria found in infections and causative risk factors.

33. Lagreca J, Hotchkiss M, Carry P, et al: Bacteriology and risk factors for development of late (greater than one year) deep infection following spinal fusion with instrumentation. *Spine Deform* 2014;2(3):186-190.

34. Gitajn I, Werth P, O'Toole RV, et al: Microbial interspecies associations in fracture-related infection. *J Orthop Trauma* 2022;36(6):309-316.

    This study analyzed the most common organisms encountered in FRIs. More specifically, the study looked at what pathogens would most likely be found together in polymicrobial infections. Level of evidence: IV.

35. Montalvo RN, Natoli RM, O'Hara NN, et al: Variations in the organisms causing deep surgical site infections in fracture patients at a Level I Trauma Center (2006-2015). *J Orthop Trauma* 2018;32(12):e475-e481.

    This study determined trends of pathogens in FRIs and how they changed over the course of 10 years. The study highlights the rising rates of treatment-resistant organisms such as MRSA in recent years. Level of evidence: III.

36. Depypere M, Morgenstern M, Kuehl R, et al: Pathogenesis and management of fracture-related infection – Author's reply. *Clin Microbiol Infect* 2020;26(5):652-653.

    This review article provides an update to diagnosing, treating, and managing FRIs. The authors highlight new international guidelines that have been put in place to help prevent and mitigate the risk of these devastating infections.

37. Kuehl R, Tschudin-Sutter S, Morgenstern M, et al: Time-dependent differences in management and microbiology of orthopaedic internal fixation-associated infections: An observational prospective study with 229 patients. *Clin Microbiol Infect* 2019;25(1):76-81.

    This study looks at the various types of pathogens and specific organisms that can be found in FRIs, along with the success rates of certain treatment strategies.

38. Rupp M, Baertl S, Walter N, Hitzenbichler F, Ehrenschwender M, Alt V: Is there a difference in microbiological epidemiology and effective empiric antimicrobial therapy comparing fracture-related infection and periprosthetic joint infection? A retrospective comparative study. *Antibiotics* 2021;10(8):921.

    The goal of this study was to identify trends in the organism profiles found in FRIs and the best ways to tackle these complications and compare with more common prosthetic joint infections.

39. O'Neill J: Antimicrobial resistance: Tackling a crisis for the health and wealth of nations. *Rev Antimicrob Resist* 2014. Available at: https://amr-review.org/sites/default/files/AMR%20Review%20Paper%20-%20Tackling%20a%20crisis%20for%20the%20health%20and%20wealth%20of%20nations_1.pdf.

40. Drago L, de Vecchi E, Cappelletti L, Mattina R, Vassena C, Romanò CL: Role and antimicrobial resistance of staphylococci involved in prosthetic joint infections. *Int J Artif Organs* 2014;37(5):414-421.

41. Siljander MP, Sobh AH, Baker KC, Baker EA, Kaplan LM: Multidrug-resistant organisms in the setting of periprosthetic joint infection – Diagnosis, prevention, and treatment. *J Arthroplasty* 2018;33(1):185-194.

    This study sheds light on the current trends of drug-resistant organisms causing prosthetic joint infections. Novel methods of circumventing antimicrobial organisms to effectively treat such patients are discussed.

42. Long DR, Bryson-Cahn C, Pergamit R, et al: 2021 Young Investigator Award Winner: Anatomic gradients in the microbiology of spinal fusion surgical site infection and resistance to surgical antimicrobial prophylaxis. *Spine (Phila Pa 1976)* 2021;46(3):143-151.

    This article underscores the importance of treatment-resistant organisms in the setting of postoperative spine infections. With more than half of the patient cohort resistant to prophylactic antibiotics, the threat of resistant organisms and the need to prevent such infections is emphasized.

43. Torbert JT, Joshi M, Moraff A, et al: Current bacterial speciation and antibiotic resistance in deep infections after operative fixation of fractures. *J Orthop Trauma* 2015;29(1):7-17.

44. Chen AF, Schreiber VM, Washington W, Rao N, Evans AR: What is the rate of methicillin-resistant staphylococcus aureus and gram-negative infections in open fractures? *Clin Orthop Relat Res* 2013;471(10):3135-3140.

45. Kapadia BH, McElroy MJ, Issa K, Johnson AJ, Bozic KJ, Mont MA: The economic impact of periprosthetic infections following total knee arthroplasty at a specialized tertiary-care center. *J Arthroplasty* 2014;29(5):929-932.

46. Parvizi J, Pawasarat IM, Azzam KA, Joshi A, Hansen EN, Bozic KJ: Periprosthetic joint infection: The economic impact of methicillin-resistant infections. *J Arthroplasty* 2010;25(6 suppl):103-107.

47. Premkumar A, Kolin DA, Farley KX, et al: Projected economic burden of periprosthetic joint infection of the hip and knee in the United States. *J Arthroplasty* 2021;36(5):1484-1489.e3.

    This article uses updated data from the National Inpatient Sample to project the number of joint procedures and subsequent infections that could be expected in the near future. The authors highlight the importance of orthopaedic surgeons preparing their future practices in anticipation of increased surgical demand.

48. Levy JF, Castillo RC, Tischler E, Huang Y, O'Hara NN: The cost of postoperative infection following orthopaedic fracture surgery. *Tech Orthop* 2020;35(2):124-128.

    The study aims to economically stratify postoperative orthopaedic infections based on the anatomic location.

49. Skibicki H, Yayac M, Krueger CA, Courtney PM: Target price adjustment for hip fractures is not sufficient in the bundled payments for care improvement initiative. *J Arthroplasty* 2021;36(1):47-53.

    This article looks at surgical reimbursement changes in light of new bundle payment programs. Discrepancies are noted in net reimbursements of joint replacements between elective and traumatic etiologies.

50. Blumberg TJ, Woelber E, Bellabarba C, Bransford R, Spina N: Predictors of increased cost and length of stay in the treatment of postoperative spine surgical site infection. *Spine J* 2018;18(2):300-306.

    This study looks at the drivers of increased costs in treating postoperative spine infections and their overall cost, along with patient-specific risk factors of cost in addition to hospital factors (ie, length of stay).

51. Daniels AH, Kawaguchi S, Contag AG, et al: Hospital charges associated with "never events": Comparison of anterior cervical discectomy and fusion, posterior lumbar interbody fusion, and lumbar laminectomy to total joint arthroplasty. *J Neurosurg Spine* 2016;25(2):165-169.

52. Padegimas EM, Maltenfort M, Ramsey ML, Williams GR, Parvizi J, Namdari S: Periprosthetic shoulder infection in the United States: Incidence and economic burden. *J Shoulder Elbow Surg* 2015;24(5):741-746.

53. Wagner ER, Ransom JE, Kremers HM, Morrey M, Sanchez-Sotelo J: Comparison of the hospital costs for two-stage reimplantation for deep infection, single-stage revision and primary total elbow arthroplasty. *Shoulder Elbow* 2017;9(4):279-284.

54. Helwig P, Morlock J, Oberst M, et al: Periprosthetic joint infection – Effect on quality of life. *Int Orthop* 2014;38(5):1077-1081.

55. Rietbergen L, Kuiper JW, Walgrave S, Hak L, Colen S: Quality of life after staged revision for infected total hip arthroplasty: A systematic review. *Hip Int* 2016;26(4):311-318.

56. Poulsen NR, Mechlenburg I, Søballe K, Lange J: Patient-reported quality of life and hip function after 2-stage revision of chronic periprosthetic hip joint infection: A cross-sectional study. *Hip Int* 2018;28(4):407-414.

    This article looks at different QoL metrics in patients treated for prosthetic joint infections. How scores may change on reinfection and subsequent revisions is investigated.

57. Henkelmann R, Glaab R, Mende M, et al: Impact of surgical site infection on patients' outcome after fixation of tibial plateau fractures: A retrospective multicenter study. *BMC Musculoskelet Disord* 2021;22(1):531.

    This article sought to assess patient QoL and function outcomes after treating postoperative infections stemming from tibial plateau fracture fixations. The authors found that functionality and QoL were greatly diminished for patients in whom infections developed compared with those with no infections after their fracture fixation.

58. Wildeman P, Rolfson O, Söderquist B, Wretenberg P, Lindgren V: What are the long-term outcomes of mortality, quality of life, and hip function after prosthetic joint infection of the hip? A 10-year follow-up from Sweden. *Clin Orthop Relat Res* 2021;479(10):2203-2213.

    The purpose of this article was to examine the long-term effects of patient QoL and functionality after prosthetic joint infections. The results of the study found that these factors were greatly diminished in patients with infection compared with those with no infection and with the general population. Level of evidence: III.

CHAPTER 2

Local Patient Risk Factors

MATTHEW J. DIETZ, MD, FAAOS • KEENAN D. ATWOOD, MD

ABSTRACT

There are numerous modifiable and nonmodifiable risk factors that must be considered before surgical intervention, which can affect the outcome of surgery, specifically the development of surgical site infections. Understanding the potential local bioburden and local risk factors present at the time of surgery can help inform surgeons how to best manage these complex patients to mitigate, if possible, the risk of surgical site infections. These risk factors include local skin/wound breakdown and ulceration, bacterial colonization, and prior trauma or surgery at or near the surgical site.

Keywords: colonization; gunshot wounds; local bacterial burden; prior surgery; skin breakdown

INTRODUCTION

Steps taken to prevent surgical site infection (SSI) and deep infection are of paramount importance, especially when considering the devastating effects these infections can have on patients' overall health and socioeconomic

---

Dr. Dietz or an immediate family member serves as a paid consultant to or is an employee of Guidepoint Consulting and Heraeus Medical; serves as an unpaid consultant to Peptilogics; has stock or stock options held in Peptilogics; and has received research or institutional support from Heraeus Medical USA and Peptilogics. Neither Dr. Atwood nor any immediate family member has received anything of value from or has stock or stock options held in a commercial company or institution related directly or indirectly to the subject of this chapter.

activity. The local surgical environment can be affected by the bacterial burden, skin colonization, skin breakdown, and prior surgeries/trauma at or near the surgical site. To reduce the risk of SSI, modification of the modifiable local risk factors is imperative, whereas the nonmodifiable risk factors pose a conundrum that warrants possible modification of the surgical procedure.

COLONIZATION WITH *STAPHYLOCOCCUS* SPECIES

A normal flora known as the human microbiome exists within the human body, but the microorganisms vary among patients and anatomic regions in each individual patient while often following geographic trends.[1] *Staphylococcus aureus* is the single most common bacterial pathogen responsible for skin and soft-tissue infections in North America, Latin America, and Europe.[1] *Pseudomonas aeruginosa*, *Enterococcus*, *Escherichia coli*, and *Klebsiella* are the next most common pathogens, but their incidence can vary depending on the geographic location of the hospital that the patient is receiving care at.[1] Staphylococci colonization in the nares has been reported in multiple studies to increase the risk of prosthetic joint infection (PJI), however it was not found to be an independent risk factor for infection.[2] Conversely, patients with nasal swabs positive for methicillin-resistant *S aureus* (MRSA) have a significantly higher risk of SSI than noncarriers.[3] A 2018 retrospective single-center review found a nasal colonization rate of 17.5% for methicillin-sensitive *S aureus* and 1.8% for MRSA, with risks for colonization attributed to diabetes, renal insufficiency, and immunosuppression.[4] Similarly, a 2020 review of the spine literature demonstrates increased relative risk (RR) of SSI (RR = 2.52) and MRSA-associated SSI (RR = 6.21) with positive

MRSA nasal colonization.[5] However, nasal colonization with methicillin-sensitive *S aureus* was not associated with an increased risk of SSI after spine surgery.[5] Other studies revealed similar results with increased rates of SSI following spine surgery when patients were colonized with MRSA compared with those who were colonized with methicillin-sensitive *S aureus* and no colonization.[6,7] Limited evidence exists in the setting of orthopaedic trauma procedures and the role of nasal colonization on postoperative SSI rate. However, some studies indicate an increased odds ratio (weighted OR, 9.9; 95% confidence interval [CI], 4.51-21.79) of SSI with a positive nasal swab.[8,9] Similarly, some studies in sports medicine have addressed this topic. Although one study reported high nasal (90%) and skin (46%) colonization rates, with coagulase-negative *Staphylococcus* as the most commonly identified organism, this has not translated into higher postoperative SSI rates.[10]

The potential for increased SSI risk in the setting of positive nasal colonization has led to the development of decolonization protocols before surgery. Some studies showed that institutional implementation of nasal decolonization programs has led to a decrease in staphylococcal SSI.[3,11,12] A meta-analysis showed that bundling both nasal decolonization and glycopeptide prophylaxis for MRSA carriers decreased SSI rates because of *S aureus* and gram-positive bacteria.[12] Although decolonization procedures have demonstrated a decreased risk for SSI in some studies, others have questioned the durability of decolonization because patients decolonized preoperatively are often recolonized after surgery.[13] Despite these rigorous decolonization protocols, it was reported that some patients remained colonized with MRSA, and in those recalcitrant cases, there was no difference in SSI rates postoperatively.[14]

BACTERIAL/FUNGAL SKIN BURDEN

The bacterial burden present on a patient varies considerably based on multiple factors including the patient's preexisting medical comorbidities.[4] Different areas of the body have different levels of bacterial burden where, for example, the ductal tissue around the periareolar region of the breast has greater bacterial load than the axilla, with the predominant bacteria being *Staphylococcus epidermidis* and *Cutibacterium acnes* (formerly *Propionibacterium acnes*). In a 2021 study, *C acnes* was often implicated in postoperative surgical shoulder infections.[15] A 2018 study and others have reported that regions of the body with a large number of sebaceous glands that can develop acne have been associated with shoulder arthroplasty SSI.[16,17] In the setting of trauma and fracture care, the presence of local bacterial load may influence wound and bone cultures obtained at the time of injury or definitive surgery, but there is little evidence associating this bioburden with postoperative complications including SSI.[18] Advances in next-generation sequencing can potentially shed light on this association and have generated new studies further exploring the effect of trauma, open fractures, and the interplay with the local microbial community on SSI rates.[19]

Skin conditions can also lead to an increased risk of infections because of increased local bacterial loads at or near the surgical site. Psoriasis and the associated psoriatic plaques have increased bacterial density compared with unaffected skin[20] and in some studies have been shown to increase the risk of PJI in total hip arthroplasty (THA).[20] Psoriasis is also thought to increase the risk of postoperative infection in elective foot and ankle surgery.[21] Patients with atopic dermatitis, defined as dryness, erythema, and pruritus, have increased rates of local colonization with *S aureus*, in which the more severe dermatitis cases and acute lesions have higher rates of colonization.[22]

Dermatophytosis, also known as tinea or ringworm, can act as a portal of entry for bacteria in the areas it is present, especially on the foot or inguinal crease. A 2018 study reported that fungal infections are rare but devastating orthopaedic complications can be exceptionally difficult to manage.[23] Reports of implant-related infections consequent to fungus-associated skin conditions are limited, although a 2022 case report highlights the concerns of dermatophytosis associated with relapsing osteomyelitis.[24]

SKIN LESIONS, BOILS, SKIN BREAKDOWNS, AND ULCERATIONS

Streptococci and staphylococci species are common causes of cutaneous infections.[25] Skin breakdown and ulceration after a skin lesion biopsy or excision have been shown to increase the risk of surgical wound infections especially in the setting of total joint arthroplasty (TJA)[26] (Figure 1). In addition, in 2018, it was reported that venous insufficiency ulcers and diabetic foot ulcers larger than 10 cm^2, with active exudate and sloughing, are all risks for postoperative infection.[27] Although there is a paucity of evidence associating skin ulceration and breakdown with increased SSI rates in other orthopaedic subspecialties, any skin openings or abnormalities should be fully evaluated and managed before surgical intervention, especially in elective cases.

PRIOR SURGERY IN JOINT/AREA

The anatomic location and extent of prior surgery at or near the surgical site that can vary from open reduction

Chapter 2: Local Patient Risk Factors

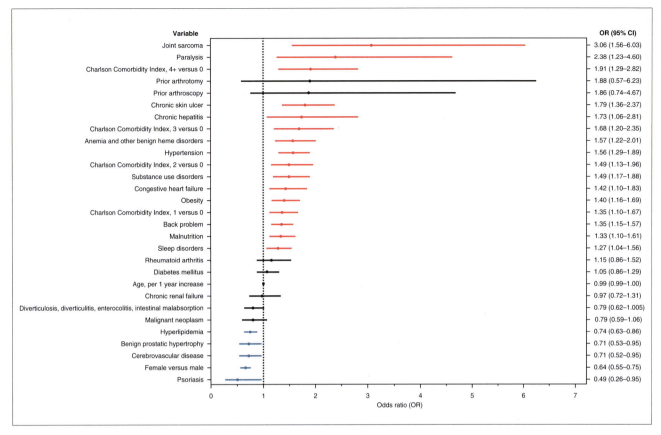

FIGURE 1 Graph showing the multivariate analysis of 147,053 patients undergoing primary total hip and knee arthroplasty, in which prosthetic joint infection (PJI) occurred in 0.5% of patients. The adjusted odds ratio of PJI increased with various skin conditions and prior surgery (CI = confidence interval). (Reprinted from Tande A, Asante D, Sangaralingham L, et al: Risk factors for early hip or knee prosthetic joint infection (PJI): Analysis of a nationwide American insurance claims dataset. *Open Forum Infect Dis* 2017;4(suppl 1):S5, by permission of Oxford University Press.)

and internal fixation (ORIF) to arthroscopic procedures have varying effects on SSI rates after definitive surgery, and in some scenarios, the data are inconclusive. Regarding the knee joint, prior trauma to the joint that leads to subsequent posttraumatic osteoarthritis can increase the risk of PJI after total knee arthroplasty (TKA) compared with TKA performed for primary knee osteoarthritis.[28] Similarly, previous ORIF around the knee with retention of hardware is associated with a significant risk factor for PJI after TKA.[29] In contrast, a 2018 study concluded that although the presence of retained hardware before a TKA in 55 patients increased the risk of postoperative mechanical complications, it did not significantly increase the risk of PJI.[30] A similar study found PJI rates of 0.9% when hardware was removed at the time of TKA after prior ORIF, which is similar to primary TKA PJI rates, therefore advocating performing these cases in a single-stage manner.[31] As described in a 2018 study, the extent of prior surgical intervention can play a key role in postoperative infections where wound complications including SSI were found to be higher in TKAs performed in patients who had undergone a previous ORIF for fracture versus patients who underwent previous knee arthroscopy for soft-tissue injury.[32] Other studies have analyzed the timing of a TKA after arthroscopy and the associated risk of postoperative infection. Studies have concluded that TKA performed within 6 months of arthroscopy can increase the risk of PJI[26,33] (**Figure 2**), whereas another study showed no difference in outcomes including PJI for TKA performed within 1 year of arthroscopy versus more than 1 year afterward.[34] Patients who underwent prior anterior cruciate ligament reconstruction have increased risks of revision surgeries after TKA for infection and other complications compared with patients without prior anterior cruciate ligament reconstruction.[32,35] A review of 35 patients who had undergone osteochondral allograft surgery concluded that this patient population is at increased risk of PJI after TKA, but it should be noted that infection developed only in two patients in the cohort and both had previously undergone multiple knee surgeries.[36]

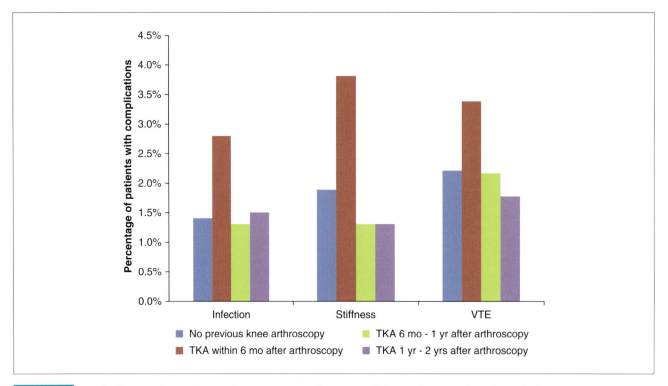

FIGURE 2 Graph showing the incidence of postoperative infection, stiffness, and venous thromboembolism (VTE) after total knee arthroplasty (TKA) with prior knee arthroscopy over specific intervals of time when compared with age-matched control patients. Patients undergoing TKA within 6 months of knee arthroscopy were at significant risk for all complications. (Reprinted from Werner BC, Burrus MT, Novicoff WM, Browne JA: Total knee arthroplasty within six months after knee arthroscopy is associated with increased postoperative complications. *J Arthroplasty* 2015;30[8]:1313-1316. Copyright 2015, with permission of Elsevier.)

Although the knee joint data show a predisposition to higher risk of infections after nonarthroscopic procedures, the hip joint literature is more conflicting and variable. Multiple studies have shown that hip arthroscopy does not increase the risk of infection after THA.[37] There has also been no increase in bacterial contamination for THA in patients who retained hardware from prior hip fracture surgery treated with intramedullary nail, screws, dynamic hip screws, or plates. In 2018, lack of bacterial contamination was evaluated with a preoperative hip aspirate and confirmed with intraoperative cultures.[38] The study also showed no increase in PJI, with only one deep infection in 109 patients.[39] Similar risks for infection were found in patients undergoing THA after rotational acetabular osteotomy compared with the respective control group.[40] Another study found that younger patients who had undergone prior hip salvage/preservation surgery such as pelvic and/or femoral osteotomies or core decompression were at increased risk of superficial infections after THA but no increase in deep infections compared with the control group.[38] In recent studies, patients undergoing a conversion THA after prior acetabular ORIF are at increased risk of PJI.[41,42] A 2022 study showed a PJI rate of 10.3% to 13.3% when hardware was retained in conversion THA after acetabular ORIF.[41] A 2020 retrospective study compared 72 conversion THAs after acetabular ORIF with 215 age-matched control patients and showed an increase in PJI rate of 6.9% compared with 0.5% in the control group.[42]

Prior shoulder surgery predisposes patients to higher risk of infection after total shoulder arthroplasty.[43] One retrospective study showed an increased risk for PJI in shoulder arthroplasty if prior shoulder surgeries such as rotator cuff repair, ORIF, and acromioplasty had been performed.[43] Another study showed that prior failed shoulder arthroplasty increased the risk of PJI for repeat shoulder arthroplasty.[44] Previous spine surgery, whether instrumented or not, has shown heterogenous results regarding infection risk after revision surgery. One study revealed that prior instrumentation has no effect on wound infection or complication rates after three-column osteotomy for thoracolumbar deformities.[45] In contrast, a 2022 report of patients undergoing spinal fusion with a history of retained hardware had increased infection rates and implant loosening compared with the control group.[46]

PRIOR LOCAL INFECTION

A history of prior superficial wound or deep infection at a surgical site can increase the 30-day risk of SSI after primary TJA (OR, 5.0 [95% CI, 2.3-10.9]).[47] Similarly, the risk of PJI after primary TJA increases to 10% if the patient had prior native septic joint.[48] A 2021 multicenter study evaluated risk factors for PJI in patients undergoing TJA who had a prior native septic joint and found that within this group, the risk of PJI after TJA increased in patients who had antibiotic-resistant organisms, who were male, or who had diabetes.[49] Both the timing of TJA from resolution of the initial septic joint infection and the number of prior surgeries to manage the initial infection can play a significant role in PJI development.[48,49] One study evaluated patients with a history of childhood septic hip who then subsequently underwent primary THA and found that all the patients in whom PJI developed had their THA performed within 10 years of them concluding treatment for the septic joint.[50] In contrast, another study concluded that the timing of TKA from resolution of the initial native knee infection was not a risk factor for PJI, but that the number of surgeries required to treat the septic knee was a predisposing factor (3.6 versus 1.6 prior surgeries, $P = 0.006$).[48] A 2021 retrospective study evaluating PJI after TJA in patients with prior septic arthritis revealed that serum markers and timing from septic arthritis to TJA did not affect rates of PJI.[51] A native septic joint can occur with or without concomitant osteomyelitis of surrounding bone and hence creates another level of complexity and poses challenges in preventing PJI after TJA. The presence of osteomyelitis in the setting of native septic joint has been shown to significantly increase the risk of PJI after TJA to approximately 15% compared with cases with isolated native septic joint infection.[52] Infections in other regions of the body distant to the surgical site including PJI of separate joints can increase the risk of PJI after a primary TJA.[53] The spine literature follows similar trends where two systematic reviews found that prior infections in the spine especially from prior surgery pose a significant risk for developing future SSIs along with modifiable risk factors including diabetes, smoking, and obesity.[54,55]

SKIN PREPARATION AND HAIR MANAGEMENT

It is a common practice to remove hair from surgical sites during skin preparation, which is often performed to aid in visualization and improve closure of the wound. However, randomized controlled studies, some of which have been underpowered, have produced conflicting data regarding the relationship between SSI and hair removal before surgery.[56,57] A 2021 study evaluated the different techniques for hair removal and concluded that using a razor increased the risk of SSI when compared with no hair removal, using clippers, or using depilatory cream, but there was no difference in SSI rates between clippers and depilatory cream compared with no hair removal.[56] Although definitive evidence is still lacking robustness for hair removal in mitigating SSI risk, hair removal from the surgical site can be performed outside of the operating room, with clippers or depilatory creams within a time frame that is reasonable and convenient before surgery.[56,57]

PREVIOUS GUNSHOT TRAUMA

Gunshot wounds (GSWs), especially intra-articular, often cause cartilage damage and may lead to posttraumatic osteoarthritis requiring TJA. Bacteria can be displaced from outside the body along the bullet track and into the joint, disproving previous concepts, including autosterilization of a bullet wound.[58] A similar study found that intra-articular low-velocity GSWs to the knee can track debris and bacteria into the joint, potentially serving as a nidus for infection.[59] The data regarding risk of SSI developing after GSW are conflicting. One study noted that posttraumatic osteoarthritis of the hip from a GSW did not increase the risk of PJI after THA,[60] whereas another study concluded that a severe GSW to the knee increased the risk of PJI.[61] GSW to the spine is associated with increased sepsis and SSI rates when colonic injury is involved, but retention of the bullet fragments does not appear to increase the likelihood of sepsis.[62] Recent studies that evaluated GSWs resulting in long bone fractures compared the complication rates of femoral fractures and tibial fractures after GSW with those of blunt trauma with open and closed femoral and tibial fractures and found that although the overall complication rates were higher for GSW, particularly compartment syndrome, the fracture-related infection risk was not significantly different.[63,64]

SUMMARY

The risk of SSI or PJI can be influenced by several local patient risk factors, some of which are modifiable including the colonization of the patient's skin and nares, changes in the overall local bacterial flora that can be influenced by prior surgeries or penetrating injuries, and prior infections at or near the surgical site. Steps to manage and mitigate these risks should be considered to reduce the risk of subsequent infection.

KEY STUDY POINTS

- Colonization with MRSA has been demonstrated to increase the risk of SSI.
- Bacterial colonization can vary depending on geography and anatomic location and is influenced by various skin conditions.
- Careful attention should be paid to local skin conditions such as ulcerations and lesions and dermatologic conditions that can increase the risk of SSI.
- Prior surgeries, GSWs, and history of infection at or near the surgical site can increase the risk of SSI.

ANNOTATED REFERENCES

1. Moet GJ, Jones RN, Biedenbach DJ, Stilwell MG, Fritsche TR: Contemporary causes of skin and soft tissue infections in North America, Latin America, and Europe: Report from the SENTRY Antimicrobial Surveillance Program (1998-2004). *Diagn Microbiol Infect Dis* 2007;57(1):7-13.

2. Maoz G, Phillips M, Bosco J, et al: The Otto Aufranc Award: Modifiable versus nonmodifiable risk factors for infection after hip arthroplasty. *Clin Orthop Relat Res* 2015;473(2):453-459.

3. Kim DH, Spencer M, Davidson SM, et al: Institutional prescreening for detection and eradication of methicillin-resistant Staphylococcus aureus in patients undergoing elective orthopaedic surgery. *J Bone Joint Surg Am* 2010;92(9):1820-1826.

4. Walsh AL, Fields AC, Dieterich JD, Chen DD, Bronson MJ, Moucha CS: Risk factors for Staphylococcus aureus nasal colonization in joint arthroplasty patients. *J Arthroplasty* 2018;33(5):1530-1533.

   This retrospective study of 716 patients undergoing TKA/THA found that 17.5% screened positive for MRSA. Diabetes, renal insufficiency, and immunosuppression were found to have increased the incidence of colonization and are known to be risk factors for infection. Level of evidence: III.

5. Ning J, Wang J, Zhang S, Sha X: Nasal colonization of Staphylococcus aureus and the risk of surgical site infection after spine surgery: A meta-analysis. *Spine J* 2020;20(3):448-456.

   A meta-analysis of seven studies including 10,650 patients who underwent nasal swab before spine surgery found that MRSA colonization is likely associated with increased risk of SSI and that decolonization may decrease this risk. Level of evidence: II.

6. Thakkar V, Ghobrial GM, Maulucci CM, et al: Nasal MRSA colonization: Impact on surgical site infection following spine surgery. *Clin Neurol Neurosurg* 2014;125:94-97.

7. Kobayashi K, Ando K, Ito K, et al: Prediction of surgical site infection in spine surgery from tests of nasal MRSA colonization and drain tip culture. *Eur J Orthop Surg Traumatol* 2018;28(6):1053-1057.

   Patients undergoing spinal instrumentation surgery had preoperative nasal swabs compared with wound drain cultures as a surrogate for SSI. Patients with nasal MRSA had higher rates of drain tip positive cultures. Level of evidence: II.

8. Wise BT, Connelly D, Rocca M, et al: A predictive score for determining risk of surgical site infection after orthopaedic trauma surgery. *J Orthop Trauma* 2019;33(10):506-513.

   This study created a predictive model using retrospective data and found that eight factors including male sex, obesity (body mass index >30 kg/m^2), diabetes, alcohol abuse, fracture region, Gustilo-Anderson type III open fracture, MRSA nasal swab testing (not tested or positive result), and the American Society of Anesthesiologists classification were found to correlate with increased risk of SSI. Level of evidence: III.

9. Berthelot P, Grattard F, Cazorla C, et al: Is nasal carriage of Staphylococcus aureus the main acquisition pathway for surgical-site infection in orthopaedic surgery? *Eur J Clin Microbiol Infect Dis* 2010;29(4):373-382.

10. Nakayama H, Yagi M, Yoshiya S, Takesue Y: Microorganism colonization and intraoperative contamination in patients undergoing arthroscopic anterior cruciate ligament reconstruction. *Arthroscopy* 2012;28(5):667-671.

11. Hacek DM, Robb WJ, Paule SM, Kudrna JC, Stamos VP, Peterson LR: Staphylococcus aureus nasal decolonization in joint replacement surgery reduces infection. *Clin Orthop Relat Res* 2008;466(6):1349-1355.

12. Schweizer M, Perencevich E, McDanel J, et al: Effectiveness of a bundled intervention of decolonization and prophylaxis to decrease Gram positive surgical site infections after cardiac or orthopedic surgery: Systematic review and meta-analysis. *BMJ* 2013;346:f2743.

13. Economedes DM, Deirmengian GK, Deirmengian CA: Staphylococcus aureus colonization among arthroplasty patients previously treated by a decolonization protocol: A pilot study. *Clin Orthop Relat Res* 2013;471(10):3128-3132.

14. Baratz MD, Hallmark R, Odum SM, Springer BD: Twenty percent of patients may remain colonized with methicillin-resistant Staphylococcus aureus despite a decolonization protocol in patients undergoing elective total joint arthroplasty. *Clin Orthop Relat Res* 2015;473(7):2283-2290.

15. Fatima N, Bjarnsholt T, Bay L: Dynamics of skin microbiota in shoulder surgery infections. *APMIS* 2021;129(12):665-674.

    This review article highlighted the characteristics of C acnes because it was related to shoulder infections, colonization of anatomic locations, and pathophysiology of the infectious process surrounding this organism. Level of evidence: V.

16. Hsu JE, Neradilek MB, Russ SM, Matsen FA: Preoperative skin cultures are predictive of Propionibacterium load in deep cultures obtained at revision shoulder arthroplasty. *J Shoulder Elbow Surg* 2018;27(5):765-770.

    In this prospective study, preoperative skin cultures were obtained from 60 patients undergoing revision shoulder arthroplasty. A positive preoperative culture was strongly predictive of positive cultures obtained at the time of surgery. Level of evidence: I.

17. Falconer TM, Baba M, Kruse LM, et al: Contamination of the surgical field with Propionibacterium acnes in primary shoulder arthroplasty. *J Bone Joint Surg Am* 2016;98(20):1722-1728.

18. Bartow-McKenney C, Hannigan GD, Horwinski J, et al: The microbiota of traumatic, open fracture wounds is associated with mechanism of injury. *Wound Repair Regen* 2018;26(2):127-135.

    Prospective collection of tissue samples was undertaken in patients with traumatic open fractures; the tissues underwent 16S ribosomal RNA sequencing to identify and characterize the local microbiota. It was found that the traumatized tissues had a microbiome that was distinct from surrounding skin but converged over time. Level of evidence: II.

19. Hannigan GD, Hodkinson BP, McGinnis K, et al: Culture-independent pilot study of microbiota colonizing open fractures and association with severity, mechanism, location, and complication from presentation to early outpatient follow-up. *J Orthop Res* 2014;32(4):597-605.

20. Drancourt M, Argenson JN, Tissot Dupont H, Aubaniac JM, Raoult D: Psoriasis is a risk factor for hip-prosthesis infection. *Eur J Epidemiol* 1997;13(2):205-207.

21. Cheleuitte E, Fleischli J, Tisa L, Zombolo R: Psoriasis and elective foot surgery. *J Foot Ankle Surg* 1996;35(4):297-302.

22. Park HY, Kim CR, Huh IS, et al: Staphylococcus aureus colonization in acute and chronic skin lesions of patients with atopic dermatitis. *Ann Dermatol* 2013;25(4):410-416.

23. Brown TS, Petis SM, Osmon DR, et al: Periprosthetic joint infection with fungal pathogens. *J Arthroplasty* 2018;33(8):2605-2612.

    In this retrospective study, 31 patients with fungal PJI demonstrated a 44% all-cause revision survivorship at 2 years. Survivorship free from infection was 38% at 2 years. This percentage was slightly improved in the TKA group compared with the THA group. Level of evidence: IV.

24. Kong P, Ren Y, Yang J, et al: Relapsed boyhood tibia polymicrobial osteomyelitis linked to dermatophytosis: A case report. *BMC Surg* 2022;22(1):156.

    This is a case report in which dermatophytosis was hypothesized to lead to reactivation of remote osteomyelitis from 29 years before. Level of evidence: IV.

25. Stevens DL, Bisno AL, Chambers HF, et al: Practice guidelines for the diagnosis and management of skin and soft-tissue infections. *Clin Infect Dis* 2005;41(10):1373-1406.

26. Tande A, Asante D, Sangaralingham L, et al: Risk factors for early hip or knee prosthetic joint infection (PJI): Analysis of a nationwide American insurance claims dataset. *Open Forum Infect Dis* 2017;4(suppl 1):S5.

27. Bui UT, Edwards H, Finlayson K: Identifying risk factors associated with infection in patients with chronic leg ulcers. *Int Wound J* 2018;15(2):283-290.

    This retrospective analysis of 561 outpatient chronic leg ulcers documented an infection prevalence of 7.8%. Multiple factors leading to increased risk of infection were identified, including depression, chronic pulmonary disease, anticoagulant use, calf:ankle circumference ratio less than 1.3, ulceration area of 10 cm^2 or larger, slough within the wound bed, and ulcers with heavy exudate. Level of evidence: IV.

28. Bala A, Penrose CT, Seyler TM, Mather RC 3rd, Wellman SS, Bolognesi MP: Outcomes after total knee arthroplasty for post-traumatic arthritis. *Knee* 2015;22(6):630-639.

29. Suzuki G, Saito S, Ishii T, Motojima S, Tokuhashi Y, Ryu J: Previous fracture surgery is a major risk factor of infection after total knee arthroplasty. *Knee Surg Sports Traumatol Arthrosc* 2011;19(12):2040-2044.

30. Manrique J, Rasouli MR, Restrepo C, et al: Total knee arthroplasty in patients with retention of prior hardware material: What is the outcome? *Arch Bone Jt Surg* 2018;6(1):23-26.

    This matched cohort study compared TKAs with retained hardware (55 patients) with 110 control patients. The TKAs with prior hardware did have higher rates of complications, but these were primarily related to mechanical issues and not PJI. Level of evidence: III.

31. Klatte TO, Schneider MM, Citak M, et al: Infection rates in patients undergoing primary knee arthroplasty with pre-existing orthopaedic fixation-devices. *Knee* 2013;20(3):177-180.

32. Ge DH, Anoushiravani AA, Kester BS, Vigdorchik JM, Schwarzkopf R: Preoperative diagnosis can predict conversion total knee arthroplasty outcomes. *J Arthroplasty* 2018;33(1):124-129.e1.

    This retrospective review of 72 conversion TKA procedures found that patients with prior fracture and fixation were at higher risk of surgical site complications and 90-day readmission than soft-tissue prior traumas. Level of evidence: III.

33. Werner BC, Burrus MT, Novicoff WM, Browne JA: Total knee arthroplasty within six months after knee arthroscopy is associated with increased postoperative complications. *J Arthroplasty* 2015;30(8):1313-1316.

34. Viste A, Abdel MP, Ollivier M, Mara KC, Krych AJ, Berry DJ: Prior knee arthroscopy does not influence long-term total knee arthroplasty outcomes and survivorship. *J Arthroplasty* 2017;32(12):3626-3631.

35. Watters TS, Zhen Y, Martin JR, Levy DL, Jennings JM, Dennis DA: Total knee arthroplasty after anterior cruciate ligament reconstruction: Not just a routine primary arthroplasty. *J Bone Joint Surg Am* 2017;99(3):185-189.

36. Steinhoff AK, Bugbee WD: Outcomes of total knee arthroplasty after osteochondral allograft transplantation. *Orthop J Sports Med* 2014;2(9):2325967114550276.

37. Haughom BD, Plummer DR, Hellman MD, Nho SJ, Rosenberg AG, Della Valle CJ: Does hip arthroscopy affect the outcomes of a subsequent total hip arthroplasty? *J Arthroplasty* 2016;31(7):1516-1518.

38. George J, Miller EM, Higuera CA, Kuivila TE, Mont MA, Goodwin RC: Influence of prior hip salvage surgery on outcomes after total hip arthroplasty in young patients. *J Arthroplasty* 2018;33(4):1108-1112.

    In this retrospective study in which young patients (younger than 30 years) undergoing THA were compared with patients who had undergone prior salvage procedure

(n = 37), it was found that the salvage group (pelvic and femoral osteotomies, core decompression) was at higher risk for wound complications, infections, and revision surgeries but with no difference in survivorship at 5 years. Level of evidence: III.

39. Klatte TO, Meinicke R, O'Loughlin P, Rueger JM, Gehrke T, Kendoff D: Incidence of bacterial contamination in primary THA and combined hardware removal: Analysis of preoperative aspiration and intraoperative biopsies. *J Arthroplasty* 2013;28(9):1677-1680.

40. Ito H, Takatori Y, Moro T, Oshima H, Oka H, Tanaka S: Total hip arthroplasty after rotational acetabular osteotomy. *J Arthroplasty* 2015;30(3):403-406.

41. Schmidutz F, Schreiner AJ, Ahrend MD, et al: Risk of periprosthetic joint infection after posttraumatic hip arthroplasty following acetabular fractures. *Z Orthop Unfall* 2022; May 23 [Epub ahead of print].

    This is a retrospective review of 67 patients who had undergone THA after acetabular fracture, with groups treated surgically compared with those treated nonsurgically and those with complete hardware removal. Increased infection rates were recognized in subgroups with retained or partially retained implants. Level of evidence: IV.

42. Aali Rezaie A, Blevins K, Kuo FC, Manrique J, Restrepo C, Parvizi J: Total hip arthroplasty after prior acetabular fracture: Infection is a real concern. *J Arthroplasty* 2020;35(9):2619-2623.

    This study reported the outcomes of 72 patients at a single center who underwent conversion to THA after prior ORIF for acetabular fracture. These patients had a higher overall complication rate, and specifically for PJI, the rate increased to 6.9% compared with 0.5% in the control group. Level of evidence: III.

43. Werthel JD, Hatta T, Schoch B, Cofield R, Sperling JW, Elhassan BT: Is previous nonarthroplasty surgery a risk factor for periprosthetic infection in primary shoulder arthroplasty? *J Shoulder Elbow Surg* 2017;26(4):635-640.

44. Morris BJ, O'Connor DP, Torres D, Elkousy HA, Gartsman GM, Edwards TB: Risk factors for periprosthetic infection after reverse shoulder arthroplasty. *J Shoulder Elbow Surg* 2015;24(2):161-166.

45. Lau D, Chan AK, Deverin V, Ames CP: Does prior spine surgery or instrumentation affect surgical outcomes following 3-column osteotomy for correction of thoracolumbar deformities? *Neurosurg Focus* 2017;43(6):E8.

46. Bratschitsch G, Puchwein P, Zollner-Schwetz I, et al: Spinal surgery site infection leading to implant loosening is influenced by the number of prior operations. *Global Spine J* 2022;12(3):458-463.

    This retrospective review of 181 patients who underwent spine surgery demonstrated that previous spinal surgery was found to be a risk factor for SSI, with *Propionibacterium* species detected in 80% of patients with multiple prior surgeries. Previous spinal surgery (OR, 1.38) and male sex (OR, 1.15) were predictive of SSI. Level of evidence: III.

47. Pugely AJ, Martin CT, Gao Y, Schweizer ML, Callaghan JJ: The incidence of and risk factors for 30-day surgical site infections following primary and revision total joint arthroplasty. *J Arthroplasty* 2015;30(9 suppl):47-50.

48. Seo JG, Moon YW, Park SH, Han KY, Kim SM: Primary total knee arthroplasty in infection sequelae about the native knee. *J Arthroplasty* 2014;29(12):2271-2275.

49. Tan T, Xu C, Kuo FC, Ghanem E, Higuera C, Parvizi J: Risk factors for failure and optimal treatment of total joint arthroplasty for septic arthritis. *J Arthroplasty* 2021;36(3):892-896.

    This is a retrospective review of the experience at five separate institutions reporting on 233 TJAs performed after prior septic arthritis. The PJI rate in this group was 12.4%, and it was found that antibiotic-resistant organisms, male gender, diabetes, and postsurgical causes of arthritis were the leading risk factors for infection. Level of evidence: III.

50. Kim YH, Oh SH, Kim JS: Total hip arthroplasty in adult patients who had childhood infection of the hip. *J Bone Joint Surg Am* 2003;85(2):198-204.

51. Tan TL, Xu C, Kuo FC, et al: When total joint arthroplasty after septic arthritis can be safely performed. *JB JS Open Access* 2021;6(2):e20.00146.

    This was an examination of 207 TJAs performed at five different institutions after prior septic arthritis. The risk of PJI was 12.1%, and there were no optimal cutoffs for serum markers or interim periods between treatment to reduce the risk of PJI. Level of evidence: III.

52. Jerry GJ Jr, Rand JA, Ilstrup D: Old sepsis prior to total knee arthroplasty. *Clin Orthop Relat Res* 1988;236:135-140.

53. Bedair H, Goyal N, Dietz MJ, et al: A history of treated periprosthetic joint infection increases the risk of subsequent different site infection. *Clin Orthop Relat Res* 2015;473(7):2300-2304.

54. Pull ter Gunne AF, Mohamed AS, Skolasky RL, van Laarhoven CJ, Cohen DB: The presentation, incidence, etiology, and treatment of surgical site infections after spinal surgery. *Spine (Phila Pa 1976)* 2010;35(13):1323-1328.

55. Xing D, Chen Y, Ma JX, et al: A methodological systematic review of early versus late stabilization of thoracolumbar spine fractures. *Eur Spine J* 2013;22(10):2157-2166.

56. Tanner J, Melen K: Preoperative hair removal to reduce surgical site infection. *Cochrane Database Syst Rev* 2021;8(8):CD004122.

    This systematic review of 19 randomized and 6 quasirandomized trials (8,919 patients) found that if hair has to be removed, clippers or depilatory cream should be used, resulting in fewer SSIs. Some small reductions were noted when hair was removed on the day of surgery versus times before the day of surgery. Level of evidence: I.

57. Lefebvre A, Saliou P, Lucet JC, et al: Preoperative hair removal and surgical site infections: Network meta-analysis of randomized controlled trials. *J Hosp Infect* 2015;91(2):100-108.

58. Grosse Perdekamp M, Kneubuehl BP, Serr A, Vennemann B, Pollak S: Gunshot-related transport of micro-organisms from

59. Tornetta P 3rd, Hui RC: Intraarticular findings after gunshot wounds through the knee. *J Orthop Trauma* 1997;11(6):422-424.

60. Naziri Q, Issa K, Rizkala A, et al: Posttraumatic arthritis from gunshot injuries to the hip requiring a primary THA. *Orthopedics* 2013;36(12):e1549-e1554.

61. Haspl M, Pećina M, Orlić D, Cicak N: Arthroplasty after war injuries to major joints. *Mil Med* 1999;164(5):353-357.

62. Velmahos G, Demetriades D: Gunshot wounds of the spine: Should retained bullets be removed to prevent infection? *Ann R Coll Surg Engl* 1994;76(2):85-87.

63. Patch DA, Levitt EB, Andrews NA, et al: Civilian ballistic femoral shaft fractures compared with blunt femur shaft fractures. *J Orthop Trauma* 2022;36(7):355-360.

This is a retrospective cohort study of 528 femoral shaft fractures, in which 140 ballistic fractures were compared with blunt trauma fractures. The overall rates of nonunion and infection were similar between all groups, but the complication rate overall was much higher for the ballistic group, which was especially concerning for thigh compartment syndrome. Level of evidence: III.

64. Prather JC, Montgomery T, Cone B, et al: Civilian ballistic tibia shaft fractures compared with blunt tibia shaft fractures: Open or closed? *J Orthop Trauma* 2021;35(3):143-148.

This is a retrospective cohort study of patients with tibial fractures categorized as ballistic or blunt or blunt/open fractures. The ballistic group had a higher number of soft-tissue reconstruction procedures and higher incidence of compartment syndrome. However, the incidence of fracture-related infection was similar between the groups (blunt 10.1% versus 9.1%, $P = 1.0$). Level of evidence: III.

CHAPTER 3

Systemic Patient Risk Factors

TEJBIR S. PANNU, MD, MS • CARLOS A. HIGUERA, MD

ABSTRACT

Infection, be it surgical site infection or prosthetic joint infection, is one of the most common and devastating complications after orthopaedic surgery. The etiology of infection is multifactorial, where patient-specific risk factors play a pivotal role. Hence, primary prevention or risk reduction might be possible with patient optimization of their systemic risk factors. Broadly, systemic patient risk factors can be divided into modifiable and nonmodifiable ones. Although the modifiable risk factors can be optimized preoperatively for risk mitigation, risk assessment of the nonmodifiable factors can assist with informed patient and surgeon decision making and set real expectations after orthopaedic surgery.

Keywords: prosthetic joint infection; risk factors; surgical site infection

---

Dr. Higuera or an immediate family member is a member of a speakers' bureau or has made paid presentations on behalf of KCI; serves as a paid consultant to or is an employee of KCI and Stryker; has stock or stock options held in PSI; has received research or institutional support from Ferring Pharmaceuticals, KCI, OREF, Osteal Therapeutics, Stryker, and Zimmer; and serves as a board member, owner, officer, or committee member of American Academy of Orthopaedic Surgeons, American Association of Hip and Knee Surgeons, and SICOT. Neither Dr. Pannu nor any immediate family member has received anything of value from or has stock or stock options held in a commercial company or institution related directly or indirectly to the subject of this chapter.

INTRODUCTION

Surgical site infection (SSI) and prosthetic joint infection (PJI) are common and devastating complications after orthopaedic surgery. Risk factors for infection are divided into patient-related (local or systemic) or surgery-related risk factors, where the patient-related factors play a significant role in outcome. Systemic patient risk factors can be divided into modifiable and nonmodifiable ones. The main modifiable risk factors include depression, smoking, anemia, malnutrition, alcohol abuse, and obesity. However, nonmodifiable factors include sex, race, diabetes, immunosuppression, renal disease, hepatitis, and liver disease, among others. Thus, thorough knowledge of both modifiable and nonmodifiable systemic patient risk factors for SSI and PJI across the different orthopaedic subspecialties can assist both the surgeon and patient in proper decision making while setting realistic expectations postoperatively.

MODIFIABLE RISK FACTORS

Depression

A national registry study has found depression to be an independent risk factor for development of PJI after total joint arthroplasty (TJA)[1] (**Table 1**). A synthesis of 66 investigations (23 prospective, 43 retrospective) with meta-analysis found depression to increase the risk of infection by an adjusted relative risk (RR) of 1.48 after TJA.[2] In a 2021 study of geriatric patients with hip fracture undergoing intramedullary nailing, preoperative depression increased the odds ratio (OR) of SSI by 1.37 and wound complications by 1.23.[3] In yet another Humana database study on patients undergoing anterior cervical diskectomy with fusion and posterior cervical fusion, patients with mental disorders had an infection rate of 4.4% at 3 months postoperatively versus 3.5% in the control group.[4]

Table 1. Systemic Patient Risk Factors for Prosthetic Joint Infection and Surgical Site Infection After Orthopaedic Surgery	
Modifiable	**Nonmodifiable**
Depression	Gender
Smoking	Race
Anemia	Diabetes
Malnutrition	Immunosuppression
Alcohol abuse	Renal disease
Obesity	Hepatitis and liver disease

Smoking

An institutional retrospective database review of more than 17,000 TJAs revealed that current smokers were twice as likely to require revision surgery for the management of infection compared with nonsmokers.[5] The same study concluded that former smokers were at similar risk of developing PJI.[5] Similarly, both current and former smokers undergoing total shoulder arthroplasty showed a significantly higher risk of infection after surgery compared with nonsmokers (respective hazard ratios [HRs], 7.27 and 4.56).[6] The spine literature also established smoking as a significant predictor of superficial and deep SSI in an analysis of more than 25,000 patients undergoing spinal decompression and fusion (OR, 1.19).[7] A 2021 meta-analysis of 19 studies on procedures performed for fractures showed that smoking was associated with an increased risk of postoperative infection (RR, 2.10).[8]

Similar results were demonstrated in yet another investigation of 1,568 patients undergoing spinal fusions showing smokers to have a more than twofold increased risk of deep infection.[9]

Anemia

When defining anemia as a hemoglobin (Hb) level of less than 12 g/dL in women and less than 13 g/dL in men, almost 20% of patients undergoing TJA were found to be anemic in one of the largest studies on this subject.[10] PJI occurred at a significantly higher rate in patients with anemia compared with those with normal preoperative Hb levels (4.3% versus 2%).[10] Furthermore, preoperative anemia has also been shown to increase the failure rate of treatment and the recurrence of infection in confirmed cases of PJI. In patients undergoing débridement, antibiotic therapy, and implant retention, Hb levels below normal values have demonstrated increased odds of failure of débridement, antibiotic therapy, and implant retention sevenfold.[11] Furthermore, a 2019 study reported that spine surgery is associated with significant blood loss even while using tranexamic acid routinely, and those requiring transfusion have a significantly higher risk of postoperative infection.[12] A 2019 meta-analysis including 34,185 patients who underwent spine surgery from eight investigations computed a pooled risk estimate of a threefold greater likelihood of postoperative infection in patients requiring a blood transfusion.[12]

Malnutrition

A study evaluating postoperative wound complications after TJA demonstrated that an albumin level of less than 3.5 mg/dL increased the complication rate sevenfold.[13] A retrospective investigation of 2,161 consecutive patients who underwent elective primary and revision TJA defined malnutrition as either serum albumin levels of 3.5 mg/dL or less or serum transferrin levels of less than 200 mg/dL.[14] In this study, malnutrition was found to increase the odds ratio of developing an acute infection within 3 months by 2.37. The effect of nutritional status has also been evaluated in patients who underwent spine surgery. In 2020, a systematic review and meta-analysis of 22 studies, involving patients undergoing spinal procedures ($n = 175,000$), exhibited a significantly higher rate of SSIs in malnourished patients (OR, 2.31).[15] On further analysis, a significant association was only found in thoracolumbar and sacral spinal surgery. In 2021, a nutritional index known as prognostic nutritional index (prognostic nutritional index = 10 × serum albumin [g/dL] + 0.005 × total lymphocyte count [µL]) was tested for SSI risk stratification after spine surgery in a retrospective study of 1,115 patients and concluded that a lower preoperative prognostic nutritional index (OR, 0.94) was a significant risk factor for SSI postoperatively.[16]

Alcohol Abuse

Alcohol use has not been definitively shown to affect the risk of infection after TJA. Most of the data linking alcohol abuse to infection after arthroplasty come from retrospective studies performed either in single medical centers or using data from registries.[17-23] A Danish study based on an anesthesia database performed risk analysis after obtaining information on the amount of alcohol consumption directly from patients.[18] This study of 30,799 patients undergoing arthroplasty demonstrated that patients who reported more than 168 g of alcohol intake per week had an increased chance of PJI compared with those who did not report any consumption (HR, 1.55). In another investigation assessing PJI risk factors after TJA, alcohol abuse did not reach statistical significance in this regard (OR, 0.98).[19] There are some data on patients undergoing spinal fusion surgery, concluding alcohol and/or drug abuse ($P = 0.034$) as significant risk factors for SSI after surgery.[20] Alcohol and drug abuse were not evaluated as separate standalone variables. However, a review of 1,010 adult patients undergoing elective spinal fusion (≥2 levels) for spinal deformities at a major academic institution did not find a significant association between preoperative alcohol consumption and 30-day postoperative complications including superficial and deep SSI.[21] With regard to trauma surgery, a 2019 retrospective analysis of 210 tibial plateau fractures treated with open reduction and internal fixation (ORIF) showed that alcohol intake of more than 13 units/wk was the only significant risk factor for postoperative infection in a multivariate model involving other patient-related variables such as smoking, diabetes, and obesity.[22] Of note, another case series looking at surgical fixation of ankle fractures in 1,045 patients failed to establish alcohol overuse as a risk factor in an adjusted multivariate model for a postoperative infection.[23]

Obesity

Obesity is one of the most extensively researched variables and unanimously accepted as a significant risk factor for postoperative infection after orthopaedic surgery.[24-28] A large study extracted data from a national insurance database and stratified patients undergoing primary total hip arthroplasty (THA) into groups: 702,360 without obesity, 123,407 with obesity (body mass index [BMI] = 30 to 30.9 kg/m^2), 62,556 with morbid obesity (BMI = 40 to 49.9 kg/m^2), and 3,244 with super obesity (BMI > 50 kg/m^2)—and compared postoperative infection rates in between the groups.[24] Although patients with super obesity were at more than 12-fold risk of infection compared with patients without obesity, they were at significant risk compared with patients with obesity (OR, 3.8) and morbid obesity (OR, 1.7) as well. The incremental infection risk was also determined in patients with obesity undergoing arthroscopic knee procedures. In an analysis of 595,083 arthroscopic knee procedures, morbid obesity was found to be the most prominent risk factor for superficial and deep SSIs (RR, 2.19).[25] The effect of obesity on postoperative infection rates also holds true for patients undergoing spine surgery. A systematic review and meta-analysis of 12 retrospective studies in patients undergoing spinal procedures showed that a 5-unit increase in BMI increased the risk of SSI by as much as 13%, which increased to 21% after adjusting for diabetes and other confounding variables.[26] Furthermore, in 2021, a systematic review of patients with obesity undergoing ORIF for pelvic or acetabular fractures revealed significantly higher rates of infection after surgery (OR range, 1.1 to 14.1) compared with patients without obesity.[27] Another study in 2019 of 724 patients who underwent ORIF of intra-articular distal femur fractures demonstrated that obesity had a 2.56-fold increased the risk of infection after surgery in an adjusted multivariate model.[28]

NONMODIFIABLE RISK FACTORS

Gender

Although gender and sex can be used interchangeably, it might not be the case always, which limits the results of different studies. In a 2018 retrospective review of 173,777 patients undergoing TJA (63.5% total knee arthroplasty [TKA] and 36.5% THA), male gender was found to significantly increase the risk of SSI (RR, 1.2) and sepsis (RR, 1.4).[29] Nevertheless, contrary results were found in a 2020 study where female gender was determined to be an independent risk factor for wound infection after THA.[30] However, males appear to be at a higher risk of postoperative infection in other orthopaedic procedures. In a retrospective investigation of 3,294 arthroscopic rotator cuff repairs in a single institution, male gender was a significant determinant of postoperative infection (OR, 23.54) in a multivariate analysis.[31] In a retrospective case-control investigation, 1,587 posterior spinal fusion procedures were analyzed, and deep SSI developed in 57 cases.[32] On a multivariate analysis, male gender was a significant risk factor for deep SSI (OR, 2.7). The role of gender in the setting of postoperative infection was also analyzed in 2021 in patients undergoing anterior cruciate ligament repair surgery. This study queried the Swedish Knee Ligament Registry to assess 26,014 primary and revision anterior cruciate ligament repairs and found male gender to be an independent risk factor of septic arthritis after surgery (OR, 1.65).[33]

Similar results, with male gender associated with 1.58 times higher risk of infection after primary ACL repair (n = 217,541).[34]

Race

In general, Hispanic and African American patients have higher rates of postoperative PJI after TJA.[35] Interestingly, the results show some variation between THAs and TKAs. For instance, one study found a significantly increased infection rate after TKAs in African American patients (OR, 1.5) but did not achieve significance in THAs. In addition, another retrospective study on TKAs compared postoperative infection rates between White and non-White patients and concluded that PJI at 90 days was significantly more prevalent in Hispanic patients (OR, 1.21) but not in African Americans.[35] Interestingly, in a retrospective review of 56,216 TKAs, contrasting findings were observed,[36] where being Hispanic was protective against postoperative infection (HR, 0.69). Adding more complexity to the debate, a review of 30,491 THAs found no significant association with being African American or Hispanic with PJI after THA.[37] Of note, these findings might not be relevant to patient race specifically, but rather may pertain to health

Diabetes Mellitus

The categorization of diabetes mellitus as nonmodifiable versus modifiable is difficult considering the lack of information on the status of disease process (controlled versus uncontrolled). Diabetes is one of the established predictors of adverse outcomes after surgery in general and orthopaedics is no different. A total of 57,575 patients undergoing primary THA were reviewed, and type 2 diabetes mellitus was found to increase the risk of deep infection by 1.5-fold, which increased to more than 2-fold if patients also had any disease-related complications.[38] Another study analyzed more than 800,000 THAs and TKAs for infection risk factors and concluded that PJI is 1.32 times more likely to develop in patients with diabetes compared with patients without diabetes.[39] Extensive research has been conducted in identifying a cutoff value for HbA1c level that would serve as a practical means for predicting PJI and setting goals for patient optimization. An HbA1c value of more than 7.7% was linked to PJI incidence postoperatively reaching 5.4% versus 0.8% in patients with values less than 7.7%.[40] Perioperative hyperglycemia with blood glucose levels of 140 mmol/L or greater has been shown to significantly correlate with the risk of PJI after surgery (HR, 1.44).[41] Serum fructosamine, which is a marker of short-term mean glycemic control, has also been proposed as a predictor of PJI risk after TJA, with values of 292 mmol/L or greater, a more than sixfold increase in the odds ratio of PJI.[42] Postoperative infection rates after spinal fusion are also affected by preoperative diabetes status. An investigation of 345 patients who underwent elective posterior instrumented thoracolumbar and lumbar arthrodesis determined the presence of diabetes mellitus to significantly increase the risk of infection after surgery (diabetes mellitus = 16.7% risk; absence of diabetes mellitus = 3.7%).[43] In addition, a 2021 analysis of 99,970 patients undergoing open and arthroscopic shoulder procedures other than arthroplasty reported diabetes to be the only independent risk factor predictive of infection (OR, 1.33) after surgery.[44] Analogous to these findings, in a national database study from 2022 on 87,169 patients who underwent ORIF for distal radius fracture, diabetes mellitus was also ascertained to increase postoperative infection risk (OR, 1.24).[45] In 2018, a systematic review and meta-analysis of ankle fracture ORIF found that the diagnoses of diabetes mellitus increased the risk of infection (OR, 2.67).[46] Similarly, the Multicenter Orthopaedic Outcomes Network study of 2,198 patients who underwent anterior cruciate ligament reconstruction found the diagnosis of diabetes mellitus to increase the likelihood of postoperative infection by 18.8-fold on adjusted multivariate analyses.[47]

Immunosuppression

Primarily, the cohort of immune-suppressed patients in orthopaedics encompasses patients with HIV infection, transplant recipients, or patients on immunosuppressive medications. A 2019 systematic review and meta-analysis that analyzed 19 studies and more than 5,000,000 arthroplasty procedures demonstrated that HIV-positive status had up to a 3.31-fold increase in the risk of PJI.[48] A review of patients who underwent transplantation for one or more solid organs, including for the pancreas, kidney, liver, and heart, before THA in the Medicare database revealed[49] a respective 1.31-, 1.56-, 1.6-, and 1.82-fold increased risk of PJI when compared with patients who did not undergo transplantation. Another study on 2,579,694 patients who underwent hip and knee arthroplasty from the Nationwide Inpatient Sample database determined that transplant recipients are at a significantly higher risk of wound healing complications (OR, 2.13).[50]

Immunosuppressive medications, such as nonbiologic and biologic disease-modifying antirheumatic drugs (DMARDs) and corticosteroids, are correlated with increased infection rates after orthopaedic surgery. A retrospective study on 420 patients with rheumatoid arthritis on DMARDs who underwent TJAs evaluated the effect on the incidence of SSI.[51] On multivariate analysis, biologic DMARDs had a 5.69-fold increase in the likelihood of SSI in these patients. More specifically, after adjusting for disease duration, tumor necrosis factor alpha (TNF-α) blockers including both infliximab and etanercept increased SSI risk more than ninefold compared with the control group. A retrospective review of more than 50,000 orthopaedic surgeries investigated the association between DMARDs and TNF-α inhibitors and the rate of postoperative infection.[52] Patients on DMARDs and TNF-α inhibitors were at an increased odds of postoperative infection, with an OR of 2.49 and 2.54, respectively. Similarly, in 2020, long-term corticosteroid use was linked to increased incidence of infection after orthopaedic surgery.[53] In 2020, a retrospective review of 403,566 patients who underwent TKA and THA concluded that patients on long-term corticosteroids had higher complication rates, including SSI, deep incisional SSI, organ space SSI, wound dehiscence, and general wound infection ($P \leq 0.0001$ for all).[54] In 2020, a retrospective cohort study of 26,734 patients who underwent lumbar decompression surgeries, including diskectomies and laminectomies, compared postoperative infection rates between patients who were on long-term corticosteroids and those who were not and established after multivariate analysis that long-term usage of corticosteroids led to significantly higher rates of sepsis complications (OR, 2.032), but not local wound infections.[53] In contrast, a prospective cohort study involving 274 patients who underwent elective thoracic or lumbar spinal surgery did not find a significant correlation between SSI and long-term corticosteroid usage.[55] A similar conclusion was reached in 2019 in a retrospective case-control study of 692 patients after undergoing ORIF for femoral neck fractures, where corticosteroid therapy was shown to significantly increase SSI rates ($P = 0.003$).[56]

Chronic Renal Disease, End-Stage Renal Disease, and Dialysis

The relationship between end-stage renal disease (ESRD) and infection as a complication after TJA has been conflicting for the most part. A review of more than 20,000 patients undergoing THA failed to find a significant correlation between SSI and chronic kidney disease and ESRD.[57] However, a larger retrospective study including more than 80,000 patients undergoing primary TKA found renal disease as a significant predictor of postoperative complications (adjusted HR = 1.38).[1] In addition to the diagnosis of ESRD, dialysis and the mode of dialysis for ESRD effect on postoperative SSI rates have been examined. In a 2019 retrospective analysis of patients who underwent TKA ($n = 531$) and THA ($n = 572$) undergoing peritoneal dialysis and hemodialysis, similar infection rates were reported in patients undergoing peritoneal dialysis compared with control patients (no dialysis) but significantly lower rates compared with patients undergoing hemodialysis.[58] A 2021 systematic review and meta-analysis did not find any significant difference in SSI rates after TJA between patients undergoing dialysis (4%) before surgery and those who underwent renal transplantation (3.7%).[59] Similarly, renal disease plays a significant role in increased SSI rates after posterolateral lumbar spine fusion (OR, 2.43) and adverse events after knee arthroscopy (OR, 7.46).[60,61] With respect to trauma surgery, a retrospective evaluation of 85,433 proximal humerus ORIFs concluded in 2022 that chronic kidney disease and ESRD are significant risk factors for postoperative SSI (OR, 1.52) and wound complications (OR, 2.67).[62]

Hepatitis and Liver Disease

For the most part, there is a strong correlation between cirrhosis/liver disease and postoperative infection after TJA. An analysis of the Danish health care TJA database revealed that the diagnosis of cirrhosis imparted a twofold greater rate of infection (HR, 2.1) after surgery.[63] Similarly, analysis of national and state databases in the United States comparing patients with and without cirrhosis undergoing THAs ($n = 306,946$) and TKAs ($n = 573,840$) revealed that cirrhosis increased the rate of PJI after THA by more than fivefold and TKA by more than threefold.[39] With respect to shoulder arthroplasty, a 2022 systematic review and meta-analysis also reported liver disease as a significant risk factor for postoperative infection (pooled OR, 1.70).[64] A study from Taiwan determined that hepatitis B infection is a risk factor for PJI, where PJI was 4.32 times more likely to develop in patients with hepatitis B compared with patients without hepatitis B.[65] In 2022, hepatitis C infection has been shown to be a significant risk factor for PJI after TKA and THA.[66] In 2019, the preoperative management of hepatitis C with oral direct-acting antiviral agents was shown to reduce infection risk threefold compared with untreated hepatitis C before TKA THA.[67] In contrast, a retrospective review in 2021 of US military veterans undergoing total shoulder arthroplasty did not show an increased risk of SSI or wound infection in patients with hepatitis C ($n = 5,774$).[68]

SUMMARY

Systemic patient risk factors for infection after orthopaedic surgery are either modifiable or nonmodifiable. Some risk factors may cross over. For example, obesity and type 2 diabetes mellitus can both be modified. Gender is also modifiable in some cases. Modifiable risk factors such as depression, smoking, anemia, malnutrition, alcohol abuse (debatable), type 2 diabetes, and obesity have all been demonstrated to increase the risk of SSI and PJI. The identification of these factors provides an opportunity for medical optimization of these patients before surgery to reduce their risk for the development of infection after surgery. Nonmodifiable risk factors, such as male gender, being African American or Hispanic (regarding social and access disparity), immunosuppression, renal disease, hepatitis, and liver disease, have shown significant association with higher postoperative infection rates. Patients eligible for orthopaedic surgeries should be counseled regarding the estimated infection risk based on their comorbidities to allow an improved informed decision-making process.

KEY STUDY POINTS

- Identification of systemic patient risk factors for infection is important for preoperative medical optimization and informing patients of their risk profile for the surgery.
- Modifiable risk factors of infection are depression, smoking, anemia, malnutrition, alcohol abuse, and obesity.
- Nonmodifiable risk factors are male gender, being African American and Hispanic, diabetes, immunosuppression, renal disease, hepatitis, and liver disease.

ANNOTATED REFERENCES

1. Bozic KJ, Lau E, Kurtz S, Ong K, Berry DJ: Patient-related risk factors for postoperative mortality and periprosthetic joint infection in medicare patients undergoing TKA. *Clin Orthop Relat Res* 2012;470(1):130-137.

2. Kunutsor SK, Whitehouse MR, Blom AW, Beswick AD, INFORM Team: Patient-related risk factors for periprosthetic joint infection after total joint arthroplasty: A systematic review and meta-analysis. *PLoS One* 2016;11(3):e0150866.

3. Broggi MS, Oladeji PO, Tahmid S, Hernandez-Irizarry R, Allen J: Depressive disorders lead to increased complications after geriatric hip fractures. *Geriatr Orthop Surg Rehabil* 2021;12:21514593211016252.

   Preoperative depression in patients undergoing hip fracture surgery increases the risk of complications. It is pertinent to identify this diagnosis during the preoperative workup. Level of evidence: IV.

4. Dedeogullari E, Paholpak P, Barkoh K, et al: Effect of mental health on post-operative infection rates following cervical spine fusion procedures. *J Orthop* 2017;14(4):501-506.

5. Tischler EH, Matsen Ko L, Chen AF, Maltenfort MG, Schroeder J, Austin MS: Smoking increases the rate of reoperation for infection within 90 days after primary total joint arthroplasty. *J Bone Joint Surg Am* 2017;99(4):295-304.

6. Hatta T, Werthel JD, Wagner ER, et al: Effect of smoking on complications following primary shoulder arthroplasty. *J Shoulder Elbow Surg* 2017;26:1-6.

7. Veeravagu A, Patil CG, Lad SP, Boakye M: Risk factors for postoperative spinal wound infections after spinal decompression and fusion surgeries. *Spine (Phila Pa 1976)* 2009;34(17):1869-1872.

8. Smolle MA, Leitner L, Böhler N, Seibert FJ, Glehr M, Leithner A: Fracture, nonunion and postoperative infection risk in the smoking orthopaedic patient: A systematic review and meta-analysis. *EFORT Open Rev* 2021;6(11):1006-1019.

   Smoking has a negative effect on the incidence of fractures and increases the risk of nonunion and postoperative infections after surgical treatment. Level of evidence: I.

9. Schimmel JJ, Horsting PP, de Kleuver M, Wonders G, van Limbeek J: Risk factors for deep surgical site infections after spinal fusion. *Eur Spine J* 2010;19(10):1711-1719.

10. Greenky M, Gandhi K, Pulido L, Restrepo C, Parvizi J: Preoperative anemia in total joint arthroplasty: Is it associated with periprosthetic joint infection? Hip. *Clin Orthop Relat Res* 2012;470(10):2695-2701.

11. Swenson RD, Butterfield JA, Irwin TJ, Zurlo JJ, Davis CM: Preoperative anemia is associated with failure of open débridement polyethylene exchange in acute and acute hematogenous prosthetic joint infection. *J Arthroplasty* 2018;33(6):1855-1860.

    Staphylococcus aureus infection and preoperative hematocrit level of 32.1 or less significantly increases failure rate of open débridement and polyethylene exchange in acute PJI. Most of these failures can be successfully managed with two-stage exchange arthroplasty. Level of evidence: I.

12. He YK, Li HZ, Lu HD: Is blood transfusion associated with an increased risk of infection among spine surgery patients?: A meta-analysis. *Medicine (Baltimore)* 2019;98(28):e16287.

    Perioperative blood transfusion significantly increases the risk of developing infection after spine surgery. However, the mechanism of this association is currently unclear. Level of evidence: I.

13. Greene KA, Wilde AH, Stulberg BN: Preoperative nutritional status of total joint patients: Relationship to postoperative wound complications. *J Arthroplasty* 1991;6(4):321-325.

14. Huang R, Greenky M, Kerr GJ, Austin MS, Parvizi J: The effect of malnutrition on patients undergoing elective joint arthroplasty. *J Arthroplasty* 2013;28(8 suppl):21-24.

15. Tsantes AG, Papadopoulos DV, Lytras T, et al: Association of malnutrition with surgical site infection following spinal surgery: Systematic review and meta-analysis. *J Hosp Infect* 2020;104(1):111-119.

    Malnutrition shows a significant association with SSI after spinal surgery. Attention must be given to preoperative nutritional status of patients undergoing spinal surgery. Level of evidence: I.

16. Ushirozako H, Hasegawa T, Yamato Y, et al: Does preoperative prognostic nutrition index predict surgical site infection after spine surgery? *Eur Spine J* 2021;30(6):1765-1773.

    Patients with a low preoperative prognostic nutrition index are at a significantly higher risk of SSI after spine surgery. Patients should be counseled regarding this increased risk in the informed consent process for surgery. Level of evidence: I.

17. Wu C, Qu X, Liu F, Li H, Mao Y, Zhu Z: Risk factors for periprosthetic joint infection after total hip arthroplasty and total knee arthroplasty in Chinese patients. *PLoS One* 2014;9(4):e95300.

18. Rotevatn TA, Bøggild H, Olesen CR, et al: Alcohol consumption and the risk of postoperative mortality and morbidity after primary hip or knee arthroplasty – A register-based cohort study. *PLoS One* 2017;12(3):e0173083.

19. Cavanaugh PK, Chen AF, Rasouli MR, Post ZD, Orozco FR, Ong AC: Complications and mortality in chronic renal failure patients undergoing total joint arthroplasty: A comparison between dialysis and renal transplant patients. *J Arthroplasty* 2016;31(2):465-472.

20. Dobran M, Marini A, Nasi D, et al: Risk factors of surgical site infections in instrumented spine surgery. *Surg Neurol Int* 2017;8:212.

21. Elsamadicy AA, Adogwa O, Vuong VD, et al: Impact of alcohol use on 30-day complication and readmission rates after elective spinal fusion (≥2 levels) for adult spine deformity: A single institutional study of 1,010 patients. *J Spine Surg* 2017;3:403-410.

22. Chan G, Iliopoulos E, Jain A, Turki M, Trompeter A: Infection after operative fixation of tibia plateau fractures. A risk factor analysis. *Injury* 2019;50(11):2089-2092.

Excessive alcohol consumption is an independent risk factor for postoperative infection after surgical management of tibial plateau fractures.

23. Olsen LL, Møller AM, Brorson S, Hasselager RB, Sort R: The impact of lifestyle risk factors on the rate of infection after surgery for a fracture of the ankle. *Bone Joint J* 2017;99-B(2):225-230.

24. Werner BC, Higgins MD, Pehlivan HC, Carothers JT, Browne JA: Super obesity is an independent risk factor for complications after primary total hip arthroplasty. *J Arthroplasty* 2017;32(2):402-406.

25. Clement RC, Haddix KP, Creighton RA, Spang JT, Tennant JN, Kamath GV: Risk factors for infection after knee arthroscopy: Analysis of 595,083 cases from 3 United States databases. *Arthroscopy* 2016;32(12):2556-2561.

26. Abdallah DY, Jadaan MM, McCabe JP: Body mass index and risk of surgical site infection following spine surgery: A meta-analysis. *Eur Spine J* 2013;22(12):2800-2809.

27. Mittwede PN, Gibbs CM, Ahn J, Bergin PF, Tarkin IS: Is obesity associated with an increased risk of complications after surgical management of acetabulum and pelvis fractures? A systematic review. *J Am Acad Orthop Surg Glob Res Rev* 2021;5(4):e21.00058.

    Obesity significantly increases the risk of complications after surgical treatment of acetabular and pelvic fractures. Infection is the most common complication.

28. Lu K, Zhang J, Cheng J, et al: Incidence and risk factors for surgical site infection after open reduction and internal fixation of intra-articular fractures of distal femur: A multicentre study. *Int Wound J* 2019;16(2):473-478.

    S aureus is the most common causative pathogen for infection after ORIF for intra-articular fractures of the distal femur. Other significant risk factors found are open fracture, obesity, smoking, and diabetes mellitus. Optimization of patients undergoing this surgery is key. Level of evidence: IV.

29. Basques BA, Bell JA, Sershon RA, Della Valle CJ: The influence of patient gender on morbidity following total hip or total knee arthroplasty. *J Arthroplasty* 2018;33(2):345-349.

    Male gender is a significant determinant of higher risk of SSI, revision surgery, and readmission in patients undergoing THA or TKA. Level of evidence: IV.

30. Patel AP, Gronbeck C, Chambers M, Harrington MA, Halawi MJ: Gender and total joint arthroplasty: Variable outcomes by procedure type. *Arthroplast Today* 2020;6(3):517-520.

    Based on the procedure type, TKA or THA, gender has a variable effect on postoperative outcomes. Gender should be included in the risk stratification models for postoperative outcomes after these procedures. Level of evidence: IV.

31. Pauzenberger L, Grieb A, Hexel M, Laky B, Anderl W, Heuberer P: Infections following arthroscopic rotator cuff repair: Incidence, risk factors, and prophylaxis. *Knee Surg Sports Traumatol Arthrosc* 2017;25(2):595-601.

32. Rao SB, Vasquez G, Harrop J, et al: Risk factors for surgical site infections following spinal fusion procedures: A case-control study. *Clin Infect Dis* 2011;53(7):686-692.

33. Kraus Schmitz J, Lindgren V, Edman G, Janarv PM, Forssblad M, Stålman A: Risk factors for septic arthritis after anterior cruciate ligament reconstruction: A nationwide analysis of 26,014 ACL reconstructions. *Am J Sports Med* 2021;49(7):1769-1776.

    The significant risk factors for septic arthritis after anterior cruciate ligament reconstruction are as follows: male gender, hamstring tendon autografts, clindamycin (versus cloxacillin), and longer surgical time. Level of evidence: IV.

34. Roecker Z, Kamalapathy P, Werner BC: Male sex, cartilage surgery, tobacco use, and opioid disorders are associated with an increased risk of infection after anterior cruciate ligament reconstruction. *Arthroscopy* 2022;38(3):948-952.e1.

    The significant risk factors for infection after anterior cruciate ligament reconstruction are male gender, obesity, tobacco use, older age, preoperative depression, and opioid use disorders. Level of evidence: IV.

35. Nwachukwu BU, Kenny AD, Losina E, Chibnik LB, Katz JN: Complications for racial and ethnic minority groups after total hip and knee replacement: A review of the literature. *J Bone Joint Surg Am* 2010;92(2):338-345.

36. Namba RS, Inacio MC, Paxton EW: Risk factors associated with deep surgical site infections after primary total knee arthroplasty: An analysis of 56,216 knees. *J Bone Joint Surg Am* 2013;95(9):775-782.

37. Namba RS, Inacio MC, Paxton EW: Risk factors associated with surgical site infection in 30,491 primary total hip replacements. *J Bone Joint Surg Br* 2012;94(10):1330-1338.

38. Pedersen AB, Svendsson JE, Johnsen SP, Riis A, Overgaard S: Risk factors for revision due to infection after primary total hip arthroplasty: A population-based study of 80,756 primary procedures in the Danish Hip Arthroplasty Registry. *Acta Orthop* 2010;81(5):542-547.

39. Jiang SL, Schairer WW, Bozic KJ: Increased rates of periprosthetic joint infection in patients with cirrhosis undergoing total joint arthroplasty. *Clin Orthop Relat Res* 2014;472(8):2483-2491.

40. Tarabichi M, Shohat N, Kheir MM, et al: Determining the threshold for HbA1c as a predictor for adverse outcomes after total joint arthroplasty: A multicenter, retrospective study. *J Arthroplasty* 2017;32(9 suppl):S263-S267.e1.

41. Chrastil J, Anderson MB, Stevens V, Anand R, Peters CL, Pelt CE: Is hemoglobin A1c or perioperative hyperglycemia predictive of periprosthetic joint infection or death following primary total joint arthroplasty? *J Arthroplasty* 2015;30(7):1197-1202.

42. Shohat N, Tarabichi M, Tischler EH, Jabbour S, Parvizi J: Serum fructosamine: A simple and inexpensive test for assessing preoperative glycemic control. *J Bone Joint Surg Am* 2017;99(22):1900-1907.

43. Hikata T, Iwanami A, Hosogane N, et al: High preoperative hemoglobin A1c is a risk factor for surgical site infection

after posterior thoracic and lumbar spinal instrumentation surgery. *J Orthop Sci* 2014;19(2):223-228.

44. Bitzer A, Mikula JD, Aziz KT, Best MJ, Nayar SK, Srikumaran U: Diabetes is an independent risk factor for infection after non-arthroplasty shoulder surgery: A national database study. *Phys Sportsmed* 2021;49(2):229-235.

    Diabetes mellitus significantly increases infection risk subsequent to shoulder surgery after adjusting for associated comorbidities in these patients. Level of evidence: IV.

45. Constantine RS, Le ELH, Gehring MB, Ohmes L, Iorio ML: Risk factors for infection after distal radius fracture fixation: Analysis of impact on cost of care. *J Hand Surg Glob Online* 2022;4(3):123-127.

    Male gender, open fracture, smoking, obesity, and comorbidities such as lung disease, chronic kidney disease, diabetes, hypertension, and liver disease are independent risk factors for developing a postoperative infection. Modifiable risk factors should be targeted for correction before surgery. Level of evidence: IV.

46. Shao J, Zhang H, Yin B, Li J, Zhu Y, Zhang Y: Risk factors for surgical site infection following operative treatment of ankle fractures: A systematic review and meta-analysis. *Int J Surg* 2018;56:124-132.

    Significant risk factors for SSI after surgical management of ankle fractures are obesity, American Society of Anesthesiologists score of 3 or greater, diabetes, alcohol consumption, open fracture, subluxation/dislocation, high-energy mechanism, chronic heart disease, history of allergy, and use of antibiotic prophylaxis. Level of evidence: I.

47. Brophy RH, Wright RW, Huston LJ, Nwosu SK, MOON Knee Group, Spindler KP: Factors associated with infection following anterior cruciate ligament reconstruction. *J Bone Joint Surg Am* 2015;97(6):450-454.

48. O'Neill SC, Queally JM, Hickey A, Mulhall KJ: Outcome of total hip and knee arthroplasty in HIV-infected patients: A systematic review. *Orthop Rev (Pavia)* 2019;11(1):8020.

    Patients with HIV infection are a unique patient population at a significantly higher risk of infection and revision after THA and TKA.

49. Klement MR, Penrose CT, Bala A, et al: Complications of total hip arthroplasty following solid organ transplantation. *J Orthop Sci* 2017;22(2):295-299.

50. Cavanaugh PK, Chen AF, Rasouli MR, Post ZD, Orozco FR, Ong AC: Total joint arthroplasty in transplant recipients: In-hospital adverse outcomes. *J Arthroplasty* 2015;30:840-845.

51. Momohara S, Kawakami K, Iwamoto T, et al: Prosthetic joint infection after total hip or knee arthroplasty in rheumatoid arthritis patients treated with nonbiologic and biologic disease-modifying antirheumatic drugs. *Mod Rheumatol* 2011;21(5):469-475.

52. Scherrer CB, Mannion AF, Kyburz D, Vogt M, Kramers-De Quervain IA: Infection risk after orthopedic surgery in patients with inflammatory rheumatic diseases treated with immunosuppressive drugs. *Arthritis Care Res (Hoboken)* 2013;65(12):2032-2040.

53. Tihista M, Gu A, Wei C, Weinreb JH, Rao RD: The impact of long-term corticosteroid use on acute postoperative complications following lumbar decompression surgery. *J Clin Orthop Trauma* 2020;11(5):921-927.

    The use of corticosteroid over a long term significantly increases the risk of acute postoperative complications, such as urinary tract infection, sepsis and septic shock, thromboembolic complications, and longer length of hospital stay, but not with superficial or deep infection in patients undergoing lumbar decompression procedures. Level of evidence: IV.

54. Kittle H, Ormseth A, Patetta MJ, Sood A, Gonzalez MH: Chronic corticosteroid use as a risk factor for perioperative complications in patients undergoing total joint arthroplasty. *J Am Acad Orthop Surg Glob Res Rev* 2020;4(7):e2000001.

    Chronic corticosteroid use and resultant immunosuppressive status significantly increases the risk of infection in the setting of TJA. Such association must be discussed with the patient before surgery. Level of evidence: IV.

55. Spatenkova V, Bradac O, Jindrisek Z, Hradil J, Fackova D, Halacova M: Risk factors associated with surgical site infections after thoracic or lumbar surgery: A 6-year single centre prospective cohort study. *J Orthop Surg Res* 2021;16(1):265.

    Corticosteroids, diabetes mellitus, or transfusions are not significant risk factors for the development of SSI; however, wound complications and warm seasons are significant. Level of evidence: II.

56. Ji C, Zhu Y, Liu S, et al: Incidence and risk of surgical site infection after adult femoral neck fractures treated by surgery: A retrospective case-control study. *Medicine (Baltimore)* 2019;98(11):e14882.

    Diabetes, obesity, corticosteroid use, anemia, and preoperative anemia are significant risk factors of SSI after surgical management of femoral neck fractures. Level of evidence: III.

57. Miric A, Inacio MCS, Namba RS: The effect of chronic kidney disease on total hip arthroplasty. *J Arthroplasty* 2014;29(6):1225-1230.

58. Browne JA, Casp AJ, Cancienne JM, Werner BC: Peritoneal dialysis does not carry the same risk as hemodialysis in patients undergoing hip or knee arthroplasty. *J Bone Joint Surg Am* 2019;101(14):1271-1277.

    The mode of dialysis has a significant effect on the risk of complications in patients dependent on dialysis who are undergoing THA/TKA. Compared with peritoneal dialysis, hemodialysis significantly increases the risk of infection. Level of evidence: IV.

59. Chou TA, Ma HH, Tsai SW, Chen CF, Wu PK, Chen WM: Dialysis patients have comparable results to patients who have received kidney transplant after total joint arthroplasty: A systematic review and meta-analysis. *EFORT Open Rev* 2021;6(8):618-628.

    In patients with ESRD, the type of renal replacement therapy (dialysis versus kidney transplantation) did not have a significant effect on the postoperative infection rate. Level of evidence: I.

60. Puvanesarajah V, Jain A, Hess DE, Shimer AL, Shen FH, Hassanzadeh H: Complications and mortality after lumbar spinal fusion in elderly patients with late stage renal disease. *Spine (Phila Pa 1976)* 2016;41(21):E1298-E1302.

61. Kothandaraman V, Kunkle B, Reid J, et al: Increased risk of perioperative complications in dialysis patients following rotator cuff repairs and knee arthroscopy. *Arthrosc Sports Med Rehabil* 2021;3(6):e1651-e1660.

    Patients on dialysis undergoing rotator cuff repair and knee arthroscopy are at a significantly higher risk of short-term complications after surgery. Patients should be counseled appropriately on this matter. Level of evidence: IV.

62. Ahlquist S, Hsiue PP, Chen CJ, et al: Renal disease is a risk factor for complications and mortality after open reduction internal fixation of proximal humerus fractures. *JSES Int* 2022;6(5):736-742.

    Patients with baseline renal disease are at a significantly increased risk of postoperative complications after surgical fixation of proximal humerus fractures. Level of evidence: IV.

63. Deleuran T, Vilstrup H, Overgaard S, Jepsen P: Cirrhosis patients have increased risk of complications after hip or knee arthroplasty: A Danish population-based cohort study. *Acta Orthop* 2015;86(1):108-113.

64. Seok HG, Park JJ, Park SG: Risk factors for periprosthetic joint infection after shoulder arthroplasty: Systematic review and meta-analysis. *J Clin Med* 2022;11(14):4245.

    The significant risk factors of PJI after shoulder arthroplasty are diabetes mellitus, liver disease, alcohol abuse, iron deficiency anemia, and rheumatoid arthritis. These specific factors shall be considered for risk stratification and counseling before surgery. Level of evidence: I.

65. Kuo SJ, Huang PH, Chang CC, et al: Hepatitis B virus infection is a risk factor for periprosthetic joint infection among males after total knee arthroplasty: A Taiwanese nationwide population-based study. *Medicine (Baltimore)* 2016;95(22):e3806.

66. Ross AJ, Ross BJ, Lee OC, Weldy JM, Sherman WF, Sanchez FL: A missed opportunity: The impact of hepatitis C treatment prior to total knee arthroplasty on postoperative complications. *J Arthroplasty* 2022;37(4):709-713.e2.

    Patients with hepatitis C virus have a significantly increased risk of PJI and revision arthroplasty following TKA. Antiviral treatment before TKA significantly decreases the risk of PJI postoperatively. Level of evidence: IV.

67. Schwarzkopf R, Novikov D, Anoushiravani AA, et al: The preoperative management of Hepatitis C may improve the outcome after total knee arthroplasty. *Bone Joint J* 2019;101-B(6):667-674.

    The management of hepatitis C before surgery again significantly reduces complications, including infection. Therefore, an appropriate preoperative optimization of patients is critical. Level of evidence: IV.

68. Su F, Cogan CJ, Bendich I, Zhang N, Whooley MA, Kuo AC: Hepatitis C infection and complication rates after total shoulder arthroplasty in United States veterans. *JSES Int* 2021;5(4):699-706.

    US military veterans with a history of hepatitis C virus are at a significantly higher risk of medical complications after total shoulder arthroplasty. Level of evidence: IV.

CHAPTER 4

Operating Room Environmental Risk Factors

GRAHAM S. GOH, MD • YALE A. FILLINGHAM, MD, FAAOS

ABSTRACT

Orthopaedic device–related infection is one of the most devastating complications in orthopaedic and trauma surgery. Infections occur when the microbial burden of a given tissue site exceeds the immune threshold of a host. Bioburden may arise from the patient's microbiome, skin flora of the perioperative team, particles in the air, or contamination of surgical instruments and the surgical field. Although the quantification of airborne particles and causal links between airborne transmission of pathogens and surgical wound contamination remain highly controversial topics in medical literature, the reduction of particles in operating room air and surfaces nonetheless remains a top priority for orthopaedic surgeons, dating back to the initial days of joint arthroplasty and other orthopaedic procedures. It is important to review the common sources of contamination within the operating room environment as well as examine the effectiveness of common interventions in addressing these sources of contamination.

Keywords: environmental contamination; operating room; prosthetic joint infection; sterility; surgical site infection

---

Dr. Goh or an immediate family member has received research or institutional support from American Academy of Orthopaedic Surgeons, American Association of Hip and Knee Surgeons, Hip Society and Musculoskeletal Infection Society, Knee Society, and Orthopaedic Research and Education Foundation. Dr. Fillingham or an immediate family member has received royalties from Exactech, Inc. and Medacta; serves as a paid consultant to or is an employee of Exactech, Inc., Johnson & Johnson, Medacta, and Zimmer; has stock or stock options held in Parvizi Surgical Innovations; and serves as a board member, owner, officer, or committee member of American Academy of Orthopaedic Surgeons and American Association of Hip and Knee Surgeons.

INTRODUCTION

Device-related infection is perhaps the most devastating complication in orthopaedic surgery. Its negative effect on patients' physical function, psychological wellbeing and overall life expectancy cannot be understated. Environmental factors play an important and often modifiable role in the pathogenesis of infection following implant or hardware insertion.

DEVICE-RELATED INFECTION

Infection rates can range between 5% and 10% in orthopaedic trauma, depending on the type of fracture as well as the site and severity of the injury.[1,2] Data from the 2021 American Joint Replacement Registry annual report have shown that infection was the primary reason to perform 20.1% of hip revisions and 25.2% of knee revisions.[3] Many modifiable and nonmodifiable risk factors for surgical site infection (SSI) and prosthetic joint infection (PJI) have been identified, one of which being an ultraclean operating room environment to reduce intraoperative environmental contamination.[4]

Bioburden on the surgical site may arise from the patient's microbiome, skin flora of the perioperative team, particles in the air, or contamination of surgical instruments and the surgical field. As the conceptual formula of the Centers for Disease Control and Prevention states, infections occur when microbial burden of a given tissue site exceeds the immune threshold of a host.[5] This has been confirmed in studies showing that the traditional presentation of a postoperative infection in a clean surgical wound required a microbial burden of approximately 105 colony-forming units (CFUs), whereas the presence of a foreign body significantly reduced the contaminating burden necessary to establish an infection.[6] Therefore, the reduction of particles in room air to produce ultraclean air has been a priority for orthopaedic surgeons, dating back to the initial days of joint arthroplasty and other orthopaedic procedures requiring implant insertion.

AIRBORNE ORGANISM LOAD

Monitoring Air Quality

To establish causal links between airborne transmission of pathogens and surgical wound contamination, an accurate determination of air quality in the operating room must be first established. Although particulate air sampling is less demanding and more standardized compared with microbiologic isolation, it remains an indirect measure of air quality that may not necessarily predict microbial contamination in all instances.[7]

Traditionally, microbial air sampling can be divided into passive (settling particles on agar plates) or active (cascade impactors or impingers) methods. However, different active air sampling devices often produce highly variable results, even when sampling is performed at the same place and time.[8] Over the past decade, the advent of laser real-time bacterial enumeration has permitted researchers to distinguish between viable and nonviable airborne particulates, yet few hospitals have incorporated these modern techniques into routine operating room air sampling, citing reasons such as high capital costs, lack of a standardized testing strategy, and failure to recognize airborne microbes as key factors in surgical infections.[9]

Airborne Particles as a Source of Contamination

Convection airflow in the operating room can spread airborne particles including dust, textile fibers, skin scales, and respiratory aerosols, all of which may contain viable microbes and settle onto environmental surfaces, the surgical wound, and instruments.[10] The assertion that airborne contamination accounts for a proportion of SSIs has been further supported by studies documenting the isolation of the same molecular strains of coagulase-negative staphylococci and *Staphylococcus aureus* from operating room air samples as well as nasopharyngeal samples from members of the surgical team during the same surgical cases.[11] The converse was also shown in a classic study that demonstrated the effect of increasing the rate of air changes on bacteria counts in the operating room,[12] underscoring the importance of minimizing airborne organism load in the operating room environment. It is now widely accepted that air in the operating room may play an important role in transmitting pathogens to the surgical site, and a significant correlation between bacterial CFU in the operating room environment and the incidence of SSI has been demonstrated.[13]

Organism Profile

Gram-positive organisms, such as *Staphylococcus* spp., *Bacillus* spp., and *Micrococcus* spp., are common in the operating room environment, followed by gram-negative organisms including *Acinetobacter* spp., *Moraxella* spp., *Pseudomonas* spp., and *Stenotrophomonas* spp.[14] Among these organisms, *S aureus* has been found to have the highest bacterial counts at all locations in the operating room and is frequently resistant to methicillin and ampicillin.[15] Concerns regarding contaminated ventilation ductwork in hospital buildings have surfaced, which have resulted in increased environmental contamination and the spread of gram-negative bacterial infections.[16]

Interventions to Reduce Air Contamination

Current SSI prevention strategies for reducing air contamination can be broadly divided into four approaches: dilution (15 to 20 air changes per hour), filtration (high-efficiency particulate arrestance [HEPA] filtration), pressurization (positive pressure), and disinfection.[4,17] Temperature and humidity should also be controlled. In addition to limiting door openings and the number of personnel during a surgical case to reduce operating room traffic, other common strategies include the use of surgical helmet systems (SHSs); ultraviolet light (UVL) plus heating, ventilation, and air conditioning systems; and ultraclean ventilation. These methods will be discussed in subsequent sections. Most hospitals follow the Centers for Disease Control and Prevention guidelines for the prevention of SSI, which recommend that airflow in the operating room be controlled and regulated to filter airborne microorganisms.[18,19] One report suggested that an acceptable bacterial limit for a working operating room should be below 180 CFU/m^3,[20,21] although the lack of consistency in operating room settings, sampling methods (eg, absorption of the medium, the amount of air drawn, size of sampling tool), sampling locations, and study periods may account for differences in microbial concentrations in different studies.

REDUCING OPERATING ROOM TRAFFIC

A higher number of door openings and operating room personnel have been identified as key factors influencing the bioburden in operating room air.[21] Multiple studies, including one from 2018, have shown that unnecessary operating room traffic increases the risk of SSI.[22-24] Consequently, the 2018 International Consensus Meeting (ICM) on musculoskeletal infections reached 98% agreement that the number of individuals in the operating room and door openings during total joint arthroplasty (TJA) should be limited because of its positive relationship with the number of airborne particles in the operating room.[25] Interestingly, the activity level of personnel in the operating room has also been shown to correlate with bacteria fallout into the sterile field.[26] Frequency of door openings has been estimated to be 0.19/min to 0.65/min for primary TJA and 0.84 per minutes for revision TJA, with the highest percentage of door openings occurring during preincision[22] or postincision periods.[7]

Door openings result in turbulent airflow, disrupting the positive laminar airflow (LAF) of the operating room and accelerating the spread of airborne particles toward the surgical field.[27] For example, this disturbance in airflow can overwhelm the positive operating room pressure in TJA cases, causing a transient reversal of airflow from the hallway into the operating room, but the time needed for the recovery of pressurization has not been determined.[28]

Multiple strategies have been implemented to limit operating room traffic and reduce contamination with the goal of decreasing the incidence of PJI.[22,29,30] One study showed that systemic and behavioral measures such as limiting unnecessary activity and personnel in the operating room led to a significant decrease in the incidence of prolonged wound drainage and superficial infections postoperatively, as well as a nonsignificant reduction in deep infections.[30] Some measures proposed in the literature have been summarized in **Table 1**.

ULTRACLEAN VENTILATION SYSTEMS, HEPA AIR FILTERS, AND LAF

Airflow systems play a major role in maintaining sterility in the operating room. Ventilated air was first introduced in 1964 by Sir John Charnley, who suggested that airborne particles could be blown away from the sterile field using clean air during total hip arthroplasty.[31] Ultraclean air in the operating room can significantly reduce the rate of SSI, as demonstrated in a multicenter randomized controlled trial involving more than 8,000 patients undergoing arthroplasty.[32] Ultraclean ventilation has now become the gold standard within orthopaedic operating rooms, reducing airborne contamination by providing a constant and uniform flow of high-velocity (0.3 to 0.5 m/s), highly filtered air that passes through a HEPA filter, which removes 99.97% of all particles that are larger than 0.3 μm. Modern airflow systems create more than 500 air changes per hour and help to reduce bacterial CFUs from 5.4/ft^2 to 0.45/ft^2.[33]

In combination with advanced filtration, positive-pressure ventilation systems now constitute an essential component of any operating room, with the two main types of airflow systems being conventional turbulent airflow and LAF systems.[27] In theory, LAF systems create a clean air environment in the operating room by increasing the rate of air exchange within the room from 30 times per hour to more than 300 times per hour.[34] The Medical Research Council showed that the use of LAF could decrease the infection rate by almost one-half.[35]

Despite strong evidence by the Medical Research Council, a growing body of evidence has questioned the effectiveness of LAF systems in reducing rates of SSI or PJI.[36-38] Registry data from the New Zealand Joint Registry[34,39] and the German national surveillance system for nosocomial infections (Krankenhaus Infektions Surveillance System)[36] have also questioned the usefulness of LAF systems in preventing deep infection. These reports have culminated in a meta-analysis, the results of which suggested that there was no additional benefit in using LAF compared with conventional turbulent ventilation in the prevention of SSIs following TJA.[37] The Centers for Disease Control and Prevention[40] and the World Health Organization have recommended that LAF ventilation systems should not be used to reduce the risk of SSI for patients undergoing TJA (conditional recommendation, low to very low quality of evidence).[41] It is important to consider that advances in surgical technique and perioperative protocols over the past few decades may have diminished the importance of LAF in preventing SSIs. These include the improved use of perioperative prophylactic antibiotics, patient optimization, and modern operating room filtration methods.

UVL DECONTAMINATION

Current evidence has shown that manual cleaning and disinfection of the operating room environment may be inadequate because of human error,[42] which can

Table 1

Measures to Limit Operating Room Traffic and Reduce Contamination

1. Restricting the number of people who can be present during an implant procedure (especially observers, researchers, and external vendors)
2. Storing commonly used instruments in the OR
3. Educating OR personnel on the potential association between OR traffic and infection
4. Using verbal interventions to warn staff of unjustified OR traffic
5. Detailed preoperative planning and templating to ensure that all necessary instruments and implants are ready before starting a case
6. Opening instrument trays as close as possible to the time of incision so as to reduce exposure to OR traffic
7. Locking the external OR door immediately after wheeling in the patient and allowing entrance only via the inner doors
8. Using an intercom for communication with the outer door
9. Using door alarms to prohibit DOs
10. Minimizing staff rotation during each case, ideally to zero
11. Disallowing DOs for social reasons, discussions, or preparing anesthetic supplies for the next case

DO = door opening, OR = operating room

then result in only one-half of surfaces being disinfected after terminal manual cleaning. In the inpatient setting, residual pathogens on contaminated surfaces have been associated with an increased risk of contracting a hospital-acquired infection,[43] and this relationship may hold true for patients undergoing surgery in the operating room.

In 2018, it was reported that no-touch disinfection technologies such as UVL disinfection systems and hydrogen peroxide vapor systems are increasingly used as adjuncts to manual cleaning at health care institutions in an effort to enhance disinfection and limit SSI incidence.[44] In a 2022 meta-analysis of 13 studies on UVL systems, significant reductions in *Clostridium difficile* infection (relative risk [RR], 0.64) and vancomycin-resistant enterococci infection rates (RR, 0.42) were noted, although only one study applied UVL in the operating room setting and there was no difference in the rate of methicillin-resistant *S aureus* or gram-negative multidrug-resistant pathogens compared with manual disinfection. Given the limited evidence, the Association of periOperative Registered Nurses guidelines state that emerging no-touch technologies may be considered as an adjunct to terminal manual cleaning processes, but additional research is needed.[17]

OPERATING ROOM TEMPERATURE AND PATIENT NORMOTHERMIA

Patient exposure to the cold air of the operating room (due to continuous air changes with the use of ultraclean ventilation systems) coupled with vasodilation following anesthesia induction may cause a decrease in core body temperature and perioperative hypothermia, defined as a core temperature of less than 36°C. Similarly, infusion of cool intravenous fluids and prewashing patients may increase this risk.[45]

Studies have shown that a reduction in core temperature of 2°C or greater was associated with a threefold increase in SSI risk[46] that has been attributed to impaired oxygen perfusion because of vasoconstriction and decreased collagen deposition. Other detriments of perioperative hypothermia include prolonged length of stay, increased blood loss, and higher mortality rates,[45] enforcing the role of intraoperative warming as standard of care.

Forced air warming (FAW) devices were previously a common type of patient warming device used in orthopaedic surgery.[47] However, as FAW devices expel warm air that is approximately 20°C higher than the temperature of operating room air, the difference in temperature generates convection currents, which have been shown to interfere with the effectiveness of LAF.[48] One popular alternative to FAW devices is conductive fabric warming devices that are more thermally efficient and release less heat into the surroundings while mitigating the risk of perioperative hypothermia.[49] Although the 2018 ICM concluded that there was no definite link between FAW devices and an increased risk of surgical infection, delegates advised that alternative methods of warming should be used.[25]

PERSONAL PROTECTION SUITS

Personal protection suits such as body exhaust suits (BES) and SHSs have been widely used in orthopaedic practice. The main difference between the two systems is that negative intrasuit pressure is maintained by aspiration tubing in BES, whereas SHS uses a fan on a helmet to maintain a positive-pressure environment within the suit.[50] A systematic review[51] identified multiple suit designs, materials, and filtering systems in different commercially available BESs and SHSs.[51] When PJI rates were compared between BES and conventional gowns, the pooled PJI rate was 0.17% (3 of 1,795 patients) compared with 1.0% (16 of 1,604 patients) at a mean of 2.5 years, respectively ($P < 0.01$). In contrast, three registry-based studies of 175,018 patients found that SHS was associated with a higher rate of deep infections (RR, 1.67) after adjustment for covariates, although this difference did not reach statistical significance ($P = 0.09$). Subsequently, data from 2018 obtained from the New Zealand Joint Registry found no difference in revision surgery or infection when surgical helmets were used in both total hip and total knee arthroplasty at 6-month and 1-year follow-up.[52]

Given the inconsistent evidence, the 2018 ICM report on musculoskeletal infections reached an 87% agreement that the use of personal protection suits is not associated with a decreased rate of subsequent SSI or PJI.[53] However, for surgeons who choose to use SHS, greater consideration should be given toward gowning systems that minimize the leakage of particles at the gown-glove interface.[54] In addition, it was reported in 2019 that airflow systems should not be activated before scrubbing in to reduce hand contamination,[55] and the SHS should ideally be activated only after complete surgical gowning.[56] Given that surgical helmets are also often contaminated with pathogens known to cause SSI, a study from 2022 reported that regular disinfection with a hypochlorite spray may be necessary to eliminate contaminants.[57]

LIGHT HANDLES, BACK TABLE, SPLASH BASINS, AND INSTRUMENT TRAYS

Operating Room Lights and Light Handles

Although the operating room light is considered a low-touch area in the operating room, it has been shown to be contaminated with bacteria, growing a maximum of 2.84 CFU/cm² in one report.[58] Using an adenosine triphosphate bioluminescence assay, light handles were also demonstrated to contain 647.8 ± 903.7 relative light units of localized bioburden.[59] Although no intraoperative measures to prevent contamination of the operating room light surface or light handle have been proposed to date, surgeons should nonetheless be cognizant of this source of contamination.

Splash Basins

Splash basins filled with sterile water in the operating room have been traditionally used to store, wash, and clear instruments of debris before reuse during an orthopaedic procedure. However, increasing evidence from a 2018 study has suggested that splash basins are a pertinent source of intraoperative bacterial contamination, with contamination rates varying widely between 2.2% and 74.4%.[60] In view of this, the 2018 ICM reached a 91% agreement advocating against the use of splash basins in orthopaedic procedures until further evidence becomes available.[61] Some studies, including one from 2020, have suggested using a dilute antiseptic solution such as chlorhexidine gluconate or dilute povidone-iodine instead of sterile water to decrease intraoperative contamination.[60,62]

Back Table

Although traditionally thought to be sterile, the back table has been identified as a potential source of microbial contamination in some studies, demonstrating a higher bioburden compared with the sterile field.[63] In a 2022 report, germicidal UVL-emitting diode was introduced to address this contamination potential, which is a smaller device compared with UVL systems that can be used for local disinfection in contrast to disinfection of the entire room.[64] Another strategy reported on in 2022 to reduce back table contamination involves fitting the back table inside a ventilation-rich zone.[65] Notwithstanding, further studies are needed to evaluate the cost-effectiveness and efficacy in reducing SSI of these emerging technologies.

Instrument Trays

Because surgical instruments are most commonly contaminated by airborne particles in the operating room, this may allow the transmission of bacteria into the surgical wound despite maintaining sterility of the surgical field. Contamination of surgical instruments was found to be time dependent in a study that reported a 4% tray contamination rate after 30 minutes of exposure compared with 30% after 4 hours.[66] The direct correlation between exposure timing of opened instrument trays was, however, minimized to a certain degree when implants were covered with a sterile towel.[66] Contamination of surgical instruments and trays has been shown to increase the incidence of deep infections.[67] It is thus recommended that instrument trays should be opened as close to the time of surgery as possible, and when not in use, these trays should then be covered with a sterile towel or drape.[61]

SUMMARY

Orthopaedic device–related infection is one of the most devastating complications in orthopaedic and trauma surgery. Despite all efforts, it is extremely difficult to maintain an operating room environment free from particles. Bioburden may arise from the patient's own microbiome, skin flora of the perioperative team, particles in the air, or contamination of surgical instruments and the surgical field. If the bioburden exceeds the immune threshold of the host, this may result in a subsequent infection. Although the quantification of airborne particles and causal links between airborne transmission of pathogens and surgical wound contamination remain highly controversial topics in medical literature, the reduction of particles in operating room air and surfaces nonetheless remains a top priority for orthopaedic surgeons, dating back to the initial days of joint arthroplasty and other orthopaedic procedures. Air quality must be maintained in any operating room via the use of ultraclean ventilation systems, which often involve the use of HEPA filters and conventional turbulent airflow or LAF systems. Operating room traffic, including the number of operating room personnel and door openings during the surgical case, should be kept to a minimum. Perioperative hypothermia should be avoided with the use of reflective blankets, and FAW devices should be avoided because of the risk of upward convection currents that increase airborne contamination. Surgeons should be cognizant of other sources of surface contamination, such as operating room light handles, the back table, and splash basins. Some emerging technologies involve the use of UVL in operating room disinfection and sterile processing. These methods may circumvent the potential for human error in manual cleaning using chemical disinfectants. Although many engineering methods and antiseptic products have been designed to decrease SSI rates by minimizing intraoperative and postoperative direct environmental wound contamination, a greater awareness of these environmental factors by the operating room team remains paramount. Knowledge of how to maintain high air quality within the operating room and the factors affecting air quality should be imparted to all members of the surgical team. Despite these measures, to suggest that most SSIs are due to intraoperative contamination would ultimately require matching the exact microorganism present at the surgical wound at the end of the case to the causative pathogen in SSI. Therefore, molecular methods such as metagenomics and RNA sequencing at the strain level may help to track microbial movement across the operating room environment, to the hair and skin of personnel, to the exposed surgical wound and surgical field, and finally, to the clinically evident SSI. Until such evidence emerges, surgeons and perioperative teams should still uphold sterile techniques to minimize bioburden and potentially avoid bacterial transmission within the operating room environment.

KEY STUDY POINTS

- Although the quantification of airborne particles and causal links between airborne transmission of pathogens and surgical wound contamination remain highly controversial topics, the reduction of particles in operating room air and surfaces nonetheless remains a top priority for orthopaedic surgeons.
- Current SSI prevention strategies for reducing airborne contamination can be broadly classified into four approaches: dilution, filtration, pressurization, and disinfection.
- A higher number of door openings and operating room personnel has been identified as key factors influencing the bioburden in operating room air. Perioperative protocols should be set up to minimize these occurrences.
- Ultraclean ventilation has become the gold standard within orthopaedic operating rooms, reducing airborne contamination by providing a constant and uniform flow of high-velocity, highly filtered air that passes through a HEPA filter. However, the utility of LAF remains highly controversial.
- SHSs have not been shown to reduce infection rates. However, they protect from splash contact with patient blood, and this reason alone may be enough to justify its added costs.
- Surgeons should be cognizant of other sources of surface contamination, such as operating room light handles, the back table, and splash basins. These sources should be addressed through thorough disinfection.

ANNOTATED REFERENCES

1. Patzakis MJ, Wilkins J: Factors influencing infection rate in open fracture wounds. *Clin Orthop Relat Res* 1989;243:36-40.

2. Richards JE, Kauffmann RM, Obremskey WT, May AK: Stress-induced hyperglycemia as a risk factor for surgical-site infection in nondiabetic orthopedic trauma patients admitted to the intensive care unit. *J Orthop Trauma* 2013;27(1):16-21.

3. American Joint Replacement Registry (AJRR): 2021 Annual Report, 2021. Available at: https://www.aaos.org/globalassets/registries/ajrr-2021-annual-report-preview.pdf.

    This report demonstrates that infection has overtaken aseptic loosening as the main cause of failure in TJA.

4. Sehulster L, Chinn R, Arduino M, et al: Guidelines for environmental infection control in health-care facilities. *Recommendations from CDC and the Healthcare Infection Control Practices Advisory Committee (HICPAC)*, 2004. Available at: https://www.cdc.gov/infectioncontrol/pdf/guidelines/environmental-guidelines-P.pdf.

5. Rutala W, Weber D, Healthcare Infection Control Practices Advisory Committee (HICPAC): Bioburden of Surgical Devices. Guideline for Disinfection and Sterilization in Healthcare Facilities, 2008. Available at: https://www.cdc.gov/infectioncontrol/pdf/guidelines/disinfection-guidelines-H.pdf.

6. Zimmerli W, Trampuz A, Ochsner PE: Prosthetic-joint infections. *N Engl J Med* 2004;351(16):1645-1654.

7. Cristina ML, Spagnolo AM, Sartini M, et al: Can particulate air sampling predict microbial load in operating theatres for arthroplasty? *PLoS One* 2012;7(12):e52809.

8. Pasquarella C, Albertini R, Dall'aglio P, Saccani E, Sansebastiano GE, Signorelli C: Air microbial sampling: The state of the art. *Ig Sanita Pubbl* 2008;64(1):79-120.

9. Parvizi J, Barnes S, Shohat N, Edmiston CE: Environment of care: Is it time to reassess microbial contamination of the operating room air as a risk factor for surgical site infection in total joint arthroplasty? *Am J Infect Control* 2017;45(11):1267-1272.

10. Stocks GW, Self SD, Thompson B, Adame XA, O'Connor DP: Predicting bacterial populations based on airborne particulates: A study performed in nonlaminar flow operating rooms during joint arthroplasty surgery. *Am J Infect Control* 2010;38(3):199-204.

11. Edmiston CEJ, Seabrook GR, Cambria RA, et al: Molecular epidemiology of microbial contamination in the operating room environment: Is there a risk for infection? *Surgery* 2005;138(4):573-579.

12. Goddard KR: *Design of air handling systems. Tech. Proc. Inst. Control Infect. Hosp.*, University of Michigan, 1965, pp 158-162.

13. Darouiche RO, Green DM, Harrington MA, et al: Association of airborne microorganisms in the operating room with implant infections: A randomized controlled trial. *Infect Control Hosp Epidemiol* 2017;38(1):3-10.

14. Wan GH, Chung FF, Tang CS: Long-term surveillance of air quality in medical center operating rooms. *Am J Infect Control* 2011;39(4):302-308.

15. Tang CS, Wan GH: Air quality monitoring of the post-operative recovery room and locations surrounding operating theaters in a medical center in Taiwan. *PLoS One* 2013;8(4):e61093.

16. Beggs C, Knibbs LD, Johnson GR, Morawska L: Environmental contamination and hospital-acquired infection: Factors that are easily overlooked. *Indoor Air* 2015;25(5):462-474.

17. AORN Guidelines for Perioperative Practice – AORN n.d. Available at: https://www.aorn.org/guidelines/about-aorn-guidelines. Accessed July 29, 2022.

18. Mangram AJ, Horan TC, Pearson ML, Silver LC, Jarvis WR: Guideline for prevention of surgical site infection, 1999. Hospital infection control practices advisory committee. *Infect Control Hosp Epidemiol* 1999;20:247-280.

19. Anderson DJ, Podgorny K, Berríos-Torres SI, et al: Strategies to prevent surgical site infections in acute care hospitals: 2014 update. *Infect Control Hosp Epidemiol* 2014;35(6):605-627.

20. Dai C, Zhang Y, Ma X, et al: Real-time measurements of airborne biologic particles using fluorescent particle counter to evaluate microbial contamination: Results of a comparative study in an operating theater. *Am J Infect Control* 2015;43(1):78-81.

21. Scaltriti S, Cencetti S, Rovesti S, Marchesi I, Bargellini A, Borella P: Risk factors for particulate and microbial contamination of air in operating theatres. *J Hosp Infect* 2007;66(4):320-326.

22. Panahi P, Stroh M, Casper DS, Parvizi J, Austin MS: Operating room traffic is a major concern during total joint arthroplasty. *Clin Orthop Relat Res* 2012;470(10):2690-2694.

23. Hamilton WG, Balkam CB, Purcell RL, Parks NL, Holdsworth JE: Operating room traffic in total joint arthroplasty: Identifying patterns and training the team to keep the door shut. *Am J Infect Control* 2018;46:633-636.

    In this three-phase observational study, an educational seminar for operating room staff and vendors successfully reduced door openings during surgery. Level of evidence: II.

24. Teter J, Guajardo I, Al-Rammah T, Rosson G, Perl TM, Manahan M: Assessment of operating room airflow using air particle counts and direct observation of door openings. *Am J Infect Control* 2017;45(5):477-482.

25. Baldini A, Blevins K, Del Gaizo D, et al: General assembly, prevention, operating room - personnel: Proceedings of international consensus on orthopedic infections. *J Arthroplasty* 2019;34(2 suppl):S97-S104.

    This document contains several consensus statements from world experts describing various methods of infection prevention within the operating room environment. Level of evidence: V.

26. Quraishi ZA, Blais FX, Sottile WS, Adler LM: Movement of personnel and wound contamination. *AORN J* 1983;38(1):146-147, 150-156.

27. Smith EB, Raphael IJ, Maltenfort MG, Honsawek S, Dolan K, Younkins EA: The effect of laminar air flow and door openings on operating room contamination. *J Arthroplasty* 2013;28(9):1482-1485.

28. Mears SC, Blanding R, Belkoff SM: Door opening affects operating room pressure during joint arthroplasty. *Orthopedics* 2015;38(11):e991-e994.

29. Pada S, Perl TM: Operating room myths: What is the evidence for common practices. *Curr Opin Infect Dis* 2015;28(4):369-374.

30. Knobben BA, van Horn JR, van der Mei HC, Busscher HJ: Evaluation of measures to decrease intra-operative bacterial contamination in orthopaedic implant surgery. *J Hosp Infect* 2006;62(2):174-180.

31. Charnley J: A clean-air operating enclosure. *Br J Surg* 1964;51:202-205.

32. Lidwell OM, Elson RA, Lowbury EJ, et al: Ultraclean air and antibiotics for prevention of postoperative infection: A multicenter study of 8,052 joint replacement operations. *Acta Orthop Scand* 1987;58(1):4-13.

33. Nelson JP, Glassburn AR Jr, Talbott RD, McElhinney JP: The effect of previous surgery, operating room environment, and preventive antibiotics on postoperative infection following total hip arthroplasty. *Clin Orthop Relat Res* 1980;147:167-169.

34. Hooper GJ, Rothwell AG, Frampton C, Wyatt MC: Does the use of laminar flow and space suits reduce early deep infection after total hip and knee replacement? *J Bone Joint Surg Br* 2011;93(1):85-90.

35. Lidwell OM, Lowbury EJ, Whyte W, Blowers R, Stanley SJ, Lowe D: Effect of ultraclean air in operating rooms on deep sepsis in the joint after total hip or knee replacement: A randomised study. *Br Med J* 1982;285(6334):10-14.

36. Brandt C, Hott U, Sohr D, Daschner F, Gastmeier P, Rüden H: Operating room ventilation with laminar airflow shows no protective effect on the surgical site infection rate in orthopedic and abdominal surgery. *Ann Surg* 2008;248(5):695-700.

37. Bischoff P, Kubilay NZ, Allegranzi B, Egger M, Gastmeier P: Effect of laminar airflow ventilation on surgical site infections: A systematic review and meta-analysis. *Lancet Infect Dis* 2017;17(5):553-561.

38. Gastmeier P, Breier AC, Brandt C: Influence of laminar airflow on prosthetic joint infections: A systematic review. *J Hosp Infect* 2012;81(2):73-78.

39. Tayton ER, Frampton C, Hooper GJ, Young SW: The impact of patient and surgical factors on the rate of infection after primary total knee arthroplasty: An analysis of 64,566 joints from the New Zealand Joint Registry. *Bone Joint J* 2016;98-B(3):334-340.

40. Berríos-Torres SI, Umscheid CA, Bratzler DW, et al: Centers for disease control and prevention guideline for the prevention of surgical site infection, 2017. *JAMA Surg* 2017;152(8):784-791.

41. Leaper DJ, Edmiston CE: World Health Organization: Global guidelines for the prevention of surgical site infection. *J Hosp Infect* 2017;95(2):135-136.

42. Munoz-Price LS, Birnbach DJ, Lubarsky DA, et al: Decreasing operating room environmental pathogen contamination through improved cleaning practice. *Infect Control Hosp Epidemiol* 2012;33(9):897-904.

43. Huang SS, Datta R, Platt R: Risk of acquiring antibiotic-resistant bacteria from prior room occupants. *Arch Intern Med* 2006;166(18):1945-1951.

44. Marra AR, Schweizer ML, Edmond MB: No-touch disinfection methods to decrease multidrug-resistant organism infections: A systematic review and meta-analysis. *Infect Control Hosp Epidemiol* 2018;39(1):20-31.

    UVL led to a significant reduction in *C difficile* infection and vancomycin-resistant enterococci infection rates, although no differences were found in rates of methicillin-resistant *S aureus* or gram-negative multidrug-resistant pathogens. Level of evidence: III.

45. Bush HL, Hydo LJ, Fischer E, Fantini GA, Silane MF, Barie PS: Hypothermia during elective abdominal aortic aneurysm repair: The high price of avoidable morbidity. *J Vasc Surg* 1995;21(3):392-400.

46. Kurz A, Sessler DI, Lenhardt R: Perioperative normothermia to reduce the incidence of surgical-wound infection and shorten hospitalization. Study of Wound Infection and Temperature Group. *N Engl J Med* 1996;334(19):1209-1215.

47. Mahoney CB, Odom J: Maintaining intraoperative normothermia: A meta-analysis of outcomes with costs. *AANA J* 1999;67(2):155-163.

48. McGovern PD, Albrecht M, Belani KG, et al: Forced-air warming and ultra-clean ventilation do not mix: An investigation of theatre ventilation, patient warming and joint replacement infection in orthopaedics. *J Bone Joint Surg Br* 2011;93(11):1537-1544.

49. Ng V, Lai A, Ho V: Comparison of forced-air warming and electric heating pad for maintenance of body temperature during total knee replacement. *Anaesthesia* 2006;61(11):1100-1104.

50. Young SW, Chisholm C, Zhu M: Intraoperative contamination and space suits: A potential mechanism. *Eur J Orthop Surg Traumatol* 2014;24(3):409-413.

51. Young SW, Zhu M, Shirley OC, Wu Q, Spangehl MJ: Do "surgical helmet systems" or "body exhaust suits" affect contamination and deep infection rates in arthroplasty? A systematic review. *J Arthroplasty* 2016;31(1):225-233.

52. Vijaysegaran P, Knibbs LD, Morawska L, Crawford RW: Surgical space suits increase particle and microbiological emission rates in a simulated surgical environment. *J Arthroplasty* 2018;33(5):1524-1529.

    Space suits cause increased particle and microbiologic emission rates compared with standard surgical clothing. This finding provides mechanistic evidence to support the increased PJI rates observed in clinical studies. Level of evidence: III.

53. Abouljoud MM, Alvand A, Boscainos P, et al: Hip and knee section, prevention, operating room environment: Proceedings of international consensus on orthopedic infections. *J Arthroplasty* 2019;34(2 suppl):S293-S300.

    This document contains several consensus statements from world experts describing various methods of infection prevention within the operating room environment when performing total joint arthroplasty cases. Level of evidence: V.

54. Fraser JF, Young SW, Valentine KA, Probst NE, Spangehl MJ: The gown-glove interface is a source of contamination: A comparative study. *Clin Orthop Relat Res* 2015;473:2291-2297.

55. Moores TS, Khan SA, Chatterton BD, Harvey G, Lewthwaite SC: A microbiological assessment of sterile surgical helmet systems using particle counts and culture plates: Recommendations for safe use whilst scrubbing. *J Hosp Infect* 2019;101(3):354-360.

    Bacterial count increased 3.7-fold with the fan switched on, and all helmets had positive cultures (mean 36 CFU/m^2). There were no positive cultures with the standard arthroplasty hood or the SHS with the fan switched off. Level of evidence: II.

56. Hanselman AE, Montague MD, Murphy TR, Dietz MJ: Contamination relative to the activation timing of filtered-exhaust helmets. *J Arthroplasty* 2016;31(4):776-780.

57. Tarabichi S, Chisari E, Van Nest DS, Krueger CA, Parvizi J: Surgical helmets used during total joint arthroplasty harbor common pathogens: A cautionary note. *J Arthroplasty* 2022;37(8):1636-1639.

    Surgical helmets worn during orthopaedic procedures were frequently contaminated with common pathogens. This contamination can be avoided when disinfected with a hypochlorite spray. Level of evidence: II.

58. Link T, Kleiner C, Mancuso MP, Dziadkowiec O, Halverson-Carpenter K: Determining high touch areas in the operating room with levels of contamination. *Am J Infect Control* 2016;44(11):1350-1355.

59. Richard RD, Bowen TR: What orthopaedic operating room surfaces are contaminated with bioburden? A study using the ATP bioluminescence assay. *Clin Orthop Relat Res* 2017;475(7):1819-1824.

60. Lindgren KE, Pelt CE, Anderson MB, Peters CL, Spivak ES, Gililland JM: A chlorhexidine solution reduces aerobic organism growth in operative splash basins in a randomized controlled trial. *J Arthroplasty* 2018;33(1):211-215.

    Addition of chlorhexidine gluconate could eliminate bacterial growth within the splash basin (zero versus 9% in sterile water). Level of evidence: I.

61. Alsadaan M, Alrumaih HA, Brown T, et al: General assembly, prevention, operating room – Surgical field: Proceedings of international consensus on orthopedic infections. *J Arthroplasty* 2019;34(2 suppl):S127-S130.

    This document contains several consensus statements from world experts describing various methods of infection prevention within the surgical field. Level of evidence: V.

62. Nazal MR, Galloway JL, Dhaliwal KK, Nishiyama SK, Shields JS: Dilute povidone-iodine solution prevents intraoperative contamination of sterile water basins during total joint arthroplasty. *J Arthroplasty* 2020;35(1):241-246.

    Addition of dilute povidone-iodine could eliminate bacterial growth within the splash basin (zero versus 48% in sterile water). Level of evidence: I.

63. Gormley T, Markel TA, Jones HW 3rd, et al: Methodology for analyzing environmental quality indicators in a dynamic operating room environment. *Am J Infect Control* 2017;45(4):354-359.

64. Jennings JM, Miner TM, Johnson RM, Pollet AK, Brady AC, Dennis DA: A back table ultraviolet light decreases

environmental contamination during operative cases. *Am J Infect Control* 2022;50(6):686-689.

A UVL emitting diode on the contamination level of a back table in the operating room could reduce CFUs at 24 and 48 hours, effectively decreasing contamination near the surgical field. Level of evidence: I.

65. Seth Caous J, Svensson Malchau K, Petzold M, et al: Instrument tables equipped with local unidirectional airflow units reduce bacterial contamination during orthopedic implant surgery in an operating room with a displacement ventilation system. *Infect Prev Pract* 2022;4(3):100222.

Local unidirectional airflow above the surgical instruments significantly reduced the bacterial count in the air above assistant table and instrument table, as well as on the instrument dummies from the assistant table. Level of evidence: II.

66. Dalstrom DJ, Venkatarayappa I, Manternach AL, Palcic MS, Heyse BA, Prayson MJ: Time-dependent contamination of opened sterile operating-room trays. *J Bone Joint Surg Am* 2008;90:1022-1025.

67. Dancer SJ, Stewart M, Coulombe C, Gregori A, Virdi M: Surgical site infections linked to contaminated surgical instruments. *J Hosp Infect* 2012;81(4):231-238.

CHAPTER 5

Perioperative Strategies to Reduce Surgical Site Infection

JEREMY M. GILILLAND, MD, FAAOS • VICTOR R. CARLSON, MD
PATRICK J. KELLAM, MD • JAMES P. REYNOLDS, MD

ABSTRACT

Multiple perioperative strategies have been used to reduce the risk of surgical site infection with varying levels of evidence. Given the significant burden surgical site infections place on patients and health care systems at large, it is imperative that surgeons are aware of the strategies that are available to combat these devastating postoperative complications. Timely administration of antibiotics remains one of the most important modalities to prevent surgical site infections. Skin site preparation, soft-tissue handling, wound closure, and dressing are additional important adjuncts.

Keywords: local measures; perioperative infection reduction; periprosthetic infection; surgical site infection

---

Dr. Gililland or an immediate family member has received royalties from MiCare Path and OrthoGrid; serves as a paid consultant to or is an employee of DJ Orthopaedics, OrthoGrid, and Stryker; has stock or stock options held in CoNextions and OrthoGrid; has received research or institutional support from Biomet, Stryker, and Zimmer; and serves as a board member, owner, officer, or committee member of American Academy of Orthopaedic Surgeons, American Association of Hip and Knee Surgeons, Hip Society, and Knee Society. None of the following authors or any immediate family member has received anything of value from or has stock or stock options held in a commercial company or institution related directly or indirectly to the subject of this chapter: Dr. Carlson, Dr. Kellam, and Dr. Reynolds.

INTRODUCTION

Substantial effort has been made to reduce the number of postoperative complications from surgical site infections (SSIs) within all orthopaedic subspecialties. In response, multiple perioperative local measures have been investigated in hopes of decreasing the risk of SSI and may serve as strategies for all musculoskeletal surgeries. Appropriate administration of antibiotics, skin site preparation, nasal decolonization, barrier draping, wound closure, and dressing are all areas in which attention to detail can potentially decrease the risk of SSI.

PREOPERATIVE STRATEGIES

In 2010, approximately 48 million surgical and nonsurgical procedures were performed in the United States.[1] Despite many advances in surgery, it is estimated that an SSI will develop in 2% to 4% of the postoperative patients, imparting significant morbidity and mortality to patients.[2] Although the severity of the SSIs vary, they represent a substantial cost to the US health care system, with estimates of up to $10 billion annually.[3-5] Timely administration of antibiotics is perhaps the most powerful modality to reduce the risk of SSI[6] (**Table 1**). Several studies, including one from 2019, have reported that cephalosporins, and cefazolin in particular, have an established record of effective prophylaxis for musculoskeletal procedures.[7-9] Caution should be exercised when transitioning to other agents in the setting of a reported penicillin allergy. A 2019 study on total joint arthroplasty (TJA) found that 97% of patients with an initial allergy-related contraindication to cephalosporins were cleared to receive cephalosporins based on skin allergy testing, highlighting the low rate of true penicillin allergy positivity.[7] In patients who do require a different agent, vancomycin and clindamycin are appropriate

Table 1

Preoperative Strategies

Appropriately timed antibiotic administration, ideally cefazolin

Methicillin-resistant *Staphylococcus aureus* colonization screening and treatment when indicated

Delaying elective procedures in patients with open wounds or poor dentition

Surgical site cleansing agents and antiseptic soap

Avoiding hair removal with razors

---

alternatives. To maximize the effect of antibiotic prophylaxis, drug levels must achieve bactericidal levels at the time of incision and continue at this level throughout the procedure. Several studies on prophylaxis, including one from 2018, reported that for cefazolin, appropriate weight-based dosage, administration within 60 minutes of incision, and redosing during extended procedures are critical.[10-12] Redosing of cefazolin should be considered when surgical duration exceeds 4 hours or when estimated blood loss exceeds 1.5 L.[13] The practice of redosing the patient with antibiotics for 24 hours postoperatively is less clear. According to a 2019 systematic review on TJA, there was no difference in SSI/prosthetic joint infection (PJI) rates between patients receiving surgical antibiotic prophylaxis for 24 hours or less and for longer than 24 hours postoperatively.[14] However, the overall body of evidence supporting this conclusion was deemed low, necessitating the need for further level I studies with adequate power to fortify this conclusion. A 2021 study of the spine literature found no difference in the rate of SSI between patients who did and those who did not receive 24 hours of postoperative antibiotics.[15]

Skin Integrity

Caution should be exercised in proceeding with elective surgery for patients with inflamed open wounds or remote SSIs because of elevated risk of SSI.[16,17] This is most evident in trauma because open fractures have consistently been found to have higher infection rates than closed fractures, regardless of location.[18,19] Furthermore, open reduction and internal fixation is associated with increased rates of infection when fasciotomy wounds are present, despite these being performed in a sterile environment.[20,21]

Skin Preparation and Decolonization

Virtually no evidence supporting one skin preparation over another exists. Various techniques have been proposed to prepare the surgical site for surgery, including chlorhexidine cleansing agents and antiseptic soaps. These agents decrease a patient's overall bacterial load and may reduce the risk of SSI. Although endorsed by the International Consensus Meeting on PJI, chlorhexidine does not have proven superiority over other antimicrobial agents.[22] In a study on TJA, no difference in PJI rates was noted on transitioning to a protocol in which chlorhexidine wipes were routinely applied in the preoperative holding area.[23] Similar outcomes have been observed in a 2020 shoulder study following a chlorhexidine wash and benzoyl peroxide soap.[24] A 2022 multinational randomized controlled trial focused on orthopaedic trauma patients looked at the difference between skin preparation solutions and found no difference between those used in reducing infection rate.[25] In the spine literature, there is conflicting evidence. A Cochrane review of randomized controlled trials studying the effect of preoperative chlorhexidine skin preparation found no difference.[26] A 2019 study of 4,266 consecutive patients demonstrated reduction in SSI rates in patients undergoing all spinal procedures after the implementation of preoperative chlorhexidine skin preparation.[27] However, for patients undergoing fusion procedures, there was no difference in the rate of SSI.

Skin Hair Removal

Hair removal directly over or around the incision area before surgery likely does not affect the risk of SSI. The World Health Organization, Society for Healthcare Epidemiology of America, and National Institute for Health and Care Excellence do not recommend hair removal before TJA to reduce SSI rates.[28-30] When necessary, the International Consensus Meeting recommends removal with clippers performed as close to the time of surgery as possible.[22] Razors should be avoided because of epidermal microabrasions that may welcome bacteria into the adjacent skin and soft tissue.[31] Little evidence exists in the trauma literature regarding hair removal; however, clipping of axillary hair has been found to increase the bacterial burden around the shoulder.[32]

Nasal Decolonization

For elective procedures, there are multiple preoperative modalities that can decrease bacterial load. Two studies, including one published in 2020, reported that nasal and skin colonization with methicillin-resistant *Staphylococcus aureus* are associated with increased risk of SSI.[33,34] Standardized screening and appropriate treatment with mupirocin with or without preoperative vancomycin have been found to lower the risk of SSI up to 69% after elective TJA.[35,36] Similarly, methicillin-resistant *S aureus* screening and treatment with confirmation of decolonization has demonstrated lower risk of developing SSI following elective spinal surgery.[34,37] A similar result was found in a 2018 report on orthopaedic trauma, with infection rates significantly decreasing following the addition of povidone-iodine nasal antiseptic agent.[38]

INTRAOPERATIVE STRATEGIES

Surgical Techniques

Various intraoperative techniques have been proposed for wound management during musculoskeletal procedures beginning with barriers to contamination (**Table 2**). Using two pairs of surgical gloves is recommended given the high rates of perforation during musculoskeletal procedures.[39] Sterile draping technique with impermeable material is critical. Multiple studies, including one from 2020, reported that despite decreasing bacterial counts on the field and initial scalpel, antimicrobial adhesive plastic adjuncts to draping have not been found to reduce rates of PJI.[40-42] When used, sealed plastic drapes should remain in place during the case, including during closure, after one study found a sixfold increase in rates of SSI when plastic adhesives were lifted off.[43] Changing the scalpel after skin incision is common practice. However, a study from 2021 reported that no difference in contamination rates has been observed using this technique.[44] For surgeons using intraoperative fluoroscopy, limiting contact with the C-arm drapes can help limit contamination because it was observed that they become contaminated a mean of 20 minutes after surgery for fracture begins.[45]

Wound Closure

For skin closure, a randomized controlled trial published in 2020 evaluated the risk of SSI after closure for total hip arthroplasty with staples versus suture. Staples were associated with approximately a threefold increase in the risk of superficial SSI and wound drainage; however, no difference was observed in rates of PJI.[46] A meta-analysis from 2022 supported sutures over staples for decreasing SSI following TJA.[47] This same analysis did not find a difference in PJI rate between continuous and interrupted suture. In the trauma literature, although it is well known that different sutures affect skin perfusion, no studies have shown a difference in infection rates based on suture type or technique.[48,49]

Similarly, a randomized controlled trial published in 2022 reported no difference in complications following closure with staples compared with a 2-octyl cyanoacrylate (Dermabond) mesh.[50] These combined sealant–polyester mesh dressings have also recently become more common for use in TJA. However, only retrospective data on TJA, such as that published in 2020, compared the risk of SSI for wound closure with and without topical sealants and subcuticular suture or mesh.[51] There is evidence that 2-octyl cyanoacrylate (Dermabond) provides intrinsic bactericidal properties at the wound edges as well as a physical barrier to bacterial inoculation.[52]

Sliver-impregnated dressings remain supported in the literature for elective TJA, including a randomized controlled trial from 2021 and a review from 2018, with growing evidence for negative-pressure devices in high-risk patients.[53-55] In two studies on orthopaedic trauma patients, including one from 2020, the use of incision negative-pressure dressings has not been found to help reduce infection rates.[56,57] As reported in 2021, negative-pressure wound therapy devices have been found to be associated with a lower incidence of SSI, superficial dehiscence, and seroma following spinal fusion surgeries.[58]

SUMMARY

A host of strategies have been developed and extensively studied to reduce the risk of musculoskeletal SSI. A comprehensive understanding of these strategies and appropriate implementation are vital given the devastating effect of SSI on patients, clinicians, and the health care system. Examination of each phase of the perioperative workflow is encouraged to minimize the risk of SSI and maximize patient outcomes.

Table 2

Intraoperative Strategies

- Sterile draping techniques and wearing two pairs of surgical gloves
- Avoiding adhesive plastic lift-off
- Closing wounds with suture
- Impregnated dressings or negative-pressure devices in high-risk patients

KEY STUDY POINTS

- Appropriately timed and retimed perioperative antibiotics, ideally cefazolin, remain the most important factor in preventing SSI following many musculoskeletal procedures.
- Screening for methicillin-resistant *S aureus* and appropriate treatment in colonized patients is encouraged.
- Skin site preparation protocols may reduce the risk of SSI in certain contexts.
- Intraoperative modifications to the surgical workflow may reduce the risk of SSI including barrier draping techniques, proper closure techniques, and sterile dressing.

Annotated References

1. Hall MJ, Schwartzman A, Zhang J, Liu X: Ambulatory surgery data from hospitals and ambulatory surgery centers: United States, 2010. *Natl Health Stat Report* 2017;102:1-15.

2. Berríos-Torres SI, Umscheid CA, Bratzler DW, et al: Centers for disease control and prevention guideline for the prevention of surgical site infection, 2017. *JAMA Surg* 2017;152(8):784-791.

3. Ban KA, Minei JP, Laronga C, et al: American College of Surgeons and Surgical Infection Society: Surgical site infection guidelines, 2016 update. *J Am Coll Surg* 2017;224(1):59-74.

4. Shepard J, Ward W, Milstone A, et al: Financial impact of surgical site infections on hospitals: The hospital management perspective. *JAMA Surg* 2013;148(10):907-914.

5. Kurtz SM, Lau E, Watson H, Schmier JK, Parvizi J: Economic burden of periprosthetic joint infection in the United States. *J Arthroplasty* 2012;27(8 suppl):61-65.e1.

6. Rezapoor M, Parvizi J: Prevention of periprosthetic joint infection. *J Arthroplasty* 2015;30(6):902-907.

7. Wyles CC, Hevesi M, Osmon DR, et al: 2019 John Charnley Award: Increased risk of prosthetic joint infection following primary total knee and hip arthroplasty with the use of alternative antibiotics to cefazolin – The value of allergy testing for antibiotic prophylaxis. *Bone Joint J* 2019;101-B(6 suppl B):9-15.

   In this retrospective review assessing the risk of PJI with various prophylactic antibiotic regimens, cefazolin was found to be associated with a 1.19% higher infection-free survival at 10 years compared with noncefazolin antibiotics. Level of evidence: IIIB.

8. Ponce B, Raines BT, Reed RD, Vick C, Richman J, Hawn M: Surgical site infection after arthroplasty: Comparative effectiveness of prophylactic antibiotics – Do surgical care improvement project guidelines need to be updated? *J Bone Joint Surg Am* 2014;96(12):970-977.

9. Rubinstein E, Findler G, Amit P, Shaked I: Perioperative prophylactic cephazolin in spinal surgery. A double-blind placebo-controlled trial. *J Bone Joint Surg Br* 1994;76(1):99-102.

10. Rondon AJ, Kheir MM, Tan TL, Shohat N, Greenky MR, Parvizi J: Cefazolin prophylaxis for total joint arthroplasty: Obese patients are frequently underdosed and at increased risk of periprosthetic joint infection. *J Arthroplasty* 2018;33(11):3551-3554.

    In this retrospective study of 17,393 primary total joint arthroplasties receiving cefazolin as perioperative prophylaxis from 2005 to 2017 was performed, it was found that patients weighing greater than 120 kg were underdosed 95.9% of the time and the underdosed patients were more likely to develop PJI. Level of evidence: IIIB.

11. Kasatpibal N, Whitney JD, Dellinger EP, Nair BG, Pike KC: Failure to redose antibiotic prophylaxis in long surgery increases risk of surgical site infection. *Surg Infect* 2017;18(4):474-484.

12. Steinberg JP, Braun BI, Hellinger WC, et al: Timing of antimicrobial prophylaxis and the risk of surgical site infections: Results from the trial to reduce antimicrobial prophylaxis errors. *Ann Surg* 2009;250(1):10-16.

13. Swoboda SM, Merz C, Kostuik J, Trentler B, Lipsett PA: Does intraoperative blood loss affect antibiotic serum and tissue concentrations? *Arch Surg* 1996;131(11):1165-1171.

14. Siddiqi A, Forte SA, Docter S, Bryant D, Sheth NP, Chen AF: Perioperative antibiotic prophylaxis in total joint arthroplasty: A systematic review and meta-analysis. *J Bone Joint Surg Am* 2019;101(9):828-842.

    This is a systematic review of 51,627 patients assessing risk of PJI after various administrations of intravenous antibiotics. The analysis found no significant difference in risk of PJI after a single preoperative dose of antibiotics compared with 24 hours of prophylaxis. Level of evidence: IIA.

15. Abola MV, Lin CC, Lin LJ, et al: Postoperative prophylactic antibiotics in spine surgery: A propensity-matched analysis. *J Bone Joint Surg Am* 2021;103(3):219-226.

    This is a propensity-matched analysis of 2,672 patients undergoing spine surgery with 24 hours of postoperative antibiotics matched to 1,782 patients who did not receive antibiotics showing no difference in rates of SSI. Level of evidence: IIIB.

16. Edwards LD: The epidemiology of 2056 remote site infections and 1966 surgical wound infections occurring in 1865 patients: A four year study of 40,923 operations at Rush-Presbyterian-St. Luke's Hospital, Chicago. *Ann Surg* 1976;184(6):758-766.

17. Valentine RJ, Weigelt JA, Dryer D, Rodgers C: Effect of remote infections on clean wound infection rates. *Am J Infect Control* 1986;14(2):64-67.

18. Gustilo RB, Anderson JT: Prevention of infection in the treatment of one thousand and twenty-five open fractures of long bones: Retrospective and prospective analyses. *J Bone Joint Surg Am* 1976;58(4):453-458.

19. Southeast Fracture Consortium: LCP versus LISS in the treatment of open and closed distal femur fractures: Does it make a difference? *J Orthop Trauma* 2016;30(6):e212-e216.

20. Blair JA, Stoops TK, Doarn MC, et al: Infection and nonunion after fasciotomy for compartment syndrome associated with tibia fractures: A matched cohort comparison. *J Orthop Trauma* 2016;30(7):392-396.

21. Dubina AG, Paryavi E, Manson TT, Allmon C, O'Toole RV: Surgical site infection in tibial plateau fractures with ipsilateral compartment syndrome. *Injury* 2017;48(2):495-500.

22. Parvizi J, Gehrke T, Chen AF: Proceedings of the international consensus on periprosthetic joint infection. *Bone Joint J* 2013;95-B(11):1450-1452.

23. Farber NJ, Chen AF, Bartsch SM, Feigel JL, Klatt BA: No infection reduction using chlorhexidine wipes in total joint arthroplasty. *Clin Orthop Relat Res* 2013;471(10):3120-3125.

24. Hsu JE, Whitson AJ, Woodhead BM, Napierala MA, Gong D, Matsen FA 3rd: Randomized controlled trial of chlorhexidine wash versus benzoyl peroxide soap for home surgical preparation: Neither is effective in removing Cutibacterium

from the skin of shoulder arthroplasty patients. *Int Orthop* 2020;44(7):1325-1329.

In this 2020 randomized controlled trial comparing skin *Cutibacterium acnes* colonization before shoulder surgery, neither chlorhexidine washes nor benzoyl peroxide soaps were found to decrease colonization, with 100% of patients having positive test results on skin swabs with similar bacterial load. Level of evidence: IB.

25. PREP-IT Investigators: Aqueous skin antisepsis before surgical fixation of open fractures (Aqueous-PREP): A multiple-period, cluster-randomised, crossover trial. *Lancet* 2022;400(10360):1334-1344.

In this 2022 cluster-randomized, crossover trial assessing rates of SSI in the setting of open fractures, equivalent 7% rates of infection were observed following preparation with aqueous 10% povidone-iodine or aqueous 4% chlorhexidine gluconate. Level of evidence: IB.

26. Webster J, Osborne S: Preoperative bathing or showering with skin antiseptics to prevent surgical site infection. *Cochrane Database Syst Rev* 2015;2015(2):CD004985.

27. Chan AK, Ammanuel SG, Chan AY, et al: Chlorhexidine showers are associated with a reduction in surgical site infection following spine surgery: An analysis of 4266 consecutive surgeries. *Neurosurgery* 2019;85(6):817-826.

In this cohort study of 4,266 patients undergoing spinal surgery comparing rates of SSI before and after implementation of a preoperative chlorhexidine shower, the study reported a significant reduction in the rates of SSI after starting the protocol on multivariate analysis. Level of evidence: IIIB.

28. Anderson DJ, Podgorny K, Berríos-Torres SI, et al: Strategies to prevent surgical site infections in acute care hospitals: 2014 update. *Infect Control Hosp Epidemiol* 2014;35(6):605-627.

29. Leaper D, Burman-Roy S, Palanca A, et al: Prevention and treatment of surgical site infection: Summary of NICE guidance. *BMJ* 2008;337:a1924.

30. WHO Global guidelines on the prevention of surgical site infection. Available at: https://www.who.int/teams/integrated-health-services/infection-prevention-control/surgical-site-infection. Accessed August 23, 2023.

31. Tanner J, Woodings D, Moncaster K: Preoperative hair removal to reduce surgical site infection. *Cochrane Database Syst Rev* 2006;(3):CD004122.

32. Marecek GS, Weatherford BM, Fuller EB, Saltzman MD: The effect of axillary hair on surgical antisepsis around the shoulder. *J Shoulder Elbow Surg* 2015;24(5):804-808.

33. Perl TM: Prevention of Staphylococcus aureus infections among surgical patients: Beyond traditional perioperative prophylaxis. *Surgery* 2003;134(5 suppl):S10-S17.

34. Ning J, Wang J, Zhang S, Sha X: Nasal colonization of Staphylococcus aureus and the risk of surgical site infection after spine surgery: A meta-analysis. *Spine J* 2020;20(3):448-456.

This 2020 meta-analysis evaluating rates of SSI in patients with nasal colonization of *Staphylococcus* species found that methicillin-resistant *S aureus* colonization significantly increases the risk of SSI, whereas methicillin-susceptible *S aureus* colonization does not. Level of evidence: IIIA.

35. Rao N, Cannella B, Crossett LS, Yates AJ Jr, McGough R 3rd: A preoperative decolonization protocol for staphylococcus aureus prevents orthopaedic infections. *Clin Orthop Relat Res* 2008;466(6):1343-1348.

36. Sporer SM, Rogers T, Abella L: Methicillin-resistant and methicillin-sensitive Staphylococcus aureus screening and decolonization to reduce surgical site infection in elective total joint arthroplasty. *J Arthroplasty* 2016;31(9 suppl):144-147.

37. Thakkar V, Ghobrial GM, Maulucci CM, et al: Nasal MRSA colonization: Impact on surgical site infection following spine surgery. *Clin Neurol Neurosurg* 2014;125:94-97.

38. Urias DS, Varghese M, Simunich T, Morrissey S, Dumire R: Preoperative decolonization to reduce infections in urgent lower extremity repairs. *Eur J Trauma Emerg Surg* 2018;44(5):787-793.

This retrospective review of a methicillin-resistant S aureus decolonization protocol using CHG bath/shower and PI-SNA nasal painting revealed a significant decrease in the infection rate of patients undergoing lower extremity fracture repairs. Level of evidence: IIIB.

39. Sanders R, Fortin P, Ross E, Helfet D: Outer gloves in orthopaedic procedures. Cloth compared with latex. *J Bone Joint Surg Am* 1990;72(6):914-917.

40. Webster J, Alghamdi A: Use of plastic adhesive drapes during surgery for preventing surgical site infection. *Cochrane Database Syst Rev* 2015;2015(4):CD006353.

41. Johnston DH, Fairclough JA, Brown EM, Morris R: Rate of bacterial recolonization of the skin after preparation: Four methods compared. *Br J Surg* 1987;74(1):64.

42. Scheidt S, Walter S, Randau TM, Köpf US, Jordan MC, Hischebeth GTR: The influence of iodine-impregnated incision drapes on the bacterial contamination of scalpel blades in joint arthroplasty. *J Arthroplasty* 2020;35(9):2595-2600.

This is a comparison of skin knife culture positivity among patients undergoing TJA with and without iodine-impregnated drapes showing higher rates of contamination without this technique. Level of evidence: IIIB.

43. Alexander JW: Development of a safe and effective one-minute preoperative skin preparation. *Arch Surg* 1986;121(5):615-616.

44. Smith EB, Russo KA, Maltenfort MG, Sharkey PF, Rihn J: After incision, the skin knife blade is no more contaminated than a fresh knife blade. *J Am Acad Orthop Surg* 2021;29(2):e98-e103.

This is a comparative study evaluating the risk of blade contamination during TJA, lumbar spine, and cervical spine surgeries. No significant difference in rates of contamination was observed between control blades and those used to make the initial skin incision. Level of evidence: IIIB.

45. Peters PG, Laughlin RT, Markert RJ, Nelles DB, Randall KL, Prayson MJ: Timing of C-arm drape contamination. *Surg Infect (Larchmt)* 2012;13(2):110-113.

46. Mallee WH, Wijsbek AE, Schafroth MU, Wolkenfelt J, Baas DC, Vervest T: Wound complications after total hip arthroplasty: A prospective, randomised controlled trial comparing staples with sutures. *Hip Int* 2020; July 7 [Epub ahead of print].

   In this randomized controlled trial comparing the risk of SSI using staples or suture to close the wound after total hip arthroplasty, staples were found to carry a threefold greater risk of superficial SSI and prolonged drainage; however, no difference was found in deep PJI. Level of evidence: IB.

47. van de Kuit A, Krishnan RJ, Mallee WH, et al: Surgical site infection after wound closure with staples versus sutures in elective knee and hip arthroplasty: A systematic review and meta-analysis. *Arthroplasty* 2022;4(1):12.

   This is a meta-analysis evaluating the effect of staples, continuous suture, and interrupted suture closure on SSI following elective TJA. The analysis of studies with low risk of bias found higher risk of SSI with staple closure. No difference was observed in continuous versus interrupted suture. Level of evidence: IA.

48. Sagi HC, Papp S, Dipasquale T: The effect of suture pattern and tension on cutaneous blood flow as assessed by laser Doppler flowmetry in a pig model. *J Orthop Trauma* 2008;22(3):171-175.

49. Mudd CD, Boudreau JA, Moed BR: A prospective randomized comparison of two skin closure techniques in acetabular fracture surgery. *J Orthop Traumatol* 2014;15(3):189-194.

50. Eichinger JK, Oldenburg KS, Lin J, et al: Comparing dermabond PRINEO versus dermabond or staples for wound closure: A randomized control trial following total shoulder arthroplasty. *J Shoulder Elbow Surg* 2022;31(10):2066-2075.

   In this 2022 randomized controlled trial comparing various closure techniques following total shoulder arthroplasty, no difference in complication rates was observed between staples, 2-octyl cyanoacrylate, or PRINEO. Level of evidence: IB.

51. Anderson FL, Herndon CL, Lakra A, Geller JA, Cooper HJ, Shah RP: Polyester mesh dressings reduce delayed wound healing and reoperations compared with silver-impregnated occlusive dressings after knee arthroplasty. *Arthroplast Today* 2020;6:350-353.

   In this retrospective study evaluating rates of successful wound healing with a sealant–polyester mesh dressing, there were significantly fewer instances of delayed wound healing in the sealant–polyester mesh group as well as fewer revision surgeries compared with the group with impregnated occlusive dressings. Level of evidence: IIIB.

52. Rushbrook JL, White G, Kidger L, Marsh P, Taggart TF: The antibacterial effect of 2-octyl cyanoacrylate (Dermabond®) skin adhesive. *J Infect Prev* 2014;15(6):236-239.

53. Higuera-Rueda CA, Emara AK, Nieves-Malloure Y, et al: The effectiveness of closed-incision negative-pressure therapy versus silver-impregnated dressings in mitigating surgical site complications in high-risk patients after revision knee arthroplasty: The PROMISES randomized controlled trial. *J Arthroplasty* 2021;36(7 suppl):S295-S302.e14.

   In this randomized controlled trial comparing the risk of SSI with the use of negative-pressure devices or impregnated silver dressings in high-risk patients undergoing total knee arthroplasty, the negative-pressure devices were found to significantly reduce the risk of surgical site complication (odds ratio, 0.22; 95% confidence interval, 0.08 to 0.59) and readmission rates (odds ratio, 0.30; 95% confidence interval, 0.11 to 0.86). Level of evidence: IB.

54. Katarincic JA, Fantry A, DePasse JM, Feller R: Local modalities for preventing surgical site infections: An evidence-based review. *J Am Acad Orthop Surg* 2018;26(1):14-25.

   This is a review article discussing local modalities for preventing surgical site infections.

55. Redfern RE, Cameron-Ruetz C, O'Drobinak SK, Chen JT, Beer KJ: Closed incision negative pressure therapy effects on postoperative infection and surgical site complication after total hip and knee arthroplasty. *J Arthroplasty* 2017;32(11):3333-3339.

56. Costa ML, Achten J, Knight R, et al: Effect of incisional negative pressure wound therapy vs standard wound dressing on deep surgical site infection after surgery for lower limb fractures associated with major trauma: The WHIST randomized clinical trial. *J Am Med Assoc* 2020;323(6):519-526.

   In this 2020 randomized controlled trial comparing rates of deep SSI following lower leg surgery for major trauma, no difference in infection was observed between groups treated with standard wound dressings compared with those treated with negative-pressure devices. Level of evidence: IB.

57. Crist BD, Oladeji LO, Khazzam M, Della Rocca GJ, Murtha YM, Stannard JP: Role of acute negative pressure wound therapy over primarily closed surgical incisions in acetabular fracture ORIF: A prospective randomized trial. *Injury* 2017;48(7):1518-1521.

58. Akhter AS, McGahan BG, Close L, et al: Negative pressure wound therapy in spinal fusion patients. *Int Wound J* 2021;18(2):158-163.

   This retrospective cohort analysis of 84 patients undergoing spinal surgery with and without a negative-pressure wound device found a significantly higher rate of SSI among the cohort with traditional dressings. Level of evidence: IIIB.

CHAPTER 6

Patient Optimization for Infection Prevention

CATALINA BAEZ, MD • LUIS PULIDO, MD

ABSTRACT

Bone and joint infection following orthopaedic surgery is associated with high morbidity, mortality, and socioeconomic burden to the patient and health care system. Hence, infection prevention, which includes patient optimization and perioperative risk management strategies, is critical. The patient host, perioperative care, and surgical confounders are the three fundamental areas for intervention to reduce complications and improve surgical outcomes. Elective surgery allows time for preoperative risk management strategies and host optimization. Patient-specific risk factors are considered modifiable if they can be corrected or improved with the appropriate management to lower the risk of postoperative bone and joint infection.

Keywords: patient optimization; perioperative risk management; prosthetic joint infection

INTRODUCTION

Prosthetic joint infection (PJI) is associated with severe morbidity, psychologic stress,[1] and economic burden to patients, surgeons, and health care systems.[2] Three studies, including one from 2019 and one from 2022, reported that mortality rates of patients with PJI

Neither of the following authors nor any immediate family member has received anything of value from or has stock or stock options held in a commercial company or institution related directly or indirectly to the subject of this chapter: Dr. Baez and Dr. Pulido.

following treatment with two-stage revision arthroplasty vary from 11% to 25% at 2 years and 40% to 45% at 5 years.[3-5]

The Centers for Disease Control and Prevention (CDC) guidelines for preventing surgical site infection (SSI) do not include host optimization but mostly focus on perioperative interventions, including appropriate antibiotic prophylaxis, glycemic control, normothermia, oxygenation, and antiseptic skin preparation.[6] A 2020 study reported that patient-specific risk factors associated with PJI are modifiable if they can be corrected or improved with the appropriate treatment. The most common modifiable conditions include obesity, poorly controlled diabetes mellitus, tobacco use and smoking, anemia, malnutrition, low vitamin D levels, intravenous drug use, periodontal disease, symptomatic urinary tract infections, and methicillin-resistant *Staphylococcus aureus* colonization.[7]

Optimization strategies require a team effort consisting of perioperative nurse navigators and physical therapists enabled as primary orthopaedic clinicians and creating patient-centered models with integrated practice units.[7-10] Although most programs claim evidence-based interventions,[8-10] there are limited prospective studies on the feasibility and success of optimization pathways in total joint arthroplasty (TJA) and their effect on mitigating PJI.

OBESITY

Epidemiology

A 2022 study reported that the prevalence of adult obesity in the United States increased from 30% to 41% from 2000 to 2020, and during the same period, the prevalence of morbid obesity increased from 5% to 9%.[11] In 2022, the CDC defined obesity as a body mass index (BMI) greater than 30 kg/m², where the body weight is considered unhealthy for a given height.[12] Class III, very severe or morbid obesity, occurs with BMI greater than 40 kg/m², after which the comorbidities and surgical risks exponentially increase.[12]

Optimization Strategy

Lifestyle interventions including a healthy diet rich in protein, caloric restriction, correction of obesity paradoxical protein malnutrition, low-impact aerobic exercise, and strengthening effectively reduce patients' weight almost 10% of initial body weight at 1 year,[13] and 50% of patients with morbid obesity maintain their weight loss at 4 years[14] (**Figure 1**). This 2018 report analyzed the Intensive Diet and Exercise for Arthritis randomized controlled clinical trial on obese patients with knee osteoarthritis that included 240 participants with significant dose responses to weight loss for pain, function, 6-minute walk distance, physical and mental health-related quality of life, knee joint compression force, and inflammation (interleukin 6).[15] The group of patients with the highest weight loss (≥20% of body weight loss) had 25% less pain, better function than the 10% to 20% group, and better physical health–related quality of life.[15]

However, there is limited evidence for the success of optimization strategies in weight reduction for patients with morbid obesity in arthroplasty and the effects on PJI. A 2020 study analyzed 125 patients with a BMI greater than 40 kg/m² who were initially denied TJA until a target BMI of 40 kg/m² was met or were offered arthroplasty if they reached the target or at least two-thirds of their weight loss goal was demonstrated.[16] Only 24 patients (19%) met their target goals and underwent TJA. A 2019 study prospectively evaluated 289 patients with a BMI greater than 40 kg/m² and end-stage hip and knee osteoarthritis over a 2-year period who were encouraged to achieve weight loss through lifestyle modifications or bariatric surgery.[17] One-third (29%) of these patients refused further contact. Most patients (52%) had no change in BMI and no additional surgery was offered. Only 19% (56 of 289 patients) ultimately underwent TJA and achieved their weight loss target through lifestyle modifications or bariatric surgery.[17]

The relative indications of bariatric surgery reported in 2023 include individuals with BMI greater than 35 kg/m², regardless of the presence, absence, or severity of comorbidities; individuals with type 2 diabetes with BMI greater than 30 kg/m²; and individuals with BMI of 30 to 34.9 kg/m² who do not achieve substantial or durable weight loss or comorbidity improvement using nonsurgical methods.[18] However, in 2019, it was reported that bariatric surgery before TJA has not been shown to reduce the risk of superficial or deep infection.[19] A 2022 study of 205 patients who underwent bariatric surgery before total knee arthroplasty (TKA), showed that patients who underwent bariatric surgery had a greater risk of revision surgery for infection and instability compared with patients with BMI greater than 40 kg/m².[20] Similarly, a 2022 study reported that patients undergoing total hip arthroplasty (THA) after bariatric surgery sustained a greater risk for revision and dislocation but similar PJI risks compared with those who did not.[21]

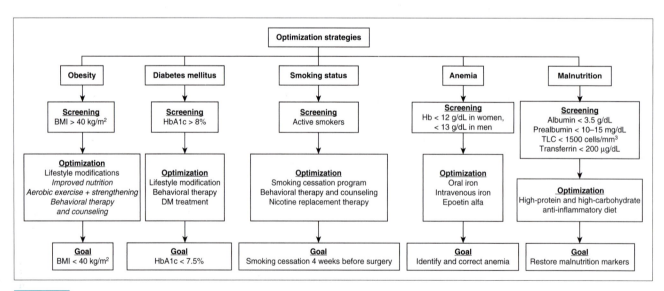

FIGURE 1 Flowchart showing patient optimization strategies. BMI = body mass index, DM = diabetes mellitus, TLC = total lymphocyte count

DIABETES MELLITUS AND HYPERGLYCEMIA

Epidemiology

Type 2 diabetes mellitus accounts for more than 90% of diabetes cases and is characterized by insulin resistance and/or abnormal insulin secretion that causes glucose intolerance and secondary hyperglycemia.[22] The prevalence of diabetes in Medicare patients undergoing TJA is 15% for THA[23] and 24% for TKA.[24]

Optimization Strategy

Type 2 diabetes occurs in conjunction with obesity, and the term diabesity has been proposed for diabetes that is obesity dependent.[25] Modest weight loss improves glycemia and reduces the need for glucose-lowering medications.[26] A goal to achieve and maintain weight loss of 5% or more is associated with improved glucose levels.[27] The Look AHEAD (Action for Health in Diabetes) randomized trial evaluated the long-term health effects of intensive lifestyle interventions, including behavioral therapy versus usual diabetes care, in 5,145 persons with type 2 diabetes and obesity.[28] Approximately 50% of intensive lifestyle intervention participants lost and maintained 5% or more of their initial body weight, whereas 27% lost and maintained 10% or more at 8 years.[28] Patients with diabetes and obesity managed with bariatric surgery and pharmacotherapy have better results than medical therapy alone in decreasing hyperglycemia and body weight and improving quality of life.[29] However, bariatric surgery has not been proven to decrease the risk of PJI after TJA.[20,21]

In 2023, it was reported that preoperative hemoglobin A1c (HbA1c) is routinely measured for patients with diabetes and/or obesity, considered as candidates for TJA as part of an optimization strategy.[30] The HbA1c level reflects the patient's preoperative glucose control for the past 3 months, has a strong correlation with postoperative glucose control, and has a weak positive correlation with PJI. One study from 2018 that included 773 patients with diabetes undergoing TJA showed that the average postoperative glycemia increased with increasing HbA1c levels (HbA1c < 7 = 167 mg/dL, HbA1c 7.0 to 8.0 = 240 mg/dL, and HbA1c > 8 = 276 mg/dL, $P < 0.0001$).[31] Patients with HbA1c level greater than 7.45% resulted in a greater chance of registering postoperative hyperglycemia, glucose levels greater than 200 mg/dL. Patients with diabetes who undergo TJA must achieve perioperative glucose control to mitigate complications including PJI. HbA1c targets between 7% and 8% are frequently incorporated in optimization strategies.[7-10,32,33] A 2018 study reported that the lower the target (less than 7%), the better the glycemic control,[31] but the less feasible it becomes to achieve, per a 2023 study.[34] In 2022, it was reported that elderly patients with multiple coexisting chronic illnesses, cognitive impairment, or functional dependence could benefit from more accommodating glycemic goals (ie, HbA1c 7.5% to 8%) because of their risks for hypoglycemia.[35]

SMOKING AND TOBACCO USE

Epidemiology

Smoking and tobacco use are the leading causes of preventable disease, disability, and death in the United States, resulting in more than 480,000 deaths every year, or approximately 1 in 5 of all deaths. More than 16 million people live with a smoking-related disease in the United States. In 2020, an estimated 47 million US adults (19%) reported currently using a tobacco product.[35,36] The prevalence of smoking among patients undergoing elective TJA is between 7% and 18%.[37-39] In 2019, it was reported that cigarette cessation indicators showed modest improvement over the past decade but remain unsatisfactory, with only 55% of smokers attempting to quit and only 7.5% successfully ceased smoking for more than 6 months.[40]

Optimization Strategy

Active smokers must be informed regarding their elevated risks and the reversibility of that risk with smoking cessation for at least 4 weeks before and after surgery.[41,42] Interventions, including weekly counseling, behavioral therapy, and referral to a smoking cessation program, are recommended. A 2019 retrospective analysis reported that nicotine replacement therapy in the form of gums, patches, lozenges, sprays, and inhalers increases the success rate of short-term smoking cessation.[43] A Danish multicenter trial included 120 active smokers scheduled for primary elective TJA who were randomized to smoking intervention 6 to 8 weeks before surgery looking at the effect of smoking interventions (weekly counseling and nicotine replacement) on postoperative complications.[44] There was a significant decrease in wound complications in the intervention group, 5% versus 31% in the control group, including superficial SSIs (4% versus 23%).[44] A 2020 study evaluated the 7-year experience of a voluntary smoking cessation program in TJA at an academic medical center.[45] The protocol consisted of four preoperative telephone sessions, including assessment, education, counseling, and nicotine replacement therapy, and two follow-up sessions within 30 days after surgery. The intervention group trended to higher quit rates (43% versus 33%) and lower infection rates (7% versus 12%).[45] Serum cotinine[43] and carbon monoxide[44] breath testing are commonly used methods to verify smoking cessation and improve smoking abstinence before TJA.[39,46]

ANEMIA

Epidemiology

The 2019 definition of anemia by the World Health Organization is a hemoglobin concentration of less than 12 g/dL in women and less than 13 g/dL in men.[47] Preoperative anemia is present in approximately 20% of patients undergoing elective TJA.[48,49] In 2022, it was reported that the prevalence of anemia is greater than 20% in patients aged 85 years or older and 50% in nursing home residents.[50] Some health, social, and racial factors associated with a higher risk for anemia in adults include female sex, being African American, renal failure, cancer, vegetarian diets, dementia, psychiatric illness, alcoholism, and homelessness.[50-54]

Optimization Strategy

Anemia must be identified and corrected before elective TJA.[55] Preoperative blood tests, including a complete blood count with differential, serum creatinine level, and iron levels, are used to detect and categorize anemia. Anemia in older adults is secondary to nutritional deficiencies (iron, folate, and vitamin B_{12}), renal failure, or chronic disease.[56] Anemia can be categorized using the corrected reticulocyte count, the mean corpuscular volume (MCV), and the patient's iron levels. Hypoproliferative anemias are considered when the corrected reticulocyte count is less than 2%.[50] These can be grouped into microcytic if MCV is less than 80 fL (ie, iron deficiency, chronic disease), normocytic if MCV is between 80 and 100 fL (renal failure, iron deficiency, chronic disease), and macrocytic if MCV is greater than 100 fL (ie, folate and vitamin B_{12} deficiency, alcohol use).[50]

The patient's iron levels are measured by serum ferritin and transferrin saturation levels. Low levels of serum ferritin (less than 30 ng/mL) and/or transferrin saturation (less than 20%) are indicative of iron deficiency.[57,58] Iron-deficiency anemia is corrected with iron supplementation. Severe cases of iron-deficiency anemia, patients with positive occult blood in stool, or any clinical suspicion for malignancy warrants a gastroenterologist referral. Preoperative oral iron therapy of 40 to 60 mg daily or 80 to 100 mg every 48 hours of elemental iron is recommended for mild anemia, provided there is sufficient time (6 to 8 weeks before surgery) and adequate tolerance. Oral iron therapy has reduced gastrointestinal absorption, and adverse effects are common, including constipation (33%), heartburn (14%), and abdominal pain (13%). The adherence rate of oral iron therapy is 67%.[59] A Canadian study including 3,435 patients who underwent TJA compared their blood management strategies before and after preoperative oral iron supplementation.[60] Oral iron therapy increased preoperative Hb levels by 0.6 and 0.8 g/dL in their hip and knee cohorts, respectively. The intervention reduced the need for intravenous iron from a range of 4% to 5% down to 2% and epoetin alfa from a range of 16% to 18% down to 6%.[60] Intravenous iron should be used for patients with moderate to severe anemia, for patients who do not respond or do not tolerate oral iron, or if surgery is planned for less than 6 weeks after the diagnosis of iron deficiency.[61] A prospective randomized trial in 44 patients with iron-deficiency anemia undergoing elective joint arthroplasty compared the efficacy of preoperative oral administration of 325 mg of iron sulfate daily (22 patients) versus a single intravenous dose of iron polymaltose (22 patients). The posttreatment preoperative Hb increased to 12.8 g/dL in the intravenous iron group compared with 11.8 g/dL in the oral iron group.[62]

Anemia secondary to chronic kidney disease is determined in patients with decreased Hb, normal or decreased iron levels, elevated serum creatinine levels, and low glomerular filtration rate.[63,64] These patients are referred to a nephrologist for evaluation and optimization. Vitamin B_{12} and folic acid levels are obtained for patients with normal iron levels and kidney function or macrocytic anemia (MCV > 100 fL).[50] Low levels of folic acid and vitamin B_{12} are corrected with supplemental therapy. Anemia of chronic disease is a diagnosis of exclusion when iron, kidney function, and vitamin levels are within normal range. Anemia of chronic disease benefits from a hematology referral, iron supplementation, and erythropoiesis-stimulating agent therapy.[50] In 2019, European guidelines recommended using recombinant human erythropoietin to improve preoperative Hb levels in patients undergoing elective orthopaedic surgery with Hb levels between 10 and 13 g/dL who are expected to have moderate blood loss.[65] A 2020 study from Spain analyzed the incorporation of a preoperative Hb optimization protocol in THA using intravenous ferric carboxymaltose and 40,000 IU of epoetin alfa administered 4 weeks before surgery.[66] The combination treatment produced a higher increase in Hb concentration (1.4 g/dL) versus the intravenous iron alone (0.7 g/dL), but no difference in postoperative complications was appreciated among the two cohorts.[66]

MALNUTRITION

Epidemiology

Malnutrition is an imbalance in a patient's nutritional status that predisposes an inability to achieve baseline and acute metabolic demands.[67,68] A study from 2019 reported that the prevalence of malnutrition in adults undergoing primary TJA range from 4% to 56%, from 15% to 38% for revision TJA, and from 43% to 53% for infected TJA.[69]

Optimization Strategy

Serologic markers, anthropometric measurements, and scoring tools have been proposed to measure nutritional levels. The serologic markers accepted as surrogates for poor nutritional status are albumin levels less than 3.5 g/dL, pre-albumin levels less than 10 to 15 mg/dL, total lymphocyte count less than 1,500 cells/mm^3, and transferrin levels less than 200 μg/dL.[67,69-72] A 2023 study showed that patients with high-risk characteristics, such as those with diabetes, those in the extremes of BMI, and those undergoing revision arthroplasty, must be screened for malnutrition.[73] However, the efficacy of preoperative optimization of malnutrition before TJA, and its mitigation of postoperative infection rates, requires further investigation.

A 2019 study evaluated the effectiveness of a hospital nutrition program that encouraged a high-protein, anti-inflammatory diet for malnourished patients before and for 1 month after TJA.[74] Malnourished patients with nutritional intervention at the study hospital had shorter hospital lengths of stays, lower charges associated with readmissions, and 90-day total charges.[74] A 2021 study from Brazil, including 3,019 consecutive elderly patients undergoing TJA, analyzed the effect of immunonutrition as part of the perioperative recovery protocol that included a high-calorie, protein-rich shake 3 times per day for 5 days before and 5 days after surgery.[75] The study group had shorter length of stay, decreased infectious and noninfectious complications, and lower rates of transfusion than the control group.[75]

SUMMARY

The main modifiable risk factors for optimization are obesity, uncontrolled diabetes mellitus, smoking, anemia, and malnutrition. Patient optimization requires a multidisciplinary team approach and patient activation for durable and sustainable changes to modify prevalent chronic conditions of society. There is a delicate balance between perioperative optimization using sustainable strategies and restrictive screening, which inevitably limits access to care. Improving the health of patients is the primary goal of patient optimization, allowing for infection risk reduction and better surgical outcomes.

KEY STUDY POINTS

- The patient as host, the perioperative care pathways, and the surgical technique are the fundamental areas for intervention to reduce infection risk.
- Optimization strategies focus on the preoperative identification and management of modifiable risk factors. The most common modifiable risk factors for infection include obesity, poorly controlled diabetes mellitus, smoking, anemia, and malnutrition.
- Morbid obesity is associated with a greater risk of PJI and treatment failure of PJI. Intensive diet and exercise in the patient with obesity and also with osteoarthritis is associated with weight loss, improved pain, better function, and quality of life. However, only 19% of patients with morbid obesity evaluated for arthroplasty successfully reduce their weight and proceed with surgery. Bariatric surgery increases the risks of revision surgery for infection in TKA (hazard ratio, 6).
- Diabetes mellitus, perioperative hyperglycemia, and increased glycemic variability increase the risk of PJI. Hyperglycemia affects all major components of innate immunity and impairs the ability of the host to combat infection. Perioperative glycemic control is recommended to decrease infection risk.
- Current smoking status is strongly associated with early SSI (odds ratio, 6.8) and deep PJI (odds ratio, 5.9). Smoking cessation strategies are successful (range, 60% to 70%) and are associated with a reduced risk of SSI.
- Anemia is present in 20% of patients before elective hip and knee arthroplasty. Anemia must be identified and corrected before elective TJA.
- Serologic markers accepted as surrogates for poor nutritional status are albumin levels less than 3.5 g/dL, total lymphocyte count less than 1,500 cells/mm^3, and transferrin levels less than 200 μg/dL. Hypoalbuminemia is associated with increased risk of SSI.

ANNOTATED REFERENCES

1. Andersson AE, Bergh I, Karlsson J, Nilsson K: Patients' experiences of acquiring a deep surgical site infection: An interview study. *Am J Infect Control* 2010;38(9):711-717.

2. Kurtz SM, Lau E, Watson H, Schmier JK, Parvizi J: Economic burden of periprosthetic joint infection in the United States. *J Arthroplasty* 2012;27(8 suppl):61-65.e1.

3. Zmistowski B, Karam JA, Durinka JB, Casper DS, Parvizi J: Periprosthetic joint infection increases the risk of one-year mortality. *J Bone Joint Surg Am* 2013;95(24):2177-2184.

4. Petis SM, Perry KI, Mabry TM, Hanssen AD, Berry DJ, Abdel MP: Two-stage exchange protocol for periprosthetic joint infection following total knee arthroplasty in 245 knees without prior treatment for infection. *J Bone Joint Surg Am* 2019;101(3):239-249.

   This was a retrospective study of the cumulative incidence of long-term reinfection and risk for PJI after two-stage exchange performed after TKA. It reported that little difference in cumulative incidence of reinfection between 5 and 15 years after surgery and that BMI, history of previous revision surgery, and McPherson host grade C are found to be predictive of long-term reinfection. Level of evidence: IV.

5. Kildow BJ, Springer BD, Brown TS, Lyden E, Fehring TK, Garvin KL: Long term results of two-stage revision for chronic periprosthetic hip infection: A multicenter study. *J Clin Med* 2022;11(6):1657.

   This retrospective study of cumulative incidence of long-term reinfection and risk after two-stage exchange for PJI after THA concludes high infection control after 5 years and found polymicrobial infection and antibiotic-resistant organisms to be risk factors for long-term reinfection. Level of evidence: IV.

6. Berríos-Torres SI, Umscheid CA, Bratzler DW, et al: Centers for disease control and prevention guideline for the prevention of surgical site infection, 2017. *JAMA Surg* 2017;152(8):784-791.

7. Dlott CC, Moore A, Nelson C, et al: Preoperative risk factor optimization lowers hospital length of stay and postoperative emergency department visits in primary total hip and knee arthroplasty patients. *J Arthroplasty* 2020;35(6):1508-1515.e2.

   This retrospective study comparing the effects of a patient optimization protocol for TJA against historical and contemporary control groups reported that decreased length of stay, 90-day postoperative emergency department visits, readmission rates, transfusion rates, and SSIs and increased discharge to home for patients in the optimization group versus the control groups. Level of evidence: IV.

8. Bullock MW, Brown ML, Bracey DN, Langfitt MK, Shields JS, Lang JE: A bundle protocol to reduce the incidence of periprosthetic joint infections after total joint arthroplasty: A single-center experience. *J Arthroplasty* 2017;32(4):1067-1073.

9. Feng JE, Novikov D, Anoushiravani AA, et al: Team approach: Perioperative optimization for total joint arthroplasty. *JBJS Rev* 2018;6(10):e4.

   This review of a multidisciplinary team approach to patient optimization via case presentation outlines appropriate patient optimization guidelines from a multidisciplinary panel and highlights the need for research on preoperative at-risk patient identification and optimization of modifiable risk factors and its potential to extend arthroplasty care to more high-risk patients. Level of evidence: V.

10. Bernstein DN, Liu TC, Winegar AL, et al: Evaluation of a preoperative optimization protocol for primary hip and knee arthroplasty patients. *J Arthroplasty* 2018;33(12):3642-3648.

    This retrospective cohort study comparing patients who underwent TJA after a preoperative optimization program with patients who did not undergo optimization found patients in the optimization group to have significantly shorter length of stay and direct variable cost, and although not significant, patients who underwent optimization also showed better outcomes for discharge to home and 90-day readmissions than patients who did not undergo optimization. This study focuses on the effect of patient optimization in introducing higher value care and lower resource utilization. Level of evidence: IV.

11. Centers for Disease Control and Prevention: Adult Obesity Facts – Overweight & Obesity. Available at: https://www.cdc.gov/obesity/data/adult.html. Accessed May 17, 2022.

    This CDC web page outlining adult obesity facts for the United States highlights obesity epidemiologic data and obesity-related complications and expenses and also highlights how obesity disproportionately affects individuals belonging to racial and ethnic minorities, as well as those with lower socioeconomic status.

12. Centers for Disease Control and Prevention: Defining Adult Overweight & Obesity. Available at: https://www.cdc.gov/obesity/basics/adult-defining.html. Accessed June 3, 2022.

    This CDC web page outlines adult obesity categorization using adult BMI measurements.

13. Unick JL, Beavers D, Jakicic JM, et al: Effectiveness of lifestyle interventions for individuals with severe obesity and type 2 diabetes: Results from the look AHEAD trial. *Diabetes Care* 2011;34(10):2152-2157.

14. Unick JL, Beavers D, Bond DS, et al: The long-term effectiveness of a lifestyle intervention in severely obese individuals. *Am J Med* 2013;126(3):236-242, 242.e1-e2.

15. Messier SP, Resnik AE, Beavers DP, et al: Intentional weight loss in overweight and obese patients with knee osteoarthritis: Is more better? *Arthritis Care Res (Hoboken)* 2018;70(11):1569-1575.

    This secondary analysis of data from the Intensive Diet and Exercise for Arthritis prospective randomized clinical trial comparing the diet-only and diet and exercise groups in subgroup analyses according to percentage of weight loss achieved and their effect on functional, quality of life, and inflammatory outcomes concluded that long-term weight loss that reaches 10% to 19.9% of baseline weight showed significant clinical and mechanical benefits compared with less weight loss. Level of evidence: I.

16. Shapiro JA, Narayanan AS, Taylor PR, Olcott CW, Del Gaizo DJ: Fate of the morbidly obese patient who is denied total joint arthroplasty. *J Arthroplasty* 2020;35(6 suppl):S124-S128.

    This is an observational study of patients who were initially denied arthroplasty because of morbid obesity. Pain and functional survey outcomes were compared between patients who achieved target weight and received surgery, those who did not achieve target weight and did not undergo surgery, and those who did not achieve target weight and underwent surgery at an outside institution. The study concluded that patients who achieved their target weight before surgery had better survey outcomes and those who did not meet weight requirements had similar outcomes regardless of having undergone surgery or not. Level of evidence: IV.

17. Springer BD: Management of the bariatric patient. What are the implications of obesity and total joint arthroplasty: The orthopedic surgeon's perspective? *J Arthroplasty* 2019;34(7 suppl):S30-S32.

    This is a commentary and data review on the effects of a strict BMI of 40 mg/kg² cutoff for TJA denial. Observational data are presented on the effects of bariatric surgery center referral for weight management in patients with morbid obesity denied for TJA. It was found that few patients achieved sufficient weight loss so as to be considered surgical candidates and this could possibly generate disparate access to care for patients with morbid obesity. This review also highlights the importance of developing multidisciplinary work groups to preoperatively optimize these patients and aid orthopaedic surgeons in their capacity to provide care to all patients who require it. Level of evidence: IV.

18. Eisenberg D, Shikora SA, Aarts E, et al: 2022 American Society of Metabolic and Bariatric Surgery (ASMBS) and International Federation for the Surgery of Obesity and Metabolic Disorders (IFSO) indications for metabolic and bariatric surgery. *Obes Surg* 2023;33(1):3-14.

    This is a report on the 2022 American Society for Metabolic & Bariatric Surgery and International Federation for the Surgery of Obesity and Metabolic Disorders meeting to update the 1991 National Institutes of Health Guidelines for Bariatric Surgery. Level of evidence: V.

19. Li S, Luo X, Sun H, Wang K, Zhang K, Sun X: Does prior bariatric surgery improve outcomes following total joint arthroplasty in the morbidly obese? A meta-analysis. *J Arthroplasty* 2019;34(3):577-585.

    This meta-analysis on the effect of bariatric surgery before performing TJA on complication rate, revision rate, length of stay, and surgical time included a total of nine studies and 38,728 patients. Findings reported only short-term reduction of 90-day complications, length of stay, and surgical time, without decreasing the risk for SSI or venous thromboembolism. It concluded by highlighting the need for more high-quality studies in this area. Level of evidence: IV.

20. Ryan SP, Couch CG, Duong SQ, et al: Does bariatric surgery prior to primary total knee arthroplasty improve outcomes? *J Arthroplasty* 2022;37(6 suppl):S165-S169.

    This was a retrospective analysis of the effect of bariatric surgery before TKA on revisions, reoperations, and 90-day complications. Patients who had a previous history of bariatric surgery were associated with greater numbers of revisions, reoperations, and 90-day complications, and it was concluded that patients who undergo bariatric surgery before TKA had worse implant survivorship related to infection and instability. Level of evidence: IV.

21. Ryan SP, Couch CG, Duong SQ, et al: Frank Stinchfield Award: Does bariatric surgery prior to primary total hip arthroplasty really improve outcomes? *J Arthroplasty* 2022;37(7 suppl):S386-S390.

    This was a retrospective analysis of the effect of bariatric surgery before THA on revisions, reoperations, and 90-day complications. Patients who had a history of bariatric surgery were associated with greater numbers of revisions, reoperations, and dislocation risk, and it was concluded that patients who undergo bariatric surgery before THA had worse implant survivorship and higher dislocation rate. Level of evidence: IV.

22. Zimmet P, Alberti KG, Shaw J: Global and societal implications of the diabetes epidemic. *Nature* 2001;414(6865):782-787.

23. Cram P, Lu X, Kaboli PJ, et al: Clinical characteristics and outcomes of Medicare patients undergoing total hip arthroplasty, 1991-2008. *J Am Med Assoc* 2011;305(15):1560-1567.

24. Cram P, Lu X, Kates SL, Singh JA, Li Y, Wolf BR: Total knee arthroplasty volume, utilization, and outcomes among Medicare beneficiaries, 1991-2010. *J Am Med Assoc* 2012;308(12):1227-1236.

25. Astrup A, Finer N: Redefining type 2 diabetes: "Diabesity" or "obesity dependent diabetes mellitus"? *Obes Rev* 2000;1(2):57-59.

26. Pastors JG, Warshaw H, Daly A, Franz M, Kulkarni K: The evidence for the effectiveness of medical nutrition therapy in diabetes management. *Diabetes Care* 2002;25(3):608-613.

27. Magkos F, Fraterrigo G, Yoshino J, et al: Effects of moderate and subsequent progressive weight loss on metabolic function and adipose tissue biology in humans with obesity. *Cell Metab* 2016;23(4):591-601.

28. Look AHEAD Research Group: Eight-year weight losses with an intensive lifestyle intervention: The look AHEAD study. *Obesity (Silver Spring)* 2014;22(1):5-13.

29. Schauer PR, Bhatt DL, Kirwan JP, et al: Bariatric surgery versus intensive medical therapy for diabetes - 5-year outcomes. *N Engl J Med* 2017;376(7):641-651.

30. Dlott CC, Metcalfe T, Jain S, Bahel A, Donnelley CA, Wiznia DH: Preoperative risk management programs at the top 50 orthopaedic institutions frequently enforce strict cutoffs for BMI and hemoglobin a1c which may limit access to total joint arthroplasty and provide limited resources for smoking cessation and dental care. *Clin Orthop Relat Res* 2023;481(1):39-47.

    This is an observational survey–based study on preoperative patient optimization programs for BMI, HbA1c, and smoking cessation at the top 50 orthopaedic institutions in the United States. Researchers analyzed institutions' arthroplasty risk factor screening protocols and availability of supporting programs to manage these conditions. Findings showed that most of these institutions had strict cutoffs for arthroplasty regarding these three risk factors and there was varied availability of programs to support patient's management of these. The study highlights the importance of shared decision making between the surgeon and the patient and proposes a way by which a patient's risk tolerance may better guide whether they should undergo surgery. Level of evidence: V.

31. Godshaw BM, Ojard CA, Adams TM, Chimento GF, Mohammed A, Waddell BS: Preoperative glycemic control predicts perioperative serum glucose levels in patients undergoing total joint arthroplasty. *J Arthroplasty* 2018;33(7 suppl):S76-S80.

    This retrospective study of the association between preoperative HbA1c and postoperative hyperglycemia and PJI risk showed that increased preoperative HbA1c was associated with higher postoperative glucose levels. PJI rate was not different between groups. The study concludes that there is a correlation between high preoperative HbA1c levels and postoperative hyperglycemia and suggests an HbA1c cutoff of 7.45%. Level of evidence: IV.

32. Khatod M: Kaiser permanente: Joint arthroplasty in an integrated capitated care delivery model. *J Arthroplasty* 2018;33(6):1649-1651.

    This is a quality report from the Kaiser Permanente health care system comparing patient outcomes, surgeon support, and hospital care with other national and international quality reports. The report's conclusion supports the continuation of value-driven care to achieve high-quality metrics. Level of evidence: IV.

33. Jayakumar P, Moore MLG, Bozic KJ: Team approach: A multidisciplinary approach to the management of hip and knee osteoarthritis. *JBJS Rev* 2019;7(6):e10.

    This characterization review for a multidisciplinary team approach to osteoarthritis of the hip and knee describes the organization and application of an integrated care delivery model aimed to manage lower extremity joint pain and concludes on the theoretical value of this approach and reiterates the need for future research that compares the individual effect of different models of care on health outcomes, health spending, and utilization. Level of evidence: V.

34. ElSayed NA, Aleppo G, Aroda VR, et al: 13. Older adults: Standards of care in diabetes-2023. *Diabetes Care* 2023;46(suppl 1):S216-S229.

    This is the American Diabetes Association's 2023 guidelines for diabetes management, treatment goals, and tools to evaluate the quality of care. Level of evidence: V.

35. Cornelius ME, Loretan CG, Wang TW, Jamal A, Homa DM: Tobacco product use among adults – United States, 2020. *MMWR Morb Mortal Wkly Rep* 2022;71(11):397-405.

    The CDC *Morbidity and Mortality Weekly Report* on US adult tobacco product use and epidemiologic analysis of the 2020 National Health Interview Survey tobacco use data reported a decrease in tobacco product use from 2019 and prevalence of cigarette use followed by e-cigarettes and highlighted the value in continued monitoring of tobacco product use and creation and implementation of strategies and policies to continue decreasing tobacco use. Level of evidence: IV.

36. U.S. Department of Health and Human Services: The health consequences of smoking – 50 years of progress: A report of the Surgeon general, 2014. Available at: https://www.hhs.gov/sites/default/files/consequences-smoking-exec-summary.pdf.

37. Gonzalez AI, Luime JJ, Uçkay I, Hannouche D, Hoffmeyer P, Lübbeke A: Is there an association between smoking status and prosthetic joint infection after primary total joint arthroplasty? *J Arthroplasty* 2018;33(7):2218-2224.

    This retrospective review of prospectively collected registry data from a single institution on the rates of PJI and hazard ratio of PJI after TJA according to smoking status found incidence rates to be higher in current smokers than both former smokers and nonsmokers. The review also found increased risk of infection in current and former smokers than in nonsmokers and similar risks of PJI beyond the first year after surgery and concluded that smoking increases the risk of PJI after TJA. Level of evidence: IV.

38. Sahota S, Lovecchio F, Harold RE, Beal MD, Manning DW: The effect of smoking on thirty-day postoperative complications after total joint arthroplasty: A propensity score-matched analysis. *J Arthroplasty* 2018;33(1):30-35.

    This retrospective analysis of the American College of Surgeons' National Surgical Quality Improvement Program's database on the effect of smoking status on short-term complications after TJA associated smokers to higher rates of 30-day readmission, surgical complications, and SSIs and concluded that smoking status is significantly associated with higher rates of short-term complications after TJA. Level of evidence: IV.

39. Hart A, Rainer WG, Taunton MJ, Mabry TM, Berry DJ, Abdel MP: Smoking cessation before and after total joint arthroplasty-an uphill battle. *J Arthroplasty* 2019;34(7 suppl):S140-S143.

    This retrospective database analysis at a single institution on the rate of successful smoking cessation programs for active and former smokers after TJA found active and former smokers to consistently return to active smoking status 1 and 8 years after TJA and concludes on the significance of smoking status as a challenge to arthroplasty surgeons in patient optimization. Level of evidence: III.

40. Creamer MR, Wang TW, Babb S, et al: Tobacco product use and cessation indicators among adults - United States, 2018. *MMWR Morb Mortal Wkly Rep* 2019;68(45):1013-1019.

    The CDC *Morbidity and Mortality Weekly Report* on US adult tobacco product use and the epidemiologic analysis of the 2018 National Health Interview Survey tobacco use data reported a significant increase in cessation indicators and highlights the value in continued monitoring of tobacco product use and creation and implementation of strategies and policies to continue decreasing tobacco use. Level of evidence: IV.

41. Sørensen LT, Toft B, Rygaard J, Ladelund S, Teisner B, Gottrup F: Smoking attenuates wound inflammation and proliferation while smoking cessation restores inflammation but not proliferation. *Wound Repair Regen* 2010;18(2):186-192.

42. Sørensen LT, Nielsen HB, Kharazmi A, Gottrup F: Effect of smoking and abstention on oxidative burst and reactivity of neutrophils and monocytes. *Surgery* 2004;136(5):1047-1053.

43. Hart A, Rainer WG, Taunton MJ, Mabry TM, Berry DJ, Abdel MP: Cotinine testing improves smoking cessation before total joint arthroplasty. *J Arthroplasty* 2019;34(7 suppl):S148-S151.

    This retrospective analysis of the effect of preoperative serum cotinine testing in active smokers before TJA and its effect on self-reported abstinence rate found most cotinine-tested patients to have successfully quit smoking before TJA and concluded on the clinical significance of cotinine testing to promote self-reported smoking abstinence before surgery and guide risk counseling for patients who report abstinence but test positive for active smoking. Level of evidence: III.

44. Møller AM, Villebro N, Pedersen T, Tønnesen H: Effect of preoperative smoking intervention on postoperative complications: A randomised clinical trial. *Lancet* 2002;359(9301):114-117.

45. Herrero C, Tang A, Wasterlain A, et al: Smoking cessation correlates with a decrease in infection rates following total joint arthroplasty. *J Orthop* 2020;21:390-394.

    This is a retrospective review of the effect of smoking cessation programs versus self-treatment smoking cessation on perioperative outcomes after TJA. Patients who took part in a guided smoking cessation program trended toward higher quit rates, shorter lengths of stay, decreased infection rates, and higher readmission rates, all differences not statistically significant from the control group. The review concludes by highlighting the need for more studies looking at the effect of preoperative smoking cessation on patient outcomes after TJA. Level of evidence: IV.

46. Akhavan S, Nguyen LC, Chan V, Saleh J, Bozic KJ: Impact of smoking cessation counseling prior to total joint arthroplasty. *Orthopedics* 2017;40(2):e323-e328.

47. Garcia-Casal MN, Pasricha SR, Sharma AJ, Peña-Rosas JP: Use and interpretation of hemoglobin concentrations for assessing anemia status in individuals and populations: Results from a WHO technical meeting. *Ann N Y Acad Sci* 2019;1450(1):5-14.

    The results from the 2019 World Health Organization technical meeting on the use and interpretation of hemoglobin concentrations in the assessment of anemia describe the gaps in knowledge that were identified and the next steps to be taken to develop inclusive and evidence-based anemia characterization. Level of evidence: V.

48. Greenky M, Gandhi K, Pulido L, Restrepo C, Parvizi J: Preoperative anemia in total joint arthroplasty: Is it associated with periprosthetic joint infection? *Clin Orthop Relat Res* 2012;470(10):2695-2701.

49. Saleh E, McClelland DB, Hay A, Semple D, Walsh TS: Prevalence of anaemia before major joint arthroplasty and the potential impact of preoperative investigation and correction on perioperative blood transfusions. *Br J Anaesth* 2007;99(6):801-808.

50. Turner J, Parsi M, Badireddy M: Anemia, in *StatPearls*. StatPearls Publishing, 2022.

    This is a review on the diagnosis, etiology, pathophysiology, and management of anemia.

51. Drake MA: The nutritional status and dietary adequacy of single homeless women and their children in shelters. *Public Health Rep* 1992;107(3):312-319.

52. Lee HS, Chao HH, Huang WT, Chen SC, Yang HY: Psychiatric disorders risk in patients with iron deficiency anemia and association with iron supplementation medications: A nationwide database analysis. *BMC Psychiatry* 2020;20(1):216.

    This retrospective database-matched cohort study on the risk of development of psychiatric conditions and diagnosis of iron-deficiency anemia concluded that patients who had been diagnosed with iron-deficiency anemia had higher risk of developing psychiatric conditions. The study also found that patients with iron-deficiency anemia who received iron supplementation had lower risk of developing psychiatric conditions than those who did not receive treatment. Level of evidence: IV.

53. Weiss A, Beloosesky Y, Gingold-Belfer R, et al: Association of anemia with dementia and cognitive decline among community-dwelling elderly. *Gerontology* 2022;68(12):1375-1383.

    This historical prospective registry-based cohort study on anemia as a risk factor for dementia and cognitive decline in the elderly population (older than 65 years) found that patients in whom dementia developed or those with a cognitive decline in a 10-year period had higher rates of anemia than those in whom these cognitive disorders did not develop. Anemia was found to be a risk factor for the development of dementia and cognitive decline with the risk increasing as the severity of anemia increases. The study concluded on the importance of anemia in the elderly population and highlights the need for research examining anemia as a cause of reversible dementia. Level of evidence: III.

54. White ND: Vitamin B_{12} and plant-predominant diets. *Am J Lifestyle Med* 2022;16(3):295-297.

    This review of the prevalence of megaloblastic anemia and vitamin B_{12} deficiencies in individuals who consume plant-predominant diets covers general information on megaloblastic anemia, diagnosis, clinical presentation, and prevention of vitamin B_{12} deficiencies. Level of evidence: V.

55. Goodnough LT, Maniatis A, Earnshaw P, et al: Detection, evaluation, and management of preoperative anaemia in the elective orthopaedic surgical patient: NATA guidelines. *Br J Anaesth* 2011;106(1):13-22.

56. Cappellini MD, Motta I: Anemia in clinical practice-definition and classification: Does hemoglobin change with aging? *Semin Hematol* 2015;52(4):261-269.

57. Auerbach M, Adamson JW: How we diagnose and treat iron deficiency anemia. *Am J Hematol* 2016;91(1):31-38.

58. Ogun AS, Adeyinka A: Biochemistry, transferrin, in *StatPearls*. StatPearls Publishing, 2022.

    This review of the biochemical functions of transferrin refers to the cellular and molecular characteristics of transferrin and covers the physiologic functions, laboratory testing, and clinical significance of this molecule.

59. Lachance K, Savoie M, Bernard M, et al: Oral ferrous sulfate does not increase preoperative hemoglobin in patients scheduled for hip or knee arthroplasty. *Ann Pharmacother* 2011;45(6):764-770.

60. Petis SM, Lanting BA, Vasarhelyi EM, Naudie DDR, Ralley FE, Howard JL: Is there a role for preoperative iron supplementation in patients preparing for a total hip or total knee arthroplasty? *J Arthroplasty* 2017;32(9):2688-2693.

61. Muñoz M, Acheson AG, Auerbach M, et al: International consensus statement on the peri-operative management of anaemia and iron deficiency. *Anaesthesia* 2017;72(2):233-247.

62. Khalafallah A: A prospective randomized controlled trial to assess the effect of intravenous versus oral iron therapy in the treatment of preoperative anaemia. *J Blood Disord Transfus* 2012;3(2):1-6.

63. Chapter 1: Diagnosis and evaluation of anemia in CKD. *Kidney Int Suppl (2011)* 2012;2(4):288-291.

64. Nurko S: Anemia in chronic kidney disease: Causes, diagnosis, treatment. *Cleve Clin J Med* 2006;73(3):289-297.

65. Gómez-Ramírez S, Bisbe E, Shander A, Spahn DR, Muñoz M: Management of perioperative iron deficiency anemia. *Acta Haematol* 2019;142(1):21-29.

   This review of preoperative anemia screening and management covers the prevalence and implications of preoperative anemia in surgical patients and presents multiple treatment options for iron-deficiency anemia, depending on the severity of the anemia and whether the treatment is preoperative or postoperative. It also recommends oral iron supplementation for mild anemia when diagnosed at least 6 to 8 weeks before surgery or intravenous iron supplementation when diagnosed less than 6 weeks before surgery or when anemia is moderate to severe and briefly covers erythropoietin treatment and indications for blood transfusion. Level of evidence: V.

66. Pinilla-Gracia C, Mateo-Agudo J, Herrera A, Muñoz M: On the relevance of preoperative haemoglobin optimisation within a Patient Blood Management programme for elective hip arthroplasty surgery. *Blood Transfus* 2020;18(3):182-190.

   This retrospective cohort study analyzing whether preoperative anemia optimization reduced red blood cell transfusion rates and improved outcomes in patients who underwent THA found patients in the preoperative optimization group, who received ferric carboxymaltose and epoetin alfa, to have increased hemoglobin levels at hospital admission and rates of discharge to home and decreased rates of red blood cell transfusion and length of stay. The study concluded that a preoperative anemia optimization program for THA effectively corrected preoperative anemia and decreased the requirement for transfusions. Level of evidence: IV.

67. Dubé MD, Rothfusz CA, Emara AK, et al: Nutritional assessment and interventions in elective hip and knee arthroplasty: A detailed review and guide to management. *Curr Rev Musculoskelet Med* 2022;15(4):311-322.

   This review of the relationship between diagnosis of preoperative malnutrition in patients undergoing TJA and the effect on postoperative outcomes provides an overview of biochemical and anthropometric measures of malnutrition, the relationship between malnutrition and TJA outcomes, and some studied interventions to optimize these patients. Level of evidence: V.

68. White JV, Guenter P, Jensen G, et al: Consensus statement: Academy of Nutrition and Dietetics and American Society for Parenteral and Enteral Nutrition – Characteristics recommended for the identification and documentation of adult malnutrition (undernutrition). *JPEN J Parenter Enteral Nutr* 2012;36(3):275-283.

69. Gu A, Malahias MA, Strigelli V, Nocon AA, Sculco TP, Sculco PK: Preoperative malnutrition negatively correlates with postoperative wound complications and infection after total joint arthroplasty: A systematic review and meta-analysis. *J Arthroplasty* 2019;34(5):1013-1024.

   This is a systematic review and meta-analysis of the relationship between malnutrition and postoperative wound infections and other complications following TJA. Twenty studies were included for review, and all used, at minimum, albumin levels as a marker for malnutrition. Decreased albumin levels were found to correlate to higher odds of developing a postoperative wound complication. It was concluded that there is strong evidence to associate serologic markers of malnutrition with an increased risk of postoperative complications in TJA. Level of evidence: IV.

70. Kishawi D, Schwarzman G, Mejia A, Hussain AK, Gonzalez MH: Low preoperative albumin levels predict adverse outcomes after total joint arthroplasty. *J Bone Joint Surg Am* 2020;102(10):889-895.

   This retrospective analysis of the American College of Surgeons National Surgical Quality Improvement Program's database on the effect of albumin levels on 30-day postoperative complications following TJA found patients with lower albumin levels to associate higher rates of multiple 30-day postoperative complications compared with patients with normal albumin levels. The analysis concluded on the importance of new research to determine the most effective preoperative management of hypoalbuminemia. Level of evidence: IV.

71. Ellsworth B, Kamath AF: Malnutrition and total joint arthroplasty. *J Nat Sci* 2016;2(3):e179.

72. Sayeed Z, Anoushiravani AA, Simha S, et al: Markers for malnutrition and BMI status in total joint arthroplasty and pharmaconutrient therapy. *JBJS Rev* 2019;7(5):e3.

   This review evaluates the nutritional status of the orthopaedic patient prior to total joint arthroplasty. Anthropometric measurements and laboratory tests including total lymphocyte count, serum albumin, and serum prealbumin, are correlated with postoperative outcomes after total joint arthroplasty. Level of evidence: V.

73. Phillips JLH, Ennis HE, Jennings JM, Dennis DA: Screening and management of malnutrition in total joint arthroplasty. *J Am Acad Orthop Surg* 2023;31(7):319-325.

   This review of current knowledge of malnutrition and its effects on TJA covers epidemiology and clinical presentation of malnutrition and risks associated with TJA and provides an overview of the screening tools for malnutrition and management recommendations. Level of evidence: V.

74. Schroer WC, LeMarr AR, Mills K, Childress AL, Morton DJ, Reedy ME: 2019 Chitranjan S. Ranawat Award: Elective joint arthroplasty outcomes improve in malnourished patients with nutritional intervention – A prospective population analysis demonstrates a modifiable risk factor. *Bone Joint J* 2019;101-B(7 suppl C):17-21.

   This is a prospective trial analyzing the effects of a nutritional intervention program for malnourished patients diagnosed preoperatively before undergoing TJA. Patients with low albumin levels received a high-protein, anti-inflammatory diet for a month before and after surgery. Findings showed that patients in the nutrition intervention program had decreased length of stay and lower overall hospital charges, readmissions charges, and 90-day total charges, regardless of covariates, compared with nonintervention control group.

The study concluded that preoperative malnutrition management was associated with better postoperative outcomes and also highlighted the importance and effects of patient education on malnutrition. Level of evidence: I.

75. Gonçalves TJM, Gonçalves SEAB, Nava N, et al: Perioperative immunonutrition in elderly patients undergoing total hip and knee arthroplasty: Impact on postoperative outcomes. *JPEN J Parenter Enteral Nutr* 2021;45(7):1559-1566.

    This is a retrospective cohort study of an immunonutrition intervention for elderly patients regardless of nourishment status and its effects on perioperative complications. Patients in the immunonutrition group received a high-protein, high-calorie nutritional shake 5 days before and 5 days after TJA and were compared with the control group. Findings showed that patients in the immunonutrition group had decreased length of stay, rates of infectious and noninfectious complications, and rates of intensive care unit transfer. The study concluded that perioperative immunonutrition in elderly patients undergoing TJA may decrease postoperative complications regardless of nutritional status. Level of evidence: IV.

SECTION 2

Basic Science

Section Editor:
Barry D. Brause, MD, FACP, FIDSA

CHAPTER 7

General Diagnostics

CARL DEIRMENGIAN, MD, FAAOS • YALE A. FILLINGHAM, MD, FAAOS
P. MAXWELL COURTNEY, MD, FAAOS

ABSTRACT

A standardized diagnosis of musculoskeletal infection is important for both research protocols and clinical practice. The acknowledgment and progress in understanding culture-negative infection has led to various technologies that can be used to diagnose infection, including biomarkers and imaging. Both systemic and synovial fluid biomarkers are used to diagnose infection and have been included in recently recommended definitions of musculoskeletal infection. In addition, various imaging technologies including ultrasonography, MRI, and tomography have been leveraged to aid in the diagnosis of infection. Finally, there has been recent understanding and progress in the development of in vitro and in vivo models that can aid in research pertaining to the diagnosis of infection. It is important to provide a general overview of recent trends and literature in general diagnostics for musculoskeletal infection.

Keywords: biomarkers; diagnosis; imaging research model; infection

INTRODUCTION

The results of microbiologic culture have historically dominated the diagnosis of infection for both the clinical and research efforts in orthopaedic surgery. The concept of an infection was historically equated with culture results, reflecting the underlying knowledge that infections are caused by microorganisms that can be isolated in the laboratory. However, the problem of being fully reliant on culture results has been recognized. Biomarkers and imaging have been leveraged to aid in the diagnosis of infection, inclusive of the concept of a culture-negative infection. Various in vitro and in vivo models have been used to gain further insight into infection and its diagnosis.

BIOMARKERS

A redefinition of infection has been formulated in the past several decades, dependent on identification of both the organism and the host immune response via biomarkers.[1-3] A biomarker is any patient characteristic that is indicative of a medical state, usually being normal or abnormal. With specific reference to orthopaedic infections, the term biomarker often refers to a laboratory test with a result that can be diagnostically

---

Dr. Deirmengian or an immediate family member serves as a paid consultant to or is an employee of Biostar Ventures and Zimmer; has stock or stock options held in Biostar Ventures, Domain, and Trice; and has received research or institutional support from Zimmer. Dr. Fillingham or an immediate family member has received royalties from Exactech, Inc. and Medacta; serves as a paid consultant to or is an employee of Exactech, Inc., Johnson & Johnson, Medacta, and Zimmer; has stock or stock options held in Parvizi Surgical Innovations; has received nonincome support (such as equipment or services), commercially derived honoraria, or other non–research-related funding (such as paid travel) from MicroGen Dx; and serves as a board member, owner, officer, or committee member of American Academy of Orthopaedic Surgeons and American Association of Hip and Knee Surgeons. Dr. Courtney or an immediate family member is a member of a speakers' bureau or has made paid presentations on behalf of Smith & Nephew; serves as a paid consultant to or is an employee of DePuy, a Johnson & Johnson Company, Hip Innovation Technology, Stryker, and Zimmer; has stock or stock options held in Parvizi Surgical Innovation; and serves as a board member, owner, officer, or committee member of American Academy of Orthopaedic Surgeons and American Association of Hip and Knee Surgeons.

helpful in a clinical or research context. The serum biomarkers most commonly used are general indicators of inflammation and include erythrocyte sedimentation rate (ESR), C-reactive protein (CRP), interleukin 6, D-dimer, and procalcitonin. The most commonly used synovial fluid biomarkers include white blood cell (WBC) count, polymorphonuclear cell percentage, alpha-defensin, and human neutrophil elastase.

Purpose of Orthopaedic Infection Biomarkers

The purpose of biomarkers in orthopaedic infection is twofold: to aid in the accurate diagnosis of orthopaedic infection in clinical research and to provide consistent standards by which clinicians can make the diagnosis of infection in routine practice.[3] These are very different purposes that may have very different biomarker requirements. For example, research teams can manage substantial diagnostic complexity to achieve the most accurate diagnostic classification possible. However, routine clinical practice can be overwhelmed by complexity and better served by simplicity and consistency.

There are two general types of biomarkers used in musculoskeletal infection: multipurpose tests that are not intended to diagnose infection and single-purpose tests that are intended to diagnose infection. The list of multipurpose tests offered by general laboratories to diagnose a variety of conditions across medicine includes ESR, CRP, D-dimer test, synovial fluid WBC count, and synovial fluid neutrophil percentage. These tests were not designed to diagnose infection, but rather were identified through research as being potentially useful in diagnosing infection. The main advantage of multipurpose tests is that they are usually less expensive and more available to clinicians in various medical settings. According to a 2022 study, the main disadvantage of multipurpose tests is that they are susceptible to being misinterpreted by physicians.[4] For example, CRP and D-dimer levels are reported with variable units and variable normal thresholds across the United States, requiring the ordering physician to convert units and apply an alternative threshold as recommended for musculoskeletal infection. This is a potential failure point for multipurpose tests for infection because the required unit of measure conversions and the application of recommended thresholds are complex, which may lead to clinical errors.[4]

Single-purpose diagnostic tests are tests that are specifically designed to diagnose infection, having navigated a regulatory process to demonstrate accuracy and reliability across users. For example, as discussed in 2021 studies, both the alpha-defensin test[5] and the calprotectin test[6] were designed specifically to diagnose prosthetic joint infection (PJI). The main disadvantage of single-purpose diagnostic tests is that they are often more expensive, reflecting their development process, and often less available to clinicians worldwide. However, the main advantage of single-purpose tests is that they are extremely easy to interpret because they have an intended use to diagnose PJI without the need for unit conversion or application of alternative thresholds. Therefore, although single-purpose diagnostic tests may be more expensive, they also carry a lower risk of misinterpretation by the ordering physician. Single-purpose biomarkers that are intended to diagnose infection have the potential to bring the diagnostic accuracy of experts to all clinicians in routine practice.

Several authoritative bodies including the International Consensus Meeting (ICM)[2] (**Figure 1**) and the European Bone and Joint Infection Society (EBJIS)[3] have recommended definitions of PJI, which include multiple biomarkers and criteria into one large scoring system. These scoring systems have inherent complexity, combining clinical findings with both multipurpose tests and single-purpose tests for PJI. They have successfully leveraged several biomarkers to provide a consistent standard that has substantial value in the field of research, a setting in which complexity can be properly managed. However, the complexity of these PJI scoring systems may serve as a barrier to routine clinical adoption, as has been observed in other areas of medicine.[7,8]

Blood Biomarkers

Blood biomarkers (ESR, CRP) were originally used and recommended as an initial screening to rule out infection.[9] However, it is now recognized that blood biomarkers are not sufficient to rule out for PJI because of a suboptimal specificity, yielding relatively frequent false-negative results.[10,11] Furthermore, given the frequent comorbidities among patients with painful joint replacements, blood biomarkers also have an elevated false-positive rate.[12] Therefore, blood biomarkers have an overall diagnostic accuracy that is lowest among all of the tests used to diagnose infection. As discussed in a 2018 study, serum tests should not be used in isolation to diagnose PJI when there is concern regarding PJI.[13]

ESR is a quite nonspecific functional test of systemic inflammation. Although prominent among early diagnostic strategies to diagnose PJI,[9] ESR no longer plays a prominent role in diagnosing PJI. For example, the EBJIS has not included the ESR in its 2021 definition of PJI,[3] and the 2018 ICM definition of PJI has assigned the lowest possible point score to a positive ESR.[2] CRP is another blood test that serves as an indicator of systemic inflammation, demonstrating a sensitivity of 85% and specificity of 81% at the diagnostic threshold of 10 mg/L.[14] It continues to be included in most of the recommended definitions for PJI[2,3] and is widely available in clinical laboratories. However, great care must be taken in interpreting the CRP test result because clinical

Major criteria (at least one of the following)	Decision
Two positive growth of the same organism using standard culture methods	Infected
Sinus tract with evidence of communication to the joint or visualization of the prosthesis	

Minor criteria	Threshold Acute[ε]	Threshold Chronic	Score	Decision
Serum CRP (mg/L) *or* D-dimer (ug/L)	100 / Unknown	10 / 860	2	
Elevated serum ESR (mm/hr)	No role	30	1	Combined preoperative and postoperative score:
Elevated synovial WBC (cells/µL) *or* Leukocyte esterase *or* Positive alpha-defensin (signal/cutoff)	10,000 / ++ / 1.0	3,000 / ++ / 1.0	3	≥6 Infected
Elevated synovial PMN (%)	90	70	2	3-5 Inconclusive*
Single positive culture			2	<3 Not infected
Positive histology			3	
Positive intraoperative purulence[¥]			3	

[ε] These criteria were never validated on acute infections. [¥] No role in suspected adverse local tissue reaction. *Consider further molecular diagnostics such as next-generation sequencing

FIGURE 1 Proposed 2018 International Consensus Meeting criteria for prosthetic joint infection. CRP = C-reactive protein, ESR = erythrocyte sedimentation rate, PMN = polymorphonuclear cell, WBC = white blood cell. (Reprinted from Shohat N, Bauer T, Buttaro M, et al: Hip and knee section, what is the definition of a periprosthetic joint infection (PJI) of the knee and the hip? Can the same criteria be used for both joints? Proceedings of international consensus on orthopedic infections. *J Arthroplasty* 2019;34[2 suppl]:S325-S327. Copyright 2018, with permission from Elsevier.)

laboratory thresholds for CRP may differ from the optimal levels used to diagnose PJI.[4] Furthermore, the CRP units of measure reported by clinical laboratories vary (mg/L and mg/dL), making it necessary for the clinician to convert the results to the units of mg/L before applying the PJI-optimized threshold for diagnosis (10 mg/L).[4]

The D-dimer test is also widely available and used across medicine. Although usually used in the field of coagulation and vascular medicine, the D-dimer test also reflects the body's general state of inflammation, providing some diagnostic information regarding PJI. Although early data suggested that the D-dimer test was the most accurate blood test for PJI,[15] recent studies have questioned the improved accuracy of the test.[16-18] Although included by the 2018 ICM definition of PJI, the D-dimer test has not been included in the 2021 EBJIS definition of PJI given its equivalence and redundancy to other blood tests currently used.[16] In addition, the D-dimer test is notorious for its potential to be misinterpreted even among experts[19] because it is reported with many different diagnostic thresholds and units of measure across clinical laboratories.[4] To use the D-dimer for the diagnosis of PJI, the clinician must convert the D-dimer result to nanograms per milliliter fibrinogen equivalent units and then apply a threshold of 850 ng/mL.

Synovial Fluid Biomarkers

The synovial compartment is a relatively enclosed compartment that surrounds all joints, which are often involved in musculoskeletal infection. Therefore, the synovial fluid provides what is likely the most relevant and accurate diagnostic glimpse into joint infection because the by-products of infection have a chance to concentrate in this enclosed compartment. It is no surprise that synovial fluid testing has recently taken a dominant role in both biomarker research and recommendations of authoritative bodies. The main disadvantage of synovial fluid biomarker testing for PJI evaluation is that it requires an aspiration of the joint, which varies in complexity across the human body, but this would not be a factor in evaluating musculoskeletal infections other than PJI.

The traditional synovial fluid biomarkers for PJI include the synovial fluid WBC count and the synovial fluid neutrophil percentage. Both of these tests have established a tradition of good diagnostic performance and are widely embraced by all definitions of PJI.[2,3] In general, an increasing WBC count can be considered a reflection of increasing inflammation, which corresponds to a higher probability that the cause is infectious. As discussed in a 2020 study, unexpectedly elevated automated WBC counts should be confirmed by manual counting because automated cell counts may be falsely positive.[20] The main disadvantage of the synovial fluid WBC and polymorphonuclear percentage is that the clinician interpreting them must correctly use the optimized thresholds for infection to achieve their expected accuracy. It is important to note that the diagnostic threshold for both the WBC count and the polymorphonuclear percentage has varied across institutions, even differing between definitions of PJI recommended by authoritative bodies.[2,3]

The alpha-defensin test for PJI is the first diagnostic test specifically developed for PJI, having received FDA authorization in 2019.[5] Its overall accuracy has been confirmed at many institutions and has been described in several recent biomarker meta-analyses as the most accurate individual biomarker for PJI,[14,21] with a sensitivity and specificity of 97% and 96% for PJI.[21] In addition, the test has been included in the most recent definitions of PJI as recommended by both the ICM (**Figure 1**) and the EBJIS.[2,3] The main disadvantage of the alpha-defensin test is its cost, which is higher than that of the traditional tests for infection. In addition, similar to other biomarkers in synovial fluid, the alpha-defensin test can be false-positive with an underlying adverse tissue reaction, hematoma, acute inflammatory arthritis, or crystal arthropathy.[22] The main advantage of the alpha-defensin test is its standardization in performance and reporting, which makes it less susceptible to misinterpretation by clinicians when compared with traditional tests for PJI.[4] Furthermore, there is some evidence that the alpha-defensin test may maintain accuracy in certain settings, such as PJIs with less virulent organisms[23] and after antibiotic treatment has been initiated.[24] Although the alpha-defensin test is remarkable, it is not universally available and the diagnosis of PJI is not dependent on it.

The urinary leukocyte esterase test strip has been described as a promising off-label test for PJI, with a specificity and specificity of 77% and 95%, respectively. Although the urinary leukocyte esterase test strip has a low cost and is very rapid, its appropriate use should likely be limited to major academic centers considering several barriers for clinical use. First, it is recommended that the sample is centrifuged before use,[25] which is generally not possible and often inappropriate in routine clinical settings. Second, the off-label nature and lack of standardization between brands of test strip introduce repeatability and interpretability concerns, requiring significant clinician knowledge and experience for correct usage as a PJI rule-in test. The leukocyte esterase test strip is included in the 2018 ICM definition of PJI but not the 2021 EBJIS definition because of its practical limitations.[3]

DIAGNOSTIC RADIOLOGY OF MUSCULOSKELETAL INFECTION

Plain Radiography

More than 2 million patients annually will undergo treatment in the United States for a musculoskeletal infection.[26] Evaluation of a patient with a suspected musculoskeletal infection typically begins with a patient history, physical examination, and radiographic evaluation. Although musculoskeletal infection is not commonly detected on radiographs until the disease process has become more advanced, appropriate radiographs of the affected extremity should be the initial imaging modality. Despite the nondiagnostic nature of radiographs for musculoskeletal infection, it provides valuable diagnostic information to guide the clinician's differential diagnosis because fracture, aseptic prosthetic failure, and degenerative joint disease are examples of alternative diagnoses that can be seen with plain radiographs.

Ultrasonography

Even though the quality of the ultrasonographic image is operator dependent, it can be a useful diagnostic tool under specific situations because it is low cost, is widely available, and does not use ionizing radiation. It can be a valuable cross-sectional imaging modality in the pediatric population because it does not require sedation or in the adult population with a contraindication to undergoing MRI, such as the presence of a cardiac pacemaker or other magnet-vulnerable indwelling devices. In addition, ultrasonography can aid in the diagnosis of musculoskeletal infection by guiding aspiration of the joint or abscess. Soft-tissue infections including cellulitis, septic bursitis, septic tenosynovitis, subcutaneous abscess, and pyomyositis will have unique characteristics on ultrasonography, allowing for their diagnosis.[27-29] However, caution should be used when solely relying on ultrasonography for diagnosis of these conditions because it may underestimate the extent of the infection.[27] Ultrasonography can be used to diagnose osteomyelitis in the pediatric population because it commonly involves a subperiosteal abscess, but it provides little benefit in diagnosing osteomyelitis in adults because the cortex of bone cannot be penetrated during ultrasonography.[30]

Scintigraphy

Technetium diphosphonate bone scanning is not specific to an infection because diphosphonate has increased uptake in all osseous tissues with an increased blood flow or increased bone metabolic activity to produce nonspecific positive scans, such as with overlying cellulitis or other soft-tissue infections, fractures, neuropathic arthropathy, bone tumors, and aseptic loosening of joint replacements and fixation devices.

In vitro labeled leukocyte (indium-111) is another method of radiotracer imaging that is more specific for evaluating bacterial infections because most leukocytes labeled with indium-111 are neutrophils. Although it has value in evaluation of bone infection in the peripheral skeleton, indium-111 is too unreliable in evaluating the axial skeleton (ie, spine, sternum) because of the interference by the nonspecific background bone marrow uptake. Another limitation with this method is the need for the patient to have a total WBC count of at least 2,000/μL.[28]

Magnetic Resonance Imaging

MRI is a powerful diagnostic tool for musculoskeletal infection because of its ability to evaluate the osseous structures and surrounding soft tissue without ionizing radiation and with a high degree of anatomic detail. The pitfalls of MRI are the associated cost, the presence of motion artifact, image quality dependence on strength of the magnet, and signal disruption from metallic implants. The infectious process results in the formation of inflammatory edema, which MRI is highly sensitive at detecting as a decreased signal intensity on T1-weighted sequences and increased signal intensity on T2-weighted sequences.[27] However, because MRI detects only edema fluid (sensitive but not specific), it is not helpful in many clinical situations. It is excellent for demonstrating soft-tissue involvement, and it has the ability to exclude osteomyelitis with a 100% negative predictive value when the bone marrow appears normal on all MRI sequences,[31] but it is too nonspecific for definitive diagnosis in patients with infections contiguous with bone, such as an overlying skin ulcer or cellulitis, neuropathic osteoarthropathy, recent trauma or surgery, a fracture or nonunion, or other causes of soft-tissue edema or lymphedema. MRI is capable of identifying osteomyelitis early in the disease process as soon as 1 to 2 days after the onset of symptoms,[28] but this high degree of sensitivity results in it being too nonspecific in complicated cases.

Computed Tomography

CT is widely available in the hospital setting, is rapidly obtained, and provides excellent detail of the osseous structures, but it is not considered a first-line diagnostic imaging modality for musculoskeletal infection. Although CT provides better evaluation of the surrounding soft tissue than plain radiography, MRI provides better diagnostic images without the use of ionizing radiation. Therefore, according to a 2020 study, CT is not routinely obtained in the evaluation of patients for a musculoskeletal infection with the exception of investigating for necrotizing fasciitis because of the rapidly progressing nature of the infection and ease of obtaining the CT image.[32]

Single-Photon Emission Computed Tomography

Single-photon emission computed tomography (SPECT) is similar to traditional scintigraphy, which can be performed with similar radiotracers such as technetium-99m–labeled diphosphonates, indium-111, and gallium-67.[33] Therefore, SPECT is used in a manner similar to that of traditional scintigraphy. The advantage of SPECT is that the multiplanar images allow for higher resolution, providing improved diagnostic sensitivity.[34] However, the combination of SPECT with traditional CT images has allowed for more precise anatomic localization.[35,36]

Fluorine-18-Fluorodeoxyglucose–Positron Emission Tomography

Fluorine-18-fluorodeoxyglucose (FDG) is a molecular structure taken up by cells through glucose transporters that does not undergo metabolization. Therefore, FDG–positron emission tomography (PET) is a method of measuring the cellular metabolic rate and number of glucose transporters in the local cells. Because activated lymphocytes, macrophages, monocytes, and neutrophils process a high number of glucose transporters and have an increased metabolic rate in the presence of an infection, FDG-PET better aids in the diagnosis of musculoskeletal infections compared with traditional scintigraphy, whereby aseptic conditions such as degenerative joint disease will not have an increased signal on the FDG-PET images.[27,28] The use of PET allows for quantitative imaging, which means serial imaging can be used to monitor treatment.[37]

With additional data collection on the use of FDG-PET imaging in complicated cases, it may be the definitive imaging technique for musculoskeletal infection.

IN VITRO AND IN VIVO STUDIES

With *Staphylococcus aureus* being among the most common organism in musculoskeletal infection, research has focused on the optimal antibiotic regimen to help eradicate this difficult pathogen. *S aureus* has several phenotypes that allow it to persist in osteoblasts and help facilitate chronic infection.[38] Bacteria become internalized in osteoblasts and escape a phagosome before lysosomal fusion, or survive in a phagolysosome and multiply in the osteoblast cytoplasm.[39-42] These other phenotypes unique to *S aureus* allow it to escape immunosurveillance, causing some physicians to consider chronic *S aureus* osteomyelitis as an incurable condition. An animal study with transmission electron microscopy of infected mouse bone observed *S aureus* within the canaliculi of live cortical bone, migrating toward osteocyte lacunae via proliferation at the leading edge.[43]

SUMMARY

The diagnosis of musculoskeletal infection can be quite challenging and current research continues to evolve. As more is learned about culture-negative infection, systemic and synovial fluid biomarkers are being used more frequently and have been recently included in new definitions of PJI. Imaging modalities such as ultrasonography, MRI, and other nuclear medicine studies are also important adjuncts in the diagnosis of musculoskeletal infection. With increasing bacterial resistance and challenging pathogens, recent in vitro and in vivo studies on antibiotics have helped guide systemic antimicrobial treatment for musculoskeletal infection.

KEY STUDY POINTS

- The purpose of biomarkers in orthopaedic infection is twofold: to aid in the accurate diagnosis of orthopaedic infection in clinical research and to provide consistent standards by which clinicians can make the diagnosis of infection in routine practice.
- Imaging modalities such as ultrasonography, MRI, and other nuclear medicine studies are also important adjuncts in the diagnosis of musculoskeletal infection.
- With increasing bacterial resistance and challenging pathogens, recent in vitro and in vivo studies on antibiotics have helped guide systemic antimicrobial treatment for musculoskeletal infection.

ANNOTATED REFERENCES

1. Goh GS, Parvizi J: Diagnosis and treatment of culture-negative periprosthetic joint infection. *J Arthroplasty* 2022;37(8):1488-1493.

   The authors provide a review of culture-negative PJI, including aspects of causes, diagnosis, and clinical considerations.

2. Shohat N, Bauer T, Buttaro M, et al: Hip and knee section, what is the definition of a periprosthetic joint infection (PJI) of the knee and the hip? Can the same criteria be used for both joints?: Proceedings of international consensus on orthopedic infections. *J Arthroplasty* 2019;34(2 suppl):S325-S327.

   The authors present the 2018 ICM-recommended definition of PJI, which is a high-complexity scoring system including major and minor criteria, points per category, and PJI-optimized thresholds for both chronic and acute PJI. This definition of PJI continues to use ESR as a serum biomarker and the leukocyte esterase test strip as a synovial fluid test and introduces utilization of the D-dimer test.

3. McNally M, Sousa R, Wouthuyzen-Bakker M, et al: The EBJIS definition of periprosthetic joint infection. *Bone Joint J* 2021;103-B(1):18-25.

   The authors present the EBJIS definition of PJI, which is a three-category, high-complexity scoring system based on the risk for PJI. They offer different PJI-optimized testing thresholds for each category to stratify patients based on the risk. This definition of PJI does not use the ESR, D-dimer, or leukocyte esterase test strip.

4. Forte SA, D'Alonzo JA, Wells Z, Levine B, Sizer S, Deirmengian C: Laboratory-reported normal value ranges should not be used to diagnose periprosthetic joint infection. *Cureus* 2022;14(8):e28258.

   The authors report on a study that surveyed clinical laboratories across the United States to determine the units of measure and thresholds used to report tests commonly used to diagnose PJI. The study found that there was substantial discrepancy between laboratories, especially for the units of measure and thresholds reported for CRP and D-dimer. The authors show that the use of laboratory-reported results could lead to false-positive test interpretations by clinicians diagnosing PJI.

5. Deirmengian C, Madigan J, Kallur Mallikarjuna S, Conway J, Higuera C, Patel R: Validation of the alpha defensin lateral flow test for periprosthetic joint infection. *J Bone Joint Surg Am* 2021;103(2):115-122.

   This is a prospective multicenter diagnostic validation study performed for the purpose of gaining FDA authorization of the alpha-defensin lateral flow test. The authors demonstrated that the lateral flow test for alpha-defensin has a high sensitivity and specificity for PJI, as defined by the Musculoskeletal Infection Society definition of PJI.

6. Warren J, Anis HK, Bowers K, et al: Diagnostic utility of a novel point-of-care test of calprotectin for periprosthetic joint infection after total knee arthroplasty: A prospective cohort study. *J Bone Joint Surg Am* 2021;103(11):1009-1015.

This prospective diagnostic study was one of the first to report on the diagnostic performance of a calprotectin point-of-care test to diagnose PJI. The authors demonstrated a high sensitivity and specificity in diagnosing PJI, as defined by the Musculoskeletal Infection Society definition of PJI. Level of evidence: II.

7. Cabana MD, Rand CS, Powe NR, et al: Why don't physicians follow clinical practice guidelines? A framework for improvement. *J Am Med Assoc* 1999;282(15):1458-1465.

8. Barth JH, Misra S, Aakre KM, et al: Why are clinical practice guidelines not followed? *Clin Chem Lab Med* 2016;54(7):1133-1139.

9. Della Valle C, Parvizi J, Bauer TW, et al: American Academy of Orthopaedic Surgeons clinical practice guideline on: The diagnosis of periprosthetic joint infections of the hip and knee. *J Bone Joint Surg Am* 2011;93(14):1355-1357.

10. McArthur BA, Abdel MP, Taunton MJ, Osmon DR, Hanssen AD: Seronegative infections in hip and knee arthroplasty: Periprosthetic infections with normal erythrocyte sedimentation rate and C-reactive protein level. *Bone Joint J* 2015;97-B(7):939-944.

11. Johnson AJ, Zywiel MG, Stroh A, Marker DR, Mont MA: Serological markers can lead to false negative diagnoses of periprosthetic infections following total knee arthroplasty. *Int Orthop* 2011;35(11):1621-1626.

12. Alijanipour P, Bakhshi H, Parvizi J: Diagnosis of periprosthetic joint infection: The threshold for serological markers. *Clin Orthop Relat Res* 2013;471(10):3186-3195.

13. Akgün D, Müller M, Perka C, Winkler T: The serum level of C-reactive protein alone cannot be used for the diagnosis of prosthetic joint infections, especially in those caused by organisms of low virulence. *Bone Joint J* 2018;100-B(11):1482-1486.

The authors report on a retrospective study evaluating the serum CRP test among patients with PJI. They found that many patients with PJI and a positive culture had normal serum CRP levels, especially among those with low-virulent organisms. The authors conclude that testing of CRP level alone is not an appropriate screening tool for PJI. Level of evidence: III.

14. Carli AV, Abdelbary H, Ahmadzai N, et al: Diagnostic accuracy of serum, synovial, and tissue testing for chronic periprosthetic joint infection after hip and knee replacements: A systematic review. *J Bone Joint Surg Am* 2019;101(7):635-649.

The authors performed a systematic review of biomarkers used to diagnose PJI. They found that, in general, synovial fluid tests outperformed the serum tests for PJI, with alpha-defensin demonstrating the best overall diagnostic performance in the review.

15. Shahi A, Kheir MM, Tarabichi M, Hosseinzadeh HRS, Tan TL, Parvizi J: Serum D-dimer test is promising for the diagnosis of periprosthetic joint infection and timing of reimplantation. *J Bone Joint Surg Am* 2017;99(17):1419-1427.

16. Xiong L, Li S, Dai M: Comparison of D-dimer with CRP and ESR for diagnosis of periprosthetic joint infection. *J Orthop Surg Res* 2019;14(1):240.

The authors conducted a prospective diagnostic evaluation of the D-dimer test, demonstrating a relatively poor sensitivity and specificity that was not an improvement over the serum CRP test for diagnosing PJI.

17. Wang R, Zhang H, Ding P, Jiao Q: The accuracy of D-dimer in the diagnosis of periprosthetic infections: A systematic review and meta-analysis. *J Orthop Surg Res* 2022;17(1):99.

The authors conducted a systematic review of the D-dimer test to diagnose PJI, demonstrating a sensitivity of 81% and a specificity of 74%, translating into a false-positive rate of 26%. They point out that there is scarce evidence reporting on D-dimer thresholds, sampling types, and detection methods, warranting more study to understand the clinical relevance of the D-dimer test for the diagnosis of PJI.

18. Fernandez-Sampedro M, Sanlés-González I, García-Ibarbia C, Fañanás-Rodríquez N, Fakkas-Fernández M, Fariñas MC: The poor accuracy of D-dimer for the diagnosis of prosthetic joint infection but its potential usefulness in early postoperative infections following revision arthroplasty for aseptic loosening. *BMC Infect Dis* 2022;22(1):91.

The authors conducted a prospective study evaluating the diagnostic performance of serum D-dimer for PJI. They found D-dimer to have a lower sensitivity than both CRP and ESR in the setting of PJI.

19. Favaloro EJ, Thachil J: Reporting of D-dimer data in COVID-19: Some confusion and potential for misinformation. *Clin Chem Lab Med* 2020;58(8):1191-1199.

This review of studies evaluating the D-dimer test in the setting of the COVID-19 pandemic demonstrated significant confusion in the literature because of a failure of studies to properly report important characteristics such as the detection technique, units of measure, and thresholds used. The authors also identified frank errors in reporting D-dimer results in the literature reviewed.

20. Deirmengian CA, Kazarian GS, Feeley SP, Sizer SC: False-positive automated synovial fluid white blood cell counting is a concern for both hip and knee arthroplasty aspirates. *J Arthroplasty* 2020;35(6 suppl):S304-S307.

The authors retrospectively reviewed a large cohort of synovial fluid samples that had both a manual and automated synovial fluid cell count performed, demonstrating high false-positive rates from automated cell counters compared with the manual count.

21. Lee YS, Koo KH, Kim HJ, et al: Synovial fluid biomarkers for the diagnosis of periprosthetic joint infection: A systematic review and meta-analysis. *J Bone Joint Surg Am* 2017;99(24):2077-2084.

22. Patel R: Periprosthetic joint infection. *N Engl J Med* 2023;388(3):251-262.

This article is a comprehensive review of the pathogenesis, treatment, prevention, and epidemiology of periprosthetic joint infection.

23. Deirmengian C, Kardos K, Kilmartin P, Gulati S, Citrano P, Booth RE Jr: The alpha-defensin test for periprosthetic joint infection responds to a wide spectrum of organisms. *Clin Orthop Relat Res* 2015;473(7):2229-2235.

24. Shahi A, Parvizi J, Kazarian GS, et al: The alpha-defensin test for periprosthetic joint infections is not affected by prior antibiotic administration. *Clin Orthop Relat Res* 2016;474(7):1610-1615.

25. Aggarwal VK, Tischler E, Ghanem E, Parvizi J: Leukocyte esterase from synovial fluid aspirate: A technical note. *J Arthroplasty* 2013;28(1):193-195.

26. Fayad LM, Carrino JA, Fishman EK: Musculoskeletal infection: Role of CT in the emergency department. *Radiographics* 2007;27(6):1723-1736.

27. Simpfendorfer CS: Radiologic approach to musculoskeletal infections. *Infect Dis Clin North Am* 2017;31(2):299-324.

28. Palestro CJ, Love C, Miller TT: Infection and musculoskeletal conditions: Imaging of musculoskeletal infections. *Best Pract Res Clin Rheumatol* 2006;20(6):1197-1218.

29. Bureau NJ, Chhem RK, Cardinal E: Musculoskeletal infections: US manifestations. *Radiographics* 1999;19(6):1585-1592.

30. Riebel TW, Nasir R, Nazarenko O: The value of sonography in the detection of osteomyelitis. *Pediatr Radiol* 1996;26(4):291-297.

31. Craig JG, Amin MB, Wu K, et al: Osteomyelitis of the diabetic foot: MR imaging-pathologic correlation. *Radiology* 1997;203(3):849-855.

32. Altmayer S, Verma N, Dicks EA, Oliveira A: Imaging musculoskeletal soft tissue infections. *Semin Ultrasound CT MR* 2020;41(1):85-98.

    This article provides a compilation of the characteristic findings of various types of musculoskeletal infections in cross-sectional imaging including ultrasonography, CT, and MRI.

33. Thang SP, Tong AK, Lam WW, Ng DC: SPECT/CT in musculoskeletal infections. *Semin Musculoskelet Radiol* 2014;18(2):194-202.

34. Weon YC, Yang SO, Choi YY, et al: Use of Tc-99m HMPAO leukocyte scans to evaluate bone infection: Incremental value of additional SPECT images. *Clin Nucl Med* 2000;25(7):519-526.

35. Shreve PD: Adding structure to function. *J Nucl Med* 2000;41(8):1380-1382.

36. Schillaci O: Hybrid SPECT/CT: A new era for SPECT imaging? *Eur J Nucl Med Mol Imaging* 2005;32(5):521-524.

37. Kalicke T, Schmitz A, Risse JH, et al: Fluorine-18 fluorodeoxyglucose PET in infectious bone diseases: Results of histologically confirmed cases. *Eur J Nucl Med* 2000;27(5):524-528.

38. Josse J, Velard F, Gangloff SC: Staphylococcus aureus vs. Osteoblast: Relationship and consequences in osteomyelitis. *Front Cell Infect Microbiol* 2015;5:85.

39. Marro FC, Abad L, Blocker AJ, Laurent F, Josse J, Valour F: In vitro antibiotic activity against intraosteoblastic Staphylococcus aureus: A narrative review of the literature. *J Antimicrob Chemother* 2021;76(12):3091-3102.

    This review of the literature describing the mechanisms of *S aureus* to invade and persist in osteoblasts covers intracellular pharmacokinetics, antibiotic activity, and outcomes of treatment.

40. Ellington JK, Harris M, Webb L, et al: Intracellular Staphylococcus aureus. A mechanism for the indolence of osteomyelitis. *J Bone Joint Surg Br* 2003;85(6):918-921.

41. Hudson MC, Ramp WK, Nicholson NC, Williams AS, Nousiainen MT: Internalization of Staphylococcus aureus by cultured osteoblasts. *Microb Pathog* 1995;19(6):409-419.

42. Flannagan RS, Heit B, Heinrichs DE: Intracellular replication of Staphylococcus aureus in mature phagolysosomes in macrophages precedes host cell death, and bacterial escape and dissemination. *Cell Microbiol* 2016;18(4):514-535.

43. Dupieux C, Trouillet-Assant S, Camus C, et al: Intraosteoblastic activity of daptomycin in combination with oxacillin and ceftaroline against MSSA and MRSA. *J Antimicrob Chemother* 2017;72(12):3353-3356.

CHAPTER 8

Microbiology of Musculoskeletal Infections

MICHAEL W. HENRY, MD • ANDY O. MILLER, MD

ABSTRACT

The bacterial and fungal organisms that cause orthopaedic infection—aerobes and anaerobes, yeasts and molds, mycobacteria and spirochetes—cause a diverse set of diseases with varying diagnostic and therapeutic targets. Obtaining proper diagnostic specimens in rational ways, and analyzing those specimens appropriately by culture, serologic analysis, or one of a set of newer molecular methods, are critical for accurate diagnosis and treatment. Although *Staphylococcus aureus* remains the most common of the orthopaedic pathogens, other families of pathogens are important to consider in different sets of clinical scenarios.

Keywords: bacteriological techniques; microbiology; osteomyelitis; prosthetic joint infection; *Staphylococcus*

INTRODUCTION

Musculoskeletal infections are caused by a diverse array of organisms. Traditional culture techniques remain the mainstay of pathogen detection, although advanced molecular technologies are emerging. Culture yields are decreased in biofilm-based infections and when pathogens grow with difficulty (fastidiously) in laboratory conditions. Molecular pathogen detection, particularly next-generation sequencing (NGS), shows promise in overcoming these shortcomings. However, culture-based wet-bench microbiology remains the backbone of diagnosis of musculoskeletal infections.

CONSIDERATIONS FROM THE MICROBIOLOGY LABORATORY

Culture-Based Methods

The accuracy of traditional culture techniques is dependent on specimen quality. The Infectious Disease Society of America and American Society for Microbiology established guidelines in 2018 for tissue acquisition and processing for microbiologic workup, including for bone and joint infections.[1] Regardless of the site cultured, the use of swabs is strongly discouraged because of low sample volume, entrapment and adsorption of organisms, and acquisition of extraneous organisms by swab fibers.[2,3] Instead, appropriate bone, synovium, disk, or necrotic tissue should be submitted to the laboratory in sterile containers; fluid should be obtained via aspiration. Cultures should be obtained before the start of antibiotics whenever possible. Multiple studies demonstrate the poor correlation between cultures taken from superficial sites, such as sinus tracts and open wounds, and corresponding deeper bony sites.[4]

The Gram stain is a traditional first step in the detection of bacterial pathogens and plays a limited role in orthopaedic infections. The yield is generally quite low, unless the submitted specimen is truly purulent; submission of multiple nonpurulent tissue samples for Gram stain,[5] acid-fast bacteria stain, and fungal stain generally are of very low clinical yield and unnecessarily burden the microbiology laboratory.[6]

After a specimen arrives at the microbiology laboratory, it is typically inoculated into solid and liquid media and incubated aerobically and anaerobically; separate media for fungi and mycobacteria are used, if indicated. Liquid media enhance detection of smaller populations

---

Neither of the following authors nor any immediate family member has received anything of value from or has stock or stock options held in a commercial company or institution related directly or indirectly to the subject of this chapter: Dr. Henry and Dr. Miller.

of organisms than do solid media, and provide a better environment for the isolation of anaerobes, but may have decreased specificity (more contaminants). Once growth is detected, the organism can be identified and antimicrobial sensitivities described. The duration of incubation is set to improve the chances of detecting a slower-growing pathogen while avoiding the detection of contaminants. For tissue cultures, including bone and joint specimens, most laboratory studies, both academic and commercial, generally incubate specimens for 2 to 5 days. When anaerobic orthopaedic infection is a concern, extended anaerobic cultures incubated for up to 2 weeks can improve the detection of *Cutibacterium acnes* and other slow-growing organisms.[3] Direct inoculation of tissue and synovial fluid into blood culture bottles has been shown to improve yield.[7,8]

Limitations of Culture-Based Methods

Although most musculoskeletal infectious pathogens can be readily identified with routine culture methods, there are important exceptions. Prolonged incubation periods and/or special media are required to isolate *C acnes* and *Brucella*, as well as many mycobacteria and fungi. Special handling and enriched media containing specific nutrients are required to identify specific organisms. An important example, *Neisseria gonorrhoeae*, grows preferentially on Thayer-Martin agar. To maximize culture yield, the specimen must be immediately inoculated onto the media and quickly transferred to an anaerobic, CO_2-rich environment of 35° to 37°C. Although most mycobacteria and fungi encountered in the setting of orthopaedic-related infections can be isolated using standardized protocols regarding media and duration period for incubation, there are some important exceptions. For example, although most mycobacterium grow optimally at 35° to 37°C, some grow better outside of this range; *Mycobacterium marinum* grows best at 30°C and *Mycobacterium xenopi* at 42°C. Although most microbiology laboratories will routinely incubate all mycobacterial cultures at appropriate temperature settings, clear communication with the laboratory is critical to ensure that the submitted specimens are being correctly processed. Communication with the laboratory is also critical when laboratory-transmissible pathogens, such as *Mycobacterium tuberculosis*, *Brucella*, and *Francisella tularensis* (the causative agent of tularemia), are being considered in the differential diagnosis because they can present serious threats to laboratory personnel.

Biofilms, Orthopaedic Infections, and the Microbiology Laboratory

Infections involving orthopaedic hardware present a special challenge to standard microbiologic investigation. In 2018, it was reported that 10% to 25% of prosthetic joint infections (PJIs) are reported as culture negative.[9] Refinement of traditional microbiologic testing over the decades, including optimization of specimen acquisition techniques, specimen number, biofilm culture methods, incubation techniques, improvements in culture media, and duration of incubation, has helped to improve accuracy.

Multiple prospective studies highlight the importance of obtaining multiple cultures in the setting of PJIs. A prospective trial used mathematical modeling to determine the optimal number of specimens to be five to six to maximize sensitivity and specificity, with the presence of three or more positive cultures to strongly correlate with infection.[10] With further advances in laboratory methodologies, including blood culture bottles for incubating synovial fluid specimens, longer duration of incubation, and automated laboratory systems, several studies suggest that three specimens may be the optimal amount.[7,11] Routinely ordering fungal and acid-fast bacterial cultures in routine cases is likely not warranted.[6]

Cultures should be collected when infection is being considered as a diagnosis. Specimens should routinely be sent for the detection of aerobic and anaerobic bacterial flora. Routine fungal and mycobacterial cultures can be sent when these diagnoses are being considered. In many cases, swab specimens are less likely to have positive results, and should be avoided in favor of whole-tissue or fluid specimens. Much attention has been placed on the ideal number of specimens to submit for particular disease states: sending a single culture is generally suboptimal (decreased sensitivity and specificity), but excess cultures place a burden on payers and on the microbiology laboratory. Research suggests that four to six cultures is a reasonable number for many orthopaedic infections. Negative cultures do not always mean that infection is absent, and alternative explanations include noncultivable (fastidious) microbes, recent or ongoing use of antimicrobials, and suboptimal specimen collection technique.

Biofilms can hinder microbiologic diagnosis via standard laboratory techniques. As traditional laboratory methods are optimized to grow free-living (planktonic) microbes, biofilm-bound microorganisms often grow poorly in culture. Simply scraping infected hardware has been shown to be ineffective to culture biofilms.[12] Numerous methods to disrupt biofilm have been explored, including chemical and mechanical methods of disruption, but the best-studied technique is sonication, as reported in 2020.[13] The explanted orthopaedic device of interest is transferred to a large container of sterile diluent, vortexed, and subsequently placed into an ultrasound bath. The sonicate fluid can then be cultured using traditional techniques. Inconsistent results have been reported, possibly because of variations in sonication technique, variations in subsequent culturing technique, colony-count thresholds, and application of molecular diagnostics to aid in identification of the microorganism. However, a growing body of literature including clinical guidelines increasingly supports the accuracy of sonication.[14] As reported in 2020, the role of sonication may have potential in other orthopaedic settings, including fracture-related infections[15] and spinal hardware infections,[16] but data to support its routine use are limited. Some literature has found sonication to not be of value when compared with routine intraoperative culture.[17]

Molecular Pathogen Detection in Orthopaedic Infections

Molecular diagnostics may bypass some of the limitations of traditional culture techniques. Molecular techniques, including targeted single and multiplex polymerase chain reaction (PCR), and next-generation shotgun sequencing of clinical isolates and of cell-free circulating DNA, may detect pathogens rapidly, accurately, and at decreased cost. In some cases, molecular microbiologic diagnostics have clearly led to improved diagnostics of musculoskeletal infections. In a 2020 study, the recognition of *Kingella kingae*, a fastidious gram-negative coccobacillus, as a dominant cause of osteoarticular infections in young children, was greatly aided by the use of PCR.[18] Similarly, it was reported in 2018 that the diagnosis of arthritis due to Lyme and Whipple diseases is aided by PCR testing.[19] In 2022, it was reported that NGS methods have shown promise in improving the microbiologic yield from surgical specimens, or even of circulating cell-free DNA in blood samples.[20,21] NGS is a collective term referring to a series of technologic advances that allow automated, massively paralleled, high-throughput sequencing to be performed, enabling the microbiology laboratory to simultaneously characterize millions of individual DNA fragments (or cDNA fragments from RNA) in a short period. These techniques can accomplish in a matter of hours to days what previously took large teams of laboratory technicians using more traditional methods years and sometimes decades to achieve.

The two NGS methods subject to the most evaluation in the setting of orthopaedic-related infections are 16S rRNA gene amplicon–targeted sequencing and shotgun metagenomics sequencing. Shotgun metagenomics sequencing refers to the process of sequencing all nucleic acids present in a given sample; the sample may contain mixed populations of microorganisms as well as human nucleic acid. The various microbial genomes are then recompiled and identified via software-driven analysis using comparisons with vast nucleic acid sequence databases. Amplicon-targeted sequencing limits the analysis to only the specific portions of DNA (such as the 16S rRNA region) that are amplified via PCR. This limits the analysis to a prespecified region of nucleic acid for which known PCR primers are available. The largest strength of shotgun metagenomics sequencing is that by sequencing all nucleic acid present, no prior knowledge of the infecting organism is required. It allows for an unbiased hypothesis-free approach to microbe detection, which in turn can facilitate the detection of novel organisms.[20-22] However, these advanced techniques have yet to gain common usage: issues of specificity, cost and access, turnaround time, and inability to assess comprehensive antimicrobial sensitivities remain important challenges to overcome.

IMPORTANT ORTHOPAEDIC PATHOGENS

Bacteria

Aerobic Gram-Positive Bacteria

Staphylococcus aureus

Among the pantheon of microorganisms causing musculoskeletal infection, *Staphylococcus aureus* predominates. Having coevolved with humans for millions of years, *S aureus* is persistent in the anterior nasal cavity of approximately 20% of humans; another 60% experiences intermittent colonization of the nasal mucosa, pharynx, and skin.[23] Carriage of *S aureus* increases the risk of surgical infections, and topical decolonization may be an effective tool to decrease the rate of orthopaedic surgical site infections. *S aureus* is able to adhere to nasal epithelium and extracellular matrix, to invade host cells and tissues, to modify and evade multiple arms of the human immune response, and to form and adhere to biofilm, using a wide variety of sticky surface molecules—many belonging to a family known as microbial surface components recognizing adhesive matrix molecules.[24,25] The ubiquity and pathogenicity of this complex microbe make it the most common pathogen in many orthopaedic clinical scenarios, including native bone and large joint infections in adolescents and adults, postoperative superficial and deep wound infections, and infections of orthopaedic hardware, including spinal and lower extremity PJIs.

Within 1 year of the introduction of antistaphylococcal beta-lactam antibiotics (or perhaps even before[26]), *S aureus* strains resistant to these agents emerged. A 2019 study reported that these resistant strains (collectively termed methicillin-resistant *S aureus*) thrived within and beyond the confines of healthcare, especially among certain at-risk populations, including the elderly, military, and those in underserved urban areas.[27] Methicillin-resistant *S aureus* differs from its methicillin-susceptible counterpart (methicillin-susceptible *S aureus*) in susceptibility to beta-lactam antibiotics but often harbors additional virulence factors, which may increase its pathogenicity. Accurate discernment of antimicrobial susceptibility in the microbiology laboratory is required to adequately treat these infections.

S aureus and other staphylococci have evolved mechanisms to persist in bone and on foreign materials. Biofilms allow bacteria to live in mechanically protected, immune-evading layers and even in free-floating clumps.[28] Persister cells, genotypically identical to their metabolically active counterparts, evade antibiotic action. Small colony variant staphylococci are genetically distinct mutants, which have lower pathogenicity but can persist intracellularly, and can exist in mixed population with wild-type counterparts.[29] These microbes have been noted to reside in bone canaliculi and osteocytes, encumbering cellular response to infection.[30,31]

There is substantial diversity to the clinical presentations of *S aureus* in orthopaedics. Infections can present acutely with sepsis and bacteremia or with mild, chronic symptoms. It is important to consider the potential of *S aureus* bacteremia as both a consequence and cause of orthopaedic infection; in some cohorts, the risk of subsequent PJI among patients with *S aureus* community-acquired bacteremia exceeds 35%.[32]

Coagulase-Negative Staphylococci

In the laboratory, *S aureus* is distinguished from most other staphylococcal species by the presence of coagulase, which can be readily detected with a simple biochemical test. In 2018, it was reported that coagulase-negative staphylococci (CoNS) are the most prevalent aerobic bacteria colonizing the skin surface.[33] Within this diverse group, *Staphylococcus epidermidis* is most prevalent, and *Staphylococcus lugdunensis* has been associated with somewhat more severe infections. In comparison with *S aureus*, these organisms, adapted to growth under hard skin surface conditions (exposure to sunlight, large variations in temperature and humidity, and the constant epithelial turnover and mechanical forces of life on human skin), generally do not cause sepsis but can survive durably in persistent biofilms. Although bacteremia and sepsis are rare with these bacteria, they are leading causes of orthopaedic device–related infections.

Streptococci and Enterococci

Streptococcal classification is complex, and only some of the species are classified by Lancefield grouping. Group A streptococcus (the cause of most strep throat), as well as groups C and G, generally causes acute orthopaedic wound infections, but bone and joint infections are uncommon. Group B streptococcus orthopaedic infections often mimic *S aureus* infections clinically. Other diverse streptococci (often grouped under the broad term viridans group streptococci), typically not characterized by a Lancefield group, are often normal denizens of the oral and gastrointestinal tracts, but can spread hematogenously to prostheses, vertebrae, and heart valves. Deep-seated infections with such organisms should prompt consideration of a source, which can include dentogingival disease (*Streptococcus mitis*) and gastrointestinal malignancy (*Streptococcus bovis*).

Enterococci, also native to the human gastrointestinal tract, cause orthopaedic wound and device infections, often as part of polymicrobial infections. They can be difficult to effectively treat, but in the setting of these orthopaedic-related infections, enterococci are rare causes of systemic sepsis. Treatment is highly dependent on susceptibility profile: they can be highly susceptible (penicillin-susceptible *Enterococcus faecalis*) or not (vancomycin-resistant *Enterococcus faecium*).

Aerobic Gram-Negative Bacteria

A key difference between gram-positive and gram-negative organisms is the production of endotoxin (lipopolysaccharides). Endotoxin elicits profound inflammatory responses in humans with gram-negative infections, which promote sepsis and shock (*S aureus*, lacking endotoxin, induces sepsis via different routes such as lipoteichoic acid).[34] Fundamental differences in the presence and form of the bacterial cell wall make some cell wall–active antibiotics such as vancomycin and daptomycin useless in gram-negative infection.

Many gram-negative organisms are encountered in orthopaedic infections. A growing health care concern worldwide is the development of extremely resistant strains that result in limited or no antimicrobial options. *Pseudomonas aeruginosa*, a common colonizer of open wounds, often causes osteomyelitis after penetrating trauma, or a podiatric complication of diabetes and vascular disease. A diversity of enteric gram-negative species such as *Escherichia*, *Klebsiella*, *Enterobacter*, *Morganella*, and others similarly can infect open wounds, often as part of mixed infections. Proper therapy is guided by resistance testing in the microbiology laboratory.

Pasteurella multocida is found in the oral cavity of healthy cats (and dogs) and is a frequent cause of deep infections after animal bites.[35] *Vibrio* and *Aeromonas* can cause severe infections after aqueous trauma.[36] As noted in 2021, *K kingae* is a major cause of bone and joint infections in children aged 6 to 48 months.[37]

Anaerobic Bacteria

As noted earlier, anaerobic organisms often grow slowly and under fastidious conditions and are difficult to isolate without dedicated culture techniques. *C acnes* is the only one found with great frequency. In 2021, it was reported that *C acnes* grows well using standard culture methods for anaerobes but often takes more than 6 days (and in some cases, upward of 14 days) to be isolated.[38] Although some microbiology laboratories may routinely hold all anaerobic cultures for 14 days, most do not. When a *C acnes* infection is suspected, it is crucial to provide the microbiology laboratory with specific instructions regarding incubation time. It is important, therefore, for the surgeon to recognize at the time of specimen acquisition when a *C acnes* infection may be present. *C acnes* orthopaedic hardware infections often present in a very indolent manner, typically with minimal signs or symptoms of inflammation. *C acnes* infections can also present with failed orthopaedic hardware in the absence of any clinical evidence of infection. *C acnes* orthopaedic hardware infections are most frequently encountered in the shoulder and spine but can cause infection of orthopaedic hardware regardless of location. Because *C acnes* is part of the skin flora, it is also a commonly encountered contaminant recovered from orthopaedic intraoperative cultures. It is therefore important to obtain multiple cultures from the surgical site, as it can help to determine if *C acnes* is present as a contaminant or as a pathogen. Because of its high concentration within the normal flora of the epidermis and dermis, the use of molecular diagnostics for *C acnes* is greatly limited. The ability of these techniques to detect even trace amounts of bacterial DNA leads to a very high rate of detection of *C acnes*, even in the absence of infection. *C acnes* is an extremely rare cause of bone or joint infection in the absence of foreign hardware or other material. Positive cultures for *C acnes* in this situation should be met with a high amount of skepticism.

Other important anaerobes include the *Peptostreptococcus*, a genus of anaerobic bacteria generally found in the mouth and gastrointestinal tract that hematogenously seed prosthetic joints and cause vertebral discitis/osteomyelitis. Clostridial species, such as *Clostridium perfringens* and even *Clostridium difficile*, are rare causes of often severe or fatal infections of orthopaedic structures.

Fungi

In immunocompetent hosts, fungal orthopaedic infections are uncommon. Species of the genus *Candida* can cause PJI, usually in the setting of elderly hosts, impaired wound healing, and complications of prior infections. The endemic dimorphic fungi (*Histoplasma, Coccidioides, Paracoccidioides, Blastomyces*, and others) are occasional causes of osteomyelitis and septic arthritis after environmental exposure in specific geographic regions, but with increasing domestic and international travel, patients with infection may present at great geographic distances from their inoculation event.

With increasing degrees of immunocompromise, particularly including the extreme immunodeficiencies of malignancy and bone marrow transplantation, the risk of invasive fungal orthopaedic infections increases. *Aspergillus* and *Candida* cause most of such infections, and prognosis is often dependent not only on source control and antifungal therapy but also on immune recovery.[39-42]

Mycobacteria

Mycobacterium tuberculosis causes vertebral discitis/osteomyelitis (Pott disease) in the underdeveloped world, but tuberculous orthopaedic infections are quite rare among people born in low-incidence nations. Bacillus Calmette-Guérin and *Mycobacterium bovis* strains used both as a childhood tuberculosis vaccine in some countries and as intravesical immunotherapy for bladder cancer can occasionally metastasize to cause septic arthritis and osteomyelitis. Nontuberculous mycobacteria, or atypical mycobacteria, are a diverse set of species. Some clinically relevant members of this group include *Mycobacteroides chelonae, Mycobacterium fortuitum*, and *Mycobacteroides abscessus*. *M marinum* causes a distinct syndrome of granulomatous infections of the hands and feet (including bone, joints, tendon, and soft tissues) in patients with exposure to marine environments, fish, and aquaria.

PATHOGENESIS AND MICROBIOLOGIC DIAGNOSIS

Orthopaedic infections can be divided into infections associated with native tissues (**Table 1**) and those that are associated with implanted orthopaedic devices (**Table 2**). These infections generally derive from one of the three routes: direct inoculation of a pathogen into an orthopaedic structure, extension (contiguity) of a nearby infection, and hematogenous spread. Hematogenous spread is common for some microbes (*S aureus*, viridans group streptococci) and distinctly rare for others (*C acnes, S epidermidis*); in patients with hematogenous infections, consideration must be given to concurrent bacterial endocarditis and other sites of metastatic infection.

Native Infections

Osteomyelitis

Osteomyelitis, or infection of bone, is usually caused by bacteria, very rarely by fungi, and never by viruses. Many clinical scenarios, from penetrating foot trauma to dental infection, lead to osteomyelitis; dozens of microbes have been reported as the cause, but *S aureus* remains most prevalent in most patient groups and is the most studied. However, microbiology varies significantly depending on patient characteristics and

Table 1

Major Pathogens That Infect Native Orthopaedic Tissues[a]

Syndrome	Common	Less Common
Joint Infections		
Native septic arthritis, pediatric	*Staphylococcus aureus* Streptococci *Kingella kingae*	*Borrelia burgdorferi* *Neisseria meningitidis* *Neisseria gonorrhoeae* (adolescent) *Haemophilus influenzae* *Salmonella* *Mycobacterium tuberculosis*
Native septic arthritis, adult	*S aureus* Gram-negative rods Streptococci *N gonorrhoeae* *B burgdorferi*	Oropharyngeal bacteria *Mycoplasma* *Ureaplasma* *Pasteurella multocida* (animal bites) Fungi
Bone Infections		
Acute osteomyelitis, hematogenous, pediatric	*S aureus* Streptococci *K kingae*	*N meningitidis* *Salmonella* *M tuberculosis* *H influenzae*
Acute osteomyelitis, hematogenous, adult	*S aureus* Gram-negative rods Streptococci	Oropharyngeal bacteria *P multocida* (animal bites) *Bartonella* *M tuberculosis* Fungi
Vertebral discitis/osteomyelitis	*S aureus* Gram-negative rods Streptococci *M tuberculosis*	*Corynebacterium* species Gram-negative rods *Candida* Nontuberculous mycobacteria
Other Orthopaedic Infections		
Tenosynovitis (typically of the hand or foot)	Staphylococci Streptococci *Pasteurella* (animal bite) *Mycobacterium marinum* (marine exposure)	*N gonorrhoeae* *Mycoplasma* *Sporothrix schenckii* *Eikenella* (human bite)
Pyomyositis	*S aureus*	Streptococci *Escherichia coli* Mycobacteria

[a] Only the most common pathogens are listed; many hundreds of pathogens have been reported to cause infection of bone, joint, and other native orthopaedic tissue.

---

the mode of infection (hematogenous, contiguous/adjacent, and direct inoculation). In the pediatric population, particularly in those younger than 5 years, hematogenous osteomyelitis is most common and beta-hemolytic streptococci, such as group A and B *Streptococcus*, and *K kingae*, are frequent. Pediatric hematogenous osteomyelitis preferentially infects more vascularized metaphyseal structures of the long bones.

The axial skeleton is proportionally overrepresented in adult hematogenous osteomyelitis.

A specific, extremely common form of osteomyelitis occurs in the (typically neuropathic) feet of patients with advanced diabetes mellitus. Combinations of microvascular disease, neuropathic injury, and immune dysfunction lead to breakdown of soft-tissue structures, allowing for contiguous infection of bone. These infections can

Table 2

Major Pathogens Associated With Device-Related Orthopaedic Infections[a]

Syndrome	Common	Less Common
Prosthetic joint infection	*Staphylococcus aureus* CoNS Group B *Streptococcus* Enteric gram-negative rods *Pseudomonas aeruginosa* *Cutibacterium acnes* (shoulder)	Oral streptococci Oral gram-positive anaerobes *Candida* *Corynebacterium* Nontuberculous mycobacteria
Spinal hardware infection	*S aureus* CoNS Enteric gram-negative rods *C acnes*	*Candida*
Fracture-related hardware infection	Staphylococci Streptococci Gram-negative rods *C acnes* (clavicle and upper extremity)	*Candida* and environmental fungi Mycobacteria
Infections associated with sutures, anchors, and grafts	*S aureus* CoNS Streptococci *C acnes* (shoulder)	Gram-negative rods

CoNS = coagulase-negative staphylococci
[a] Only the most common pathogens are listed; many hundreds of pathogens have been reported to cause infections of orthopaedic hardware.

be polymicrobial, but often involve *S aureus* in bone with polymicrobial communities in the overlying infected ulcer. Multidisciplinary approaches to treatment are required with judicious use of antibiotics, adequate surgical débridement, offloading of the affected area, and aggressive management of the underlying endocrine disorder.

In adults, hematogenous osteomyelitis often seeds the spine. The usual initial infective site in hematogenous vertebral osteomyelitis is the anterior vertebral body, which has the largest vascular supply. The anterior vertebral arteries bifurcate and supply two adjacent vertebrae, and the infection often involves two adjacent vertebral bodies because of the bifurcation. The disk becomes infected secondarily by the spread from the vertebral end plate. As noted in a 2021 study, blood cultures should be sent before biopsy when possible because they can elucidate a pathogen in approximately 50% of cases.[43] Iatrogenic osteomyelitis from percutaneous injections is an uncommon but serious complication that can require a high index of suspicion for diagnosis.

Septic Arthritis

Septic arthritis of native joints has analogous routes of entry and diversity of microbial offenders. As in osteomyelitis, *S aureus* remains the most prevalent pathogen among most patient groups. Important microbes to consider also include *N gonorrhoeae*, which can be difficult to grow in culture from the joint fluid, and the microbial diagnosis can be supported by molecular testing or culture from mucosal tissues of the urethra, vaginal cervix, pharynx, and rectum. Lyme arthritis, caused by the tick-borne spirochete *Borrelia burgdorferi*, is similarly not cultured in the clinical microbiology laboratory; serologic testing and synovial fluid PCR can be used.

Other Orthopaedic Infectious Syndromes

All other musculoskeletal structures are associated with distinct and diverse infectious syndromes. Infections of periarticular bursal spaces (in particular, of the knee and olecranon) are common, are usually caused by *S aureus*, and occasionally require débridement with bursectomy in addition to antibiotics. Limb-threatening infections of tendons (tenosynovitis) can be seen after trauma (such as animal bites), especially in patients with impaired immunity. In northern climates, infection of muscle (pyomyositis) is relatively uncommon, but it is an important consideration in some countries, and among immunocompromised and malnourished populations. Finally, as reported in 2022, necrotizing fasciitis is an important entity for the orthopaedic surgeon to recognize because these infections often progress much more quickly than anticipated and can be lethal.[44] Type I encompasses polymicrobial infections, largely because of gut anaerobes and *Enterobacteriaceae* and involving the abdominal wall and groin or the head and neck. Type II is usually monomicrobial, usually because of group A streptococci, and often involves the extremities. All forms require emergent, aggressive care.

Device-Related Infections
Prosthetic Joint Infections
Although PJI can be caused by diverse pathogens, most of these infections are the result of a small number of bacterial species. *S aureus* and CoNS together account for more than one-half of these infections, and *Streptococcus* spp. and *Enterococcus* spp. are found in approximately 10% of cases; microbiology varies based on the timing and route of infection.[45,46] In early postoperative infections, *S aureus* is the most frequently isolated species, found in 25% to 45% of PJIs, followed closely by CoNS.[45-48] Enterococci and gram-negative bacilli, including the *Enterobacteriaceae* and *P aeruginosa*, are also important causes of early-onset PJIs, each responsible for approximately 10% of cases. CoNS are the dominant cause of late-onset PJIs, found in 35% to 55% of cases that are not caused by late hematogenous spread.[45,47] *C acnes*, *Corynebacterium* spp., enterococci, and gram-negative bacilli together represent a significant percentage of delayed-onset infections that are not a result of CoNS. Acute-onset late infections are generally secondary to bacteremia with virulent organisms such as *S aureus* and streptococci.[49,50] Polymicrobial PJIs, 10% to 20% of all PJIs, generally present earlier than monomicrobial PJIs[47,51] and may represent up to 40% of all early-onset PJI.[48]

Less than 1% of all PJIs are secondary to fungi, with *Candida* species responsible for 80% of these cases. Fungal PJIs are most commonly a result of hematogenous seeding but can also be a result of direct inoculation or contiguous spread.[52] Mycobacteria, both *M tuberculosis* and nontuberculous mycobacteria, are also a well-documented but rare cause of PJIs.[46]

Although the literature describing the microbiology of PJIs is based almost entirely on hip and knee infections, studies of elbow and shoulder PJIs have reported comparable distributions of pathogens, except for the notable dominant role *C acnes* plays in shoulder PJI, particularly in subacute and chronic infections.[53,54]

Spinal Hardware and Infection After Fracture Fixation
Studies describing the microbiology of other types of orthopaedic hardware infections are also limited in scope and quality. Spinal hardware infections are most often the results of inoculation at the time of surgery or contiguous spread via an overlying wound infection.

More than one-half of early-onset infections are a result of staphylococci and gram-negative rods. CoNS and *C acnes* are common causes of late-onset spinal hardware infections.[55,56]

Infections after fracture fixation also develop as a result of inoculation at the time of instrumentation or as a result of overlying wound infection.[57,58] In the setting of an open fracture, the hardware can be infected by organisms introduced at the time of trauma. Staphylococci, *P aeruginosa*, and the enteric gram-negative rods are the most commonly encountered organisms. Polymicrobial infections are encountered in up to 50% of cases of infections after fracture fixation.[59,60]

SUMMARY

The microbiologic diversity of orthopaedic infections is broad and constantly increasing. Although *S aureus* is common in most clinical scenarios, the need to consider a variety of other pathogens is essential—whether *M tuberculosis* in thoracic spinal tuberculosis, *C acnes* in shoulder surgery, or fungal diseases in the patient with advanced immunodeficiency. The orthopaedic surgeon's role in the diagnosis and treatment of these infections is critical: to recognize infection, to obtain and submit suitable laboratory samples, to débride and resect infected source tissue adequately, and to enable the patient to achieve an acceptable functional outcome. Therefore, a basic understanding of microbiology laboratory concepts and practice, of the major groupings of orthopaedic pathogens, and of the relationships between these groups and the clinical syndromes seen by orthopaedic surgeons is essential.

KEY STUDY POINTS

- Orthopaedic surgeons with a better understanding of microbiology and the microbiology laboratory will improve the diagnosis and treatment of patients with orthopaedic infections.
- The frequency of different bacterial and fungal pathogens can vary, depending on the situation faced by the orthopaedic surgeon, but *S aureus* is the predominant pathogen in many such syndromes.
- Obtaining diagnostic specimens properly and understanding the possibilities and limitations of the microbiology laboratory are important for the proper care of the patient with an infection.
- New methods, including molecular pathogen detection, have great potential, but cultures remain the cornerstone of accurate diagnosis, even in the setting of more modern methods.

ANNOTATED REFERENCES

1. Miller JM, Binnicker MJ, Campbell S, et al: A guide to utilization of the microbiology laboratory for diagnosis of infectious diseases: 2018 update by the Infectious Diseases Society of America and the American Society for Microbiology. *Clin Infect Dis* 2018;67(6):e1-e94.

   This set of guidelines from the Infectious Diseases Society of America provides detailed, evidence-based instruction for clinicians to submit blood and tissue for microbiologic analysis, including a subsection dedicated to bone and joint infection. The guidelines underscore the importance of close communication between the clinician and the microbiology laboratory.

2. Buchan BW, Ledeboer NA: Emerging technologies for the clinical microbiology laboratory. *Clin Microbiol Rev* 2014;27(4):783-822.

3. Ascione T, Barrack R, Benito N, et al: General assembly, diagnosis, pathogen isolation – Culture matters: Proceedings of international consensus on orthopedic infections. *J Arthroplasty* 2019;34(2 suppl):S197-S206.

   This report provides guidance for proper pathogen isolation when diagnosing and treating orthopaedic infections as part of the proceedings of the second International Consensus Meeting on orthopaedic infections in 2018. Key issues regarding appropriate specimen collection, including the optimal number of specimens to collect, the efficacy of superficial cultures from sinus tracts, and the interpretation, were also discussed.

4. Wilson ML, Winn W: Laboratory diagnosis of bone, joint, soft-tissue, and skin infections. *Clin Infect Dis* 2008;46(3):453-457.

5. Wouthuyzen-Bakker M, Shohat N, Sebillotte M, Arvieux C, Parvizi J, Soriano A: Is Gram staining still useful in prosthetic joint infections? *J Bone Jt Infect* 2019;4(2):56-59.

   In this retrospective single-center study of patients with late acute PJI, a positive preoperative Gram stain was associated with a higher C-reactive protein level and the presence of *S aureus*, but not with a difference in clinical outcome. Level of evidence: IV.

6. Tai DBG, Wengenack NL, Patel R, Berbari EF, Abdel MP, Tande AJ: Fungal and mycobacterial cultures should not be routinely obtained for diagnostic work-up of patients with suspected periprosthetic joint infections. *Bone Joint J* 2022;104-B(1):53-58.

   Compelling analysis of the value of routine acid-fast bacteria and fungal cultures in orthopaedics suggests that they add significant cost and increase the labor required in the laboratory, with negligible clinical benefit. Level of evidence: IV.

7. Peel TN, Sedarski JA, Dylla BL, et al: Laboratory workflow analysis of culture of periprosthetic tissues in blood culture bottles. *J Clin Microbiol* 2017;55(9):2817-2826.

8. Li C, Ojeda-Thies C, Trampuz A: Culture of periprosthetic tissue in blood culture bottles for diagnosing periprosthetic joint infection. *BMC Musculoskelet Disord* 2019;20(1):299.

   This meta-analysis of four studies, comprising 1,071 patients, assessed the diagnostic accuracy of tissue cultures in blood culture bottles in the setting of PJI and reported a pooled sensitivity of 70% and specificity of 97%. The authors noted that this analysis had several limitations, including lack of a gold standard for the diagnosis of PJI and lack of comparison with conventional culture techniques.

9. Tan TL, Kheir MM, Shohat N, et al: Culture-negative periprosthetic joint infection: An update on what to expect. *JB JS Open Access* 2018;3(3):e0060.

   This retrospective review reported a prevalence of suspected culture-negative PJI of 22%, with a poor rate of treatment success (55.6%). When suspected cases were limited to those meeting the Musculoskeletal Infection Society criteria, the culture-negative rate dropped to 6.4%. Level of evidence: IV.

10. Atkins BL, Athanasou N, Deeks JJ, et al: Prospective evaluation of criteria for microbiological diagnosis of prosthetic-joint infection at revision arthroplasty. The OSIRIS Collaborative Study Group. *J Clin Microbiol* 1998;36(10):2932-2939.

11. Bémer P, Léger J, Tandé D, et al: How many samples and how many culture media to diagnose a prosthetic joint infection: A clinical and microbiological prospective multicenter study. *J Clin Microbiol* 2016;54(2):385-391.

12. Bjerkan G, Witsø E, Bergh K: Sonication is superior to scraping for retrieval of bacteria in biofilm on titanium and steel surfaces in vitro. *Acta Orthop* 2009;80(2):245-250.

13. Karbysheva S, Di Luca M, Butini ME, Winkler T, Schütz M, Trampuz A: Comparison of sonication with chemical biofilm dislodgement methods using chelating and reducing agents: Implications for the microbiological diagnosis of implant associated infection. *PLoS One* 2020;15(4):e0231389.

    Using an in vitro model, the investigators compared several methods to improve microbiologic diagnosis by disrupting the biofilm. Sonication was found to be superior to two different methods of chemical dislodgement: the chelation with ethylenediaminetetraacetic acid and the reduction of disulfide bonds and protein denaturation with dithiothreitol.

14. Abdel M, Akgün D, Akin G, et al: Hip and knee section, diagnosis, pathogen isolation, culture: Proceedings of international consensus on orthopedic infections. *J Arthroplasty* 2019;34(2 suppl):S361-S367.

    This document on the proceedings of the second International Consensus Meeting on orthopaedic infections in 2018 provides specific guidance for the diagnoses and treatment of hip and knee orthopaedic infections.

15. Govaert GAM, Kuehl R, Atkins BL, et al: Diagnosing fracture-related infection: Current concepts and recommendations. *J Orthop Trauma* 2020;34(1):8-17.

    This is detailed review of the medical literature underpinning the proposed diagnostic criteria for fracture-related infections was issued in a joint consensus document in 2018 by the AO Foundation and the European Bone and Joint Infection Society. Recommendations for microbiologic specimen acquisition and laboratory methodology are also discussed.

16. Carlson BC, Hines JT, Robinson WA, et al: Implant sonication versus tissue culture for the diagnosis of spinal implant infection. *Spine* 2020;45(9):E525-E532.

    This retrospective review of 152 patients (the largest to date) found that sonicate fluid cultures were as sensitive and specific as conventional peri-implant tissue cultures. The authors recommended the use of 20 colony-forming unites per 10 mL as the optimal threshold for diagnosis via sonicate fluid cultures. Level of evidence: IV.

17. Grosso MJ, Frangiamore SJ, Yakubek G, Bauer TW, Iannotti JP, Ricchetti ET: Performance of implant sonication culture for the diagnosis of periprosthetic shoulder infection. *J Shoulder Elbow Surg* 2018;27(2):211-216.

    This retrospective cohort study is one of the few in the literature to assess the role of implant sonication cultures in the diagnosis of shoulder prosthetic joint infection. No benefit over standard culture technique was found. Level of evidence: IV.

18. Wong M, Williams N, Cooper C: Systematic review of Kingella kingae musculoskeletal infection in children: Epidemiology, impact and management strategies. *Pediatric Health Med Ther* 2020;11:73-84.

    K kingae is an important cause of joint, bone, and tendon infection in the pediatric population and is the leading cause of septic arthritis in healthy children younger than 4 years. Clinical presentation can be subacute, necessitating a high index of suspicion in some cases.

19. Lagier JC, Raoult D: Whipple's disease and Tropheryma whipplei infections: When to suspect them and how to diagnose and treat them. *Curr Opin Infect Dis* 2018;31(6):463-470.

    Tropheryma whipplei can cause chronic localized infection in a wide array of organs, including both native and prosthetic joints. Diagnosis often depends on the use of 16S rRNA PCR.

20. Goswami K, Clarkson S, Phillips CD, et al: An enhanced understanding of culture-negative periprosthetic joint infection with next-generation sequencing: A multicenter study. *J Bone Joint Surg Am* 2022;104(17):1523-1529.

    In contrast to other studies of molecular pathogen detection, this study found that bacterial DNA was present in 66% of culture-negative infections, which may indicate a role for molecular pathogen detection in the diagnosis of PJI. Level of evidence: II.

21. Echeverria AP, Cohn IS, Danko DC, et al: Sequencing of circulating microbial cell-free DNA can identify pathogens in periprosthetic joint infections. *J Bone Joint Surg Am* 2021;103(18):1705-1712.

    Remnants of bacterial genomes, circulating from the site of PJI, can be detected in some patients with PJI. This technique quickly and noninvasively aided traditional diagnosis in this study of 53 patients, finding an organism in 87% of patients. Level of evidence: II.

22. Hong HL, Flurin L, Thoendel MJ, et al: Targeted versus shotgun metagenomic sequencing-based detection of microorganisms in sonicate fluid for periprosthetic joint infection diagnosis. *Clin Infect Dis* 2023;76(3):e1456-e1462.

    This study compared the more complex and costly shotgun sequencing with targeted sequencing and found that results did not differ significantly. Level of evidence: IV.

23. Kluytmans J, van Belkum A, Verbrugh H: Nasal carriage of Staphylococcus aureus: Epidemiology, underlying mechanisms, and associated risks. *Clin Microbiol Rev* 1997;10(3):505-520.

24. Foster TJ, Geoghegan JA, Ganesh VK, Höök M: Adhesion, invasion and evasion: The many functions of the surface proteins of Staphylococcus aureus. *Nat Rev Microbiol* 2014;12(1):49-62.

25. Kobayashi SD, Malachowa N, DeLeo FR: Pathogenesis of Staphylococcus aureus abscesses. *Am J Pathol* 2015;185(6):1518-1527.

26. Harkins CP, Pichon B, Doumith M, et al: Methicillin-resistant Staphylococcus aureus emerged long before the introduction of methicillin into clinical practice. *Genome Biol* 2017;18(1):130.

27. Turner NA, Sharma-Kuinkel BK, Maskarinec SA, et al: Methicillin-resistant Staphylococcus aureus: An overview of basic and clinical research. *Nat Rev Microbiol* 2019;17(4):203-218.

    This is a comprehensive review of current research on methicillin resistant *S aureus*, including the clinical presentation and management of MRSA bacteremia, endocarditis, osteomyelitis, pneumonia, prosthetic joint infections and skin and soft tissue infections. The authors highlighted the versatile and unpredictable nature of this organism, and the need to better understand the host-pathogen relationship, as well as the role genomics can play in improving our understanding of the epidemiology of MRSA and in improving our approach to treatment.

28. Roilides E, Simitsopoulou M, Katragkou A, Walsh TJ: How biofilms evade host defenses. *Microbiol Spectr* 2015;3(3).

29. Kahl BC, Becker K, Löffler B: Clinical significance and pathogenesis of staphylococcal small colony variants in persistent infections. *Clin Microbiol Rev* 2016;29(2):401-427.

30. de Mesy Bentley KL, Trombetta R, Nishitani K, et al: Evidence of staphylococcus aureus deformation, proliferation, and migration in canaliculi of live cortical bone in murine models of osteomyelitis. *J Bone Miner Res* 2017;32(5):985-990.

31. Garcia-Moreno M, Jordan PM, Günther K, et al: Osteocytes serve as a reservoir for intracellular persisting Staphylococcus aureus due to the lack of defense mechanisms. *Front Microbiol* 2022;13:937466.

    This cell culture studies was designed to better elucidate the mechanism by which *S aureus* can enter and remain viable within osteocytes, focusing on the role of the innate immune system. The authors found that unlike osteoblasts, osteocytes were unable to increase expression of Toll-like receptor (TLR) 2, which is the main TLR that detects the presence of *S aureus*. In addition, osteocytes where found to have a low level of expression of antimicrobial peptide, further impairing the osteocytes' host response to infection by *S aureus*. The ability for *S aureus* to persist within osteocytes contributes to the often refractory nature of *S aureus* bone infection despite optimal treatment.

32. Tande AJ, Palraj BR, Osmon DR, et al: Clinical presentation, risk factors, and outcomes of hematogenous prosthetic joint infection in patients with Staphylococcus aureus bacteremia. *Am J Med* 2016;129(2):221.e11-e20.

33. Byrd AL, Belkaid Y, Segre JA: The human skin microbiome. *Nat Rev Microbiol* 2018;16(3):143-155.

    This is an extensive and detailed review of our current understanding of the human skin microbiome, with specific focus on role of next-generation sequencing techniques have played in developing a better understanding the diversity of commensal microorganisms. The authors reviewed what is currently understood regarding the evolution of the skin microbiome in healthy hosts as well as alterations of the microbiome seen in specific disease state. In addition, the mechanisms of interactions both among the residing organism and between these organism and the host immune system was discussed.

34. Ramachandran G: Gram-positive and gram-negative bacterial toxins in sepsis: A brief review. *Virulence* 2014;5(1):213-218.

35. Wilson BA, Ho M: Pasteurella multocida: From zoonosis to cellular microbiology. *Clin Microbiol Rev* 2013;26(3):631-655.

36. Diaz JH, Lopez FA: Skin, soft tissue and systemic bacterial infections following aquatic injuries and exposures. *Am J Med Sci* 2015;349(3):269-275.

37. Yagupsky P: Review highlights the latest research in Kingella kingae and stresses that molecular tests are required for diagnosis. *Acta Paediatr* 2021;110(6):1750-1758.

    This review article reviewed the role of *Kingella kingae* as a cause of pediatric osteoarticular infections, highlighting recent advances in molecular diagnostic techniques. The authors concluded that *K kingae* is the leading cause of osteoarticular infections in children ages 6 to 48 months and strongly underscored the need for nucleic amplification techniques to establish the diagnosis.

38. Moore NF, Batten TJ, Hutton CE, White WJ, Smith CD: The management of the shoulder skin microbiome (Cutibacterium acnes) in the context of shoulder surgery: A review of the current literature. *Shoulder Elbow* 2021;13(6):592-599.

    This systematic review was designed to better understand the shoulder skin microbiome, but was ultimately limited to a review of the current knowledge and understanding of *C acnes*. Of the 813 articles identified, all but 25 were excluded; an additional 14 were identified using forward referencing. The authors found that all but 4 focused exclusively on *C acnes*. Outside of *C acnes* very little has been published regarding the microbiome of the shoulder skin.

39. Gamaletsou MN, Kontoyiannis DP, Sipsas NV, et al: Candida osteomyelitis: Analysis of 207 pediatric and adult cases (1970-2011). *Clin Infect Dis* 2012;55(10):1338-1351.

40. Rammaert B, Gamaletsou MN, Zeller V, et al: Dimorphic fungal osteoarticular infections. *Eur J Clin Microbiol Infect Dis* 2014;33(12):2131-2140.

41. Gamaletsou MN, Rammaert B, Bueno MA, et al: Aspergillus osteomyelitis: Epidemiology, clinical manifestations, management, and outcome. *J Infect* 2014;68(5):478-493.

42. Taj-Aldeen SJ, Rammaert B, Gamaletsou M, et al: Osteoarticular infections caused by non-Aspergillus filamentous fungi in adult and pediatric patients: A systematic review. *Medicine (Baltimore)* 2015;94(50):e2078.

43. Kim NJ: Microbiologic diagnosis of pyogenic spondylitis. *Infect Chemother* 2021;53(2):238-246.

    This is a review of the diagnostic considerations in discitis/osteomyelitis, including tuberculous infection.

44. Pelletier J, Gottlieb M, Long B, Perkins JC: Necrotizing soft tissue infections (NSTI): Pearls and pitfalls for the emergency clinician. *J Emerg Med* 2022;62(4):480-491.

    Necrotizing fasciitis and related infections can be catastrophic and easy to miss; prompt therapy is needed. This article reviews the presentation, diagnosis, and treatment of such infections, and although aimed at emergency medicine clinicians, it is also relevant to orthopaedic clinicians.

45. Benito N, Mur I, Ribera A, et al: The different microbial etiology of prosthetic joint infections according to route of acquisition and time after prosthesis implantation, including the role of multidrug-resistant organisms. *J Clin Med* 2019;8(5):673.

    Marked differences in microbiologic etiology were found when PJIs were stratified by the Tsukayama scheme, as well as when stratifying nonhematogenous PJIs by the time of infection onset following surgery. Multidrug-resistant organisms were three times more common in early postoperative infections than in late postoperative infection. There was also a decreasing linear trend of multidrug-resistant organisms and polymicrobial infections diagnosed in the setting of nonhematogenous PJIs as the time for surgery increased. Level of evidence: IV.

46. Tande AJ, Patel R: Prosthetic joint infection. *Clin Microbiol Rev* 2014;27(2):302-345.

47. Zeller V, Kerroumi Y, Meyssonnier V, et al: Analysis of postoperative and hematogenous prosthetic joint-infection microbiological patterns in a large cohort. *J Infect* 2018;76(4):328-334.

    Hematogenous PJIs were monomicrobial in 99% of cases. *S aureus* was the most commonly isolated bacteria, but streptococcal species, as a whole, were more commonly encountered than staphylococcal species. Fifteen percent of nonhematogenous postoperative infections were monomicrobial. Level of evidence: IV.

48. Manning L, Metcalf S, Clark B, et al: Clinical characteristics, etiology, and initial management strategy of newly diagnosed periprosthetic joint infection: A multicenter, prospective observational cohort study of 783 patients. *Open Forum Infect Dis* 2020;7(5):ofaa068.

    In this prospective cohort of 783 patients, late-onset acute infections were the most common presentation of PJIs, comprising approximately one-half of all patients. Early postoperative infections occurred in 25% of cases, and the remainder were chronic in nature. Level of evidence: II.

49. Rakow A, Perka C, Trampuz A, Renz N: Origin and characteristics of haematogenous periprosthetic joint infection. *Clin Microbiol Infect* 2019;25(7):845-850.

    The most common organisms were *S aureus*, streptococci, and enterococci. Blood cultures were positive in 61% of cases, and the primary source was identified in 68% of cases. An active search for the source of infection in all patients presenting with an acute hematogenous PJI was advocated for. Level of evidence: IV.

50. Renz N, Trampuz A, Perka C, Rakow A: Outcome and failure analysis of 132 episodes of hematogenous periprosthetic joint infections-A cohort study. *Open Forum Infect Dis* 2022;9(4):ofac094.

    Given the questions regarding the optimal surgical and medical management of hematogenous PJIs, this retrospective cohort evaluated the clinical outcomes of 132 consecutive cases. The treatment failure rate was 32%, which is consistent with other published studies. When stratified by surgical management, the failure rates were significantly lower in patients undergoing implant removal as compared to DAIR (32% versus 49%, $P = 0.033$). Level of evidence: IV.

51. Flurin L, Greenwood-Quaintance KE, Patel R: Microbiology of polymicrobial prosthetic joint infection. *Diagn Microbiol Infect Dis* 2019;94(3):255-259.

    Polymicrobial infections were more common in patients with underlying fractures and occurred closer in time to the index surgery than did monomicrobial PJIs. *S epidermidis* was the most prevalent organism overall and was more common in polymicrobial infections than monomicrobial infections. Level of evidence: IV.

52. Henry MW, Miller AO, Walsh TJ, Brause BD: Fungal musculoskeletal infections. *Infect Dis Clin North Am* 2017;31(2):353-368.

53. Paxton ES, Green A, Krueger VS: Periprosthetic infections of the shoulder: Diagnosis and management. *J Am Acad Orthop Surg* 2019;27(21):e935-e944.

    The most common causes of shoulder PJIs are *C acnes* and CoNS. Single-stage revision surgery has shown similar outcomes to two-stage revisions for these two organisms. *S aureus* and other virulent organisms are usually treated with two-stage revisions. The proper management of unexpected positive cultures for *C acnes* taken at the time of revision is still unclear and continues to be an area of investigation.

54. Achermann Y, Vogt M, Spormann C, et al: Characteristics and outcome of 27 elbow periprosthetic joint infections: Results from a 14-year cohort study of 358 elbow prostheses. *Clin Microbiol Infect* 2011;17(3):432-438.

55. de la Hera B, Sánchez-Mariscal F, Gómez-Rice A, Vázquez-Vecilla I, Zúñiga L, Ruano-Soriano E: Deep surgical-site infection following thoracolumbar instrumented spinal surgery: The experience of 25 years. *Int J Spine Surg* 2021;15(1):144-152.

    Deep surgical site infection following thoracolumbar instrumented surgery resulted in major complications and the need for additional surgeries in 14.3% of patients. *Staphylococcus* spp. and *Enterobacteriaceae* were the most commonly isolated bacteria in early infection cases. *C acnes* and CoNS were the most frequent causes of delayed and late infections. Level of evidence: IV.

56. Kasliwal MK, Tan LA, Traynelis VC: Infection with spinal instrumentation: Review of pathogenesis, diagnosis, prevention, and management. *Surg Neurol Int* 2013;4(suppl 5):S392-S403.

57. Zimmerli W: Clinical presentation and treatment of orthopaedic implant-associated infection. *J Intern Med* 2014;276(2):111-119.

58. Steinmetz S, Wernly D, Moerenhout K, Trampuz A, Borens O: Infection after fracture fixation. *EFORT Open Rev* 2019;4(7):468-475.

    Infection following fracture fixation is a complex complication that can lead to fracture nonunion, failure of hardware, and loss of function. This article summarizes recent developments and advances in the diagnosis and treatment of these infections.

59. Lu V, Zhang J, Patel R, Zhou AK, Thahir A, Krkovic M: Fracture related infections and their risk factors for treatment failure – A major trauma centre perspective. *Diagnostics (Basel)* 2022;12(5):1289.

    In this cohort, treatment failed in 23.5% of patients, defined as infection recurrence or amputation. Obesity, Gustilo-Anderson type IIIC fracture, and implant retention were all found to be independent risk factors for treatment failure. Level of evidence: IV.

60. Depypere M, Morgenstern M, Kuehl R, et al: Pathogenesis and management of fracture-related infection. *Clin Microbiol Infect* 2020;26(5):572-578.

    This is a narrative review of the current understanding of fracture-related infection pathogenesis, treatment, and outcomes, highlighting areas that still require further research. The most common bacteria causing fracture-related infections are *S aureus*, CoNS, and *Enterobacteriaceae*.

CHAPTER 9

Biofilm

NOREEN J. HICKOK, PhD • KENNETH L. URISH, MD, PHD, FAAOS, FAOA
PAUL STOODLEY, PhD, FAAM

ABSTRACT

The formation of surface-attached biofilms and biofilmlike suspended aggregates by bacterial and fungal pathogens is recognized as a major virulence factor in musculoskeletal infections, particularly in the presence of foreign body hardware. When bacteria and fungi form biofilms, they become highly recalcitrant to antibiotics, antimicrobial agents, and host immunity. Biofilm infections are often difficult to diagnose because there are no biomarkers or direct imaging modalities and there is a high rate of false-negative results from clinical cultures. An understanding of biofilms and their development is an important consideration in recognizing and managing musculoskeletal infections.

Dr. Hickok or an immediate family member serves as a paid consultant to or is an employee of Biogen and SINTX; serves as an unpaid consultant to Irrisept; has stock or stock options held in Biogen; and has received nonincome support (such as equipment or services), commercially derived honoraria, or other non–research-related funding (such as paid travel) from Irrisept. Dr. Urish or an immediate family member serves as a paid consultant to or is an employee of Adaptive Phage Therapeutics, Peptilogics, and Smith & Nephew; has stock or stock options held in Peptilogics; has received research or institutional support from Peptilogics and Smith & Nephew; and serves as a board member, owner, officer, or committee member of American Academy of Orthopaedic Surgeons and ASTM. Dr. Stoodley or an immediate family member is a member of a speakers' bureau or has made paid presentations on behalf of Biocomposites Ltd; serves as a paid consultant to or is an employee of Biocomposites, Dyson, and Zimmer; and has received research or institutional support from Azko-Nobel, Biocomposites, Colgate-Palmolive, Mondelez, Procter & Gamble, and Unilever.

Keywords: antibiotic tolerance; biofilm; biofilmlike aggregates; host immunity; treatment challenges

INTRODUCTION

Chronic device related orthopedic infections are notoriously difficult to treat. Two main factors contribute to this; biofilm formation by the infecting pathogen and lack of early and accurate microbiological diagnostics. In this chapter we explain what biofilm and biofilmlike aggregates are and how they form, specific diagnostic and treatment challenges associated with biofilm and mechanisms that biofilms use to evade clearance by host immunity. We also discuss factors that are known to influence the establishment of prosthetic joint infection and biomaterial surface modifications that could inhibit biofilm formation.

BACTERIAL CONTAMINATION

Bacterial contamination occurs in almost all surgical procedures.[1] In 2019, it was reported that successful mitigation occurs through aggressive anti-infection procedures, as evidenced by infection rates of less than 4%[2] occurring in more than 1 million joint arthroplasties per year in the United States.[3] Difficulties associated with treatment of prosthetic joint infection (PJI) appear to be intimately associated with bacterial biofilm formation and bacterial interactions with the joint environment. To this point, rapid bacterial adherence to the implant surface is a significant risk because much lower levels of bacteria are required to initiate an infection when a foreign material is present.[4] It is now accepted that formation of biofilms and biofilmlike suspended aggregates is a major factor in musculoskeletal infections.[5]

DEFINITION OF BIOFILM

There is no universal definition of what a biofilm is, but the consensus is that biofilms are surface-attached aggregates of microorganisms that are held together within a self-produced extracellular polymeric substance (EPS) slime matrix.[6] EPS composition is species dependent and generally consists of polysaccharides, extracellular DNA, proteins, and lipids, where EPS tends to be negatively charged because of anionic sugars and extracellular DNA. In addition to adherent biofilms, in the joint, nonadherent bacterial aggregates held together with EPS and/or synovial fluid components such as fibronectin, fibrinogen, and other serum proteins are also biofilmlike and referred to as biofilmlike aggregates.[7,8]

The Biofilm Life Cycle

On introduction of bacteria into a surgical site, the bacteria then aggregate, with the size determined by the host environment[9,10] (**Figure 1**). These aggregated bacteria either remain free floating or rapidly adhere to tissues or implants to initiate the biofilm life cycle: surface attachment, bacterial proliferation, EPS formation, and at maturity, dispersal of single cells by active processes or detachment of aggregates by physical forces such as fluid shear. The attachment of single planktonic (free-floating) cells or aggregates can occur within seconds. Once attached, bacteria undergo profound phenotypic changes that include production of EPS to form collections of microcolonies or aggregates. Formation of this immature biofilm can occur over minutes to hours. As biofilms grow and EPS becomes more abundant, diffusion of nutrients into the biofilm and of metabolites and waste products out of the

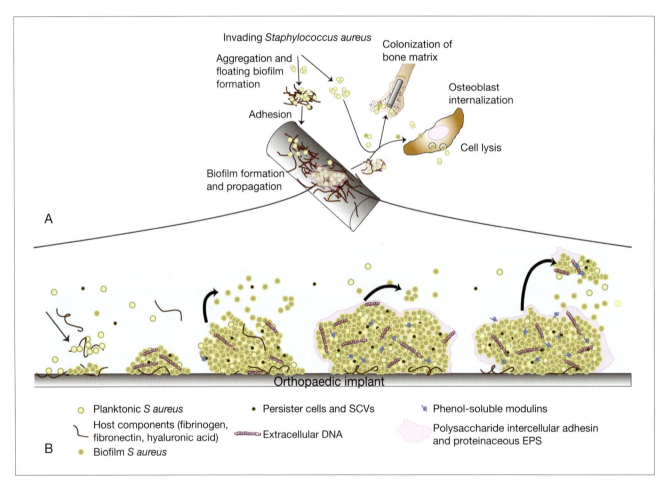

FIGURE 1 Illustration showing anatomic locations of infecting *Staphylococcus aureus* and conceptual model of the life cycle of *S aureus* biofilm. **A**, A series of events from the initial entry of *S aureus* into the surgical site followed by rapid aggregation and adherence to implants and bone and subsequent biofilm formation. *S aureus* can also invade bone tissue and host cells. **B**, A conceptual model of *S aureus* biofilm development on an implant surface. The model is redrawn from a five-stage model presented elsewhere. The five stages from left to right are: attachment to the implant mediated by electrostatic or hydrophobic interactions with the material or through microbial surface components recognizing adhesive matrix molecules binding to host components deposited on the implant (seconds to minutes); multiplication, where cells divide and produce extracellular polymeric substance (EPS) consisting primarily of extracellular DNA (eDNA) and proteinaceous polymers (minutes to hours); exodus, where a subpopulation of cells is released from the biofilm by nuclease-mediated eDNA degradation (hours); maturation, where there is more cell division and production of eDNA and proteinaceous EPS (hours to days depending on environmental conditions); and dispersal, where cells are released from the biofilm through autolysis, the production of proteases and surfactants orchestrated by Agr, the accessory gene regulator (multiple hours to days). The model has been expanded to include host component–mediated aggregation before attachment and the shedding of aggregated by the attached biofilm. SCVs = small colony variants.

biofilm is limited; further development of chemical gradients and microenvironments create phenotypic heterogeneity within the biofilm. Because of the rapid consumption of oxygen by bacteria at the outer edges and production of fermentation acids by bacteria in the biofilm interior, biofilm bacteria can create hypoxic acidic zones within the biofilm just 50 μm from the surface of the biofilm, even when the bathing physiologic fluid exists in normoxia. When the biofilm has reached steady state physically, chemically, and physiologically, it is referred to as a mature biofilm. In the laboratory, biofilms can reach maturity within a few days. The last stage is dispersion, in which cells are released from the biofilm following dissolution of the EPS, mediated by nutrient limitation and cell signaling; this can occur within minutes to hours.[11] Although this conceptual model is largely based on studies of *Pseudomonas aeruginosa* in vitro, similar stages are seen in staphylococci[12] and other species. However, as described in a 2022 study, the model was expanded to include a biofilmlike life cycle for aggregate formation in suspension, with exchange between the surface-attached and fluid phases possible at all stages of development.[13] How closely this conceptual model, based on laboratory studies largely in rich media, reflects biofilm formation in an infected artificial joint is not known because clinical samples provide only a snapshot of the process and usually only after the infection is established and after physical surgical manipulation to recover tissue and hardware specimens. Microscopic examination of clinical specimens of hardware and periprosthetic tissue reveals aggregates of approximately 10 to 20 μm,[14] much smaller than laboratory-grown biofilms. The floating aggregates in joint infection, however, range from microns to centimeters, based on in vitro and in vivo (**Figure 2**) investigations.[7]

Transition to Proteinaceous Biofilms and Aggregates in Physiologic Fluid

Biofilms are typically studied in ideal, nutrient-rich media that does not replicate the orthopaedic environment. The role of this environment is especially marked in prosthetic and native joint infections in which synovial fluid fosters the formation of dense, proteinaceous, floating, and tissue-adherent bacterial biofilmlike aggregates that can be macroscopic and have phenotypic similarity to biofilms.[9,15,16] As discussed in a 2018 study, the antibiotic tolerance of biofilms is confirmed by the persistence of infections despite aggressive treatment and the use of supratherapeutic concentration of antimicrobial agents locally.[17] Bacteria in the joint also exhibit the expected adherence to an implant, as well as invasion of the bone canalicular network[18] and perhaps, according to a 2021 study, even internalization within resident osteoblasts.[19]

Biofilmlike aggregates can be studied in vitro, where microscopic clusters are seen in serum and microscopic

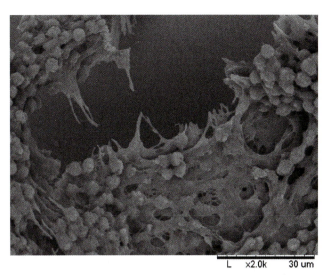

FIGURE 2 Micrograph shows mucinous biofilmlike aggregate from an infected knee: An approximately 10-cm mucinous bacterial aggregate was retrieved from the normally discarded material extracted from an infected knee. This micrograph (magnification, ×2000) shows a detail of the biofilmlike aggregate where bacteria are encased in matrix as is characteristic of biofilm. Notably, the different bacterial and host cells are aligned along a proteinaceous, fibrous network that provides strong interactions for bacterial sequestration. This use of deidentified material was classified as nonhuman research by the Thomas Jefferson University Institutional Review Board/Office of Human Research Protection. A portion of the aggregate was fixed in paraformaldehyde, dehydrated by using a graded series of ethanol incubations, dried, sputter coated, and visualized using scanning electron microscopy.

clusters as well as visible aggregates in synovial fluid.[7,10] A 2021 study reported that methicillin-sensitive and methicillin-resistant *Staphylococcus aureus*, *Escherichia coli*, and *P aeruginosa*, among other pathogens, aggregate via assembly of a proteinaceous matrix; for methicillin-sensitive and methicillin-resistant *S aureus*, fibrin[o-gen] is a critical component.[20] Methicillin-sensitive and methicillin-resistant *S aureus* biofilmlike aggregates show increased antimicrobial tolerance and are encased in a polysaccharide intercellular adhesin matrix.[7,9,15]

Biofilm Treatment Challenges

One of the hallmark features of biofilms and a major virulence factor,[21] studied most recently in 2018,[22] is the incredible tolerance (from hundreds to thousands of times) of bacteria within the biofilm to antibiotics and antimicrobial agents. The term tolerance is often favored over resistance because the reduced susceptibility is a result of emergent and adaptive properties of the biofilm phenotype, as reported in a 2022 study.[23] This is distinguished from antibiotic resistance that arises from heritable changes in the genetic makeup of the bacteria. In 2018, this tolerance was shown to be true for numerous bacterial and fungal species against numerous classes of antibiotics and antimicrobial agents by numerous laboratories.[24] There are many mechanisms for this antibiotic tolerance, including metabolic dormancy, which can be due to nutrient limitation, causing the cells to go into stationary phase, as well as the presence of small populations of persister bacteria and small colony variants that are slow growing or dormant regardless of nutrient availability. In addition, reduced antibiotic penetration into the biofilm by certain antibiotics can contribute to antibiotic inefficacy.

Reduced Penetration
The biofilm EPS creates protective microenvironments, and its constituent components of polysaccharides, nucleic acids, and protein all contribute to antibiotic tolerance.[25] Vancomycin and tobramycin, both positively charged antibiotics, have been shown to bind to EPS extracellular DNA and polysaccharides in *S aureus*[26] and *P aeruginosa*,[27] respectively. Rifampicin shows good penetration into staphylococcal biofilms and has efficacy against slow-growing cells, but frequent development of resistance through a single-point mutation suggests that it should be used in combination with other antibiotics.

Slow-Growing and Dormant Phenotypes
Antibiotics have been shown to interfere with cellular metabolic processes critical for bacterial growth[28] so that slow growth or dormancy can result in antibiotic tolerance. In addition, biofilms can harbor populations of cells with slow growth phenotypes. Small colony variants are slow-growing phenotypes that are difficult to detect via routine microbiological culture because of their long incubation times. A 2021 study showed that with *S aureus*, small colony variants can occur as a result of mutation in the electron transport system, rendering them deficient in aerobic respiration or via a reversible slow growth phenotype.[29] Antibiotic tolerance can also occur through the development of bacterial persister cells that are able to survive in the presence of antibiotics. Persister cells are small populations of cells (<1%) that are dormant, even if nutrients are available, and occur in both planktonic (nonadherent) cultures and biofilms. They are highly tolerant to antibiotics without undergoing any genetic changes.[30] It is hypothesized that they are less sensitive to antibiotics because their cellular metabolism is repressed. Their antibiotic tolerance in the biofilm state is accomplished via toxin-antitoxin systems. This system is composed of a toxin that can disrupt an important cellular process and an antitoxin that prevents toxin activation. The toxin and antitoxin form a complex in conditions of normal homeostasis. When the bacterium encounters an environmental stress (ie, antibiotic treatment), the antitoxin disassembles from the toxin. The toxin becomes activated and disrupts bacterial metabolism to induce a state of dormancy and antibiotic tolerance.[31] When treatment is stopped, the antitoxin binds to the toxin, resuming metabolic activities and antibiotic sensitivity.

Biofilm Antibiotic Susceptibility Testing
Minimum inhibitory concentration (prevents proliferation) and bactericidal concentration (≥3-log kill) are performed on rapidly growing cells in rich agar or broth media with inoculum densities of approximately 10^5 colony-forming units per mL over an 18- to 24-hour incubation period. The advantage of these tests is that they are relatively simple, cheap, and standardized; however, this also imparts limitations in extending their utility when it comes to treating biofilm infections. Biofilm cells can have much higher cell densities, exist in a nutrient-limited environment, and require extended antibiotic exposure times to exhibit susceptibility.[32] The concept of a minimum biofilm eradication concentration has been adopted to assess susceptibility when growing as a biofilm. In this case, clinical cultures are grown as biofilms and exposed to an antibiotic/antimicrobial concentration series. However, inhibition is difficult to assess if the biofilm cells are not growing because of nutrient limitation or phenotypic variation. Although minimum biofilm eradication concentration has the potential for meaningful clinical application, as of 2018, there was no standardization in terms of biofilm growth conditions, material on which the biofilm is grown, or methods; therefore, the technique remains a research tool.[33]

The Effect of Moving Fluids on Biofilm Physiology
Biofilms exhibit viscoelastic properties and are able to rearrange their macroscopic structure in response to shear stressing forces to form more draglike forms such as streamers or ripples.[34] Under different conditions, the same biofilm can behave as a fluid, a solid, or a mixture of the two.[35,36] Biofilms with ripple or wavy patterns have been found growing inside endotracheal tubes[37] and venous catheters.[38] In an elegant study, the rippling effect of the biofilm was studied using a compressed air jet.[39] These studies highlight how the extracellular matrix of the biofilm can allow it to survive irrigation in the context of orthopaedic infections. Thus, although débridement techniques such as pulse lavage remove some biofilm, in vitro assays demonstrate that significant amounts of biofilm remain on the surface.[40]

Diagnostic Challenges
In addition to therapeutic challenges in the management of biofilm infections, a definitive diagnosis is hampered by significant difficulties. In 2020, it was reported that clinical microbiology culture can produce false-negative results, and even if bacteria are cultured, the dominant or fast-growing organism may predominate, missing polymicrobial infections.[41] Negative culture results can be explained by several factors (**Table 1**).

Table 1
Factors Related to Negative Culture Results
Sampling issues—Often, synovial fluid is sampled, and that may not include bacteria residing in biofilms, on surfaces, or that which invades bone and soft tissue. Even if surfaces are swabbed, biofilm is heterogeneous and therefore might be missed.
Residual antibiotics—If the patient is not put on an antibiotic holiday before sampling, residual antibiotics in the tissue and fluid may suppress the growth of the clinical culture, even though it is not effective in killing antibiotic-tolerant biofilm bacteria.
Slow growth—Biofilm cells can be dormant or slow growing and only culture under extended incubation.
No biofilm biomarkers—To date, no specific biofilm bacterial or host response biomarkers have been identified.
Lack of imaging modalities—Dissimilar to cancer diagnostic tests, there are no approved medical imaging modalities that directly detect biofilm. Some imaging approaches rely on bone loss or immunologic reaction, but similar changes occur with trauma or foreign body reaction to an implant.

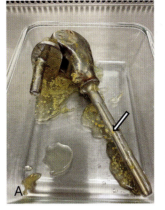
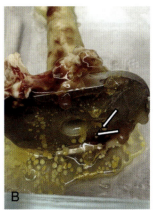
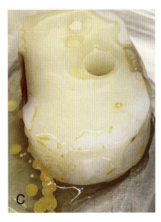
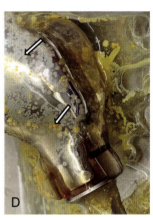

Techniques to improve clinical culture results include sonication to remove biofilm bacteria from implants or tissue biopsies[42] and, as reported in 2019, obtaining cultures directly from the implant[43,44] (**Figure 3**); however, these require specialized equipment and training because these methods have not been standardized. Culture-independent methods such as whole-genome sequencing show promise,[41] but there may be issues with contaminating DNA, and although genes associated with antibiotic resistance can be used to guide antibiotic therapy, a complete antibiogram requiring testing on a clinical isolate is not possible.

Difficulties in culturing prompted the Musculoskeletal Infection Society in 2018 to generate an algorithm based on major and minor diagnostic criteria, which were later weighted for their strength of evidence in which a diagnosis of PJI could be made solely on the basis of immunologic markers and wound characteristics at the surgical site.[45]

Surfaces That Favor Biofilm Formation

Laboratory studies and examination of clinical specimens have shown that biofilms can form to some extent on all materials used in orthopaedic surgical procedures, including different metals, polyethylene, surgical sutures, and polymethyl methacrylate bone cement. However, biofilm formation is most tenacious on rough surfaces.[46] Other physical factors include hydrophobicity and surface charge, although many of the surface properties of hardware can be masked by the adherence of host components. Although roughness from nanometer to

FIGURE 3 Photographs showing outgrowth of colonies from biofilms on surfaces of a hinged knee from a patient who underwent revision surgery for prosthetic joint infection (PJI). After explantation, the components were rinsed with sterile saline to remove loosely adhered cells and coated with cooled molten brain-heart infusion agar and incubated at 37°C, 5% CO_2 and monitored for colony development. **A**, *Staphylococcus aureus* colonies grew out from all parts of the hinge component, including the stems, which would have been inaccessible for débridement in a débridement, antibiotic therapy, implant retention procedure. Of note, colonies were found in the grooves of the stem (arrow), consistent with an in vitro study showing that biofilm preferentially accumulated on surface features such as holes, edges, and ridges. **B**, Colonies outgrew from the mating surfaces of the metal tibial tray and (**C**) the polyethylene component in the small gap between these components. There were gold and occasional white colonies (arrows in **B**). By polymerase chain reaction, these were both identified as *S aureus*, which was consistent with clinical culture. Small colony variants of *S aureus* isolated from patients with PJI have been shown to lose their golden pigment, staphyloxanthin, a carotenoid with antioxidant properties that protect against neutrophils. **D**, A close-up of the side of the femoral component grew out both gold and white colonies (arrows). (Images supplied by Jacob Brooks, BS, OSU Medical Student and collected by Douglas Chonko, DO, OSU Dept. Orthopaedics under the approved IRB protocol Study Number: 2020H0014, Study Title: Infected Orthopaedic Hardware: An analysis of pathogenic bacteria. Date of IRB Approval: 03/06/2022. Date of IRB Approval Expiration: 03/06/2023.)

millimeter scale has been well studied, these tend to be on flat, featureless surfaces. Less is known regarding how larger-scale features such as edges, ridges, grooves, holes, and threads may harbor biofilm; however, a 2022 study reported that these appear to be locations where biofilm preferentially accumulates during growth on orthopaedic implants in vitro.[47] In addition to physical interactions with the surface, bacteria such as *S aureus* express many surface adhesive proteins (microbial surface components recognizing adhesive matrix molecules) that bind to specific host matrix components such as fibrinogen and fibronectin that coat any physiologically implanted material. Microbial surface components recognizing adhesive matrix molecules are also important in synovial fluid–induced aggregation and attachment to host tissue.

Biomaterial Surface Modifications That Could Inhibit Biofilm Formation

Many implant surface modifications have been proposed such as manipulation of hydrophobicity, roughness, antimicrobial coatings, self-assembling monolayers with antimicrobial activity, and nanopatterning with the intention of inherent anti-attachment or biocidal activity, but none of these have made it to market. Animal testing is necessary to factor in the effects of the body's response to the materials, including coating by serum proteins and masking by a fibrous reaction. In addition, many bacterial pathogens found clinically may respond differently than standard strains used for screening in the laboratory. Finally, such strategies need to be economically viable, not interfere with the function of the implanted device and be noncytotoxic. A comprehensive review of various surface modification strategies is found elsewhere.[25] However, elution systems such as antibiotic-impregnated bone cement (as reported in 2020)[48] and mineral bone void fillers (as reported in 2018)[49] are used to supply high concentrations of antibiotics locally over extended periods beyond those achievable by systemic administration.

Effects of Biofilms on Host Immunity

The phenotype of the biofilm and biofilm aggregates also alters immune surveillance and response to the infection. This interplay is critical to establish the presence of PJI, and more generally, musculoskeletal infection (**Table 2**). This phenotype determines neutrophil activation and lysis (during the time that the bacteria remain ensconced in aggregates and/or biofilms). Importantly, in the presence of a staphylococcal joint infection (in mice), the macrophage response tends to be biased toward the noninflammatory M2 phenotype rather than the expected M1 response, which is classically triggered to combat an established acute infection.[50] Thus, the immune response seems to evolve depending on the stage of infection and the phenotype of the pathogens, although the understanding of this evolution is still limited. However, anecdotal evidence suggests that biofilm bacteria can survive despite an inflammatory immune response and infiltration of large numbers of neutrophils. In part, it is thought that this is because of the inability of neutrophils to fully penetrate the protective biofilm EPS as seen in a mouse biofilm catheter infection model.[51] Similarly, biofilms (in vitro) have been shown to reduce the penetration of immunoglobulin G and the efficacy of complement-mediated killing.[52] In addition, a 2018 study noted that the production of leukocidins and waste product metabolites and the consumption of oxygen by the biofilm bacteria as well as the presence of a foreign body and immune deficiencies in leukocyte infiltrates and inflammatory mediator expression, will all contribute to attenuating the efficacy of clearance by host immunity.[53]

Table 2

Factors That Are Known to Influence the Establishment of Prosthetic Joint Infection

Number of invading bacteria: The threshold for number of bacteria required to initiate an infection is markedly reduced by as much as 1,000-fold (for subdermal implants).

The type of organism: Staphylococci cause more than 70% of PJIs.

The chronic foreign body response to the implant affecting immune surveillance.

Serum protein coating of the implant that facilitates bacterial adhesion/biofilm formation.

Formation of floating biofilmlike aggregates that are antibiotic tolerant.

Suppressed bacterial metabolism and increased antibiotic tolerance, and suppressed virulence factor expression.

Limited bacterial clearance by the immune system: Biofilms and large floating biofilm aggregates that [as suggested by the authors] prevent phagocytosis and inhibit neutrophil action.

Macrophage polarization induced by changes in cytokines, nutrients, and other constituents.

Migration of bacteria into the bone as remodeling and osteointegration is initiated. At this point, bone débridement is critical, although bacterial phenotypic changes within the bone challenge all therapies.

SUMMARY

Treatment of PJI relies on the ability to decrease bacterial numbers to ranges where systemic antibiotics and the immune system can clear the infection. Although these bacteria may or may not be genotypically antibiotic resistant, their sequestration into biofilm structures confers an antibiotic tolerance that challenges the capability to remain within the therapeutic window. Knowledge of bacterial behavior within biofilms adherent to implant surfaces, as well as within fibrin[ogen]-anchored biofilmlike clusters, suggests that reduction is reliant on concentrations of antibiotics that far exceed traditional measures of the minimum inhibitory concentration, as well as the ability to target bacteria that have acquired a dormant phenotype.

KEY STUDY POINTS

- Bacterial biofilms and biofilmlike aggregates are assemblages of bacteria that can form on any orthopaedic material, form on bone and soft tissue, and reside in suspension in synovial fluid.
- All musculoskeletal pathogens can form biofilms, which can also comprise multiple species.
- Bacterial biofilm infections are difficult to diagnose because they often do not yield culture results, there are no definitive biomarkers, and no direct medical imaging modalities can detect them.
- When bacteria are present in biofilms and aggregates, they become highly tolerant of antibiotics and antimicrobials and can also evade immunity.
- Bacterial biofilms are viscoelastic, and while parts can break off, remaining layers can flow over surfaces when subjected to mechanical and fluid shear.

ACKNOWLEDGMENTS

The authors would like to thank Marc Harwood, MD (Rothman Orthopaedic Institute), and Antonia F. Chen, MD, MBA, FAAOS (Brigham and Women's Hospital), for supplying synovial fluid. Research reported in this publication was supported by the National Institutes of Health under award numbers R01GM124436 (PS), R01AR069119 (NJH), R01AR072513 (NJH), and R01AR076941 (NJH). The content is solely the responsibility of the authors and does not necessarily represent the official views of the National Institutes of Health.

ANNOTATED REFERENCES

1. Sharkey PF, Lichstein PM, Shen C, Tokarski AT, Parvizi J: Why are total knee arthroplasties failing today—has anything changed after 10 years? *J Arthroplasty* 2014;29(9):1774-1778.

2. Izakovicova P, Borens O, Trampuz A: Periprosthetic joint infection: Current concepts and outlook. *EFORT Open Rev* 2019;4(7):482-494.

    This review discusses the definition of PJI, infection rates, diagnostic challenges, and treatment options.

3. Kurtz SM, Lau E, Watson H, Schmier JK, Parvizi J: Economic burden of periprosthetic joint infection in the United States. *J Arthroplasty* 2012;27(8 suppl):61-65.e1.

4. Elek SD, Conen PE: The virulence of Staphylococcus pyogenes for man: A study of the problems of wound infection. *Br J Exp Pathol* 1957;38(6):573-586.

5. McConoughey SJ, Howlin R, Granger JF, et al: Biofilms in periprosthetic orthopedic infections. *Future Microbiol* 2014;9(8):987-1007.

6. Høiby N: A short history of microbial biofilms and biofilm infections. *APMIS* 2017;125(4):272-275.

7. Dastgheyb S, Parvizi J, Shapiro IM, Hickok NJ, Otto M: Effect of biofilms on recalcitrance of staphylococcal joint infection to antibiotic treatment. *J Infect Dis* 2015;211(4):641-650.

8. Perez K, Patel R: Biofilm-like aggregation of Staphylococcus epidermidis in synovial fluid. *J Infect Dis* 2015;212(2):335-336.

9. Dastgheyb SS, Hammoud S, Ketonis C, et al: Staphylococcal persistence due to biofilm formation in synovial fluid containing prophylactic cefazolin. *Antimicrob Agents Chemother* 2015;59(4):2122-2128.

10. Crosby HA, Kwiecinski J, Horswill AR: Staphylococcus aureus aggregation and coagulation mechanisms, and their function in host–pathogen interactions. *Adv Appl Microbiol* 2016;96:1-41.

11. Purevdorj-Gage B, Costerton W, Stoodley P: Phenotypic differentiation and seeding dispersal in non-mucoid and mucoid Pseudomonas aeruginosa biofilms. *Microbiology* 2005;151(pt 5):1569-1576.

12. Moormeier DE, Bayles KW: Staphylococcus aureus biofilm: A complex developmental organism. *Mol Microbiol* 2017;104(3):365-376.

13. Sauer K, Stoodley P, Goeres DM, et al: The biofilm life cycle: Expanding the conceptual model of biofilm formation. *Nat Rev Microbiol* 2022;20(10):608-620.

    This review article describes a simplistic developmental model for biofilm formation that is flexible enough to include all potential scenarios and microenvironments where biofilms are formed, with the ultimate purpose of understanding biofilms and anti-biofilm strategies that can be tailored to the microenvironment under investigation.

14. Nistico L, Hall-Stoodley L, Stoodley P: Imaging bacteria and biofilms on hardware and periprosthetic tissue in orthopedic infections, in *Microbial Biofilms*. Springer, 2014, pp 105-126.

15. Gilbertie JM, Schnabel LV, Hickok NJ, et al: Equine or porcine synovial fluid as a novel ex vivo model for the study of bacterial free-floating biofilms that form in human joint infections. *PLoS One* 2019;14(8):e0221012.

    The authors demonstrated that synovial fluid from horses or pigs is similar to human synovial fluid in terms of bacterial aggregation, antibiotic tolerance, and adenosine triphosphate usage; a panel of clinically relevant antibiotics are characterized, as well as several bacterial species including *S aureus*.

16. Pestrak MJ, Gupta TT, Dusane DH, et al: Investigation of synovial fluid induced Staphylococcus aureus aggregate development and its impact on surface attachment and biofilm formation. *PLoS One* 2020;15(4):e0231791.

   In vitro experiments showed that *S aureus* rapidly aggregated in the presence of bovine or artificial synovial fluid but that coating smooth glass surface with these components (principally fibrinogen and fibronectin) hindered initial attachment of single cells or aggregates, demonstrating both antagonistic and protective effects of synovial fluid.

17. Kunutsor SK, Whitehouse MR, Blom AW, et al: One- and two-stage surgical revision of peri-prosthetic joint infection of the hip: A pooled individual participant data analysis of 44 cohort studies. *Eur J Epidemiol* 2018;33(10):933-946.

   This observational pooled study suggests that a one-stage revision strategy may be as effective as a two-stage revision strategy in treating PJI of the hip. Level of evidence: III.

18. de Mesy Bentley KL, Trombetta R, Nishitani K, et al: Evidence of Staphylococcus aureus deformation, proliferation, and migration in canaliculi of live cortical bone in murine models of osteomyelitis. *J Bone Miner Res* 2017;32(5):985-990.

19. Gunn NJ, Zelmer AR, Kidd SP, et al: A human osteocyte cell line model for studying Staphylococcus aureus persistence in osteomyelitis. *Front Cell Infect Microbiol* 2021;11:781022.

   This in vitro study examined an osteoblastlike cell line that models primary osteoblasts and the same line after phosphate differentiation to an osteocyte phenotype for its ability to internalize *S aureus* within cells and persist to lay a basis for chronic infections.

20. Knott S, Curry D, Zhao N, et al: Staphylococcus aureus floating biofilm formation and phenotype in synovial fluid depends on albumin, fibrinogen, and hyaluronic acid. *Front Microbiol* 2021;12:655873.

   In vitro experiments showed that fibrin[ogen] is critical for *S aureus* aggregation in synovial fluid, and full aggregation requires at least albumin, fibrin[ogen], and hyaluronic acid; these components are used to create a pseudosynovial fluid that supports in vitro aggregation.

21. Costerton JW, Geesey GG, Cheng KJ: How bacteria stick. *Sci Am* 1978;238(1):86-95.

22. Ma D, Shanks RMQ, Davis CM 3rd, et al: Viable bacteria persist on antibiotic spacers following two-stage revision for periprosthetic joint infection. *J Orthop Res* 2018;36(1):452-458.

   In this ex vivo study, spacers from 13 patients recovered in a two-stage revision after antibiotic therapy were assessed for the presence of bacteria using 16S ribosomal DNA identified by polymerase chain reaction, a culture-independent method. Bacterial DNA was found in 53.8% (7 of 13 patients) spacers, providing evidence for the persistence of biofilm despite antibiotic therapy. Level of evidence: III.

23. Hamad C, Chowdhry M, Sindeldecker D, Bernthal NM, Stoodley P, McPherson EJ: Adaptive antimicrobial resistance, a description of microbial variants, and their relevance to periprosthetic joint infection. *Bone Joint J* 2022;104-B(5):575-580.

   This review article discusses the various known subpopulations of antibiotic-tolerant cells that may reside in biofilms formed from PJI pathogens. Several different phenotypes have been described in the literature, demonstrating that multiple mechanisms may lead to antibiotic tolerance.

24. Salisbury AM, Woo K, Sarkar S, et al: Tolerance of biofilms to antimicrobials and significance to antibiotic resistance in wounds. *Surg Technol Int* 2018;33:59-66.

   This review article discussed the various mechanisms identified that bacteria use to evade antibiotics.

25. Koo H, Allan RN, Howlin RP, Stoodley P, Hall-Stoodley L: Targeting microbial biofilms: Current and prospective therapeutic strategies. *Nat Rev Microbiol* 2017;15(12):740-755.

26. Doroshenko N, Tseng BS, Howlin RP, et al: Extracellular DNA impedes the transport of vancomycin in Staphylococcus epidermidis biofilms preexposed to subinhibitory concentrations of vancomycin. *Antimicrob Agents Chemother* 2014;58(12):7273-7282.

27. Tseng BS, Zhang W, Harrison JJ, et al: The extracellular matrix protects P seudomonas aeruginosa biofilms by limiting the penetration of tobramycin. *Environ Microbiol* 2013;15(10):2865-2878.

28. Stokes JM, Lopatkin AJ, Lobritz MA, Collins JJ: Bacterial metabolism and antibiotic efficacy. *Cell Metab* 2019;30(2):251-259.

   This review article explores the influence of antibiotics on bacterial metabolism on killing efficacy and the effect of the level of bacterial metabolism on antibiotic efficacy. It was concluded that a high level of evidence supports the statement that antibiotic efficacy is directly related to growth rate and that stationary phase confers tolerance.

29. Manasherob R, Mooney JA, Lowenberg DW, Bollyky PL, Amanatullah DF: Tolerant small-colony variants form prior to resistance within a staphylococcus aureus biofilm based on antibiotic selective pressure. *Clin Orthop Relat Res* 2021;479(7):1471-1481.

   This laboratory study shows that bacteria in biofilms were protected from vancomycin because of poor penetration into the biofilm, whereas combination therapy with rifampin significantly increased the reduction of bacteria and also resulted in the formation of antibiotic-tolerant small colony variants, demonstrating the multiple mechanisms biofilm bacteria use to evade antibiotic therapy.

30. Lewis K: Persister cells. *Annu Rev Microbiol* 2010;64:357-372.

31. Fasani RA, Savageau MA: Molecular mechanisms of multiple toxin-antitoxin systems are coordinated to govern the persister phenotype. *Proc Natl Acad Sci U S A* 2013;110(27):E2528-E2537.

32. Castaneda P, McLaren A, Tavaziva G, Overstreet D: Biofilm antimicrobial susceptibility increases with antimicrobial exposure time. *Clin Orthop Relat Res* 2016;474(7):1659-1664.

33. Coenye T, Goeres D, Van Bambeke F, Bjarnsholt T: Should standardized susceptibility testing for microbial biofilms be introduced in clinical practice? *Clin Microbiol Infect* 2018;24(6):570-572.

This article discusses issues with irreproducibility in current research laboratory methods in determining biofilm antibiotic susceptibility and making the argument for the need of standard methods such as the minimum inhibitory and bactericidal concentration assay before having clinical utility. Level of evidence: III.

34. Stoodley P, Lewandowski Z, Boyle JD, Lappin-Scott HM: Structural deformation of bacterial biofilms caused by short-term fluctuations in fluid shear: An in situ investigation of biofilm rheology. *Biotechnol Bioeng* 1999;65(1):83-92.

35. Bol M, Mohle RB, Haesner M, Neu TR, Horn H, Krull R: 3D finite element model of biofilm detachment using real biofilm structures from CLSM data. *Biotechnol Bioeng* 2009;103(1):177-186.

36. Blauert F, Horn H, Wagner M: Time-resolved biofilm deformation measurements using optical coherence tomography. *Biotechnol Bioeng* 2015;112(9):1893-1905.

37. Inglis TJ: Evidence for dynamic phenomena in residual tracheal tube biofilm. *Br J Anaesth* 1993;70(1):22-24.

38. Rusconi R, Lecuyer S, Guglielmini L, Stone HA: Laminar flow around corners triggers the formation of biofilm streamers. *J R Soc Interface* 2010;7(50):1293-1299.

39. Fabbri S, Li J, Howlin RP, et al: Fluid-driven interfacial instabilities and turbulence in bacterial biofilms. *Environ Microbiol* 2017;19(11):4417-4431.

40. Urish KL, DeMuth PW, Craft DW, Haider H, Davis CM 3rd: Pulse lavage is inadequate at removal of biofilm from the surface of total knee arthroplasty materials. *J Arthroplasty* 2014;29(6):1128-1132.

41. Goswami K, Parvizi J: Culture-negative periprosthetic joint infection: Is there a diagnostic role for next-generation sequencing? *Expert Rev Mol Diagn* 2020;20(3):269-272.

    This review focuses on the balance between the increased sensitivity of next-generation sequencing versus its weaknesses associated with contamination, uncertain use for therapeutic decisions, and cost. Randomized clinical trials are needed to adequately assess this methodology.

42. Trampuz A, Piper KE, Jacobson MJ, et al: Sonication of removed hip and knee prostheses for diagnosis of infection. *N Engl J Med* 2007;357(7):654-663.

43. Moley JP, McGrath MS, Granger JF, Sullivan AC, Stoodley P, Dusane DH: Mapping bacterial biofilms on recovered orthopaedic implants by a novel agar candle dip method. *APMIS* 2019;127(3):123-130.

    By using agar overlay coating of explants from two-stage PJI revisions with low melting temperature, agar assessment of biofilm distribution was made by observing outgrowth of colonies from the explant surfaces. Evidence of biofilm was found on all components and all materials, including hot spots such as the skirt rim of the femoral head. Level of evidence: III.

44. Sendi P, Rohrbach M, Graber P, Frei R, Ochsner PE, Zimmerli W: Staphylococcus aureus small colony variants in prosthetic joint infection. *Clin Infect Dis* 2006;43(8):961-967.

45. Parvizi J, Tan TL, Goswami K, et al: The 2018 definition of periprosthetic hip and knee infection: An evidence-based and validated criteria. *J Arthroplasty* 2018;33(5):1309-1314.e2.

    This report provides a validated definition of PJI based on expert consensus.

46. Ribeiro M, Monteiro FJ, Ferraz MP: Infection of orthopedic implants with emphasis on bacterial adhesion process and techniques used in studying bacterial-material interactions. *Biomatter* 2012;2(4):176-194.

47. Moore K, Gupta N, Gupta TT, et al: Mapping bacterial biofilm on features of orthopedic implants in vitro. *Microorganisms* 2022;10(3):586.

    Various hip and knee components were incubated with a light-producing *S aureus* SAP231, a bioluminescent USA300 methicillin-resistant *S aureus* strain. Biofilm preferentially formed on the rough surfaces and also surface features such as tapped holes, ridges, and edges.

48. Sebastian S, Liu Y, Christensen R, Raina DB, Tägil M, Lidgren L: Antibiotic containing bone cement in prevention of hip and knee prosthetic joint infections: A systematic review and meta-analysis. *J Orthop Translat* 2020;23:53-60.

    This meta-analysis of 37 studies and 9 trials showed that antibiotic-loaded bone cement used in primary joint arthroplasty reduced the risk of PJI by 20% to 84%.

49. Kallala R, Harris WE, Ibrahim M, Dipane M, McPherson E: Use of stimulan absorbable calcium sulphate beads in revision lower limb arthroplasty: Safety profile and complication rates. *Bone Joint Res* 2018;7(10):570-579.

    This is a prospective observational study to assess the safety profile of Stimulan beads when used in revision arthroplasty. Level of evidence: II.

50. Hanke ML, Kielian T: Deciphering mechanisms of staphylococcal biofilm evasion of host immunity. *Front Cell Infect Microbiol* 2012;2:62.

51. Thurlow LR, Hanke ML, Fritz T, et al: Staphylococcus aureus biofilms prevent macrophage phagocytosis and attenuate inflammation in vivo. *J Immunol* 2011;186(11):6585-6596.

52. Kristian SA, Birkenstock TA, Sauder U, Mack D, Götz F, Landmann R: Biofilm formation induces C3a release and protects Staphylococcus epidermidis from IgG and complement deposition and from neutrophil-dependent killing. *J Infect Dis* 2008;197(7):1028-1035.

53. Heim CE, Vidlak D, Odvody J, Hartman CW, Garvin KL, Kielian T: Human prosthetic joint infections are associated with myeloid-derived suppressor cells (MDSCs): Implications for infection persistence. *J Orthop Res* 2018;36(6):1605-1613.

    This study examined possible immune deficiencies in leukocyte infiltrates and inflammatory mediator expression that might help explain host factors for PJI.

CHAPTER 10

Irrigants and Irrigation

ANTONIA F. CHEN, MD, MBA, FAAOS • WILLIAM J. RUBENSTEIN, MD

ABSTRACT

Irrigation and débridement of surgical site infections is a mainstay of treatment. There are a variety of irrigant additives with antimicrobial properties that can be used in irrigation solutions to help control infection, although the optimal solution remains an open question. Questions also remain regarding the optimal delivery mechanism, volume, and duration of irrigation for surgical site infections. It is important to review the current literature to provide clarity on which irrigation protocols may best manage surgical site infections.

Keywords: irrigant additives; irrigation; surgical site infections

---

Dr. Chen or an immediate family member has received royalties from Stryker; serves as a paid consultant to or is an employee of 3M, Adaptive Phage Therapeutics, Avanos, BICMD, Convatec, Ethicon, GLG, Guidepoint, Heraeus, Irrimax, Pfizer, and Stryker; has stock or stock options held in Hyalex, IlluminOss, Irrimax, Joint Purification Systems, and Sonoran; has received research or institutional support from Adaptive Phage Therapeutics and Elute; and serves as a board member, owner, officer, or committee member of American Academy of Orthopaedic Surgeons, AJRR, and American Association of Hip and Knee Surgeons. Neither Dr. Rubenstein nor any immediate family member has received anything of value from or has stock or stock options held in a commercial company or institution related directly or indirectly to the subject of this chapter.

INTRODUCTION

Surgical site infections (SSIs) continue to be a major cause of postsurgical morbidity. As the volume of surgical procedures continues to increase both overall and among patients with increased comorbidities, it is likely that SSIs will continue to increase.[1] SSIs, especially in the presence of orthopaedic implants, are often treated with irrigation and débridement or explant. Studies have shown that as few as 10 organisms in the presence of an implant can result in an infection.[2] Thus, irrigation may be helpful for reducing contamination through the mechanical removal of particles and bacteria, eradicating biofilm, and destroying remaining bacteria. This must be performed in the context of preserving healthy tissue and minimizing both local and systemic toxicity. A wide variety of techniques are used differently among surgeons with respect to irrigation agent, technique, and volume. It is important to review the evidence around the optimal irrigation techniques for SSIs.

IRRIGATION AGENTS

There are an array of available irrigation agents used in irrigation solutions, typically grouped into one of three categories: surfactants, antibiotics, and antiseptics.

Surfactants

Surfactants function by chemically disrupting bacterial adherence to the wound or implant. Surfactants thus aid in the removal of bacteria as opposed to acting as bactericidal agents.[3] The most commonly used surfactants include castile soap (anionic) and benzalkonium chloride (cationic). Initial animal studies suggested that surfactants were potentially beneficial with few adverse effects. In two studies in rats comparing benzalkonium with normal saline, the surfactant solution was found to be superior.[4,5] Although castile soap was not more effective than normal saline when used for a *Staphylococcus* infection, it did appear superior when *Pseudomonas* was the infecting bacteria.[4] In addition, a 1% soap solution was shown to have greater preservation of alkaline phosphatase activity, bone nodule formation, and osteoclast preservation compared with other irrigation additives including povidone-iodine, bacitracin, and chlorhexidine gluconate (CHG).[6]

However, more recent surfactant studies have shown less-promising results. Although castile soaps appeared to cause an initial reduction in *Pseudomonas* counts in a goat model, there was a subsequent rebound effect to 120% of pretreatment levels at 48 hours posttreatment, in contrast to 68% in the normal saline group.[7] In the clinical setting, the Fluid Lavage of Open Wounds trial randomized 2,447 patients with open fractures to a castile soap irrigation group versus a normal saline irrigation group, and reoperation rates were higher in the castile soap group.[8]

There is some evidence that surfactant use in combination with additional antiseptics may have increased effectiveness. One in vitro study found that a combination of an antiseptic and a detergent was most effective at reducing bacterial colony counts compared with a detergent alone.[9] A 2021 in vitro study assessed the effect of various irrigant additives on reductions in methicillin-resistant *Staphylococcus aureus* (MRSA) biofilms and found that Bactisure (Zimmer Biomet), a proprietary solution that includes the surfactant benzalkonium chloride, had the greatest reduction in *Pseudomonas* biofilm in the study.[10] However, it is not clear from these studies what effect the surfactant itself has on the positive reported results in contrast to the other antiseptics in the solution. Given the available evidence, as of 2020, the routine use of surfactants is not currently recommended in the irrigation of musculoskeletal infections.[11]

Antibiotics

Antibiotics have historically been an additive to irrigation solutions. The ideal antibiotic contains bactericidal and fungicidal activity against biofilm-associated microbes with minimal host toxicity. The most commonly used antibiotics are bacitracin, polymyxin, and neomycin.[3,12]

The basic science literature on the effectiveness of antibiotic-laden irrigation solutions is mixed. One study using a canine model found that applying bacitracin solution lowered the number of wound cultures that were positive for *S aureus*.[13] Another study subsequently recommended a triple antibiotic solution including neomycin, polymyxin, and bacitracin to remain in the wound for a minimum of 1 minute to help reduce wound infections.[14] However, a 2019 study exposing *S aureus* and *Escherichia coli* to a variety of different irrigation solutions for 1- and 3-minute intervals found that irrigation with a polymyxin-bacitracin solution was ineffective in eradicating bacteria.[15]

The limited data from the orthopaedic literature do not show any major benefit to the use of antibiotic irrigation solutions. A prospective randomized study compared the irrigation of open fractures with irrigation using detergent with antibiotics. There were no significant differences in infection rates between the two groups, although there were increased wound healing issues in the group irrigated with bacitracin.[16] In clinical studies looking at the use of antibiotic irrigation for prosthetic joint infections (PJIs) being treated using débridement, antibiotics, and implant retention, success rates ranged from 31% to 44%.[17-19] In a 2021 study, this was not significantly different from the historically reported rate of success with saline irrigation of approximately 50%.[20]

Setting aside the questionable clinical efficacy of antibiotic irrigation, consideration must also be given to the potential harm associated with antibiotic irrigation. There are risks related to hypersensitivity, anaphylaxis, and antibiotic resistance, not to mention the increased cost.[3,21,22] Currently, the World Health Organization, UK National Institute for Health and Care Excellence, and US Centers for Disease Control and Prevention do not recommend routine use of antibiotic irrigation in the prevention or treatment of surgical infections (**Table 1**). This is in accordance with two reviews on the topic that also saw no indication for routine usage of antibiotic irrigation in light of the questionable efficacy, adverse effect profile, and cost.[11,20]

Antiseptics

Antiseptics are a class of irrigant additives that indiscriminately target cell walls and membranes, increasing permeability and resulting in cell death. Although these can be effective against bacteria, fungi, and viruses, the effects can also affect and damage host cells.[23] There are several available antiseptics currently used for the prevention of SSIs (**Table 2**).

Acetic Acid

Acetic acid is a weak organic acid prevalent in vinegar. Its antimicrobial properties have been known for thousands of years, and it has been recently used for a variety of treatment strategies including burns and catheter-associated urinary tract infections.[24] In a 2021 study, it was reported that acetic acid is thought to affect bacteria by lowering intracellular pH and inhibiting adenosine triphosphate formation, although its precise mechanism of action needs further investigation.[25] Its effect is concentration dependent with concentrations less than 5% thought to be noncytotoxic to host tissue.

Table 1
Institutional Guidelines for Irrigation to Prevent Surgical Site Infection

Institution	Antibiotics	Normal Saline	Acetic Acid	Povidone-Iodine	CHG
WHO	Against level of evidence: Very low	Neither for nor against level of evidence: Very low	No data	For level of evidence: Data low	No data
CDC	No recommendation level of evidence: Low	No data	No data	For level of evidence: Moderate	No data
ICM	Against level of evidence: Moderate; strong consensus	No data	Neither for nor against[a] level of evidence: Limited; no consensus	For level of evidence: Strong consensus	No data

CDC = Centers for Disease Control and Prevention, CHG = chlorhexidine gluconate, ICM = International Consensus Meeting, WHO = World Health Organization

[a]The ICM evaluated acetic acid in the management of prosthetic joint infection and not specifically with prevention of surgical site infection.

Reprinted from Siddiqi A, Abdo ZE, Rossman SR, et al: What is the optimal irrigation solution in the management of periprosthetic hip and knee joint infections? *J Arthroplasty* 2021;36(10):3570-3583. Copyright 2021, with permission from Elsevier.

Acetic acid has been shown to be effective against a variety of both gram-positive and gram-negative bacteria. An in vitro study looking at bacteria commonly found in burns showed a 3% acetic acid solution to be effective against all bacteria tested, including MRSA and *Pseudomonas*.[26] In vitro studies have also shown acetic acid to be effective against mycobacterium as well as *Pseudomonas aeruginosa* and *S aureus* biofilms.[27,28] An in vitro study using a methicillin-sensitive *S aureus* (MSSA) biofilm model found that a 5% solution of acetic acid eliminated 96.1% of the biofilm after a 20-minute treatment. For shorter treatment intervals, a 2018 study reported that higher concentrations were required to eliminate the biofilm.[29] Clinically, a 20-minute 3% acetic acid soak was used as part of a débridement protocol in 23 patients with PJI after total knee arthroplasty with an overall success rate of 87%. The study showed no adverse effects but did note that in concurrent in vitro testing, acetic acid was only bactericidal against 40% of the isolates.[30]

Overall, acetic acid is relatively inexpensive and readily available. There is good in vitro evidence regarding its clinical efficacy against a wide array of pathogens. However, the 20-minute time period necessary for it to have an effect may limit widespread adoption.

Povidone-Iodine

Povidone-iodine is a commonly used antiseptic in clinical medicine. Povidone-iodine consists of free iodine conjugated to a hydrophilic compound. The iodine oxidizes the cell membrane and intracellular components resulting in cell death in a concentration-dependent manner.[20]

There have been both in vitro and clinical studies assessing the effect of povidone-iodine on infectious pathogens. A 2019 study comparing commonly used irrigation solutions found that povidone-iodine was effective against both *S aureus* and *E coli* with minimal cytotoxicity.[15] Other studies have found similar efficacy of povidone-iodine against additional pathogens including MRSA, *Staphylococcus epidermidis*, *Haemophilus influenzae*, and *Pseudomonas*.[31,32] In one of the initial clinical studies assessing the use of povidone-iodine in orthopaedic surgery, patients undergoing lumbar fusion showed a decrease in infection rate when irrigated with a povidone-iodine solution without any effect on wound healing, bone union, or clinical outcomes.[33] Most recent clinical studies have focused on PJI prevention. One study showed an infection rate of 0.97% before the institution of a dilute povidone-iodine lavage and a 0.15% infection rate after institution of a 3-minute povidone-iodine wash.[34] A randomized controlled trial from 2020 focused on aseptic revisions for total hip and knee arthroplasty and also noted a significant decrease in infection rate after a 3-minute dilute povidone-iodine lavage.[35] However, two studies performed at a different institution did not find the same effect. One 2019 study focusing on primary total hip and knee arthroplasty examined more than 2,800 primary joints and found no advantage to using povidone-iodine irrigation at 3 or 12 months postoperatively.[36] Another 2019 study that analyzed approximately 12,000 revision arthroplasties also did not find any differences in the rate of reoperation at 3 or 12 months.[37]

There remain some concerns regarding the use of povidone-iodine. Several studies have shown cytotoxic effects on tissue and articular cartilage.[38] Rare cases of iodine allergies and anaphylaxis have been reported.[39] Nonsterile povidone-iodine has been found to be

Table 2

Common Antiseptic Mechanism and Activity

Antiseptic	Mechanism of Action	Bacteria	Mycobacteria	Spores	Fungi	Viruses	Biofilm
Acetic acid	Anion production that denatures proteins and enzymes resulting in increased cell wall permeability	Bactericidal	—	—	Fungicidal	—	Some effect
CHG	Attacks inner bacterial cytoplasmic membranes or yeast plasma membranes with resultant cytoplasmic clumping	Bactericidal	Mycobacteriostatic	Sporostatic	—	Viricidal	Some effect
Hydrogen peroxide	Acts as an oxidant-producing hydroxyl-free radicals that attack lipids, protein, and DNA	Bactericidal (gram-positive more than gram-negative)	—	Sporostatic	Fungicidal	—	Limited effect
Sodium hypochlorite	Oxidizing agent destroys cellular proteins	Bactericidal	—	Sporicidal at higher levels	—	Viricidal	No effect
Povidone-iodine	Delivers free iodine to cells, which attacks proteins, nucleotides, and fatty acids	Bactericidal	Mycobactericidal	Sporicidal	Fungicidal	Viricidal	Limited effect

CHG = chlorhexidine gluconate

Reprinted with permission from Kavolus JJ, Schwarzkopf R, Rajaee SS, Chen AF: Irrigation fluids used for the prevention and treatment of orthopaedic infections. *J Bone Joint Surg Am* 2020;102(1):76-84.

contaminated with pathogens, though there is now a commercially available sterile povidone-iodine for use intraoperatively.[40] Liposomal bupivacaine is lysed by povidone-iodine, so it should not be used before a povidone-iodine lavage. Recognizing these potential limitations, given the evidence in support of its clinical efficacy and relatively strong safety profile, the International Consensus Meeting 2019 statement on orthopaedic infections recommended the use of dilute povidone-iodine irrigation during clean orthopaedic procedures.[41] Povidone-iodine concentrations vary by institution, but typically a 0.2% to 0.3% povidone-iodine solution is used.

Chlorhexidine Gluconate

CHG is another antiseptic with a broad spectrum of action against a wide array of pathogens. CHG is a cationic bisbiguanide that binds to cell walls and interferes with osmotic cellular equilibrium.[20] At lower concentrations (<0.5%), it is bacteriostatic, whereas at higher levels, it causes intracellular coagulation and is bactericidal.[25]

CHG is active against many common pathogens including MSSA, MRSA, coagulase-negative *Staphylococcus*, gram-negative bacteria, and fungi.[42]

Intrawound irrigation of CHG has been noted to be safe at concentrations of 0.05% and produce a 5-log reduction in bacteria colony-forming units after 60 seconds.[43] Additional in vitro studies highlighted the efficacy of CHG on reducing biofilm from a titanium alloy.[9,44] Mechanical scrubbing with CHG was effective in eradicating biofilm in a PJI model at a concentration of 2%, a level that may be cytotoxic to host tissue based on other in vitro studies.[9,45] In fact, CHG may be cytotoxic even at concentrations as low as 0.02%.[46] Few high-level clinical studies have been performed assessing the efficacy of CHG. One retrospective study compared povidone-iodine irrigation with a 0.05% CHG solution in hip and knee arthroplasty and found no differences in infection rates or complications.[44] Similarly, a 2020 study found equivalent PJI rates using CHG or povidone-iodine.[47]

The FDA currently has approved a 0.05% CHG preparation in sterile water for use in joint irrigation. Although current studies suggest this solution is safe to use in total joint arthroplasty, its clinical efficacy has not been proven in randomized controlled trials.[44] CHG has broad-spectrum antimicrobial capabilities and is not affected by bodily fluids such as blood (unlike povidone-iodine), making it a potentially powerful tool in fighting infection. Given the current lack of high-level clinical studies, further investigation is required to determine the appropriate concentration for clinical use that will provide the desired bactericidal effect while minimizing cytotoxicity to host tissue.

Hydrogen Peroxide

Hydrogen peroxide occurs naturally in human tissues and serves a variety of roles, including in the inflammatory response to infection. Hydrogen peroxide produces free radicals that result in cell death via oxidative damage of DNA, lipids, and proteins. Hydrogen peroxide is considered to be more effective against gram-positive organisms.[48,49] It is efficacious at a concentration of 3%, though its effectiveness is hindered by catalase, which can be present in blood and other body fluids and can be produced by some bacteria.[48]

Multiple in vitro studies have shown hydrogen peroxide to have antimicrobial activity including effectiveness against biofilm.[48,50] One study suggested that hydrogen peroxide was more effective than povidone-iodine in treating *S epidermidis* biofilm.[50] Interestingly, hydrogen peroxide appears to have a synergistic effect when used in concert with additional antiseptics. A combination of hydrogen peroxide and sodium hypochlorite was bactericidal against *P aeruginosa* and removed biofilms from both stainless steel and aluminum surfaces.[51] A similar synergistic effect against *Saccharomyces cerevisiae*, *E coli*, *S aureus*, and *P aeruginosa* was seen when hydrogen peroxide was used in conjunction with povidone-iodine.[52] Although limited, there have been clinical studies on hydrogen peroxide with mixed results. In the general surgery literature, hydrogen peroxide did not result in decreased infection rate in appendectomies or bacterial load of skin wounds, but did increase the rate of skin graft acceptance in chronically infected burn wounds.[53-55] The orthopaedic literature has also shown mixed results with some studies showing no benefits to infection or sarcoma recurrence, with possible reduction in infection of external fixation pin sites.[56-58] Two clinical studies, one in patients undergoing spine surgery and one in patients with PJI, showed a reduced rate of infection when using a combined hydrogen peroxide and povidone-iodine lavage.[59,60]

As with most antiseptic solutions, there is concern regarding cytotoxicity, although no in vivo studies have shown negative effects on wound healing or host tissues. In addition, because of its bubble-forming nature, there is risk of immediate air embolism if hydrogen peroxide is used in enclosed spaces such as the medullary canal; thus, this is not recommended.[48]

Sodium Hypochlorite

Sodium hypochlorite is commercially known as Dakin solution (full strength, 0.5%) and works by inhibiting protein synthesis and lipids in the bacterial cell membrane through oxidization by reactive chloride ions.[61] Its effect is maximized at a lower pH level.[49] Unlike many of the other antiseptics, this is a time-dependent rather than a concentration-dependent process. In addition to its antimicrobial properties, it also has the capability to dissolve necrotic tissue.[62]

There is limited literature regarding the effect of sodium hypochlorite both in vitro and clinically. A 2018 in vitro study found that sodium hypochlorite significantly reduced the colony-forming units on metal disks with *S aureus* but did not result in complete bacterial eradication.[63] Another 2018 study reported that sodium hypochlorite was ineffective in reducing bioburden in validated rat and goat model studies involving *P aeruginosa* and *S aureus* and showed rapid degradation when exposed to soft tissues.[64] There have been very few clinical studies on sodium hypochlorite performed in orthopaedics, as sodium hypochlorite is often part of a heterogenous protocol involving other antiseptic and antibiotic modalities.[65] Of note, sodium hypochlorite should never be combined with acetic acid as this can create lethal chlorine gas, and sodium hypochlorite should not be mixed with CHG as this can result in combustible oxygen.[25]

Section 2: Basic Science

Hypochlorous Acid

Hypochlorous acid is produced naturally in the body by white blood cells and a variety of other anti-inflammatory cells. It has a similar mechanism to sodium hypochlorite, with chloride ions oxidizing bacterial cells, and plays a key role in the innate immunity pathway, as reported in a 2020 review.[66]

Hypochlorous acid is available as a commercial solution and has historically been used for superficial wound management.[67] It has demonstrated efficacy against *S aureus* biofilm, although there is concern regarding its effect on erosion of metal implants.[68,69] Clinical studies show its use in orthopaedics is limited thus far.

Commercial Antiseptics

There are numerous commercially available antiseptic agents containing the irrigant additives mentioned previously (Table 3). These include Irrisept (0.05% CHG solution, Irrimax Corporation), Vashe Wound Solutions (hypochlorous acid, SteadMed Medical), Prontosan (betadine and polyhexanide, B. Braun Medical), Bactisure (ethanol, acetic acid, and benzalkonium chloride, Zimmer Biomet), and Surgiphor (povidone-iodine, BD). These

Table 3

Preparation of Most Common Irrigation Solutions

Solution	Additive Category	Irrigation Preparation
0.45% Castile soap	Surfactant	80 mL of castile soap in a 3-L NS bag
0.03% Benzalkonium chloride	Surfactant	5.2 mL of 17% aqueous stock solution in a 3-L NS bag
Polymyxin-bacitracin solution	Antibiotic	Polymyxin 500,000 units and bacitracin 50,000 units in a 3-L NS bag
Vancomycin	Antibiotic	1 g/L in 3-L NS bag
Gentamicin	Antibiotic	80 mg/L in 3-L NS bag
Povidone-iodine	Antiseptic	Dilute (0.5%) sterile formulation is commercially available as Surgiphor or made by combining 17.5 mL of 10% PI in 500 mL NS
		10% = nondiluted
0.05% Chlorhexidine gluconate	Antiseptic	Commercially available as Irrisept (Innovation Technologies, Inc.)
3% Acetic acid	Antiseptic	Available in 3% concentration without further dilution
Sodium hypochlorite	Antiseptic	Commercially available as Dakin solution (dilute sodium hypochlorite 0.5%)
		Can be further diluted with 500 mL NS for 0.25% concentration
Hypochlorous acid	Antiseptic	Commercially available as Vashe Wound Therapy Solution (SteadMed Medical LLC)
0.1% Polyhexamethylene biguanide	Antiseptic-surfactant combination	Commercially available as Prontosan Wound Irrigation Solution (B. Braun Medical Inc.)
0.1% betadine		
Ethanol	Antiseptic-surfactant combination	Commercially available as Bactisure Wound Lavage Solution (Next Science R&D, distributed by Zimmer Biomet)
Acetic acid		
Sodium acetate		
Benzalkonium chloride		
Sterile water		

NS = normal saline 0.9%, PI = povidone-iodine

Reprinted from Siddiqi A, Abdo ZE, Rossman SR, et al: What is the optimal irrigation solution in the management of periprosthetic hip and knee joint infections? *J Arthroplasty* 2021;36(10):3570-3583. Copyright 2021, with permission from Elsevier.

premixed solutions can help eliminate potential mixing errors by the pharmacy and operating room staff, and there are data suggesting they are potentially effective in preventing infection.[70,71] Of course, these commercial solutions are often more costly than other available solutions and may not be more clinically effective compared with alternatives.[25]

DELIVERY

Delivery method of the chosen irrigation solution is an important consideration[19] (**Table 4**). Several studies have analyzed the difference between high-pressure (15 to 35 psi) and low-pressure (1 to 15 psi) delivery systems. High-pressure irrigation is typically delivered by a

Table 4
Irrigation Recommendations

	Prophylactic Irrigation	Irrigation for Contaminated and/or Infected Wounds	Description
Volume	≤2 L	≤9 L	On the basis of recent studies from the general surgery literature, there is likely a point of diminishing returns in terms of irrigation volume, tempering the adage that the solution to pollution is dilution. For grossly infected wounds, surgical débridement should likely be the mainstay for the removal of infected materials with judicious subsequent irrigation, such that all gross contamination is removed and remaining bacterial count is diminished.
Delivery	Preference	Initial low pressure followed by preference	Given the equivocal results of clinical comparison investigations, the use of pulsed lavage or low flow is at the discretion of the surgeon. However, in light of higher bacterial rebound and the possibility of spreading infection with higher-pressure delivery, it is thought that contaminated and/or infected wounds should initially be débrided and irrigated with a low-pressure system before using high-pressure systems, which may be more expeditious and practical when irrigating with volumes of >2 L.
Additives			
Antibiotics	Never	Never	As the mechanism of action of antibiotics requires a longer duration than irrigation affords, there is concern for resistance and clinical investigations have never demonstrated a benefit.
Surfactants	Never	Never	Basic science studies have found a significant rebound when used, whereas the FLOW study found higher reoperation rates for open fractures.
Antiseptics	Likely CHG or povidone-iodine	Consider acetic acid, povidone-iodine, or CHG (or some combination)	Dakin solution and hydrogen peroxide carry marked risk without advantage over other antiseptics, so their use is not currently advised. Acetic acid demonstrates promise in the setting of biofilm but requires a longer duration of exposure, so use in presumed clean wounds is unlikely to confer advantage over povidone-iodine or CHG. CHG and povidone-iodine have both proven effective for prophylaxis and infected wounds with limited risk and likely provide a reduced risk of infection. For infected wounds, certain antiseptics confer different advantages; therefore, combinations may be advisable but caution in terms of mixing these compounds in patient wounds is advised.

CHG = chlorhexidine gluconate, FLOW = Fluid Lavage of Open Wounds

Reprinted with permission from Kavolus JJ, Schwarzkopf R, Rajaee SS, Chen AF: Irrigation fluids used for the prevention and treatment of orthopaedic infections. *J Bone Joint Surg Am* 2020;102(1):76-84.

mechanical pulse lavage, whereas low-pressure delivery systems include bulb irrigation, cysto tubing, or simply pouring of irrigation over a wound from a sterile container. In theory, high pressure can help mechanically remove microbes and associated biofilm while delivering the irrigation solution. There is evidence from several studies that pulse lavage results in a greater decrease in bacterial burden.[7,72,73] However, there is also evidence to suggest that these high-pressure systems are damaging to surrounding tissues and may serve to drive bacteria deeper into soft tissue and bone where they can continue to result in infection.[74-76]

One of the largest trials to date is the Fluid Lavage of Open Wounds trial, where 2,447 patients with open fractures were randomized to high-pressure, low-pressure, and very-low-pressure groups. There were no differences in reoperation rates among the three groups; thus, low-pressure irrigation was recommended as it is more cost effective.[8] It remains to be seen if the results of this trial are applicable to other situations, especially those involving chronic infections as well as implants with biofilm.

VOLUME

The optimal irrigation volume remains an unresolved question. Historically, it was suggested that increased irrigation in multiple volumes of 3 L each should be used for each open fracture graded increasingly on the Gustilo-Anderson classification. This was based on the underlying theory that the more open/contaminated the wound bed, the more irrigation would be required, and 3-L bags of normal saline are routinely available.[3] This theory is supported by one study that found decreased bacterial burden as irrigation volume increased to 9 L in both low- and high-pressure systems.[73] However, a 2018 study found increased SSI rates when more than 2 L of saline irrigation was used following appendectomy.[77] Further studies are required to determine optimal irrigation volumes for musculoskeletal infections.

DURATION

Duration of wound irrigation is another recent focus of investigation. Many of the irrigant additives discussed require a certain amount of contact time with the microbes to have the desired clinical effect. If a certain irrigation solution requires a lavage time of upward of 20 minutes to have a bactericidal effect, this may make its use in the operating room impractical.[31] Past studies have shown that povidone-iodine may be effective with a 3-minute lavage.[34] A 2022 in vitro study found that povidone-iodine, sodium hypochlorite, and acetic acid eradicated all bacterial growth after 2 minutes.[78] The required duration of irrigation is likely affected by the presence of biofilm, which requires a longer duration of irrigation, as noted in a 2018 study.[79] Further clinical studies are required as duration of irrigation is likely greatly affected by the presence of bodily fluids such as blood, which may affect the efficacy of irrigation solutions.

SUMMARY

Musculoskeletal infections in orthopaedics remain a difficult clinical complication, and irrigation is a key part of management. There are a wide variety of irrigant additives both off-label and commercially available that have antimicrobial effects and may be useful in combating infection. However, there remain significant unknowns regarding the most effective additive or additive combinations, ideal delivery system, volume, and duration of irrigation. Future research should include well-designed randomized clinical trials to help answer these questions, with results including both clinical outcomes and complications associated with the various irrigation options.

KEY STUDY POINTS

- Intrawound irrigation is a necessary and effective means of controlling SSIs.
- Irrigation solutions are often supplemented with antibiotics, surfactants, or antiseptics.
- The literature does not currently support the addition of antibiotics or surfactants to irrigation solution. The efficacy of antiseptics and the optimal antiseptic selection/combination remains an open question.
- A low-pressure delivery system should be used to irrigate wounds with increasing volumes of solution for wounds with a higher burden of contamination or infection.
- Further prospective randomized controlled trials are required to determine optimal irrigation solutions and protocols.

ANNOTATED REFERENCES

1. DeFrances CJ, Podgornik MN: 2004 National Hospital discharge survey. *Adv Data* 2006;371:1-19.

2. Lidwell OM, Lowbury EJ, Whyte W, Blowers R, Stanley SJ, Lowe D: Airborne contamination of wounds in joint replacement operations: The relationship to sepsis rates. *J Hosp Infect* 1983;4(2):111-131.

3. Anglen JO: Wound irrigation in musculoskeletal injury. *J Am Acad Orthop Surg* 2001;9(4):219-226.

4. Conroy BP, Anglen JO, Simpson WA, et al: Comparison of castile soap, benzalkonium chloride, and bacitracin as irrigation solutions for complex contaminated orthopaedic wounds. *J Orthop Trauma* 1999;13(5):332-337.

5. Tarbox BB, Conroy BP, Malicky ES, et al: Benzalkonium chloride. A potential disinfecting irrigation solution for orthopaedic wounds. *Clin Orthop Relat Res* 1998;346:255-261.

6. Bhandari M, Adili A, Schemitsch EH: The efficacy of low-pressure lavage with different irrigating solutions to remove adherent bacteria from bone. *J Bone Joint Surg Am* 2001;83(3):412-419.

7. Owens BD, White DW, Wenke JC: Comparison of irrigation solutions and devices in a contaminated musculoskeletal wound survival model. *J Bone Joint Surg Am* 2009;91(1):92-98.

8. FLOW Investigators, Bhandari M, Jeray KJ, et al: A trial of wound irrigation in the initial management of open fracture wounds. *N Engl J Med* 2015;373(27):2629-2641.

9. Schwechter EM, Folk D, Varshney AK, Fries BC, Kim SJ, Hirsh DM: Optimal irrigation and debridement of infected joint implants: An in vitro methicillin-resistant Staphylococcus aureus biofilm model. *J Arthroplasty* 2011;26(6 suppl):109-113.

10. O'Donnell JA, Wu M, Cochrane NH, et al: Efficacy of common antiseptic solutions against clinically relevant microorganisms in biofilm. *Bone Joint J* 2021;103-B(5):908-915.

    This in vitro study examined the efficacy of several antiseptic solutions against both nascent and mature microorganisms. Bactisure and povidone-iodine had the best overall effectiveness.

11. Kavolus JJ, Schwarzkopf R, Rajaee SS, Chen AF: Irrigation fluids used for the prevention and treatment of orthopaedic infections. *J Bone Joint Surg Am* 2020;102(1):76-84.

    This review article summarizes literature around optimal irrigation solutions, volume, and delivery. Level of evidence: II.

12. Crowley DJ, Kanakaris NK, Giannoudis PV: Irrigation of the wounds in open fractures. *J Bone Joint Surg Br* 2007;89(5):580-585.

13. Rosenstein BD, Wilson FC, Funderburk CH: The use of bacitracin irrigation to prevent infection in postoperative skeletal wounds. An experimental study. *J Bone Joint Surg Am* 1989;71(3):427-430.

14. Dirschl DR, Wilson FC: Topical antibiotic irrigation in the prophylaxis of operative wound infections in orthopedic surgery. *Orthop Clin North Am* 1991;22(3):419-426.

15. Goswami K, Cho J, Foltz C, et al: Polymyxin and bacitracin in the irrigation solution provide no benefit for bacterial killing in vitro. *J Bone Joint Surg Am* 2019;101(18):1689-1697.

    This in vitro study found that polymyxin-bacitracin irrigation solution was ineffective against *S aureus* and *E coli*. Povidone-iodine appeared to be the most effective.

16. Anglen JO: Comparison of soap and antibiotic solutions for irrigation of lower-limb open fracture wounds. A prospective, randomized study. *J Bone Joint Surg Am* 2005;87(7):1415-1422.

17. Azzam KA, Seeley M, Ghanem E, Austin MS, Purtill JJ, Parvizi J: Irrigation and debridement in the management of prosthetic joint infection: Traditional indications revisited. *J Arthroplasty* 2010;25(7):1022-1027.

18. Deirmengian C, Greenbaum J, Stern J, et al: Open debridement of acute gram-positive infections after total knee arthroplasty. *Clin Orthop Relat Res* 2003;416:129-134.

19. Koyonos L, Zmistowski B, Della Valle CJ, Parvizi J: Infection control rate of irrigation and débridement for periprosthetic joint infection. *Clin Orthop Relat Res* 2011;469(11):3043-3048.

20. Siddiqi A, Abdo ZE, Rossman SR, et al: What is the optimal irrigation solution in the management of periprosthetic hip and knee joint infections? *J Arthroplasty* 2021;36(10):3570-3583.

    This review article summarizes the optimal irrigant additives in the management of PJI based on the current literature. Level of evidence: II.

21. Antevil JL, Muldoon MP, Battaglia M, Green R: Intraoperative anaphylactic shock associated with bacitracin irrigation during revision total knee arthroplasty. A case report. *J Bone Joint Surg Am* 2003;85(2):339-342.

22. Damm S: Intraoperative anaphylaxis associated with bacitracin irrigation. *Am J Health Syst Pharm* 2011;68(4):323-327.

23. Ortega-Peña S, Hidalgo-González C, Robson MC, Krötzsch E: In vitro microbicidal, anti-biofilm and cytotoxic effects of different commercial antiseptics. *Int Wound J* 2017;14(3):470-479.

24. Halstead FD, Rauf M, Moiemen NS, et al: The antibacterial activity of acetic acid against biofilm-producing pathogens of relevance to burns patients. *PLoS One* 2015;10(9):e0136190.

25. Plate JF, Zuskov A, Seyler TM: Use of adjunct antiseptic agents in periprosthetic joint infections. *J Am Acad Orthop Surg* 2021;29(23):e1151-e1158.

    This review article outlines the current literature on the use of antiseptic irrigant additives in PJI. Level of evidence: II.

26. Ryssel H, Kloeters O, Germann G, Schäfer T, Wiedemann G, Oehlbauer M: The antimicrobial effect of acetic acid – An alternative to common local antiseptics? *Burns* 2009;35(5):695-700.

27. Bjarnsholt T, Alhede M, Jensen PØ, et al: Antibiofilm properties of acetic acid. *Adv Wound Care (New Rochelle)* 2015;4(7):363-372.

28. Cortesia C, Vilchèze C, Bernut A, et al: Acetic Acid, the active component of vinegar, is an effective tuberculocidal disinfectant. *mBio* 2014;5(2):e00013-e00014.

29. Tsang STJ, Gwynne PJ, Gallagher MP, Simpson AHRW: The biofilm eradication activity of acetic acid in the management of periprosthetic joint infection. *Bone Joint Res* 2018;7(8):517-523.

    This study assesses the efficacy of acetic acid solutions used at various times of application and concentrations on a strain of

30. Williams RL, Ayre WN, Khan WS, Mehta A, Morgan-Jones R: Acetic acid as part of a debridement protocol during revision total knee arthroplasty. *J Arthroplasty* 2017;32(3):953-957.

31. Cichos KH, Andrews RM, Wolschendorf F, Narmore W, Mabry SE, Ghanem ES: Efficacy of intraoperative antiseptic techniques in the prevention of periprosthetic joint infection: Superiority of betadine. *J Arthroplasty* 2019;34(7 suppl):S312-S318.

   This study assesses the effect of povidone-iodine, CHG, and vancomycin against a number of different bacteria. All seven bacterial isolates were killed by povidone-iodine at all time points.

32. Gilotra M, Nguyen T, Jaffe D, Sterling R: Dilute betadine lavage reduces implant-related bacterial burden in a rabbit knee prosthetic infection model. *Am J Orthop (Belle Mead NJ)* 2015;44(2):E38-E41.

33. Chang FY, Chang MC, Wang ST, Yu WK, Liu CL, Chen TH: Can povidone-iodine solution be used safely in a spinal surgery? *Eur Spine J* 2006;15(6):1005-1014.

34. Brown NM, Cipriano CA, Moric M, Sporer SM, Della Valle CJ: Dilute betadine lavage before closure for the prevention of acute postoperative deep periprosthetic joint infection. *J Arthroplasty* 2012;27(1):27-30.

35. Calkins TE, Culvern C, Nam D, et al: Dilute betadine lavage reduces the risk of acute postoperative periprosthetic joint infection in aseptic revision total knee and hip arthroplasty: A randomized controlled trial. *J Arthroplasty* 2020;35(2):538-543.e1.

   This randomized controlled trial determines the effectiveness of dilute betadine lavage versus normal saline lavage in aseptic revision total hip and knee arthroplasties. There was a significant reduction in PJI in the betadine lavage group. Level of evidence: I.

36. Hart A, Hernandez NM, Abdel MP, Mabry TM, Hanssen AD, Perry KI: Povidone-iodine wound lavage to prevent infection after revision total hip and knee arthroplasty: An analysis of 2,884 cases. *J Bone Joint Surg Am* 2019;101(13):1151-1159.

   In this comparison of revision total hip and total knee arthroplasty, with cohorts using a povidone-iodine lavage protocol against a baseline group, no significant differences in infection rates were found between the groups. Level of evidence: III.

37. Hernandez NM, Hart A, Taunton MJ, et al: Use of povidone-iodine irrigation prior to wound closure in primary total hip and knee arthroplasty: An analysis of 11,738 cases. *J Bone Joint Surg Am* 2019;101(13):1144-1150.

   In this comparison of primary total hip and total knee arthroplasty, with cohorts using a povidone-iodine lavage protocol against a baseline group, no significant differences in infection rates were found between the groups. Level of evidence: III.

38. von Keudell A, Canseco JA, Gomoll AH: Deleterious effects of diluted povidone-iodine on articular cartilage. *J Arthroplasty* 2013;28(6):918-921.

39. Waran KD, Munsick RA: Anaphylaxis from povidone-iodine. *Lancet* 1995;345(8963):1506.

40. Chang CY, Furlong LA: Microbial stowaways in topical antiseptic products. *N Engl J Med* 2012;367(23):2170-2173.

41. Blom A, Cho J, Fleischman A, et al: General assembly, prevention, antiseptic irrigation solution: Proceedings of international consensus on orthopedic infections. *J Arthroplasty* 2019;34(2 suppl):S131-S138.

   The International Consensus Meeting group summarized their 2019 findings and recommendations related to antiseptic irrigation solutions in orthopaedic infections. Level of evidence: IV.

42. George J, Klika AK, Higuera CA: Use of chlorhexidine preparations in total joint arthroplasty. *J Bone Jt Infect* 2017;2(1):15-22.

43. Edmiston CE, Bruden B, Rucinski MC, Henen C, Graham MB, Lewis BL: Reducing the risk of surgical site infections: Does chlorhexidine gluconate provide a risk reduction benefit? *Am J Infect Control* 2013;41(5 suppl):S49-S55.

44. Frisch NB, Kadri OM, Tenbrunsel T, Abdul-Hak A, Qatu M, Davis JJ: Intraoperative chlorhexidine irrigation to prevent infection in total hip and knee arthroplasty. *Arthroplast Today* 2017;3(4):294-297.

45. Liu JX, Werner J, Kirsch T, Zuckerman JD, Virk MS: Cytotoxicity evaluation of chlorhexidine gluconate on human fibroblasts, myoblasts, and osteoblasts. *J Bone Jt Infect* 2018;3(4):165-172.

   This study investigating in vitro effects of CHG on fibroblasts, myoblasts, and osteoblasts found that clinically used concentrations significantly reduced the survival of all cell types.

46. van Meurs SJ, Gawlitta D, Heemstra KA, Poolman RW, Vogely HC, Kruyt MC: Selection of an optimal antiseptic solution for intraoperative irrigation: An in vitro study. *J Bone Joint Surg Am* 2014;96(4):285-291.

47. Driesman A, Shen M, Feng JE, et al: Perioperative chlorhexidine gluconate wash during joint arthroplasty has equivalent periprosthetic joint infection rates in comparison to betadine wash. *J Arthroplasty* 2020;35(3):845-848.

   In this retrospective study comparing the use of a CHG wash with that of a betadine wash, no significant differences in rate of PJI or wound complications were found between the two groups. Level of evidence: III.

48. Lu M, Hansen EN: Hydrogen peroxide wound irrigation in orthopaedic surgery. *J Bone Jt Infect* 2017;2(1):3-9.

49. McDonnell G, Russell AD: Antiseptics and disinfectants: Activity, action, and resistance. *Clin Microbiol Rev* 1999;12(1):147-179.

50. Presterl E, Suchomel M, Eder M, et al: Effects of alcohols, povidone-iodine and hydrogen peroxide on biofilms of Staphylococcus epidermidis. *J Antimicrob Chemother* 2007;60(2):417-420.

51. DeQueiroz GA, Day DF: Antimicrobial activity and effectiveness of a combination of sodium hypochlorite and hydrogen peroxide in killing and removing Pseudomonas aeruginosa biofilms from surfaces. *J Appl Microbiol* 2007;103(4):794-802.

52. Zubko EI, Zubko MK: Co-operative inhibitory effects of hydrogen peroxide and iodine against bacterial and yeast species. *BMC Res Notes* 2013;6:272.

53. Lau WY, Wong SH: Randomized, prospective trial of topical hydrogen peroxide in appendectomy wound infection. High risk factors. *Am J Surg* 1981;142(3):393-397.

54. Leyden JJ, Bartelt NM: Comparison of topical antibiotic ointments, a wound protectant, and antiseptics for the treatment of human blister wounds contaminated with Staphylococcus aureus. *J Fam Pract* 1987;24(6):601-604.

55. Mohammadi AA, Seyed Jafari SM, Kiasat M, Pakyari MR, Ahrari I: Efficacy of debridement and wound cleansing with 2% hydrogen peroxide on graft take in the chronic-colonized burn wounds; a randomized controlled clinical trial. *Burns* 2013;39(6):1131-1136.

56. Egol KA, Paksima N, Puopolo S, Klugman J, Hiebert R, Koval KJ: Treatment of external fixation pins about the wrist: A prospective, randomized trial. *J Bone Joint Surg Am* 2006;88(2):349-354.

57. Patterson MM: Multicenter pin care study. *Orthop Nurs* 2005;24(5):349-360.

58. Wooldridge AN, Kolovich GP, Crist MK, Mayerson JL, Scharschmidt TJ: Predictors of local recurrence in high-grade soft tissue sarcomas: Hydrogen peroxide as a local adjuvant. *Orthopedics* 2013;36(2):e207-e215.

59. George DA, Konan S, Haddad FS: Single-stage hip and knee exchange for periprosthetic joint infection. *J Arthroplasty* 2015;30(12):2264-2270.

60. Ulivieri S, Toninelli S, Petrini C, Giorgio A, Oliveri G: Prevention of post-operative infections in spine surgery by wound irrigation with a solution of povidone-iodine and hydrogen peroxide. *Arch Orthop Trauma Surg* 2011;131(9):1203-1206.

61. Levine JM: Dakin's solution: Past, present, and future. *Adv Skin Wound Care* 2013;26(9):410-414.

62. Keyes M, Jamal Z, Thibodeau R: *Dakin Solution*. StatPearls, 2022.

    This article reviews the use of Dakin solution including use in the clinical setting, adverse events, different formulations/strengths, and administration of the solution. Level of evidence: III.

63. Ernest EP, Machi AS, Karolcik BA, LaSala PR, Dietz MJ: Topical adjuvants incompletely remove adherent Staphylococcus aureus from implant materials. *J Orthop Res* 2018;36(6):1599-1604.

    In this assessment of the effect of adjuvant treatment strategies on *S aureus* biofilm, it was found that although betadine, Dakin solution, and hydrogen peroxide all reduced *S aureus* biofilm, none completely eradicated it.

64. Mangum LC, Franklin NA, Garcia GR, Akers KS, Wenke JC: Rapid degradation and non-selectivity of Dakin's solution prevents effectiveness in contaminated musculoskeletal wound models. *Injury* 2018;49(10):1763-1773.

    This study evaluated the effectiveness of Dakin solution in a rat and goat model. There was no evidence of therapeutic benefit in either of these animal models.

65. Duque AF, Post ZD, Lutz RW, Orozco FR, Pulido SH, Ong AC: Is there still a role for irrigation and debridement with liner exchange in acute periprosthetic total knee infection? *J Arthroplasty* 2017;32(4):1280-1284.

66. Block MS, Rowan BG: Hypochlorous acid: A review. *J Oral Maxillofac Surg* 2020;78(9):1461-1466.

    This is review reports on the use and efficacy of hypochlorous acid in a variety of settings. Level of evidence: III.

67. Niezgoda JA, Sordi PJ, Hermans MH: Evaluation of Vashe Wound Therapy in the clinical management of patients with chronic wounds. *Adv Skin Wound Care* 2010;23(8):352-357.

68. Kubacki GW, Gilbert JL: The effect of the inflammatory species hypochlorous acid on the corrosion and surface damage of Ti-6Al-4V and CoCrMo alloys. *J Biomed Mater Res A* 2018;106(12):3185-3194.

    In this investigation of the effect of hypochlorous acid on titanium and cobalt chrome alloys, extensive surface damage was visualized after exposure to the irrigation solution for 5 days.

69. Wang L, Bassiri M, Najafi R, et al: Hypochlorous acid as a potential wound care agent: Part I. Stabilized hypochlorous acid – A component of the inorganic armamentarium of innate immunity. *J Burns Wounds* 2007;6:e5.

70. Atkin L, Stephenson J, Cooper DM: Wound bed preparation: A case series using polyhexanide and betaine solution and gel-a UK perspective. *J Wound Care* 2020;29(7):380-386.

    In this case series, the use of a polyhexanide and betadine wound irrigation solution in chronic wounds was found to improve outcomes and chances of wound healing. Level of evidence: IV.

71. Day A, Alkhalil A, Carney BC, Hoffman HN, Moffatt LT, Shupp JW: Disruption of biofilms and neutralization of bacteria using hypochlorous acid solution: An in vivo and in vitro evaluation. *Adv Skin Wound Care* 2017;30(12):543-551.

72. Bhandari M, Schemitsch EH, Adili A, Lachowski RJ, Shaughnessy SG: High and low pressure pulsatile lavage of contaminated tibial fractures: An in vitro study of bacterial adherence and bone damage. *J Orthop Trauma* 1999;13(8):526-533.

73. Svoboda SJ, Bice TG, Gooden HA, Brooks DE, Thomas DB, Wenke JC: Comparison of bulb syringe and pulsed lavage irrigation with use of a bioluminescent musculoskeletal wound model. *J Bone Joint Surg Am* 2006;88(10):2167-2174.

74. Boyd JI, Wongworawat MD: High-pressure pulsatile lavage causes soft tissue damage. *Clin Orthop Relat Res* 2004;427:13-17.

75. Hassinger SM, Harding G, Wongworawat MD: High-pressure pulsatile lavage propagates bacteria into soft tissue. *Clin Orthop Relat Res* 2005;439:27-31.

76. Kalteis T, Lehn N, Schröder HJ, et al: Contaminant seeding in bone by different irrigation methods: An experimental study. *J Orthop Trauma* 2005;19(9):591-596.

77. Hernandez MC, Finnesgard EJ, Aho JM, Jenkins DH, Zielinski MD: Association of postoperative organ space infection after intraoperative irrigation in appendicitis. *J Trauma Acute Care Surg* 2018;84(4):628-635.

In this report, irrigation volumes of greater than 2 L were associated with postoperative organ space infection in patients after undergoing appendectomy. Level of evidence: IV.

78. Christopher ZK, Tran CP, Vernon BL, Spangehl MJ: What is the duration of irrigation? An in vitro study of the minimum exposure time to eradicate bacteria with irrigation solutions. *J Arthroplasty* 2022;37(2):385-389.e2.

    In this in vitro study examining a variety of irrigation solutions and their effect on different bacterial species, all antiseptic solutions with the exception of CHG successfully eradicated bacterial growth with exposure times of less than 2 minutes.

79. Schmidt K, Estes C, McLaren A, Spangehl MJ: Chlorhexidine antiseptic irrigation eradicates Staphylococcus epidermidis from biofilm: An in vitro study. *Clin Orthop Relat Res* 2018;476(3):648-653.

    In this in vitro *study* examining whether commonly used antibacterials and antiseptics kill bacteria in a biofilm model at clinically relevant concentrations/exposure times, CHG was the only tested irrigant capable of eradicating *S aureus* from biofilm.

SECTION 3

Antibiotics

Section Editor:
Sandra B. Nelson, MD

CHAPTER 11

Antibiotics: General Principles of Use in Orthopaedic Infections

JULIE E. REZNICEK, DO • JIHYE KIM, PHARMD

ABSTRACT

Surgical advancements, such as those in total joint arthroplasties and spinal fusions, have allowed patients to regain function and improve quality of life, but unfortunately they are also associated with an inherent risk of infection. Management of these infections is complicated by unique obstacles, such as biofilm formation, isolation of multidrug-resistant pathogens, or inability to safely remove an implant. Bone and joint infections in the absence of indwelling hardware also require a complex, multidisciplinary approach. Treatment of bone and joint infections typically consists of adjunctive antimicrobial therapy after surgical débridement. Antimicrobial selection, including route of administration, is dependent on multiple host and microbial factors, all of which must be taken into consideration.

Keywords: bactericidal/bacteriostatic; bioavailability; biofilm; definitive and suppressive; prophylactic

INTRODUCTION

The basic principles for choosing the appropriate antimicrobial therapy for a bone and joint infection (BJI) are very similar to those used for other infections. Knowledge of the host and disease state is essential when identifying the most common pathogens associated with certain BJIs. The chronicity of the infection must also be taken into consideration, especially when hardware is present. This is classically seen in prosthetic joint infections (PJIs) where an acute infection is more likely to be secondary to a more virulent pathogen such as *Staphylococcus aureus*, as opposed to a chronic infection where *Staphylococcus epidermidis* is commonly the causative pathogen.

There are some unique aspects to antibiotic management in the orthopaedic patient. The presence of hardware that cannot be feasibly removed often indicates the need for long-term antibiotic suppression. Depending on the resistance panel of the organism, there may be limited options that meet all the necessary criteria including (1) a narrow spectrum of activity, (2) long-term tolerability, and (3) limited significant drug interactions. Intravenous antibiotics are typically preferred for the treatment of BJIs; however, more recently, the pendulum is shifting toward oral antibiotics initially or at least a quicker transition from intravenous to oral therapy. Duration of treatment of a BJI is longer, in comparison with treatment courses for skin and soft-tissue infections and other common infections seen in practice. The data to support this recommendation are weak and it may be possible to shorten treatment duration especially in scenarios in which an adequate surgical débridement was obtained.

Very often, the clinician has multiple antimicrobial options based on the desired spectrum of activity, but this list can be further narrowed down based on penetration into the infected target site, the patient's allergies or intolerances, and even socioeconomic factors, such as ability to afford home intravenous antibiotics. Ideally, the orthopaedic surgeon will work hand in hand with an infectious diseases specialist and/or clinical pharmacist who can advise on optimal dosing regimens based on the host, causative pathogen, and target site.

DEFINITIONS

It has been almost a century since the monumental discovery of mold juice inhibiting staphylococcal growth

---

Neither of the following authors nor any immediate family member has received anything of value from or has stock or stock options held in a commercial company or institution related directly or indirectly to the subject of this chapter: Dr. Reznicek and Dr. Kim.

on Petri dishes, thereby launching the antibiotic era, and now there are more than 100 antibiotics beyond penicillin to choose from, with varying modes of delivery. Multiple factors go into the selection of an antibiotic, but the guiding principles remain the same. Prescribers must choose agents that cover all known and/or potential pathogens, while also being cognizant of antibiotic overuse, selection of antimicrobial resistance, and potential adverse effects experienced by the patient.

Historically, antibiotics have been administered for prophylaxis, empiric therapy, or definitive treatment of an infection (**Table 1**). With the advent of indwelling medical devices, chronic suppression therapy has now become a relatively common indication for prolonged antibiotics. Prophylactic antibiotics can be further delineated as primary, secondary, or eradication. They are typically administered before a high-risk situation to prevent a primary infection, recurrent infection, or elimination of colonizing organisms, respectively.[1] Current recommendations for primary antibiotic prophylaxis in orthopaedic surgery include administration of a preoperative antibiotic within 60 to 120 minutes before the first incision, depending on which drug is chosen. The antibiotic should be redosed for prolonged surgeries or in those patients who experience significant blood loss, and antibiotics should be continued for no more than 24 hours after skin closure.[2]

Empiric antibiotic therapy is initiated when the suspicion of infection is high but when infection has not yet been confirmed. It is based on experience and knowledge of potential causative organisms. This community of microorganisms, the surrounding environment, and the unique interplay between the two is termed the microbiome.[3] Clinicians must always keep in mind that microbiomes are not stagnant, and the composition may change with age, antibiotic use, anatomic location, and even diet. Empiric therapy will often transition to definitive (directed) therapy once the microorganisms are identified. Treatment may involve oral or intravenous antibiotics or a combination of the two.

There are currently many terms in the BJI literature that have similar meaning and are often used interchangeably despite some variability in the duration of treatment. For example, in one study chronic antibiotic suppression was defined as treatment with oral antibiotics for at least 6 months after the initial intravenous antibiotic course.[4] Regarding the optimal oral antibiotic treatment course after a débridement, antibiotics, and implant retention procedure, the term extended antibiotic prophylaxis was used in a 2020 study to mean any oral antibiotic use, regardless of duration, that was started after the completion of a 6-week intravenous antibiotic course.[5] The indication for extended oral antibiotic therapy may also vary depending on the procedure involved: prevention of infection in primary joint arthroplasties; suppressive therapy after a débridement, antibiotics, and implant retention procedure; or long-term prophylaxis after a two-stage revision. As the amount of research on extended antibiotic use continues to grow, physicians must be aware of these subtle, yet possibly clinically relevant, variations in definitions.

The optimal duration of therapy for these clinical scenarios where extended oral antibiotics are used has not been agreed on. Inflammatory markers such as

Table 1

Definitions of Antibiotic Indications

	Indication/Timing	Clinical Example
Prophylaxis	Administered before a high-risk situation	Not applicable
Primary	Prevention of an initial infection	Surgical prophylaxis to prevent a surgical site infection
Secondary	Prevention of the recurrence of an infection	Administration of oral penicillin to prevent recurrent cellulitis in a patient with lymphedema
Eradication	Elimination of colonizing organisms to prevent infection	Antibiotics given before an elective cystoscopy for urinary colonization
Empiric	High clinical suspicion of infection	Diabetic foot ulcer with foul-smelling drainage and surrounding erythema
Definitive	Microorganism-directed therapy	Prosthetic joint infection with all intraoperative cultures positive for methicillin-sensitive *Staphylococcus aureus*
Suppression	Oral antibiotics used to delay or prevent the progression of a known infection, when curative strategies are not feasible	Intraoperative cultures are positive during a second-stage procedure, but no additional surgeries are recommended

erythrocyte sedimentation rate and C-reactive protein level can be used as an indirect measurement of ongoing infection, but despite high sensitivity, these laboratory tests lack specificity. Many other variables are typically taken into consideration, such as risk of relapse based on causative pathogen, extent of previous surgical débridements, and risk of amputation if antibiotics were stopped. Most importantly, the continuation or cessation of oral antibiotics should be periodically discussed with the patient, with a remainder of the ongoing risks and benefits associated with that specific clinical scenario.

In addition, not all clinical scenarios are suitable for chronic antibiotic suppression. This occurs if the causative organism has limited oral antibiotics options (eg, *Pseudomonas aeruginosa*) or the selected oral antibiotics are not tolerable for an extended period. During these specific situations, communication between the surgeon and infectious diseases specialist is essential.

The use of extended oral antibiotic suppression is one of the criteria used to determine success or failure in the management of PJI; therefore, this data point should always be collected. A Delphi-based international multidisciplinary consensus did not include this variable when considering infection eradication;[6] however, other studies have considered long-term antibiotic suppression therapy as a data point to define success or failure.[7,8]

Most orthopaedic surgeons and infectious disease specialists would agree that treatment of a PJI is not uniform for all patients, and the benefit of lifelong oral antibiotics often outweighs the risk of additional surgeries in certain scenarios.

ANTIMICROBIAL SELECTION

Antibiotic Spectrum

The process of selecting antibiotics in BJIs takes into consideration the disease state and its potential causative pathogens as well as the host status. Common pathogens such as *Staphylococcus* species still account for most BJIs, but even within this genus, nuances do occur.[9] For example, *S epidermidis*, typically a commensal organism with little pathogenicity, is much more likely to cause infection in the setting of indwelling hardware. If the infection occurs in a patient who is immunocompromised or has had extensive exposure to antibiotics in the past, the pathogen differential will expand to include less common organisms such as fungi, mycobacteria, and multidrug-resistant pathogens. The antimicrobial regimen should have a narrow spectrum of activity and limited toxicity. This may not be feasible initially, but regimens should be tailored as additional data are collected.

In the past decade, significant efforts have been made to develop novel antibiotics to combat multidrug-resistant organisms.[10] Some of the newer agents such as ceftaroline, ceftolozane/tazobactam, ceftazidime/avibactam, and omadacycline bring additional treatment options to the current armamentarium of antibiotics.[11-15] However, treating patients with BJIs with multidrug-resistant organisms can present additional challenges to clinicians because most of these newer agents are being used off-label and current available data for the use of these agents in the treatment of BJIs are based on case reports and observational studies. Therapeutic drug monitoring for beta-lactam antibiotics and other antibiotics is not a widely used strategy in current practice because of limited availability and cost. However, this could be the future direction of treatment of patients with BJIs to help ensure that newer agents have adequate drug concentration, because interpatient variability and physicochemical characteristics of different drug classes can play a significant role in bone concentration and bone-to-serum concentration ratio.[16]

Antibiotics in Biofilm

Although the biofilm concept was first introduced in the 1930s with the characterization of water bacteria, it is not until recently that physicians have started to understand the strong interplay between biofilms and human disease.[17] By definition, a biofilm is an "aggregate of microorganisms in which cells are frequently embedded in a self-produced matrix of extracellular polymeric substances (EPS) that are adherent to each other and/or a surface."[18] Orthopaedic biofilm infections can involve innate matter, such as sequestrum in the setting of chronic osteomyelitis, or in the form of an implant-related infection. Regardless of the substrate, efficacious treatment typically involves both surgical débridement and antimicrobial therapy.

The ability to eradicate bacteria from a biofilm is much more complex than once thought and has evolved significantly over the past 2 decades. Reduced bacterial penetration is no longer the sole mechanism, and this is supported by studies showing that even with excellent penetration into the extracellular matrix, the biofilm bacteria are able to survive.[19] The ideal antimicrobial agent would not only penetrate the biofilm but also be able to overcome the unique resistance mechanisms of biofilm bacteria.

Evaluating the efficacy of an antibiotic against biofilm bacteria has proved to be difficult on many levels. Results from research using planktonic bacteria typically do not correlate with biofilm-growing bacteria for numerous reasons.[20] A dynamic biofilm model that mimics in vivo conditions and can be easily reproduced is currently lacking. Traditional minimum inhibitory concentration (MIC) values cannot be applied to biofilm bacteria, spawning new pharmacodynamic parameters, such as minimum biofilm inhibitory concentration and minimum biofilm eradication concentration.[21]

Rifampin is likely the most studied antibiotic agent against orthopaedic implant-related infections. After years of in vitro and animal model data showing rifampin's efficacy against biofilm infection, the first randomized controlled clinical trial was performed in 1998, showing the benefits of a ciprofloxacin and rifampin combination after initial débridement.[22-24] Rifampin, the most commonly used member of the rifamycin class, inhibits bacterial transcription by inhibiting DNA-dependent RNA polymerase.[25] Its efficacy on biofilm bacteria likely stems from its ability to enter the biofilm and bactericidal activity that is independent of active bacterial division, but the exact mechanism has not been elucidated.[26] Additional studies are needed to determine when a rifampin-containing regimen should be started because some studies have shown that success may depend on the age of the biofilm and bacterial load,[27] whereas others, including studies in 2020 and 2021, have shown little benefit in the addition of rifampin.[28,29]

Decades before the advent of the biofilm concept, local antibiotics were used in orthopaedic infections.[30] Shortly after that landmark study that looked at the addition of gentamicin to bone cement, gentamicin-containing polymethyl methacrylate (PMMA) beads were produced and the use of local antibiotics quickly became a common adjuvant to surgical débridement and systemic antibiotics. This method of antibiotic delivery has multiple advantages, including minimal risk of systemic toxicity despite reaching local antibiotic concentrations that can be 10 to 100 times greater than concurrent serum concentration.[31,32] These higher local levels are needed to overcome the higher MICs and minimum bactericidal concentrations (MBCs) of sessile biofilm bacteria. There are recommendations for the type and dose of local antibiotics used in BJIs,[33] and clinicians must be aware that multiple variables affect the rate of antibiotic elution, including the dose and combination of the chosen antibiotic or antibiotics, and also the type and porosity of the carrier. In addition, antibiotic elution is a finite process, and bacterial colonization of spacers can occur.[34]

BONE PENETRATION

When considering antibiotics for treatment, antibiotic penetration at the site of infection is one of the most critical characteristics that needs to be considered, especially for BJIs, with the goal being to achieve a bone concentration that exceeds the organism's MBC (**Table 2**). The MBC is defined as the lowest concentration of antibiotic required to kill 99.9% of the bacterial inoculum.

If the antibiotic is bactericidal, the MBC will be very close to the MIC, defined as the lowest concentration (mg/L or µg/µL) of antibiotic that inhibits visible in vitro growth of the organism. The difference between these two values will be slightly more for bacteriostatic drugs.[35] Specific antibiotic characteristics may lead to greater bone tissue penetrations, including a larger volume of distribution, ability to bind to calcium in inorganic bone material, lower protein binding, greater lipophilicity, and a more rapid equilibration rate of antibiotic concentration between bone and serum.[35] However, the relevance and interplay of these factors is not fully understood. For example, some studies have found unexpectedly lower bone-to-serum concentration with clavulanic acid despite its small molecule size and with ceftriaxone despite it being highly protein bound.[36,37] Population pharmacokinetic analysis has been suggested to be the most appropriate method to calculate antibiotic penetration in bone tissues because it incorporates the dose, duration of infusion, time of sample collection, and other interpatient variability.[35] Although population pharmacokinetic analysis has been proposed as optimal for understanding bone penetration, most studies use simplified pharmacokinetics/pharmacodynamic analyses to calculate the bone-to-serum concentration at a certain time after antibiotic administration.[35]

Low bone concentration relative to serum levels may still be overcome if the serum concentration is sufficiently high. For example, beta-lactam antibiotics have a serum-to-bone penetration ratio of 5% to 20%; however, patients with BJIs have been successfully treated with this class of antibiotics when administered intravenously, because the absolute bone concentration is still well above MICs.[38] Similarly, vancomycin has a comparable serum-to-bone penetration ratio as beta-lactam antibiotics, but availability of vancomycin therapeutic drug monitoring ensures that adequate drug concentrations needed to exceed MIC are reached.[38,39] As discussed in a 2019 study, antibiotics such as amoxicillin/clavulanate, piperacillin/tazobactam, cephalosporins, carbapenems, aztreonam, aminoglycosides, fluoroquinolones, tetracyclines, vancomycin, linezolid, daptomycin, clindamycin, trimethoprim/sulfamethoxazole, rifampin, dalbavancin, and oritavancin have been demonstrated to possess sufficient bone and joint tissue penetrations[40] (**Table 3**). Even though there are limitations on the available data used to evaluate the bone penetration of these antibiotics (which are further hampered by small sample size, variation in dosing strategies and timing of bone sampling, and sampling of healthy bone without vascular insufficiency), these antibiotics have been used successfully to treat BJIs.[38]

Table 2

Summary of Antibiotic Concentrations in Spongy Bone, Cortical Bone, and Joints

Antibiotic	Average Spongy Bone Concentration (µg/mL)	Average Cortical Bone Concentration (µg/mL)	Average Joint Concentration (µg/mL)
Penicillin G	Undetectable		NA
Amoxicillin/clavulanate	27.8/2.5	37.4/3.6	NA
Oxacillin	NA	4	3.4
Cloxacillin	NA	3.8	0.5
Dicloxacillin	NA	3.8	NA
Flucloxacillin	89.5	Detectable	NA
Piperacillin/tazobactam	40.5/Detectable	35.5/Detectable	69.9/7.7
Cefazolin	75.4	Detectable	112.2
Cephalexin	4.2		15.8
Cefadroxil	5.1		NA
Ceftriaxone	10.7		NA
Ceftazidime	32.1		NA
Cefepime	99.8	67.6	NA
Imipenem	NA	NA	13.8
Meropenem	10.6		12.5
Ertapenem	9.9	6.1	19.8
Aztreonam	16		83
Amikacin	Detectable		Detectable
Gentamicin	Detectable		Detectable
Ciprofloxacin	13.8		NA
Levofloxacin	10	4.6	8.9
Moxifloxacin	2.8		3.4
Doxycycline	3		NA
Vancomycin	3.8	4.5	NA
Daptomycin	21.4		21.6
Linezolid	6.4		> 4
Clindamycin	6.9		2
Trimethoprim/sulfamethoxazole	6.8/35.8		Detectable
Fosfomycin	NA		NA
Rifampin	6.5	1.3	NA
Metronidazole	5.6	5.7	5.6
Dalbavancin	13.4	4.2	NA
Oritavancin	27	65.6	NA

NA = not applicable

Modified with permission of International Society of Infectious Diseases from Thabit AK, Fatani DF, Bamakhrama MS, Barnawi OA, Basudan LO, Alhejaili SF: Antibiotic penetration into bone and joints: An updated review. *Int J Infect Dis* 2019;81:128-136.

Table 3

Oral Antibiotics With Good Bone Penetration

Amoxicillin
Amoxicillin/clavulanate
Dicloxacillin
Cephalexin
Ciprofloxacin
Levofloxacin
Moxifloxacin
Doxycycline
Clindamycin
Sulfamethoxazole/trimethoprim
Linezolid
Rifampin

Data from Thabit AK, Fatani DF, Bamakhrama MS, Barnawi OA, Basudan LO, Alhejaili SF: Antibiotic penetration into bone and joints: An updated review. *Int J Infect Dis* 2019;81:128-136.

BACTERICIDAL VERSUS BACTERIOSTATIC ANTIMICROBIAL THERAPY

Certain antibiotics are more likely to have bactericidal activity, killing the offending bacteria, whereas other antibiotics are considered to be bacteriostatic in vitro, defined as inhibiting the growth of organisms.[41] This has historically been one of the key factors to consider when selecting an antimicrobial regimen to treat patients with serious infections. However, according to a 2018 study, the meaning of bactericidal and bacteriostatic may be misunderstood by many clinicians: in fact, all antibiotics can be bactericidal if the drug concentrations are well above the MIC.[42] Furthermore, these characteristics are determined in vitro and can be influenced by the inoculum size, bacterial growth conditions, and test duration. Therefore, bactericidal and bacteriostatic activity may not be reproducible in vivo; antibiotics may exhibit different activity depending on drug concentration and organisms.[41]

BJIs have been considered to be severe infections for which antibiotics with known bactericidal activity would lead to better outcome in clinical practice.[41] However, this belief has been based on assumptions and on extrapolation of its misunderstood concept without clinical data.[43] There are two systematic review articles that evaluated the hypothesis of this theory. Between the two studies, severe infections such as endocarditis, meningitis, pneumonia, and bacteremia were included and demonstrated that there was no significant superiority in clinical outcomes when using antibiotics with bactericidal activity.[42,43] Therefore, clinicians should not solely focus on this concept but should consider other drug characteristics and factors such as pharmacokinetic/pharmacodynamic properties, dosing, and bone penetration to maximize treatment outcome.

ANTIBIOTIC ALLERGY

Choosing the ideal antibiotic or antibiotics for a patient requiring prophylaxis or treatment of a BJI is sometimes complicated by allergy, most commonly a listed penicillin allergy. Despite being self-reported in almost 10% of hospitalized patients, up to 90% of these patients are able to tolerate penicillins.[44-46] Unfortunately, the downstream negative effect of an unsubstantiated or antiquated penicillin allergy can be significant. In a 2018 large retrospective cohort study of more than 9,000 procedures, including hip and knee arthroplasties, the risk of a surgical site infection was 1.5 times higher in patients with a reported penicillin allergy, compared with their matched cohorts.[47] Patients with a reported penicillin allergy received possible suboptimal surgical prophylaxis with antibiotics such as vancomycin or clindamycin, instead of the standard-of-care beta-lactam antibiotics. The trend toward higher PJI rates in patients with a reported penicillin allergy has now been seen in multiple recent studies, including one cohort of more than 1.27 million patients.[48,49] Multiple tools have been used to successfully delabel a penicillin allergy, including skin testing, oral challenge, and allergy consultation.[50,51] A detailed evaluation of a patient's allergy list is essential to ensure that optimal therapy is selected whenever feasible.

OUTPATIENT PARENTERAL ANTIMICROBIAL THERAPY

Although intravenous antibiotic therapy historically necessitated long hospital stays, since its inception in the 1970s outpatient parenteral antimicrobial therapy (OPAT) has revolutionized the way infections are medically managed. The treatment of BJIs lends itself to the utilization of OPAT because the patients are relatively healthy with no need for an acute care setting other than antibiotic administration. Multiple studies have cited the wide-ranging benefits of an OPAT program. Patients report increased satisfaction with their plan of care when they can recover in their home environment and possibly return to work. Recent studies have reported that health care systems with OPAT programs have routinely demonstrated reduced lengths of stay, decreased total health care spending, and lower readmission rates.[52-54]

Although the most common indication for OPAT continues to be skin and soft-tissue infection, BJIs including osteomyelitis, septic arthritis, and PJIs account for the highest number of treatment days because each of these disease states typically require many weeks of therapy.[55] Multiple studies have demonstrated that success rates are high for BJIs managed through OPAT, and those poor treatment results (diabetic osteomyelitis) in BJIs are likely to occur because of the disease state itself.

SUMMARY

Treatment of BJIs requires not only knowledge about the potential causative organisms but also specific nuances about antibiotic bone penetration, effectiveness against biofilm organisms, possible altered vascular supply, and the presence of indwelling hardware. These complex cases often benefit from an interdisciplinary approach.

KEY STUDY POINTS

- Beyond the spectrum of activity, factors such as biofilm activity and bone penetration may affect antibiotic selection in BJIs.
- In general, antibiotics have limited efficacy against organisms contained in biofilm, necessitating higher antibiotic concentrations and surgical débridement.
- The understanding of bone penetration is limited, but data suggest that most antibiotics achieve bone levels sufficient for infection eradication.
- Most patients with a listed penicillin allergy can tolerate a cephalosporin.

ANNOTATED REFERENCES

1. Bratzler DW, Dellinger EP, Olsen KM, et al: Clinical practice guidelines for antimicrobial prophylaxis in surgery. *Surg Infect (Larchmt)* 2013;14(1):73-156.

2. Prokulski L: Prophylactic antibiotics in orthopaedic surgery. *J Am Acad Orthop Surg* 2008;16:283-293.

3. Young VB: The role of the microbiome in human health and disease: An introduction for clinicians. *BMJ* 2017;356:j831.

4. Siqueira MB, Saleh A, Klika AK, et al: Chronic suppression of periprosthetic joint infections with oral antibiotics increases infection-free survivorship. *J Bone Joint Surg Am* 2015;97(15):1220-1232.

5. Shah NB, Hersh BL, Kreger A, et al: Benefits and adverse events associated with extended antibiotic use in total knee arthroplasty periprosthetic joint infection. *Clin Infect Dis* 2020;70(4):559-565.

   Patients who received oral antibiotics after a débridement, antibiotics, and implant retention procedure for a total knee arthroplasty PJI had superior infection-free survival with no increase in adverse events. The ideal duration of oral antibiotics was 1 year. Level of evidence: III.

6. Diaz-Ledezma C, Higuera CA, Parvizi J: Success after treatment of periprosthetic joint infection: A Delphi-based international multidisciplinary consensus. *Clin Orthop Relat Res* 2013;471(7):2374-2382.

7. Bradbury T, Fehring TK, Taunton M, et al: The fate of acute methicillin-resistant Staphylococcus aureus periprosthetic knee infections treated by open debridement and retention of components. *J Arthroplasty* 2009;24(6 suppl):101-104.

8. Estes CS, Beauchamp CP, Clarke HD, Spangehl MJ: A two-stage retention débridement protocol for acute periprosthetic joint infections. *Clin Orthop Relat Res* 2010;468(8):2029-2038.

9. Tsai Y, Chang CH, Lin YC, Lee SH, Hsieh PH, Chang Y: Different microbiological profiles between hip and knee prosthetic joint infections. *J Orthop Surg (Hong Kong)* 2019;27(2):2309499019847768.

   S aureus is the most common causative pathogen in both hip and knee PJIs. Polymicrobial infections are more common in the hip and tend to occur in the early postoperative period. Level of evidence: IV.

10. Infectious Diseases Society of America: The 10 × '20 initiative: Pursuing a global commitment to develop 10 new antibacterial drugs by 2020. *Clin Infect Dis* 2010;50(8):1081-1083.

11. Bloem A, Bax HI, Yusuf E, Verkaik NJ: New-generation antibiotics for treatment of gram-positive infections: A review with focus on endocarditis and osteomyelitis. *J Clin Med* 2021;10(8):1743.

    In this review article, nine antibiotic agents with mostly gram-positive activity were evaluated. It is promising to have these novel agents as alternative options; however, clinical data on their use in osteomyelitis and PJI are lacking.

12. Johnson LB, Ramani A, Guervil DJ: Use of ceftaroline fosamil in osteomyelitis: CAPTURE study experience. *BMC Infect Dis* 2019;19(1):183.

    This is a retrospective registry study that was extended from a phase 4, multicenter, retrospective cohort study called Clinical Assessment Program and Teflaro Utilization Registry (CAPTURE). Of 150 patients with gram-positive osteomyelitis, overall clinical success was seen in 92.7% of patients who were treated with ceftaroline. In addition, 92.5% of patients with methicillin-resistant *S aureus* infection were successfully treated with ceftaroline and only two patients had adverse events that led to discontinuation of therapy. Level of evidence: IV.

13. Rodvold KA, Pai MP: Pharmacokinetics and pharmacodynamics of oral and intravenous omadacycline. *Clin Infect Dis* 2019;69(suppl 1):S16-S22.

    This study describes the pharmacokinetic and pharmacodynamic characteristics of a novel aminomethylcycline agent, omadacycline. This agent has been shown to have high tissue-to-blood ratio and is a promising alternative option in the management of BJI.

14. Jolliff JC, Ho J, Joson J, Heidari A, Johnson R: Treatment of polymicrobial osteomyelitis with ceftolozane-tazobactam: Case report and sensitivity testing of isolates. *Case Rep Infect Dis* 2016;2016:1628932.

15. Gentile I, Buonomo AR, Maraolo AE, et al: Successful treatment of post-surgical osteomyelitis caused by XDR pseudomonas aeruginosa with ceftolozane/tazobactam monotherapy. *J Antimicrob Chemother* 2017;72(9):2678-2679.

16. Fratoni AJ, Nicolau DP, Kuti JL: A guide to therapeutic drug monitoring of β-lactam antibiotics. *Pharmacotherapy* 2021;41(2):220-233.

17. Henrici AT: Studies of freshwater bacteria: I. A direct microscopic technique. *J Bacteriol* 1933;25(3):277-287.

18. Vert M, Doi Y, Hellwich KH, et al: Terminology for biorelated polymers and applications (IUPAC recommendations 2012). *Pure Appl Chem* 2012;84(2):377-410.

19. Rodríguez-Martínez JM, Ballesta S, Pascual Á: Activity and penetration of fosfomycin, ciprofloxacin, amoxicillin/clavulanic acid and co-trimoxazole in Escherichia coli and Pseudomonas aeruginosa biofilms. *Int J Antimicrob Agents* 2007;30(4):366-368.

20. Lebeaux D, Ghigo JM, Beloin C: Biofilm-related infections: Bridging the gap between clinical management and fundamental aspects of recalcitrance toward antibiotics. *Microbiol Mol Biol Rev* 2014;78(3):510-543.

21. Brady AJ, Laverty G, Gilpin DF, Kearney P, Tunney M: Antibiotic susceptibility of planktonic- and biofilm-grown staphylococci isolated from implant-associated infections: Should MBEC and nature of biofilm formation replace MIC? *J Med Microbiol* 2017;66(4):461-469.

22. Widmer AF, Frei R, Rajacic Z, Zimmerli W: Correlation between in vivo and in vitro efficacy of antimicrobial agents against foreign body infections. *J Infect Dis* 1990;162(1):96-102.

23. Zimmerli W, Frei R, Widmer AF, Rajacic Z: Microbiological tests to predict treatment outcome in experimental device-related infections due to Staphylococcus aureus. *J Antimicrob Chemother* 1994;33(5):959-967.

24. Zimmerli W, Widmer AF, Blatter M, Frei R, Ochsner PE: Role of rifampin for treatment of orthopedic implant-related staphylococcal infections: A randomized controlled trial. Foreign-Body Infection (FBI) Study Group. *J Am Med Assoc* 1998;279(19):1537-1541.

25. Phillips I: Clinical uses and control of rifampicin and clindamycin. *J Clin Pathol* 1971;24(5):410-418.

26. Zheng Z, Stewart PS: Penetration of rifampin through Staphylococcus epidermidis biofilms. *Antimicrob Agents Chemother* 2002;46(3):900-903.

27. Barberán J, Aguilar L, Carroquino G, et al: Conservative treatment of staphylococcal prosthetic joint infections in elderly patients. *Am J Med* 2006;119(11):993.e7-e10.

28. Karlsen ØE, Borgen P, Bragnes B, et al: Rifampin combination therapy in staphylococcal prosthetic joint infections: A randomized controlled trial. *J Orthop Surg Res* 2020;15(1):365.

This multicenter randomized controlled trial of 99 patients with acute staphylococcal PJIs did not show a benefit in the use of rifampin as a companion drug to standard antibiotic regimens.

29. Aydın O, Ergen P, Ozturan B, Ozkan K, Arslan F, Vahaboglu H: Rifampin-accompanied antibiotic regimens in the treatment of prosthetic joint infections: A frequentist and Bayesian meta-analysis of current evidence. *Eur J Clin Microbiol Infect Dis* 2021;40(4):665-671.

Thirteen observational studies were included in this random-effects meta-analysis to look at the evidence to support the use of rifampin in PJI caused by gram-positive organisms. This analysis was limited by the lack of randomized controlled trials, but the current evidence did not support the use of adjunctive rifampin.

30. Wahlig H, Buchholz HW: Experimental and clinical studies on the release of gentamicin from bone cement. *Chirurg* 1972;43(10):441-445.

31. Stravinskas M, Nilsson M, Horstmann P, Petersen MM, Tarasevicius S, Lidgren L: Antibiotic containing bone substitute in major hip surgery: A long term gentamicin elution study. *J Bone Jt Infect* 2018;3(2):68-72.

The elution of gentamicin from a ceramic bone substitute is compared to the elution from gentamicin containing poly bone cement.

32. Mutimer J, Gillespie G, Lovering AM, Porteous AJ: Measurements of in vivo intra-articular gentamicin levels from antibiotic loaded articulating spacers in revision total knee replacement. *Knee* 2009;16(1):39-41.

33. Porteus A, Squire MW, Geriner J: Question 3: What is the optimal antibiotic(s) dosage to be used in cement during reimplantation that does not significantly interfere with the mechanical strength of cement used for fixation? in Parvizi J, Gehrke T, eds: *Proceedings of the Second International Conference on Musculoskeletal Infection*. Data Trace Publishing Company, 2018, pp 304-307.

34. Nelson CL, Jones RB, Wingert NC, Foltzer M, Bowen TR: Sonication of antibiotic spacers predicts failure during two-stage revision for prosthetic knee and hip infections. *Clin Orthop Relat Res* 2014;472(7):2208-2214.

35. Landersdorfer CB, Bulitta JB, Kinzig M, Holzgrabe U, Sörgel F: Penetration of antibacterials into bone pharmacokinetic, pharmacodynamic and bioanalytical considerations. *Clin Pharmacokinet* 2009;48(2):89-124.

36. Adam D, Heilmann HD, Weismeier K: Concentrations of ticarcillin and clavulanic acid in human bone after prophylactic administration of 5.2 g of timentin. *Antimicrob Agents Chemother* 1987;31(6):935-939.

37. Lovering A, Walsh T, Bannister G, MacGowan A: The penetration of ceftriaxone and cefamandole into bone, fat and haematoma and relevance of serum protein binding to their penetration into bone. *J Antimicrob Chemother* 2001;47(4):483-486.

38. Spellberg B, Lipsky BA: Systemic antibiotic therapy for chronic osteomyelitis in adults. *Clin Infect Dis* 2012;54(3):393-407.

39. Rybak MJ, Le J, Lodise TP, et al: Therapeutic monitoring of vancomycin for serious methicillin-resistant Staphylococcus aureus infections: A revised consensus guideline and review by the American Society of Health-System Pharmacists, the Infectious Diseases Society of America, the Pediatric Infectious Diseases Society, and the Society of Infectious Diseases Pharmacists. *Am J Health Syst Pharm* 2020;77(11):835-864.

The updated consensus guideline for vancomycin monitoring strategies to treat serious methicillin-resistant *S aureus* infections including osteomyelitis suggested a goal area under the curve/MIC ratio of 400 to 600 to optimize efficacy and minimize nephrotoxicity instead of trough-based monitoring.

40. Thabit AK, Fatani DF, Bamakhrama MS, Barnawi OA, Basudan LO, Alhejaili SF: Antibiotic penetration into bone and joints: An updated review. *Int J Infect Dis* 2019;81:128-136.

    This review article evaluated the clinical outcomes and extent of bone and joint tissue penetration of more than 30 antibiotics. Most antibiotics showed good bone and joint tissue penetration based on pharmacokinetics studies; however, not all antibiotics reviewed in this study had clinical studies in osteomyelitis and septic arthritis.

41. Pankey GA, Sabath LD: Clinical relevance of bacteriostatic versus bactericidal mechanisms of action in the treatment of Gram-positive bacterial infections. *Clin Infect Dis* 2004;38(6):864-870.

42. Wald-Dickler N, Holtom P, Spellberg B: Busting the myth of "static vs cidal": A systemic literature review. *Clin Infect Dis* 2018;66(9):1470-1474.

    This systematic review article evaluated the clinical efficacy and outcome of treating infections with bacteriostatic compared with bactericidal agents. Of 56 published trials, 49 studies (87.5%) were found to have no significant difference in efficacy.

43. Nemeth J, Oesch G, Kuster SP: Bacteriostatic versus bactericidal antibiotics for patients with serious bacterial infections: Systematic review and meta-analysis. *J Antimicrob Chemother* 2015;70(2):382-395.

44. Macy E: Penicillin and beta-lactam allergy: Epidemiology and diagnosis. *Curr Allergy Asthma Rep* 2014;14(11):476-477.

45. Apter AJ, Schelleman H, Walker A, Addya K, Rebbeck T: Clinical and genetic risk factors of self-reported penicillin allergy. *J Allergy Clin Immunol* 2008;122(1):152-158.

46. Joint Task Force on Practice Parameters, American Academy of Allergy Asthma and Immunology, American College of Allergy, Asthma and Immunology, Joint Council of Allergy, Asthma and Immunology: Drug allergy: An updated practice parameter. *Ann Allergy Asthma Immunol* 2010;105(4):259-273.

47. Blumenthal KG, Ryan EE, Li Y, Lee H, Kuhlen JL, Shenoy ES: The impact of a reported penicillin allergy on surgical site infection risk. *Clin Infect Dis* 2018;66(3):329-336.

    In this study of 8,385 patients undergoing various surgical procedures, 922 (11%) reported a penicillin allergy. When adjusting for age, race, surgery type, American Society of Anesthesiologists score, procedure duration, and wound class, the reported penicillin allergy was associated with increased odds of a surgical site infection. Level of evidence: III.

48. Wyles CC, Hevesi M, Osmon DR, et al: 2019 John Charnley Award: Increased risk of prosthetic joint infection following primary total knee and hip arthroplasty with the use of alternative antibiotics to cefazolin – The value of allergy testing for antibiotic prophylaxis. *Bone Joint J* 2019;101-B(6 suppl B):9-15.

    A total of 2,576 patients with a reported penicillin allergy who were undergoing primary arthroplasties underwent preoperative antibiotic testing. Of the total, 97% of these patients were cleared to take a cephalosporin. The risk of a PJI was 32% lower in patients who were able to be treated with cefazolin. Level of evidence: III.

49. Wu VJ, Iloanya MC, Sanchez FL, et al: Is patient-reported penicillin allergy independently associated with increased risk of prosthetic joint infection after total joint arthroplasty of the hip, knee, and shoulder? *Clin Orthop Relat Res* 2020;478(12):2699-2709.

    Patients who report a penicillin allergy have an increased risk of a PJI after total knee arthroplasty and total shoulder arthroplasty. This trend was not seen after total hip arthroplasty. Level of evidence: III.

50. Ramsey A: Penicillin allergy and perioperative anaphylaxis. *Front Allergy* 2022;3:903161.

    This review discusses the epidemiology of penicillin allergy, how to treat the patient with penicillin allergy, and various techniques that can be used to successfully delabel a patient with penicillin allergy.

51. Savic L, Gurr L, Kaura V, et al: Penicillin allergy de-labelling ahead of elective surgery: Feasibility and barriers. *Br J Anaesth* 2019;123(1):e110-e116.

    Incorporation of a direct oral challenge can be successful in delabeling penicillin allergies in a surgical preassessment clinic.

52. Mahoney MV, Ryan KL, Alexander BT: Evaluation of OPAT in the age of antimicrobial stewardship. *Curr Treat Options Infect Dis* 2020;12(2):158-177.

    This review examines antimicrobial stewardship and OPAT and highlights principles that are relevant to both.

53. Matthews PC, Conlon CP, Berendt AR, et al: Outpatient parenteral antimicrobial therapy (OPAT): Is it safe for selected patients to self-administer at home? A retrospective analysis of a large cohort over 13 years. *J Antimicrob Chemother* 2007;60(2):356-362.

54. Schrank GM, Wright SB, Branch-Elliman W, Lasalvia MT: A retrospective analysis of adverse events among patients receiving daptomycin versus vancomycin during outpatient parenteral antimicrobial therapy. *Infect Control Hosp Epidemiol* 2018;39(8):947-954.

    In this single-center, retrospective observational cohort study, patients received either daptomycin or vancomycin via an OPAT program. Patients receiving vancomycin had a higher rate of adverse drug events, but rates of readmission were similar between the two groups. Level of evidence: III.

55. Tice A: The use of outpatient parenteral antimicrobial therapy in the management of osteomyelitis: Data from the outpatient parenteral antimicrobial therapy outcomes registries. *Chemotherapy* 2001;47(suppl 1):5-16.

CHAPTER 12

Local Antibiotic Delivery Methods

NIALL COCHRANE, MD • TAYLOR STAUFFER, BS • JONATHON M. FLORANCE, MD
PATRICK KELLY, MD • THORSTEN M. SEYLER, MD, PhD, FAAOS

ABSTRACT

The use of local antibiotic delivery systems has become an accepted treatment method that continues to evolve. These systems can achieve high local concentrations of antibiotics, which is desirable in the typical infected, avascular wound environment. Certain delivery systems also have osteoinductive and osteoconductive materials that can aid in bone regeneration. Despite their rapid acceptance in recent years, there remain many unanswered questions related to their use. First and most importantly, both local tissue and systemic toxicity have been associated with high antibiotic levels in the tissue. Additional research to standardize the types of antibiotics, loading doses, mixing methods, and elution kinetics will improve antimicrobial efficacy in these systems going forward.

Keywords: antibiotics; cement; local delivery; orthopaedic infections

---

Dr. Seyler or an immediate family member has received royalties from Pattern Health and Restor3d; serves as a paid consultant to or is an employee of Heraeus, Smith & Nephew, and Total Joint Orthopedics, Inc.; has received research or institutional support from Next Science and Zimmer; and serves as a board member, owner, officer, or committee member of American Association of Hip and Knee Surgeons and Musculoskeletal Infection Society. None of the following authors or any immediate family member has received anything of value from or has stock or stock options held in a commercial company or institution related directly or indirectly to the subject of this chapter: Dr. Cochrane, Taylor Stauffer, Dr. Florence, and Dr. Kelly.

INTRODUCTION

Several techniques for local antibiotic delivery exist including the implantation of both bioabsorbable and nonbioabsorbable carriers. Antibiotic cement, including spacers and beads, comprise most of the nonbiodegradable implants used, whereas antibiotic-impregnated calcium sulfate beads and chitosans are degradable implants that can be left in the surgical wound. The basic principles of local antibiotic delivery, including different carriers used for local delivery, their mechanism of action, and indications and contraindications are highlighted.

ORTHOPAEDIC INFECTIONS

Infections are a devastating complication in the field of orthopaedic surgery, with a 2019 study reporting incidences varying from less than 1% to more than 15%, depending on the surgical procedure performed.[1] They can occur after both elective and nonelective surgery and are commonly seen with the use of orthopaedic implants. Infections require significant time and resources to control and are associated with high rates of morbidity and mortality.[2] As the number of surgeries using implantable hardware continues to increase, the relative infection rates will increase as well.[3] Treatment of orthopaedic infections is both invasive and expensive and commonly includes surgical débridement, implant removal, systemic antibiotic therapy, and local antibiotic delivery.[1,2,4] Local antibiotic therapy can be a critical component in the treatment of certain orthopaedic infections and may be necessary for the delivery of therapeutic levels of antibiotics to the target tissue, particularly in settings of reduced vascularity.[5-7]

HISTORY

There is a long history of local antibiotic use in the treatment of orthopaedic infections.[8] The first study that described the use of antibiotic beads used gentamicin-impregnated cement to create antibiotic beads and temporarily fill dead space created after the débridement of infected bone, reporting a 91.4% cure rate in patients treated for chronic osteomyelitis.[9] After this report, interest in the use of antibiotic-impregnated cement beads increased precipitously, despite persistent controversy regarding their proof of efficacy and safety.[8] Currently, antibiotic beads are used in conjunction with systemic antibiotic therapy to provide high local antibiotic concentrations in patients with orthopaedic infections. Although nonbiodegradable systems of local antibiotic delivery are widely used, there is some concern they can attract glycocalyx-producing bacteria and act as a surface for bacterial colonization. Thus, there has more recently been an effort to develop biodegradable antibiotic carrier systems, including the use of antibiotic-containing calcium sulfate preparations and chitosans in the surgical wound.

CARRIERS AND MECHANISMS

Polymethyl Methacrylate

Nonbiodegradable polymethyl methacrylate (PMMA) cement is the most common carrier used for antibiotic delivery and has been the gold standard for decades. PMMA is fabricated by mixing a polymer powder with a monomer liquid, resulting in an exothermic polymerization reaction that creates solid cement.[10] It can be used as a solid spacer or broken up into smaller antibiotic beads to be placed in a soft-tissue void. The antibiotic used in the cement must be water soluble, available as powder, and able to remain intact during the exothermic polymerization reaction. Antibiotic-impregnated PMMA has been an effective method for providing sustained high concentrations of antibiotics locally. The success of these carriers stems from the lack of any immune response from the host and the rapid yet sustained release of antibiotics from the cement.

After the PMMA cement is deployed in tissues, antibiotic release occurs in two phases.[1] The initial release of antibiotics, called burst release, occurs minutes to hours after implantation. This burst release is a surface phenomenon where the antibiotics in the surface dissolve out of the cement and into the surrounding tissue. It results in a high concentration of antibiotics in the surrounding tissue. The second phase, called sustained release, occurs for at least several days after implantation. Water-soluble antibiotics diffuse out of the PMMA after depth penetration of the water containing body fluids, which results in prolonged, lower concentration of antibiotics.[1,11]

Many studies have demonstrated that the pharmacokinetic release profiles of PMMA can be optimized by adjusting several properties of the PMMA. First, increasing the surface roughness and the porosity of the PMMA results in an expansion of the surface area, leading to an increased antibiotic release.[12] Second, hand mixing the PMMA instead of vacuum mixing increases its porosity, which leads to a more robust release of antibiotics.[13] Finally, adding polymeric fillers (eg, xylitol and glycine) and using highly water-soluble substances both increase the dissolution capacity of antibiotics from PMMA.[14]

Antibiotic-impregnated PMMA can be used in either antibiotic spacers or bead molds. Bead molds are available in a variety of sizes, ranging from 2 to 8 mm. Consistency in size and shape of the beads facilitates their passage into tight spaces, including the medullary canal. In vitro and in vivo studies have shown that smaller PMMA beads increase the release of antibiotics by increasing the surface area of cement. These so-called minibeads (3 × 5 mm instead of 7 × 7 mm) release up to 93% of the added antibiotics (versus 24% in normal PMMA beads) and achieve antibiotic concentrations up to seven times higher compared with normal PMMA beads. These minibeads have a similar antibiotic release period with sufficient release concentrations in comparison with the normal PMMA beads.[9]

One study demonstrated that wound closure after implantation of gentamicin-PMMA chains increases the local concentrations of antibiotic achieved by 200 times when compared with systemic antibiotic administration alone.[15] In contrast, use of the beads in an open system or in combination with suction irrigation has been shown to lower local antibiotic concentrations and diminish their therapeutic advantage. PMMA beads also allow the surgeon to fill the infected cavity and reduce dead space. This increases surface area for antibiotic release when compared with a solid PMMA plug.[16,17] It also reduces hematoma collection, which results in a higher local antibiotic concentration.

Calcium Sulfate

Calcium sulfate has been used extensively as a bioabsorbable bone substitute for more than 90 years.[18] It was first used in the form of plaster of paris in 1892 by Dreesmann to pack bone defects. Water-soluble antibiotics can be incorporated into its crystalline structure and delivered in vivo.

Its advantages include its low cost, ready availability, and unlimited supply. In addition, it has inherent osteoconductive properties and may facilitate bone growth. Other advantages of calcium sulfate beads are that, unlike the PMMA type, they typically dissolve and do not need to be removed surgically. Furthermore, they do not generate heat when formed, allowing antibiotics to be used, which otherwise would not survive the exothermic reaction that occurs in PMMA. They have been shown in the literature to be effective in the treatment of osteomyelitis, PJI, and the prevention of infection after open fractures.

Calcium sulfate is a carrier composed of a few trace elements with a uniform crystalline structure similar to bone and predictable antibiotic elution rates.[19] The main advantage of calcium sulfate as a carrier lies in its osteoconductive properties, allowing normal physiologic $CaSO_4$ absorption with concomitant deposition of autogenous cancellous bone. Specifically, the precipitation of calcium with local phosphate ions creates an osteoconductive microscaffold for bone deposition. In addition, dissolution of the substrate leads to local acidification, conferring antimicrobial action that can be further augmented with incorporation of antibiotics.[20] A 2021 study of in vitro draining knee model found that elution kinetics of calcium sulfate might improve with addition of PMMA, increasing the area under the curve after 2 hours.[21]

Chitosans

Chitosan, a polymerized D-glucosamine polysaccharide, is able to act as a drug carrier and also has intrinsic antibacterial and antifungal activity. Chitosan is obtained by alkaline deacetylation of chitin and is one of the most abundant polysaccharides in nature, second only to cellulose. It has two types of antibacterial property. First, its positive charge reacts with negatively charged molecules at the surface of cells, altering cell permeability and thereby preventing the material from entering the intracellular space. Second, chitosan is able to bind to DNA to inhibit RNA synthesis.[22,23]

The antimicrobial activity of chitosan is based on electrostatic interactions between positively charged chitosan and the negatively charged components of the bacterial cell membrane, such as the anionic cell wall of glycans and proteins or phospholipids in the cytoplasmic membrane. Chitosan adheres to the anionic macromolecules of the bacterial cell wall (found in gram-positive organisms), forming an impermeable layer around the cell and preventing transport of nutrients into and out of the cell. In contrast, among gram-negative organisms, chitosan interacts with the bacterial cell membrane constituents, altering its permeability and leading to the leakage of intracellular electrolytes, glucose, enzymes, and other cytoplasmic materials.[22] Drug elution from chitosans is determined by the amount of cross-linkage, the size of the implant, and the initial drug content. The speed at which cross-linked chitosan gel degrades has been shown to be several times slower than that of non–cross-linked chitosan.[22]

Antibiotic Powder

The use of antibiotic powder administered locally without a carrier is a low-cost intervention that can be used for both infection prophylaxis and treatment. It can be used with several antibiotic combinations and has been used as an adjunct to many other local delivery mechanisms detailed in this chapter. The use of antibiotic powder for both infection prevention and treatment has been shown to be effective without significant adverse effects for many orthopaedic conditions including open fractures, osteomyelitis, prevention of surgical site infections after spine surgery, and PJI.

ANTIBIOTIC SELECTION

Antibiotic selection for local delivery is complicated, and available in vitro studies provide contradictory results. In general, the surgeon should select an antibiotic to which the known or likely pathogen is susceptible. However, bacterial sensitivities are based on systemic administration and consider whether the drug when administered systemically can achieve levels sufficient to exceed the minimum inhibitory concentration for that organism at the site of infection. There are limited data on organism sensitivity when antibiotics are administered locally and on how the high initial concentration of antibiotics followed by sustained lower levels seen after initial elution affects bacterial resistance patterns.[24,25]

Each antibiotic has a different pharmacokinetic release profile from PMMA. Certain antibiotics are not heat stable and thus do not release in an intact bioactive form after the exothermic hardening process of PMMA.[26-28] The literature has consistently demonstrated good release rates for aminoglycosides and glycopeptides.[29]

Aminoglycosides such as gentamicin and tobramycin are the most commonly used antibiotics in PMMA. They are effective against aerobic gram-negative bacilli and staphylococci, with more limited activity against streptococci and enterococci.[30] There is extensive information on the elution patterns of aminoglycosides from cement in a variety of clinical scenarios.[31] Studies have shown that between 13% and 29% of gentamicin is eluted from antibiotic cement.[28] Vancomycin should be considered when there is a risk a gram-positive infection. Vancomycin is available in powder form and in a 2020 review was not neutralized by the heat of PMMA polymerization.[32] In 2019, the addition of vancomycin to aminoglycoside in cement spacers was shown to reduce the rate of positive cultures at reimplantation.[33] A comprehensive list of antibiotics used in beads can be found in **Table 1**.

If the infecting organisms are known before surgery, organism sensitivities should be considered in antibiotic selection. In addition, consultation with infectious disease and pharmacy colleagues is recommended when choosing the proper drug and dosing to use in the local delivery system of choice.

Table 1

Commonly Used Antibiotics in Polymethyl Methacrylate and Calcium Sulfate Beads

	Spectrum	Suggested Doses[a]	Notes
Aminoglycosides			
Tobramycin[b], Gentamicin[b]	Gram-negative aerobic bacteria	1-4.8 g	Commonly used in the United States
Glycopeptides			
Vancomycin[b]	Gram-positive	0.5-4.0 g	—
Cephalosporins			
Cefazolin	Spectrum varies by generation and specific antimicrobial, with greater gram-positive activity in earlier generation cephalosporins and greater gram-negative activity in third-generation and fourth-generation cephalosporins	1.0-2.0 g	Not commonly used in cement
Macrolides			
Clindamycin	Many gram-positives; anaerobes	1.0-2.0 g	Commonly used with gentamicin
Monobactams			
Aztreonam	Aerobic gram-negative organisms	4.0 g	—
Fluoroquinolones			
Ciprofloxacin	Gram-negative and some gram-positive organisms	0.2-3.0 g	Some concerns for osteocyte toxicity
Antifungal Agents			
Amphotericin	Most yeast and molds	100-200 mg	During production, covalent cross-linkage may result in poor drug release from the bone cement
Voriconazole	Most yeast forms	200-1,000 mg	Not water soluble

[a]Dosing for calcium sulfate is less well established; however, typical administration is per 40 g PMMA pack and 10 mL of calcium sulfate.
[b]Most common in polymethyl methacrylate (PMMA) beads.
Data from Schwarz EM, Parvizi J, Gehrke T, et al: 2018 International consensus meeting on musculoskeletal infection: Research priorities from the general assembly questions. *J Orthop Res* 2019;37(5):997-1006.

CLINICAL SCENARIOS

Antibiotic cement can be used in multiple different applications. Typical indications include infection prevention after open fractures, treatment of established bone infection (ie, acute and chronic osteomyelitis), treatment of prosthetic joint infections (PJIs), and dead space management in patients after débridement with large soft-tissue voids.[34] A complete list of indications and contraindications can be found in **Table 2**.

Orthopaedic Trauma

There is significant evidence in the literature suggesting that local antibiotic delivery systems are effective in preventing infection after orthopaedic trauma, with both animal and clinical studies demonstrating benefits of the use of antibiotics after open fractures.[34-37] These systems can be used both for infection prevention at the time of surgery and if a wound becomes infected after initial treatment. Antibiotics can be administered through coating of an implant (intramedullary nail or plate), antibiotic beads, antibiotic powder before closure, or a two-stage foreign-body membrane technique.

One study demonstrated a 90% prevention rate in the development of osteomyelitis following contamination with *Staphylococcus aureus* after insertion of gentamicin-loaded cement.[37] Another study reported a significant reduction in the bacterial count of *S aureus* after the

Table 2

Clinical Applications for the Use of Local Antibiotic Delivery Systems

Trauma
Open fractures (infection prevention)
Limb salvage

Infection
Prosthetic joint infection
Osteomyelitis
Biofilm
Soft-tissue infection

Other
Large soft-tissue defects
Prevention of infection in spine surgery

---

insertion of tobramycin-loaded beads in a canine model.[38] Finally, a study comparing the addition of an antibiotic bead pouch versus systemic antibiotics alone in preventing infection in 1,085 open fractures reported infection rates of 3.7% in patients treated with the antibiotic bead pouch in addition to systemic antibiotics, compared with 12% in patients treated with systemic antibiotics alone.[36]

Antibiotic powder can also be used for infection prevention after open fractures. An open-label randomized clinical trial performed in 2021 at 36 US trauma centers enrolled adult patients with a surgically treated tibial plateau or pilon fracture who met the criteria for a high risk of infection.[39] Patients enrolled were given vancomycin powder at the time of definitive fracture fixation. Within 182 days, deep surgical site infection was observed in only 29 of 481 patients in the treatment group and 46 of 499 patients in the control group, and the authors concluded that use of antibiotic-laden powder decreased the risk of a gram-positive deep surgical site infection. Additional studies evaluating results of local antibiotic delivery in orthopaedic trauma[17,18,32,35,40-45] can be found in **Table 3**.

Because critical-sized segmental defects continue to pose significant clinical challenges for both patients and clinicians, an innovative technique has been increasingly studied for the treatment of bony defects caused by resection of infected tissue. The Masquelet technique capitalizes on the existing foreign-body reaction in the presence of a PMMA spacer to induce formation of a pseudosynovial fibrous membrane that expresses multiple bone morphogenic proteins.[46,47] This not only promotes osseous healing but also provides a physical barrier against microbes to aid in infection resolution. Although the employment of a foreign-body membrane that supports tissue regeneration has the potential to shift patient care paradigms, the scientific study of this technique is just beginning.

Osteomyelitis

The infective nidus of osteomyelitis harbors a bacterial matrix that is relatively impermeable to antibiotics and requires radical débridement for treatment. Radical débridement often leaves a tissue void that, if not filled, will lead to fluid accumulation that can become a nidus for repeat bacterial contamination.[39] Studies have demonstrated the utility of antibiotic beads in the management of chronic osteomyelitis. One study further corroborated the effectiveness of PMMA beads after demonstrating a 100% union rate in patients with chronic osteomyelitis and bony defects who underwent débridement, systemic antibiotics, and bead placement.[48] Another article compared three treatment modalities for chronic osteomyelitis as follows: débridement with placement of antibiotic beads alone, débridement with systemic antibiotic therapy alone, and débridement with both placement of antibiotic beads and systemic antibiotic therapy.[49] A 100% cure rate was reported in patients who underwent débridement with placement of antibiotic beads and systemic antibiotic therapy, although this was not significantly superior to either treatment administered alone.

Biodegradable implants can also be used for local delivery of antibiotics and have shown promising early results in animal studies. Chitosan alone has been shown to reduce the rate of infection of *S aureus* in experimental models of osteomyelitis. Borate glass in combination with chitosans has also provided some interesting data. One author implanted a teicoplanin-loaded borate glass–chitosan composite in rabbits with methicillin-resistant *S aureus* osteomyelitis and showed that infection was cleared in 85%, compared with 43% in patients treated with a 4-week course of intravenous teicoplanin. Of note is the fact that a borate glass–chitosan composite without antibiotics cleared infection in only 21% of cases, adding weight to the argument that antibiotics and chitosan work synergistically.[50] Additional studies evaluating results of local antibiotic delivery in osteomyelitis can be found in **Table 3**.

Calcium sulfate beads have also been demonstrated to be of use in osteomyelitis because of the osteoconductive scaffold, which is beneficial for concomitant bone defects. A 2022 meta-analysis demonstrated that antibiotic-loaded calcium sulfate leads to a 92% overall eradication rate of chronic osteomyelitis, with no difference between tobramycin or vancomycin and gentamicin with regard to eradication and postoperative complications.[40]

Prosthetic Joint Infections

Antibiotic-loaded cement is used in total joint arthroplasty as both a prophylactic strategy to prevent PJI and a method of local antibiotic delivery for the treatment of

Table 3

Outcomes of Local Antibiotic Delivery

	Type of Study	Objective	Major Findings
Prosthetic Joint Infection			
Abosala and Ali 2020	Systematic review	Review the use of $CaSO_4$ beads in knee and hip PJI	$CaSO_4$ beads can accommodate heat-stable and non–heat-stable antibiotics and have favorable outcomes when used as an adjuvant to PJI revision rather than DAIR. Higher complication rates are associated with increased bead use.
Calanna et al 2019	Report on surgical technique	Explain novel DAPRI technique in knee PJI	The DAPRI technique, using absorbable $CaSO_4$ beads and other augmenting procedures, allows for prolonged antibiotic concentration and can help fight biofilm, which might represent a safe, nonsurgical treatment for acute PJI.
Chung et al 2019	Retrospective review	Determine success rate of two-stage DAIR with antibiotic beads for hip and knee PJI compared with single-stage DAIR ($n = 83$)	The two-stage DAIR protocol resulted in a success rate of 86.7% infection control at a mean follow-up of 41.8 months, which is higher than that reported for single-stage DAIR procedures (52%).
Tarity et al 2022	Matched retrospective cohort	Compare postoperative infection rate after DAIR for hip and knee PJI in patients with and without antibiotic $CaSO_4$ beads ($n = 40$)	No significant differences between the use of dissolvable $CaSO_4$ beads and matched control group for infection-related failure at 2 years or 90 days postoperatively.
Osteomyelitis			
Patel et al 2021	Retrospective review	Explore efficacy of PMMA beads in patients with osteomyelitis ($n = 82$)	Antibiotic-loaded PMMA beads are effective in treatment of chronic osteomyelitis and in preventing infection recurrence, with only 7.9% recurrence in patients with gentamicin- and cefuroxime-loaded beads.
Thahir et al 2022	Systematic review	Evaluate the use of $CaSO_4$ beads in osteomyelitis of the femur and tibia	Cumulative infection recurrence rates for $CaSO_4$ beads were 6.9% versus 21.2% in PMMA beads. Wound drainage complication rates were higher in treatment of tibial osteomyelitis.
Shi et al 2022	Meta-analysis	Gather evidence on infection eradication rate with the use of antibiotic-loaded $CaSO_4$ beads for osteomyelitis	Antibiotic-loaded $CaSO_4$ leads to a 92% overall eradication rate of chronic osteomyelitis, with no difference between tobramycin or vancomycin and gentamicin.
Trauma			
Burtt et al 2020	Retrospective review	Evaluate efficacy of NPWT versus antibiotic beads in open lower extremity fractures requiring soft-tissue coverage ($n = 73$)	Antibiotic beads were associated with a decreased risk of infection compared with NPWT (6.4% versus 30.7%, $P = 0.01$). NPWT was associated with increased risk of complications (45.7% versus 4.2%, $P = 0.001$).
Fernando et al 2020	Retrospective review	Assess outcomes in patients with PMMA beads after retention versus removal in extremity or pelvic fracture ($n = 51$)	Of the 35 patients who did not undergo bead removal (73%), there were no wound complications at long-term follow-up (mean, 35 weeks). Routine removal of PMMA beads is not necessary in most patients with pelvis or extremity fractures.

Table 3

Outcomes of Local Antibiotic Delivery (Continued)

Soft Tissue	Type of Study	Objective	Major Findings
Gorvetzian et al 2019	Retrospective review	Determine the use of absorbable $CaSO_4$ antibiotic beads in chronic wound soft-tissue infection (n = 60)	There is diminished all-cause repeat surgical burden for wounds following surgery using antibiotic beads, possibly attributed to reduced biofilm formation. Rate of revision surgery decreased from 1.7 before $CaSO_4$ bead surgery to 0.05 after $CaSO_4$ bead surgery ($P < 0.001$).

DAIR = débridement, antibiotics, and implant retention, DAPRI = débridement, antibiotic pearls, and retention of implant, NPWT = negative pressure wound therapy, PJI = prosthetic joint infection, PMMA = polymethyl methacrylate

PJI. In European countries, the use of antibiotic-loaded cement is common in both primary and revision arthroplasty for infection prevention; however, in the United States, it is only approved for revision arthroplasty.[1] In the setting of infection prophylaxis in arthroplasty, a lower concentration of antibiotics is typically used when compared with treatment applications. Because antibiotics decrease the biomechanical strength of PMMA, the use of antimicrobial cement may interfere with optimal prosthesis fixation.[51] In the treatment of PJI, however, the purpose of antibiotics within the cement is local delivery and infection eradication. As the device is not used for definitive implant fixation and long-term weight bearing, the antibiotic concentrations within temporary cement spacers are much higher.[52] Antibiotics can be used in both cement spacers and within beads that are left within the surgical wound after débridement.

Antibiotic cement spacers can be either static or articulating. Static spacers in the knee provide for a relatively firm arthrodesis between the distal femur and proximal tibia. After removal of the infected components, two to four packages of PMMA (with variable amounts of admixed heat-stable antibiotics, usually tobramycin and vancomycin) are prepared on the back table. This cement is then placed in the manually held gap between the distal femur and proximal tibia and is then gently compressed to form an arthrodesis. Before this, two antibiotic cement dowels are prepared by hand, with or without a metal rod within the cement dowel, and placed into the intramedullary canals of the femur and tibia. In contrast, a 2020 review reported that articulating spacers enable range of motion; a wide variety of modern articulating or mobile spacers are available including handmade cement-on-cement spacer, premolded articulating spacers, surgical molds for intraoperative fabrication, and cement-on–new metal and polyethylene components.[53]

Antibiotic beads not only assist with local antimicrobial therapy but are also useful for proper dead space and soft-tissue management. Two 2019 publications reported that antibiotic beads can fill both bony and soft-tissue defects after surgery, which aids in the reduction of hematoma burden, and ultimately increases tissue penetration of the local antibiotics.[41,42] A 2020 meta-analysis reviewed the use of antibiotic beads in the treatment of PJI and reported favorable outcomes when used as an adjuvant to revision arthroplasty in PJI.[32] However, there was an increase in complications when a higher volume of beads was used, especially in subcutaneous structures in high-risk patients. Another study reviewed a novel technique of two-stage débridement with implant retention for PJI.[42] In this technique, antibiotic beads were placed during the first stage and retained until the second stage. A higher likelihood of infection control was reported with this novel technique when compared with single-stage débridement with implant retention. These results were contrasted by a study that demonstrated that the addition of antibiotic beads did not improve infection eradication after irrigation and débridement with implant retention.[54] Additional studies evaluating results of local antibiotic delivery in PJI can be found in **Table 3**.

Contraindications

Despite their wide use currently in the treatment of orthopaedic infections, contraindications to the use of local antibiotic delivery systems do exist. First, the surgeon must ensure that there are no known allergies to the antimicrobials being used within the local carrier system. With respect to antibiotic beads, patients with small wounds that cannot accommodate the size of cement beads or with incisions that cannot be closed should not have beads placed. In infections due to highly resistant organisms, local antibiotic delivery may not be feasible if a suitable drug to which the organism is sensitive cannot be identified. Finally, antibiotic beads should be removed after several weeks as the concentration of antibiotics decreases and as the beads themselves can form a local substratum for bacterial inoculation.[55,56] Although this is not an absolute contraindication, patients who are not candidates for a second surgery should not have antibiotic beads placed. Antibiotics themselves also pose a risk to patients with preexisting comorbidities. For example, the nephrotoxic effects of vancomycin, gentamicin, and other aminoglycosides have been demonstrated, even when in local delivery forms.[57,58] Although there are limited data and no clear contraindications, it has been suggested proceed cautiously with patients with preexisting kidney disease.

COMPLICATIONS

As with any orthopaedic procedure, complications related to the use of local antibiotic delivery systems have been reported. The highest risk of complications associated with local antibiotic delivery stems from the antibiotics themselves. The optimal dose, duration of treatment, and relative efficacy of various antibiotic classes when used in bone cement are not known. Although cement produced by manufacturers are usually premade with one antibiotic agent, surgeons will often mix additional antibiotics into the cement batch intraoperatively. The variability in cement construction practices can result in high antibiotic concentrations in the cement and lead to both local and systemic toxicity.

Spacers

There are several complications related to the use of antibiotic cement spacers. Spacer fracture and dislocation have both been reported in the literature. In addition, radiographic mechanical failure has been reported in several studies. The surgical technique for cementing mobile spacers requires adequate stability for weight-bearing ambulation and range of motion but avoids such deep penetration of cement into the bone. Adequate fixation to bone is necessary to avoid extrusion of the components, which can make removal in the second stage of the procedure very difficult.[42] Finally, supratherapeutic aminoglycoside levels have been demonstrated to cause nephrotoxicity in several studies evaluating the use of antibiotic cement spacers.[59]

Beads

Complications regarding the use of antibiotic beads are also uncommon. There are reports in the literature that the difficulty of bead removal increases significantly when beads are left in place too long. In addition, beads do not always cure infection, and recurrence after bead removal is a possibility. There are reports of fragmentation or dislodgement of beads when they are subjected to excessive loading through an extremity.[18] A 2021 study reported that fluoroquinolones are widely associated with tendinopathy when used systemically, and the same mechanism of action has been shown to cause local tissue toxicity when used in a surgical wound.[60] Furthermore, vancomycin use has been documented to cause a variety of adverse reactions resulting from both immunoglobulin E–mediated and acute histamine release after delivery of the antibiotic. Two case reports from 2018 showed that, when used locally, the results were hypersensitivity, ototoxicity, and nephrotoxicity.[61,62] Finally, beads should not be implanted for longer than 3 weeks as it makes their removal more difficult, and there is a theoretical risk that after the cement stops eluting antibiotics, it can become a nidus for infection itself.[10]

Calcium Sulfate

Complications after the use of calcium sulfate include failure of union, infection recurrence, wound drainage, hypercalcemia, and heterotopic ossification.[32,43,44] Another postulated complication with the use of higher volumes of beads includes acceleration or wear rate and possible arthritis due to surface abrasion; however, this has not been demonstrated to date.[54]

Chitosans

There is relatively little literature reporting on systemic complications of chitosan when used in human subjects. Some animal and oncologic studies have associated complications of chitosan; however, their translation to orthopaedic indications remains unclear.

FUTURE DIRECTIONS

Scientific development has continued to expand the field of local antibiotic delivery. New methods of sterilization for vancomycin-tobramycin antibiotic PMMA beads do not impede their elution properties. This allows for bead storage for up to 6 months with preserved bioactivity. Calcium sulfate beads have recently been manufactured with new antibiotic options (amikacin, meropenem, and dalbavancin) for use in the orthopaedic setting. Their elution kinetics show similar profiles to that of vancomycin and tobramycin, which are currently considered to be the gold standard.

In addition, because of the necessity for second surgery and concern of biofilm development on the delivery system, the development of biodegradable carriers is being quickly explored. These are seen as theoretically advantageous because of the potential reduction in the

Chapter 12: Local Antibiotic Delivery Methods

Table 4
Future Directions of Local Antibiotic Delivery

Study	Major Findings
Hasan et al 2021	Antibiotic-releasing bone void filling putty with bioactive glass is a substrate-based, biodegradable, and press-fitting alternative treatment option for osteomyelitis in in vivo rat models. It can simultaneously support infection eradication and bone healing through osteoconduction.
Levack et al 2021	By quantifying elution kinetics in a $CaSO_4$ bead model, this study demonstrates the utility of new antibiotic options (amikacin, meropenem, and dalbavancin) as alternatives for $CaSO_4$ beads in the orthopaedic setting. Their elution kinetics show profiles similar to that of vancomycin and tobramycin, which are currently considered to be the gold standard.
Rajendran et al 2021	The synthesis and use of hydroxyapatite bone cement in nanoform is suitable for the treatment of osteomyelitis, providing a more slow, sustained delivery of antibiotics for 8 weeks.
Shaw et al 2020	Autoclaving, ethylene oxide gas, or ultraviolet light sterilization methods for vancomycin-tobramycin antibiotic PMMA beads do not impede their elution properties and can allow bead storage for up to 6 months with equal bioactivity.
He et al 2021	In vivo experiments using porous tricalcium phosphate beads loaded with ε-polylysine (PL) and silver (Ag) instead of antibiotics serve as a viable local delivery system for managing osteomyelitis, especially sequestrum-débrided osteomyelitis. The Ag/PL beads show strong antibacterial activity and osteoconductivity with low toxicity.
Fang et al 2019	A new biocomposite bone cement composed of chitosan/tricalcium phosphate/PMMA biocomposites can create rougher surfaces beneficial to cell adherence and growth, suggesting osteoconductive and osteointegrative properties of the chitosan scaffold.
Wu et al 2021	$CaSO_4$ cement microbeads impregnated with chitosan and penicillin create a novel, nontoxic scaffold with injectability, good strength, strong antibacterial effects, and good biocompatibility to support stem cell viability for osteogenesis.
Wang et al 2021	First report on the efficacy of custom-made antibiotic cement-coated intramedullary nails through a 3D printing technique for the treatment of infected long bones in a retrospective cohort of 19 patients.
Kaplan et al 2021	Demonstrates that sodium borate and calcium borate mineral loading into antibiotic cements enhances antibacterial activity and cell integration without compromising mechanical properties when compared with plain bone cement.
Qiao et al 2022	PLLA and pearl composite scaffolds prepared with 3D printing and loaded with rifampicin/moxifloxacin microspheres promote adhesion, proliferation, and differentiation of mesenchymal stem cells. When used in vivo in rabbit models of infected bone defects, this was the only scaffold to demonstrate both anti-infection and osteoconductive properties compared with PLLA and PLLA + Pearl scaffolds alone.

3D = three-dimensional, PLLA = poly-L-lactic acid, PMMA = polymethyl methacrylate

risk of secondary infection and the need for removal of the implant. Several of these studies evaluating future directions of local antibiotic delivery systems have been summarized[60,63-71] in **Table 4**. One study from 2021 postulated the use of antibiotic-relapsing bone void filling putty with bioactive glass as a treatment alternative for osteomyelitis to both mitigate infection and promote bone healing.[63] Another investigation from 2021 was the first report on the efficacy of custom-made antibiotic cement–coated intramedullary nails through a three-dimensional printing technique for the treatment of infected long bones.[64]

SUMMARY

The use of local antibiotic delivery systems has become an accepted treatment method that continues to evolve. These systems can achieve high local concentrations of antibiotics, which is desirable in the typical infected, avascular wound environment. Certain delivery systems also have osteoinductive and osteoconductive materials that can aid in bone regeneration. Scientific development has continued to expand the field of local antibiotic delivery; however, additional research to standardize the methods of local delivery will improve their efficacy going forward.

KEY STUDY POINTS

- Local antibiotic delivery systems can achieve high local concentrations of antibiotics, which is desirable in the typical infected, avascular wound environment.
- There may be both local tissue and systemic toxicity that are associated with the high antibiotic levels in the tissue.
- Additional research to standardize the types of antibiotics, loading doses, mixing methods, and their elution profiles will improve antimicrobial efficacy in these systems going forward.

ANNOTATED REFERENCES

1. Van Vugt TA, Arts JJ, Geurts JA: Antibiotic-loaded polymethylmethacrylate beads and spacers in treatment of orthopedic infections and the role of biofilm formation. *Front Microbiol* 2019;10:1626.

   This review article demonstrated that $CaSO_4$ remains an inexpensive, safe, reliable bone void filler that can also serve as a absorbable delivery vehicle for antibiotics or other compounds. Level of evidence: I.

2. Zmistowski B, Karam JA, Durinka JB, Casper DS, Parvizi J: Periprosthetic joint infection increases the risk of one-year mortality. *J Bone Joint Surg Am* 2013;95(24):2177-2184.

3. Dale H, Hallan G, Espehaug B, Havelin LI, Engesæter LB: Increasing risk of revision due to deep infection after hip arthroplasty: A study on 97,344 primary total hip replacements in the Norwegian Arthroplasty Register from 1987 to 2007. *Acta Orthop* 2009;80(6):639-645.

4. Zimmerli W, Trampuz A, Ochsner PE: Prosthetic-joint infections. *N Engl J Med* 2004;351(16):1645-1654.

5. Gogia JS, Meehan JP, Di Cesare PE, Jamali AA: Local antibiotic therapy in osteomyelitis, in *Seminars in Plastic Surgery*. © Thieme Medical Publishers, 2009, vol 23, No. 02, pp 100-107.

6. Hake ME, Young H, Hak DJ, Stahel PF, Hammerberg EM, Mauffrey C: Local antibiotic therapy strategies in orthopaedic trauma: Practical tips and tricks and review of the literature. *Injury* 2015;46(8):1447-1456.

7. O'Toole RV, Joshi M, Carlini AR, et al: Local antibiotic therapy to reduce infection after operative treatment of fractures at high risk of infection: A multicenter, randomized, controlled trial (VANCO study). *J Orthop Trauma* 2017;31(suppl 1):S18-S24.

8. Tsourvakas S: Local antibiotic therapy in the treatment of bone and soft tissue infections, in *Selected Topics in Plastic Reconstructive Surgery*. Intech Open, 2012.

9. Klemm K: The use of antibiotic-containing bead chains in the treatment of chronic bone infections. *Clin Microbiol Infect* 2001;7(1):28-31.

10. DeCoster TA, Bozorgnia S: Antibiotic beads. *J Am Acad Orthop Surg* 2008;16(11):674-678.

11. van de Belt H, Neut D, Schenk W, van Horn JR, van der Mei HC, Busscher HJ: Gentamicin release from polymethylmethacrylate bone cements and Staphylococcus aureus biofilm formation. *Acta Orthop Scand* 2000;71(6):625-629.

12. Rasyid HN, van der Mei HC, Frijlink HW, et al: Concepts for increasing gentamicin release from handmade bone cement beads. *Acta Orthop* 2009;80(5):508-513.

13. Walenkamp G: Small PMMA beads improve gentamicin release. *Acta Orthop Scand* 1989;60(6):668-669.

14. Wahlig H, Dingeldein E, Bergmann R, Reuss K: The release of gentamicin from polymethylmethacrylate beads. An experimental and pharmacokinetic study. *J Bone Joint Surg Br* 1978;60-B(2):270-275.

15. Walenkamp GH: Antibiotic loaded cement: From research to clinical evidence, in *Infection and Local Treatment in Orthopedic Surgery*. Springer, 2007, pp 170-175.

16. Anagnostakos K, Hitzler P, Pape D, Kohn D, Kelm J: Persistence of bacterial growth on antibiotic-loaded beads: Is it actually a problem? *Acta Orthop* 2008;79(2):302-307.

17. Fernando N, Werner S, Elhaddad M, Davies J, Firoozabadi R: Do antibiotic beads need to be removed? *Arch Bone Jt Surg* 2020;8(4):502-505.

    This retrospective review of 51 patients with an extremity or pelvic fracture and implantation of PMMA beads over a 5-year period reported the utility of PMMA beads in delivering high-dose antibiotics. This study also demonstrated that beads do not have to be removed in all patients, as 73% of patients did not have complications necessitating removal. Level of evidence: II.

18. Patel KH, Bhat SN, Mamatha H: Outcome analysis of antibiotic-loaded poly methyl methacrylate (PMMA) beads in musculoskeletal infections. *J Taibah Univ Med Sci* 2021;16(2):177-183.

    This is longitudinal study of 82 patients with chronic osteomyelitis treated for more than 6 years demonstrated effectiveness of PMMA beads for the management of chronic osteomyelitis and prevention of reinfection. Level of evidence: II.

19. Beuerlein MJ, McKee MD: Calcium sulfates: What is the evidence? *J Orthop Trauma* 2010;24(suppl 1):S46-S51.

20. Boyan BD, Baker MI, Lee CSD, et al: Bone tissue grafting and tissue engineering concepts, in Ducheyne P, ed: *Comprehensive Biomaterials*. Elsevier, 2011, pp 237-255.

21. Moore K, Os RW, Dusane DH, et al: Elution kinetics from antibiotic-loaded calcium sulfate beads, antibiotic-loaded polymethacrylate spacers, and a powdered antibiotic bolus for surgical site infections in a novel in vitro draining knee model. *Antibiotics (Basel)* 2021;10(3):270.

    This is in vitro study of a draining knee model found that the combination of PMMA with $CaSO_4$ beads presented an effective combination for killing biofilm bacteria. Level of evidence: I.

22. Zapata MEV, Tovar CDG, Hernandez JHM: The role of chitosan and graphene oxide in bioactive and antibacterial properties of acrylic bone cements. *Biomolecules* 2020;10(12):1616.

This review article reported the advantages and disadvantages of chitosan as a bioactive filler in cement in multiple disciplines. Level of evidence: I.

23. Ueno H, Mori T, Fujinaga T: Topical formulations and wound healing applications of chitosan. *Adv Drug Deliv Rev* 2001;52(2):105-115.

24. Calhoun JH, Mader JT: Antibiotic beads in the management of surgical infections. *Am J Surg* 1989;157(4):443-449.

25. Hoff SF, Fitzgerald RH Jr, Kelly PJ: The depot administration of penicillin G and gentamicin in acrylic bone cement. *J Bone Joint Surg Am* 1981;63(5):798-804.

26. Picknell BA, Mizen LI, Sutherland R: Antibacterial activity of antibiotics in acrylic bone cement. *J Bone Joint Surg Br* 1977;59(3):302-307.

27. Walenkamp GH: *Gentamicin-PMMA Beads: A Clinical, Pharmacokinetic and Toxicological Study*. Netherlands, Radboud University Nijmegen, 1983. Doctoral dissertation.

28. Chang Y, Tai CL, Hsieh PH, Ueng SW: Gentamicin in bone cement: A potentially more effective prophylactic measure of infection in joint arthroplasty. *Bone Joint Res* 2013;2(10):220-226.

29. Anagnostakos K, Meyer C: Antibiotic elution from hip and knee acrylic bone cement spacers: A systematic review. *Biomed Res Int* 2017;2017:4657874.

30. Chang Y, Chen WC, Hsieh PH, et al: In vitro activities of daptomycin-vancomycin-and teicoplanin-loaded polymethylmethacrylate against methicillin-susceptible, methicillin-resistant, and vancomycin-intermediate strains of Staphylococcus aureus. *Antimicrob Agents Chemother* 2011;55(12):5480-5484.

31. Kendoff DO, Gehrke T, Stangenberg P, Frommelt L, Bösebeck H: Bioavailability of gentamicin and vancomycin released from an antibiotic containing bone cement in patients undergoing a septic one-stage total hip arthroplasty (THA) revision: A monocentric open clinical trial. *Hip Int* 2016;26(1):90-96.

32. Abosala A, Ali M: The use of calcium sulphate beads in periprosthetic joint infection, a systematic review. *J Bone Jt Infect* 2020;5(1):43-49.

This systematic review demonstrated the utility of CaSO$_4$ beads for hip and knee revision for PJI rather than as an adjuvant to débridement, antibiotics, and implant retention procedure. This study also reported increased complications with higher bead volume. Level of evidence: I.

33. Wouthuyzen-Bakker M, Kheir MM, Moya I, et al: Failure after 2-stage exchange arthroplasty for treatment of periprosthetic joint infection: The role of antibiotics in the cement spacer. *Clin Infect Dis* 2019;68(12):2087-2093.

This is retrospective study evaluated two-stage exchange for PJI found that the addition of glycopeptide to cement spacer reduces the rate of positive cultures during reimplantation and is associated with a lower failure rate because of coagulase-negative staphylococci. Level of evidence: II.

34. Cancienne JM, Burrus MT, Weiss DB, Yarboro SR: Applications of local antibiotics in orthopedic trauma. *Orthop Clin North Am* 2015;46(4):495-510.

35. Burtt KE, Badash I, Leland HA, et al: The efficacy of negative pressure wound therapy and antibiotic beads in lower extremity salvage. *J Surg Res* 2020;247:499-507.

This retrospective review of patients with traumatic lower extremity open fractures who received negative-pressure wound therapy and/or antibiotic beads before soft-tissue reconstruction demonstrated that negative-pressure wound therapy may contribute to greater complication rates. Level of evidence: II.

36. Ostermann PA, Seligson D, Henry SL: Local antibiotic therapy for severe open fractures. A review of 1085 consecutive cases. *J Bone Joint Surg Br* 1995;77(1):93-97.

37. Keating JF, Blachut PA, O'Brien PJ, Meek RN, Broekhuyse H: Reamed nailing of open tibial fractures: Does the antibiotic bead pouch reduce the deep infection rate? *J Orthop Trauma* 1996;10(5):298-303.

38. Fitzgerald RH Jr: Experimental osteomyelitis: Description of a canine model and the role of depot administration of antibiotics in the prevention and treatment of sepsis. *J Bone Joint Surg Am* 1983;65(3):371-380.

39. Major Extremity Trauma Research Consortium (METRC), O'Toole RV, Joshi M, et al: Effect of intrawound vancomycin powder in operatively treated high-risk tibia fractures: A randomized clinical trial. *JAMA Surg* 2021;156(5):e207259.

This randomized control trial evaluated the outcomes after pilon fracture using vancomycin powder, demonstrating reduced risk of gram-positive deep surgical site infection among a cohort of 980 patients. Level of evidence: I.

40. Shi X, Wu Y, Ni H, et al: Antibiotic-loaded calcium sulfate in clinical treatment of chronic osteomyelitis: A systematic review and meta-analysis. *J Orthop Surg Res* 2022;17(1):104.

This is a systematic review of the use of CaSO$_4$ for osteomyelitis. Level of evidence: I.

41. Calanna F, Chen F, Risitano S, et al: Debridement, antibiotic pearls, and retention of the implant (DAPRI): A modified technique for implant retention in total knee arthroplasty PJI treatment. *J Orthop Surg* 2019;27(3):2309499019874413.

This surgical technique guide shows novel technique for the management of PJI, including the use of antibiotic beads. Level of evidence: IV.

42. Chung AS, Niesen MC, Graber TJ, et al: Two-stage debridement with prosthesis retention for acute periprosthetic joint infections. *J Arthroplasty* 2019;34(6):1207-1213.

This retrospective study of 83 patients undergoing two-stage débridement with implant retention revealed a higher likelihood of infection control with a two-stage retention protocol compared with prior reports of single-stage débridement and modular part exchange. Level of evidence: II.

43. Thahir A, Lim JA, West C, Krkovic M: The use of calcium sulphate beads in the management of osteomyelitis of femur and tibia: A systematic review. *Arch Bone Jt Surg* 2022;10(4):320-327.

This is systematic review evaluated the use of antibiotic-impregnated CaSO$_4$ beads for the management of infected tibia and femur, demonstrating higher infection remission compared with PMMA. Level of evidence: I.

44. Tarity TD, Xiang W, Jones CW, et al: Do antibiotic-loaded calcium sulfate beads improve outcomes after debridement, antibiotics, and implant retention? A matched cohort study. *Arthroplast Today* 2022;14:90-95.

    This retrospective cohort study of 20 patients undergoing débridement, antibiotics, and implant retention procedures with antibiotic beads for acute hematogenous PJI demonstrated no significant differences between patients and control patients for overall infection-related failure at 2 years or early infection-related failure at 90 days. Level of evidence: II.

45. Gorvetzian JW, Kunkel RP, Demas CP: A single center retrospective evaluation of a surgical strategy to combat persistent soft tissue wounds utilizing absorbable antibiotic beads. *Adv Wound Care* 2019;8(2):49-57.

    This retrospective analysis of surgical cases using $CaSO_4$ antibiotic beads demonstrated decreased infection and all-cause reoperation rates among 60 patients and 84 total surgeries. Level of evidence: II.

46. Christou C, Oliver RA, Yu Y, Walsh WR: The Masquelet technique for membrane induction and the healing of ovine critical sized segmental defects. *PLoS One* 2014;9(12):e114122.

47. Alford AI, Nicolaou D, Hake M, McBride-Gagyi S: Masquelet's induced membrane technique: Review of current concepts and future directions. *J Orthop Res* 2021;39(4):707-718.

    This is a review of current indications and studies surrounding the Masquelet technique. Level of evidence: IV.

48. Patzakis MJ, Mazur K, Wilkins JE, Sherman RA, Holtom PA: Septopal beads and autogenous bone grafting for bone defects in patients with chronic osteomyelitis. *Clin Orthop Relat Res* 1993;295:112-118.

49. Evans RP, Nelson CL: Gentamicin-impregnated polymethylmethacrylate beads compared with systemic antibiotic therapy in the treatment of chronic osteomyelitis. *Clin Orthop Relat Res* 1993;295:37-42.

50. Jia WT, Zhang X, Luo SH, et al: Novel borate glass/chitosan composite as a delivery vehicle for teicoplanin in the treatment of chronic osteomyelitis. *Acta Biomater* 2010;6(3):812-819.

51. Lautenschlager EP, Marshall GW, Marks KE, Schwartz J, Nelson CL: Mechanical strength of acrylic bone cements impregnated with antibiotics. *J Biomed Mater Res* 1976;10(6):837-845.

52. Chen AF, Parvizi J: Antibiotic-loaded bone cement and periprosthetic joint infection. *J Long Term Eff Med Implants* 2014;24(2-3):89-97.

53. Lachiewicz PF, Wellman SS, Peterson JR: Antibiotic cement spacers for infected total knee arthroplasties. *J Am Acad Orthop Surg* 2020;28(5):180-188.

    This is a review article of antibiotic cement spacers for infected knee arthroplasties, discussing advantages and disadvantages of static versus mobile spacers and the complications of high-dose spacers. Level of evidence: IV.

54. Flierl MA, Culp BM, Okroj KT, Springer BD, Levine BR, Della Valle CJ: Poor outcomes of irrigation and debridement in acute periprosthetic joint infection with antibiotic-impregnated calcium sulfate beads. *J Arthroplasty* 2017;32(8):2505-2507.

55. Nelson CL, Griffin FM, Harrison BH, Cooper RE: In vitro elution characteristics of commercially and noncommercially prepared antibiotic PMMA beads. *Clin Orthop Relat Res* 1992;284:303-309.

56. Van de Belt H, Neut D, Uges DR, et al: Surface roughness, porosity and wettability of gentamicin-loaded bone cements and their antibiotic release. *Biomaterials* 2000;21(19):1981-1987.

57. Rybak MJ, Albrecht LM, Boike SC, Chandrasekar PH: Nephrotoxicity of vancomycin, alone and with an aminoglycoside. *J Antimicrob Chemother* 1990;25(4):679-687.

58. Ma AH, Hoffman C, Mcneil JI: Acute tubular necrosis associated with high serum vancomycin and tobramycin levels after revision of total knee arthroplasty with antibiotic-containing calcium sulfate beads. *Open Forum Infect Dis* 2019;6(4):ofz141.

    This is a case report of a patient with acute tubular necrosis following revision total knee arthroplasty with $CaSO_4$ beads. Level of evidence: IV.

59. Hall MM, Finnoff JT, Smith J: Musculoskeletal complications of fluoroquinolones: Guidelines and precautions for usage in the athletic population. *PM R* 2011;3(2):132-142.

60. Rajendran M, Iraivan G, Ghayathri BL, et al: Antibiotic loaded nano rod bone cement for the treatment of osteomyelitis. *Recent Pat Nanotechnol* 2021;15(1):70-89.

    This patented work studied hydroxyapatite bead synthesis in nanoform for sustained release and evaluated release kinetics. Level of evidence: I.

61. Nagahama Y, VanBeek MJ, Greenlee JDW: Red man syndrome caused by vancomycin powder. *J Clin Neurosci* 2018;50:149-150.

    This is a case report of vancomycin powder use in local surgical wounds for infection prophylaxis leading to red man syndrome. Level of evidence: IV.

62. Chen CT, Ng KJ, Lin Y, Kao MC: Red man syndrome following the use of vancomycin-loaded bone cement in the primary total knee replacement: A case report. *Medicine (Baltimore)* 2018;97(51):e13371.

    This is a case report of red man syndrome following total knee arthroplasty with the use of vancomycin bone cement. Level of evidence: IV.

63. Hasan R, Schaner K, Mulinti P, Brooks A: A bioglass-based antibiotic (Vancomycin) releasing bone void filling putty to treat osteomyelitis and aid bone healing. *Int J Mol Sci* 2021;22(14):7736.

    This in vivo laboratory study reports that a bioactive glass substrate–based, press-fitting antibiotic-releasing bone void filling putty provides effective local antibiotic release for up to 6 weeks, in addition to support for bone regeneration. Level of evidence: I.

64. Wang G, Luo W, Zhou Y, et al: Custom-made antibiotic cement-coated nail for the treatment of infected bone defect. *Biomed Res Int* 2021;2021:6693906.

    This is retrospective study reported the efficacy of custom intramedullary nails coated with antibiotic cement made with three-dimensional printing for long bone infection. Level of evidence: II.

65. Levack AE, Turajane K, Yang X, et al: Thermal stability and in vitro elution kinetics of alternative antibiotics in polymethylmethacrylate (PMMA) bone cement. *J Bone Joint Surg Am* 2021;103(18):1694-1704.

    This is an in vitro study demonstrating notable differences in the thermal stability and pharmacodynamics of amikacin, meropenem, minocycline, and PMMA beads, specifically finding that tobramycin, amikacin, and meropenem were orders of magnitude higher than minocycline and fosfomycin in elution concentrations, rates, and cumulative drug mass throughout the 7-day study period. Level of evidence: I.

66. He W, Wu Z, Wu Y, et al: Construction of antimicrobial material-loaded porous tricalcium phosphate beads for treatment of bone infections. *ACS Appl Bio Mater* 2021;4(8):6280-6293.

    This is an in vitro and in vivo study evaluating tricalcium phosphate beads for management of osteomyelitis demonstrating strong antibacterial activity and good osteoconductivity, with enhanced performance and low toxicity when loaded with ε-polylysine and silver. Level of evidence: I.

67. Shaw J, Gary J, Baker A, et al: Effects of sterilization techniques on bioactivity of polymethyl methacrylate antibiotic beads containing vancomycin and tobramycin. *J Orthop Trauma* 2020;34(4):e109-e113.

    This laboratory study demonstrates that sterile PMMA beads with vancomycin and tobramycin stored for up to 6 months have the same efficacy as current bead standards synthesized in a sterile manner and used immediately. This study also found that the elution of the antibiotic beads are not negatively affected by different sterilization methods. Level of evidence: I.

68. Fang CH, Lin YW, Sun JS, Lin FH: The chitosan/tri-calcium phosphate bio-composite bone cement promotes better osteo-integration: An in vitro and in vivo study. *J Orthop Surg Res* 2019;14(1):162.

    A new biocomposite bone cement composed of chitosan/tricalcium phosphate/PMMA biocomposites can create rougher surfaces beneficial to cell adherence and growth, suggesting osteoconductive and osteointegrative properties of the chitosan scaf. Level of evidence: I.

69. Wu S, Lei L, Bao C, et al: An injectable and antibacterial calcium phosphate scaffold inhibiting Staphylococcus aureus and supporting stem cells for bone regeneration. *Mater Sci Eng C Mater Biol Appl* 2021;120:111688.

    $CaSO_4$ cement microbeads impregnated with chitosan and penicillin create a novel, nontoxic scaffold with injectability, good strength, strong antibacterial effects, and good biocompatibility to support stem cell viability for osteogenesis. Level of evidence: I.

70. Kaplan M, Özgür E, Ersoy O, Kehribar L, İdil N, Uzun L: Borate mineral loading into acrylic bone cements to gain cost-effectivity, enhanced antibacterial resistivity, and better cellular integration properties. *J Biomater Sci Polym Ed* 2021;32(8):980-993.

    Demonstrates that sodium borate and calcium borate mineral loading into antibiotic cements enhances antibacterial activity and cell integration without compromising mechanical properties when compared with plain bone cement. Level of evidence: I.

71. Qiao Z, Zhang W, Jiang H, Li X, An W, Yang H: 3D-printed composite scaffold with anti-infection and osteogenesis potential against infected bone defects. *RSC Adv* 2022;12(18):11008-11020.

    PLLA and pearl composite scaffolds prepared with 3D printing and loaded with rifampicin/moxifloxacin microspheres promote adhesion, proliferation, and differentiation of mesenchymal stem cells. Level of evidence: I.

CHAPTER 13

Systemic Antibiotic Therapy

JESSICA L. SEIDELMAN, MD, MPH • MARJAN WOUTHUYZEN-BAKKER, MD, PhD
ALEX SORIANO, MD

ABSTRACT

Clinicians have historically preferred to treat bone and joint infections with intravenous antibiotics as opposed to oral antibiotics, with treatment regimens often lasting 4 to 6 weeks or longer. However, over recent years, mounting evidence is emerging to support the use of oral antibiotics to treat bone and joint infection. In addition, pharmacokinetic data indicate that many oral antibiotics achieve adequate concentrations in bone. Current American and European practices pertaining to route and duration of treatment for bone and joint infections diverge. There is still considerable concern in the United States about the generalizability of newer, primarily European studies' conclusions given the heterogeneity of infections, organisms, and surgical management. Therefore, the treatment route and duration for bone and joint infections remain an area of active investigation and debate. Specific knowledge on the types of antimicrobial agents, their potential interactions, and adverse events is necessary to select the optimal therapy for each individual patient.

Keywords: antibiotics; antibiotic-associated adverse events; drug-drug interactions; intravenous antibiotics; joint infection; oral antibiotics

INTRODUCTION

Bone and joint infections (BJIs) are complex and frequently require a multidisciplinary approach, including orthopaedic and trauma surgeons for débridement and removal of necrotic bone or foreign bodies while preserving function, and infectious diseases physicians, microbiologists, and pharmacists to select and optimize antibiotic treatment to control bacteria to avoid relapses. In addition, many other specialties are necessary to help patients with BJI, including in diagnosis (eg, radiology), soft-tissue coverage (plastic surgeons), and functional recovery (physical and occupational therapists) to improve patient outcomes and to minimize the effect on patients' quality of life. These infections require a substantial amount of healthcare resources with a high economic burden. However, the annual number of patients with BJI treated at an individual institution is relatively small in comparison with other common infections such as pneumonia or urinary tract infections. This fact coupled with the different behavior of bacteria within the bone environment and/or within biofilm, not evaluated by classic microbiologic methods, may explain why the acquisition of important data on antibiotic therapy for treatment of BJIs has been slow and mainly based on expert opinion. Indeed, the number of randomized trials looking at the treatment of BJIs is limited. In contrast to other infections with similarities to BJIs such as endocarditis, international collaboration for developing large prospective databases has been absent except for some

---

Dr. Wouthuyzen-Bakker or an immediate family member serves as an unpaid consultant to Zimmer. Dr. Soriano or an immediate family member is a member of a speakers' bureau or has made paid presentations on behalf of Angelini, Menarini, Merck, Pfizer, and Shionogi; serves as a paid consultant to or is an employee of Pfizer; and serves as a board member, owner, officer, or committee member of European Bone and Joint Infection Society. Neither Dr. Seidelman nor any immediate family member has received anything of value from or has stock or stock options held in a commercial company or institution related directly or indirectly to the subject of this chapter.

efforts based on retrospective collection of data from different centers. According to the progression of BJI management, there have been two main currents: one from the United States and the other from Europe, particularly in the context of implant-related infections. The US information was based on the Infectious Diseases Society of America guidelines.[1] The US guidelines currently favor the use of standard antibiotics (intravenous beta-lactams [β-lactams] for susceptible and glycopeptides for resistant microorganisms) with implant removal. In cases of implant retention, the US current favors several weeks of initial intravenous therapy with prolonged oral antibiotic therapy thereafter. The current from Europe is based on experimental animal models developed in Switzerland during the 1990s. This model of foreign body infection showed that glycopeptides fail to constrain the infection in a high percentage of cases when the implant is not removed.[2] In contrast, the use of rifampin was associated with a significantly higher eradication rate and the rate was even higher when it was combined with ciprofloxacin but not when combined with glycopeptides.[2] The fact that both rifampin and fluoroquinolones (particularly levofloxacin and moxifloxacin) have a high oral bioavailability (≥90%) opened the opportunity for early switch from intravenous to oral regimens. One of the most cited clinical trials in BJIs compared the use of ciprofloxacin alone versus the combination of ciprofloxacin plus rifampin in patients with metalwork or prosthetic joint infection (PJI) with implant retention.[3] These results prompted the use of shorter oral rifampin-based combinations for PJI particularly in Europe. The differences between both currents were exposed in the Infectious Diseases Society of America guidelines, which were written in collaboration with a European expert. In recent years, there has been a closer collaboration between American and European centers to elaborate common recommendations, to do collaborative research and develop prospective databases that should be supported to increase knowledge about BJIs and optimize best treatment practices.

TRENDS IN ORAL VERSUS INTRAVENOUS THERAPY

Historically, most clinicians in the United States have treated BJIs with intravenous antibiotics based on the concept that oral antibiotics are less efficacious compared with intravenous antibiotics for this indication.[4] Although historically intravenous therapy has been used more often than oral therapy for BJI, there have never been data to support its use over oral antibiotics, only expert opinion and in some cases anecdotal studies. Nine earlier studies concluded that oral and intravenous antibiotics had similar cure rates for BJIs. However, these studies were all small in size, and only one was randomized.[5]

However, the Oral Versus Intravenous Antibiotics for Bone and Joint Infection (OVIVA) trial published in 2019 challenged this paradigm.[6] This study included 1,054 patients with osteomyelitis, native joint infection, PJI, or infections involving orthopaedic fixation devices. Patients were randomized to intravenous or oral antibiotics within 1 week of starting antibiotic therapy. The type and dosing of antibiotic was left up to the judgment of the treating infectious diseases clinician. Based on blind adjudication 1 year after infection treatment, the study concluded that oral antibiotic treatment was noninferior to the intravenous treatment.

More recent studies have reported on real-world experience with application of the OVIVA trial treatment protocol. For example, a 2021 study of a single orthopaedic hospital in the United Kingdom examined patient outcomes during a 12-month period, implementing the OVIVA protocol's expeditious switch to oral antibiotics, and compared these results with patient outcomes during the preceding 12-month period.[7] The investigators found that BJIs treated in the postimplementation group had a median reduction in hospital length of stay of 4 days and a median cost reduction of £2,764.28 ($3,517) per patient compared with the preimplementation group. However, approximately one in three patients in the postimplementation group could not be treated with oral antibiotics because of multidrug resistance, the lack of a defined pathogen, and/or preexisting allergies or intolerances to oral antibiotics. More complications related to intravenous access occurred in the preimplementation phase than the postimplementation phase.

For several reasons, many clinicians and patients would prefer to treat BJIs with oral antibiotics instead of intravenous antibiotics when feasible. The use of oral antibiotics can decrease the duration of hospital stays and cost of treatment.[7] A 2023 single-center retrospective study found that oral therapy could have resulted in an estimated mean savings per patient of $3,270.69 versus intravenous therapy.[8] Administering parenteral antibiotic therapy via intravascular devices increases the risk of secondary infection and thromboembolic events.[9] Oral therapy also avoids issues with maintaining patent venous access and insurance approval and obviates the need for admission to assisted-care facilities for prolonged intravenous therapy.[6] Therefore, oral antibiotic treatment avoids catheter-related complications, shortens hospital stay, lowers cost, and improves patient comfort.

However, oral antibiotic treatment for the management of BJIs also has inherent concerns. First, oral antibiotics can still lead to adverse events, but patients on oral therapy may not be monitored as closely as patients who are receiving parenteral therapy. Although the events were not necessarily related to the antibiotics, one in four patients in both arms of the OVIVA study experienced a serious adverse event.[6,10] Second, oral antibiotics are not always an option when the infection is deemed to be caused by multidrug-resistant pathogens. In fact, oral antibiotics were not an option because of organism resistance in 31 of the 183 patients (16.9%) in the post-implementation group in the implementation study, and this was the most common reason (49.2%) for requiring intravenous therapy.[7] In addition, fewer than half of patients screened for the OVIVA study were ultimately randomized, leading to concerns about its generalizability. In addition, achieving adequate drug levels using oral antibiotics may be challenging in patients with particular comorbidities that affect gastrointestinal absorption or obesity. Moreover, some patients may forget to take oral antibiotics. Nonadherence to oral antibiotics has been linked to poor clinical outcomes such as infection relapses, need for new antibiotics, and additional medical procedures. Although in the OVIVA trial adherence was lower in the oral antibiotic group, this group did not have poorer outcomes compared with the intravenous group. However, one study found that antibiotics taken one, two, or three times daily had adherence rates of 80%, 69%, and 38%, respectively.[11] This is in comparison with intravenous antibiotics that have been found in a 2020 study to have an adherence rate of closer to 90%.[12] In addition, much of the data examining the efficacy of oral to intravenous therapy use fluoroquinolones as the oral antibiotic (often paired with rifampin). Therefore, the success of this antibiotic class may not be generalizable to all other antibiotic classes. Although antibiotics are critical in the treatment of BJIs, other factors that are independent from antibiotic therapy and may differ across centers (eg, surgical débridement quality) also contribute to outcomes of infection and potentially confound the effect of antibiotic route.

Although oral antibiotics offer some clear advantages over parenteral antibiotics for treatment of BJIs, it is still not clear whether oral antibiotics are optimal for treatment of all BJIs.[5] Clinicians need to be aware of the pitfalls and caveats of oral therapy and decide on an individual basis if oral treatment is right for the patient.

SPECIFIC ANTIBIOTICS AND THEIR CONSIDERATIONS

Multiple antibiotics may be used to treat BJI. Important antimicrobials are reviewed, and key findings are summarized in **Table 1**.

Rifamycins

Rifampin has become an increasingly important part of the therapeutic armamentarium against BJI. Adjunctive therapy is an additional treatment used to increase the efficacy of the primary treatment. Adjunctive rifampin has been studied for a variety of BJIs: chronic osteomyelitis, diabetic foot infections, and PJIs.[13-15]

Rifampin has some unique antimicrobial properties that make it an attractive adjunctive agent for treating BJIs. Specifically, rifampin penetrates osteoblasts and remains active within these cells compared with β-lactam antibiotics and glycopeptides, which have slower uptake and few intracellular activities.[16] In addition, rifampin breaches biofilms and also retains its activity within these layers, whereas standard antibiotics may not be as efficacious in breaching biofilms or retaining activity against bacteria in planktonic state.[17]

Rifampin must always be paired with another active agent to avoid development of resistance; according to a 2021 study, the strongest data for treatment of staphylococcal BJIs with adjunctive rifampin are in conjunction with fluoroquinolones.[18] A small trial found higher failure rates for treatment of PJIs using rifampin in combination therapy with linezolid, cotrimoxazole, and clindamycin.[19] This finding was explained by the fact that rifampin reduces the serum concentration of these antibiotics.[20] Other studies found that higher doses of clindamycin in conjunction with rifampin actually had outcomes similar to those of fluoroquinolones.[18] One of the most significant considerations when prescribing rifampin is the number of drug-drug interactions. Rifampin is a potent inducer of cytochrome P450 enzyme, P-glycoprotein, and phase II metabolic processes (glucuronidation and sulfation). Cytochrome P450 proteins are the main enzymes that metabolize many medications, such as the commonly used drug classes of beta blockers, antidepressants, antiepileptic drugs, statins, and anticoagulants. P-glycoprotein and phase II metabolic processes in the liver are responsible for elimination and metabolization of other group of drugs. Therefore, the major consideration when prescribing rifampin is its interaction with concurrent medications metabolized or eliminated by these different hepatic pathways. Pharmacists and/or interaction checkers are essential when prescribing rifampin.

The safety profile of rifampin is similar to that of other antibiotics used to treat staphylococcal BJIs. However, adverse effects may be more frequent when higher doses are used to treat patients. Serious non–dose-dependent adverse effects specifically associated with rifampin include anaphylaxis, hemolytic anemia, thrombocytopenia, acute renal failure, hepatotoxicity, gastrointestinal symptoms, and rash.[21] Although not a harmful adverse effect, rifampin also causes orange-red discoloration of body fluids such as tears, sweat, saliva, urine, and feces because of its excretion in these fluids. Although no dosage adjustments are needed for hepatic impairment, rifampin is commonly avoided in patients with liver disease because of hepatotoxicity risk.

Table 1

List of Specific Antibiotics With Their Associated Drug-Drug Interactions, Dosing Considerations, Adverse Events, and Other Considerations

Antibiotic	Drug-Drug Interaction	Dosing Considerations	Adverse Events	Other Considerations
Rifampin	Potent inductor of P450 cytochrome (CYP3A4, CYP2C, CYP2D6), P-glycoprotein, and phase II metabolic processes (glucuronoconjugation and sulfatation). Reduces the serum levels of all drugs that are substrate of CYP450, P-glycoprotein, or phase II reactions	Dose reduction in severe hepatic dysfunction (Child-Pugh class C)	Nausea/vomiting Hepatotoxicity Bone marrow toxicity Orange/red body fluid discoloration	Rapid emergence of resistance when used as monotherapy
Fluoroquinolones	Oral absorption is reduced with antacids containing Al or Mg or multivitamins with Fe, Zn, or Ca Concurrent rifampin will lower the concentration of moxifloxacin	Dose reduction in renal failure (eGF ≤ 30 mL/min) for ciprofloxacin and levofloxacin	Diarrhea/nausea/vomiting Tendinopathy Aortic aneurysm and dissection Alterations of central nervous system Phototoxicity QTc prolongation (moxifloxacin) *Clostridioides difficile* infection	Emergence of resistance when used as monotherapy for staphylococcal infections, particularly with ciprofloxacin
Nafcillin/oxacillin	Nafcillin is a moderate inducer of CYP3A4	May need to increase dose in individuals with obesity	Nafcillin: Cholestasis, neurotoxicity Oxacillin: Acute interstitial nephritis, acute renal tubular disease	Contains a significant amount of sodium, should be used with caution in patients with heart failure or concomitant renal and liver failure
Penicillin/ampicillin	—	Dose reduction in renal failure (eGF ≤ 50 mL/min)	Penicillin: Acute interstitial nephritis, renal tubular disease (high doses)	Should be used with caution in patients with a history of seizure disorder
Piperacillin-tazobactam	—	Dose reduction in renal failure (eGF ≤ 50 mL/min)	Acute kidney injury, acute interstitial nephritis, nephrotoxicity	Contains a significant amount of sodium, should be used with caution in patients with renal impairment
Cefazolin	—	Dose reduction in renal failure (eGF ≤ 30 mL/min)	Hepatitis Eosinophilia, leukopenia, neutropenia, thrombocytopenia	May be associated with elevated INR Should be used with caution in patients with reported penicillin allergies

Table 1

List of Specific Antibiotics With Their Associated Drug-Drug Interactions, Dosing Considerations, Adverse Events, and Other Considerations (Continued)

Antibiotic	Drug-Drug Interaction	Dosing Considerations	Adverse Events	Other Considerations
Ceftriaxone	—	—	Hepatitis	Should be used with caution for infections with *Enterobacter*, indole-positive *Proteus*, *Serratia*, and *Citrobacter* even if these organisms are susceptible to cephalosporins given potential for inducible beta-lactamase May be associated with elevated INR
Ceftaroline	May enhance the anticoagulant effect of vitamin K antagonists	Dose reduction in renal failure (eGF ≤ 50 mL/min)	Skin reactions of hypersensitivity Eosinophilia and eosinophilic pneumonia Interstitial nephritis Diarrhea and nausea Coombs test positive in 10% of patients without hemolysis Neutropenia beyond 2 weeks of treatment	Beta-lactam with activity against methicillin resistant *Staphylococcus aureus* and CoNS
Cefepime	May enhance the anticoagulant effect of vitamin K antagonists	Dose reduction in renal failure (eGF ≤ 60 mL/min)	Confusion, myoclonus, tremor, and seizures particularly in older patients and/or those with renal failure	Active against *Pseudomonas aeruginosa*
Vancomycin	The risk of acute kidney injury increases when used with concurrent piperacillin-tazobactam and semisynthetic penicillins (cloxacillin, nafcillin)	Dose reduction in renal failure (eGF ≤ 50 mL/min)	Skin reaction (pruritic erythema) common when infused in less than 1 hour Acute kidney injury Ototoxicity (rare)	Requires serum concentration monitoring
Dalbavancin	—	Dose reduction in renal failure (eGF ≤ 30 mL/min)	Nausea/diarrhea Skin reaction (similar to that of vancomycin) if it is rapidly infused	Infusion time 1 hour Weekly or biweekly administration Broad spectrum for gram-positive cocci except VRE Needs more clinical data to define the dose and success rate in BJIs

(continued)

Table 1

List of Specific Antibiotics With Their Associated Drug-Drug Interactions, Dosing Considerations, Adverse Events, and Other Considerations (Continued)

Antibiotic	Drug-Drug Interaction	Dosing Considerations	Adverse Events	Other Considerations
Oritavancin	False prolongation of prothrombin time and activated partial thromboplastin time (consider to avoid sodium heparin) Weak inhibitor of CYP2C9 and CYP2C19, so it could increase warfarin levels	None (no data with an eGF < 20 mL/min)	Phlebitis Nausea/vomiting Headache Skin reaction (similar to that of vancomycin) if it is rapidly infused	Infusion time 3 hours Weekly or biweekly administration Broad spectrum for gram-positive cocci including VRE Needs more clinical data to define the dose and success rate in BJIs
Daptomycin	May increase the risk of myopathy with concurrent statin use	Dose reduction in renal failure (eGF ≤ 30 mL/min)	Myopathy and rhabdomyolysis Eosinophilic pneumonia	Broad spectrum for gram-positive cocci including VRE has no activity in the lungs as it is inactivated by surfactant
Linezolid	Concurrent administration of linezolid with serotonergic or adrenergic agents or inhibitors of serotonin reuptake can result in serotonin syndrome Rifampin reduces linezolid serum concentration probably by P-glycoprotein induction	None	Gastrointestinal events (nausea/vomiting) Myelosuppression (thrombocytopenia and anemia) more common in patients with renal failure Optic and peripheral neuropathy Lactic acidosis Serotonin syndrome	Oral option for resistant gram-positive cocci including MRSA and VRE Tolerance for greater than 4 weeks is limited by adverse events
Tedizolid	No association with serotonin syndrome	None	Less frequent myelosuppression than with linezolid Peripheral neuropathy but not optic neuropathy	Oral option for resistant gram-positive organisms including MRSA and VRE. More active than linezolid, but the total dose is lower Minimal data for use in treating BJIs particularly in prolonged treatment strategies
Minocycline	Oral absorption is reduced with antacids containing Al or Mg or multivitamins with Fe, Zn, or Ca	None. Avoid in hepatic failure	Nausea/vomiting Vertigo, instability, and tinnitus Skin hyperpigmentation	Retains good activity for methicillin-resistant staphylococci Good experience in BJI as suppressive therapy (months or years)

Table 1

List of Specific Antibiotics With Their Associated Drug-Drug Interactions, Dosing Considerations, Adverse Events, and Other Considerations (*Continued*)

Antibiotic	Drug-Drug Interaction	Dosing Considerations	Adverse Events	Other Considerations
Doxycycline	Oral absorption is reduced with antacids containing Al or Mg or multivitamins with Fe, Zn, or Ca, although the effect is less than that with other tetracyclines Substrate of CYP3A4. Rifampin can decrease the serum levels	None	Nausea/vomiting Phototoxicity Esophagitis	Higher MIC among staphylococci compared with minocycline
Clindamycin	Substrate of CYP3A4. Rifampin can decrease serum levels	None. Avoid high doses in liver cirrhosis (Child-Pugh class C)	Diarrhea/nausea/vomiting *C difficile* infection	do not use if organism is erythromycin resistant without confirming the target organism has no inducible resistance
Trimethoprim/sulfamethoxazole	Rifampin can decrease the serum levels probably by inducing the hepatic metabolism Increased risk of hyperkalemia in case of concomitant treatment with ACE inhibitors, angiotensin receptor blockers, beta-blockers, and spironolactone	Dose reduction in renal failure (eGF ≤ 30 mL/min) In liver cirrhosis (Child-Pugh class C), the dose should be reduced or avoided	Bone marrow suppression Skin rash Nausea/vomiting Hyperkalemia by blocking the sodium canals at distal tubule. The risk is higher in older patients or those with renal failure	Failure rate is higher in the setting of necrotic tissue, abscess, or other locations with high thymidine concentration Retains good activity for methicillin-resistant staphylococci Good experience in BJI as suppressive therapy (months or years) Falsely elevates creatinine

ACE = angiotensin-converting enzyme, Al = aluminum, BJIs = bone and joint infections, Ca = calcium, CoNS = coagulase-negative staphylococci, eGF = estimated glomerular filtration, Fe = iron, INR = International Normalized Ratio, Mg = magnesium, MIC = minimum inhibitory concentration, MRSA = methicillin-resistant *Staphylococcus aureus*, QTc = corrected QT interval, VRE = vancomycin-resistant enterococci, Zn = zinc

Clinicians should be aware of the rapid emergence of resistance of bacteria to rifampin, particularly when the bacterial inoculum (before or early after débridement) is high and rifampin is administered alone.[22] Even in combination, a 2021 study found that one predictor of failure for the management PJI was starting rifampin within 5 days after surgical débridement.[18] Potential explanations for this finding could be that rifampin works antagonistically with other antibiotics when there are still bacteria in the planktonic phase (acute phase)[23] or that early rifampin treatment even in combination with other antibiotics with poor diffusion to tissues (eg, vancomycin) may expose bacteria for several hours to monotherapy with rifampin, which adds to the risk for selection of resistant strains.

In some individuals, adverse drug reactions and adverse effects may preclude the use of rifampin. Although rifampin has been studied and used for decades in the treatment of BJIs, rifabutin may be a reasonable substitute, though data on its use are still very limited. Rifabutin and rifampin are structurally similar, but rifabutin has fewer drug-drug interactions and adverse effects. A 2021 study found that among 132 staphylococcal species isolated from clinical BJIs, rifabutin had a lower minimum biofilm eradication concentration compared with that of rifampin in all strains tested.[24] Several small retrospective case series, including a 2022 study, suggest favorable outcomes when rifabutin is used,[25] but larger studies are needed to confirm these findings.

Fluoroquinolones

Fluoroquinolones have been a mainstay of treatment for BJIs because of their ability to penetrate bones and joints, oral bioavailability, and spectrum of activity. Commonly used fluoroquinolones for the treatment of BJIs include ciprofloxacin, levofloxacin, and moxifloxacin. Fluoroquinolones may be used for both staphylococcal BJI (usually in combination with rifampin) and gram-negative BJIs.

Levofloxacin and moxifloxacin tend to have lower minimum inhibitory concentrations for gram-positive pathogens compared with ciprofloxacin and have a higher barrier to the emergence of resistance.[26] In addition, ciprofloxacin used alone in staphylococcal infections may select resistant mutants, which is why this older fluoroquinolone should always be used in combination with another agent.[27] Conversely, fluoroquinolone-resistant mutants did not emerge in animal models with moxifloxacin or levofloxacin.[28] Delafloxacin is the newest member of the fluoroquinolone class that is active in vitro against methicillin-sensitive *Staphylococcus aureus* (MSSA), methicillin-resistant *S aureus* (MRSA), coagulase-negative staphylococci (CoNS), and streptococci. Delafloxacin even retains activity against strains of *S aureus* that are resistant to other fluoroquinolones.[29] Because it has unique structural characteristics, some typical adverse events are less prevalent (prolongation of corrected QT interval or phototoxicity). Delafloxacin's safety profile and good in vitro activity against biofilms make it a promising alternative to other fluoroquinolones, though minimal data have been published on the clinical use of delafloxacin for BJI. The most common adverse events are gastrointestinal (diarrhea, nausea, vomiting), but fluoroquinolones are also associated with particular but uncommon adverse events including tendon rupture, aortic aneurysm, aortic dissection, central nervous system perturbations (headache, dizziness, confusion, and convulsions), photosensitivity, and prolongation of corrected QT interval prolongation (most frequent with moxifloxacin). Last, there has been some hesitancy in prescribing fluoroquinolones in the United States as a result of multiple black box warnings reported by the FDA in a 2018 study.[30] The absorption of fluoroquinolones is impaired by coadministration of antacids containing aluminum or magnesium and with multivitamin products containing iron, calcium, or zinc. If these supplements are necessary, fluoroquinolones should be administered 2 hours before or 4 to 6 hours after the mineral supplement.

Beta-Lactams

β-Lactam antibiotics are widely used to treat BJIs because of MSSA, enterococci, streptococci, *Cutibacterium*, and gram-negative pathogens when susceptibility testing support their use. The β-lactam antibiotic class is broad, but clinicians should be aware of a few adverse effects associated with this class of therapeutic agents: immunoglobulin E–mediated allergic reactions, dermatologic reactions, central nervous system toxicity or seizures, kidney complications, and hematologic issues. There is wide support and experience for treatment of BJIs with β-lactams, including nafcillin, oxacillin, ampicillin, penicillin, piperacillin-tazobactam, cefazolin, and ceftriaxone. A few specific β-lactam antibiotics with special interest for the treatment of BJIs are discussed in the following paragraphs.

Ceftaroline

Ceftaroline is the first β-lactam with activity against MRSA thanks to a novel mechanism of action. Based on an allosteric interaction that changes the three-dimensional structure of the penicillin-binding protein PBP2A, ceftaroline is able to bind to and inhibit PBP2A, which encodes methicillin resistance among *S aureus*. In addition, ceftaroline is active against methicillin-susceptible and methicillin-resistant CoNS and streptococci, but like other cephalosporins has low or no activity against *Enterococcus* species. Ceftaroline is well-tolerated and its safety profile is reflective of other cephalosporin antibiotics, but it should be noted that low neutrophil count (<1,500 cells/mm^3) has been described more frequently with ceftaroline than with ceftriaxone (18% versus 6%) in patients receiving the drug for more than 2 weeks, according to a 2019 study.[31] There have been few studies examining ceftaroline as monotherapy in the treatment of BJIs; however, it may be useful when vancomycin is contraindicated or in polymicrobial infection including MRSA, if susceptible.

Cefepime

Cefepime is a fourth-generation cephalosporin that is commonly used for its activity against *Pseudomonas aeruginosa* and other gram-negative BJIs. Clinicians should be cautious in prescribing high doses of cefepime to elderly patients with renal dysfunction or underlying central nervous system disease because cefepime has been associated with both seizures and neurotoxicity. The incidence of cefepime neurotoxicity is rare: 2% to 3%.[32] Although cefepime was previously the only antibiotic implicated in neurotoxicity, newer literature, including a 2022 study, indicates that this can occur with all antipseudomonal β-lactam antibiotics.[32]

Vancomycin

In a 2021 study, vancomycin is described as a glycopeptide antibiotic agent that is the mainstay of treatment for a multitude of infections, including those caused by MRSA.[33] Vancomycin carries the greatest cumulative clinical experience for treating MRSA BJIs, but it may be surprising to learn that there are no controlled trials evaluating vancomycin as a treatment of MRSA BJIs.[34]

The main adverse effects of vancomycin are phlebitis, infusion reactions, acute kidney injury, and ototoxicity. Vancomycin-induced infusion reaction is a common histamine-mediated reaction of the skin during or immediately following infusion. This reaction is not a contraindication to vancomycin use; it typically can be ameliorated by prolonging the infusion time and with premedication administration of antihistamines. As discussed in a 2020 study, vancomycin nephrotoxicity is caused by accumulation of vancomycin within the proximal tubular epithelial cells, prompting apoptosis.[35] Vancomycin-associated acute kidney injury is associated with vancomycin trough levels of 15 to 20 mg/L, previous renal failure, and coadministration with other nephrotoxic agents.[36] Of particular interest, because of its common administration, there is an increased risk of acute kidney injury when vancomycin is combined with piperacillin/tazobactam and other semisynthetic penicillins (cloxacillin, nafcillin). Therefore, serum concentrations of vancomycin and renal function should be routinely monitored, and the coadministration of other nephrotoxic medications such as aminoglycosides, piperacillin/tazobactam, and NSAIDs should be avoided when possible. Patients should be regularly asked about tinnitus or decreased hearing while taking vancomycin. Potential risk factors for the development of ototoxicity are renal dysfunction and preexisting hearing abnormalities.

Lipoglycopeptides

Dalbavancin and oritavancin are prolonged half-life lipoglycopeptides that can be administered in weekly or longer interval regimens. Although they are attractive for treatment of BJIs given their broad spectrum of gram-positive activity and infrequent dosing, their use is limited by a paucity of clinical data, medication cost, and insurance barriers. Dalbavancin has in vitro activity against MSSA, MRSA, vancomycin-intermediate *S aureus*, CoNS, streptococci, and enterococci, but not enterococci with a *vanA* mutation. Oritavancin's spectrum of activity is similar to that of dalbavancin but offers the additional coverage of *vanA*-containing vancomycin-resistant enterococci (VRE). However, only limited data exist for using oritavancin and dalbavancin in the management of BJI.

Given the recent development of these two long-acting lipoglycopeptides, the data on adverse effects and interactions are scarce particularly when they are used for longer treatments. Dalbavancin is well-tolerated and early evidence suggests that it has less nephrotoxicity than vancomycin. Oritavancin does not yet have many reportable adverse effects. However, oritavancin does interact with several laboratory tests, including activated partial thromboplastin time and prothrombin time. Recent preliminary retrospective data and one 2019 clinical trial on patients with osteomyelitis are encouraging in the use of new lipoglycopeptides to treat BJI,[37-39] but larger trials are needed.

Daptomycin

Daptomycin is a cyclic lipopeptide with activity against a broad range of gram-positive organisms, and there are reasonable data to support its use in the treatment of BJI. Daptomycin is often substituted for vancomycin when toxicities preclude its use or in the setting of VRE.[40] The target dosage of daptomycin for treatment of BJIs is not clear, although the efficacy of daptomycin is thought to be dose dependent. Guidelines have suggested doses of 6 mg/kg, but doses upward of 10 mg/kg per day are well tolerated.

Daptomycin in combination with other antibiotics has been investigated in vitro and in experimental models of foreign-body infection. The most frequently evaluated combinations were daptomycin with rifampin or with a β-lactam. In general, these studies documented that combination therapy increased daptomycin efficacy.[41] Recent in vitro studies, including a 2019 study, show that daptomycin plus ceftaroline is a potent and synergistic combination against MRSA;[42] however, there is no clinical evidence to support this combination for BJI specifically.

As with other agents, daptomycin does have important toxicities. Daptomycin may elevate creatinine phosphokinase, which can be accompanied by rhabdomyolysis. Patients receiving daptomycin should be monitored for muscle pain or weakness. Concurrent statin therapy, renal failure, and a trough serum concentration of 25 mg/L or more have been reported in a 2018 study to increase the risk of rhabdomyolysis.[43] Clinicians may discontinue statin therapy if warranted based on cardiovascular risk, if the planned treatment duration is prolonged (>154 days), and if the patient is receiving a higher dose of daptomycin (>8 mg/kg per day). Eosinophilic pneumonia has been rarely described during prolonged use of daptomycin, although no risk factors have been identified.

Oxazolidinones

Linezolid is an oxazolidinone antibiotic agent that inhibits protein synthesis by binding the bacterial 23S rRNA subunit; it has in vitro activity against MSSA, MRSA, CoNS, streptococci, and enterococci, including VRE. Linezolid has been shown to be an effective treatment for gram-positive BJIs, likely in part because of its excellent bioavailability and tissue and bone penetration.[44]

Despite its favorable spectrum and tissue penetration, adverse reactions and medication interactions limit the widespread and extended use of linezolid. The underlying mechanism for adverse events is due to mitochondrial toxicity, given the similarity between bacterial 23S ribosomal RNA and human mitochondrial 16S RNA.[45] Major adverse events include gastrointestinal effects, myelosuppression, and lactic acidosis, particularly with treatment courses beyond 2 weeks, and neuropathy in courses beyond 3 months.[46] Linezolid-associated myelosuppression is dose and duration dependent, with thrombocytopenia being the most common presentation; fortunately, this condition reverses on cessation of therapy.[47] Renal impairment is an important risk factor for myelosuppression. Linezolid is associated with both an optic and peripheral stocking glove neuropathy[48] with prolonged treatment, but the incidence is not known. Although optic neuropathy is likely reversible, peripheral neuropathy may be irreversible in some cases.[48]

Drug-drug interactions also affect the use of linezolid. Linezolid coadministration with monoamine oxidase inhibitors, selective serotonin reuptake inhibitors, serotonin norepinephrine reuptake inhibitors, or bupropion can dangerously increase the amount of serotonin within synapses, causing serotonin syndrome. For patients taking interacting medications, options are to monitor closely for serotonin syndrome or to lower the dosage of or stop the interaction medication if feasible, optimally 2 weeks before initiation of linezolid.

Tedizolid is a newer oxazolidinone with a spectrum of activity similar to that of linezolid but with lower minimum inhibitory concentrations (up to fourfold) than with linezolid. Tedizolid has the benefit of being administered once per day, has not been associated with lactic acidosis or serotonin syndrome, and has a lower rate of thrombocytopenia than with linezolid.[49] At this time, there are no data on any clinical trials evaluating the use of tedizolid to specifically treat BJI, and experience with tedizolid is still limited compared with that of linezolid in BJIs.

Tetracyclines

Minocycline and doxycycline are tetracyclines with good tissue penetration, oral bioavailability, and antistaphylococcal activity.[50] Moreover, both minocycline and doxycycline are relatively well-tolerated and do not require dose adjustment for renal or liver dysfunction. Minocycline is approximately twice as lipophilic as doxycycline and would be expected to have a higher concentration in tissue.[51] However, no head-to-head comparison of minocycline and doxycycline in BJI currently exists.

Interactions and adverse effects from tetracyclines are relatively mild. Common adverse effects include nausea, vomiting, and anorexia. Notably, doxycycline is more frequently associated with esophagitis compared with minocycline.[52] Similar to fluoroquinolones, the absorption of tetracyclines can be impaired by coadministration of specific minerals (calcium, magnesium, iron), which are commonly found in antacids and dairy products, and dose separation is also advised. Prescribers should also counsel patients on skin changes while on tetracyclines. Minocycline turns black when oxidized, which can lead to hyperpigmentation of the skin, nails, and teeth with chronic therapy.[53] Hyperpigmentation may take months to years to resolve after drug discontinuation, but pigmentation may never completely disappear.[54] According to a 2019 study, patients taking doxycycline should be advised about skin photosensitivity that can occur while on this medication and should minimize direct sun exposure.[55]

As discussed in a 2019 study, omadacycline is a new member of the tetracycline antibiotics, with in vitro activity against tetracycline-resistant strains including MSSA, MRSA, CoNS, streptococci, and enterococci including VRE,[56] with a similar safety profile as other tetracyclines. Unfortunately, omadacycline remains associated with high costs and there is a paucity of data on treatment of BJIs.

Clindamycin

Clindamycin is a lincosamide antibiotic with excellent bioavailability (approximately 90%) and bone penetration that is commonly used for treatment of BJIs. However, clindamycin is not recommended without additional testing if the target organism is erythromycin resistant because 50% of these strains have an inducible expression of a methylase (MLS_B mechanism) that leads to full clindamycin resistance on exposure to clindamycin. Inducible resistance should be assessed before the use of clindamycin.

The most common adverse events are gastrointestinal (diarrhea, nausea, and vomiting), present in up to 20% of cases. Although any antibiotic agent may be implicated in *Clostridioides difficile* infection, clindamycin has historically been the antimicrobial therapy associated with *C difficile* infection, leading to some at higher risk to avoid its use.

Trimethoprim/Sulfamethoxazole

Trimethoprim/sulfamethoxazole (TMP-SMX) is a sulfonamide commonly used to treat BJIs.[57] Because the availability of exogenous thymidine may bypass the blockage of TMP-SMX, it should not be used in the setting of necrotic tissue or abscess.[57]

TMP-SMX is generally well-tolerated, although important toxicities do merit counseling and in some cases laboratory safety monitoring. The most commonly reported adverse effects with TMP-SMX are gastrointestinal tract (nausea and vomiting) and skin (rash and pruritus) reactions.[58] True nephrotoxicity is uncommon, but TMP-SMX can decrease the tubular secretion of creatinine, which can lead to an increase in serum creatinine.[59] This increase in creatinine is not a true reduction in glomerular filtration rate. Conversely, the trimethoprim component can cause a true hyperkalemia, which may need to be monitored.[60] This drug should be used only with caution in persons at risk for hyperkalemia, including those on certain medications. Trimethoprim inhibits human dihydrofolate reductase, which is needed for folate recycling; therefore, TMP-SMX should be used with caution in patients with folate deficiency or those at risk for complications of folate deficiency such as pregnancy or chronic hemolytic anemia.[61] As discussed in a 2019 study, clinicians should screen patients for allergy to sulfonamide or TMP-SMX and counsel about the development of rash, given the high incidence of allergy in the population.[62]

SUMMARY

The treatment of BJI is complex and requires a multidisciplinary approach. Antimicrobial treatment should ideally have features that include antibiofilm activity, adequate bone penetration, excellent oral bioavailability, and a good safety profile. In cases in which these criteria are fulfilled, an early switch from intravenous to oral treatment may be justified and safe, although shifting the mindset away from intravenous therapy has been challenging. Because the duration of antimicrobial treatment is long (at least 6 weeks), knowledge about common adverse effects and drug-drug interactions is needed to deliver safe care.

KEY STUDY POINTS

- Oral antibiotic are appropriate to treat BJIs when there is good bioavailability, adequate bone penetration, and antibiofilm activity.
- Clinicians should be aware of the drug-drug interactions and monitor for adverse effects of antibiotics used to treat BJIs.
- The European and American approaches to the management of BJI differ in that Europeans tend to use oral antibiotics in conjunction with rifampin and treatment duration is typically shorter.

ANNOTATED REFERENCES

1. Osmon DR, Berbari EF, Berendt AR, et al: Diagnosis and management of prosthetic joint infection: Clinical practice guidelines by the Infectious Diseases Society of America. *Clin Infect Dis* 2013;56(1):e1-e25.

2. Zimmerli W, Frei R, Widmer AF, Rajacic Z: Microbiological tests to predict treatment outcome in experimental device-related infections due to Staphylococcus aureus. *J Antimicrob Chemother* 1994;33(5):959-967.

3. Zimmerli W, Widmer AF, Blatter M, Frei R, Ochsner PE: Role of rifampin for treatment of orthopedic implant-related staphylococcal infections: A randomized controlled trial. Foreign-Body Infection (FBI) Study Group. *J Am Med Assoc* 1998;279(19):1537-1541.

4. Li HK, Agweyu A, English M, Bejon P: An unsupported preference for intravenous antibiotics. *PLoS Med* 2015;12(5):e1001825.

5. Seidelman J, Sexton DJ: Is long-term oral therapy for treatment of bone and joint infections ready for prime time? *Clin Infect Dis* 2021;73(9):e2589-e2591.

   Although treating BJIs with oral antibiotics is reasonable, parenteral antibiotics should remain the first-line therapy for such infections at this time.

6. Li HK, Rombach I, Zambellas R, et al: Oral versus intravenous antibiotics for bone and joint infection. *N Engl J Med* 2019;380(5):425-436.

   Oral antibiotic therapy was noninferior to intravenous antibiotic therapy when used during the first 6 weeks for complex orthopaedic infection, as assessed by treatment failure at 1 year.

7. Azamgarhi T, Shah A, Warren S: Clinical experience of implementing oral versus intravenous antibiotics (OVIVA) in a specialist orthopedic hospital. *Clin Infect Dis* 2021;73(9):e2582-e2588.

   Implementation of OVIVA trail in clinical practice led to reduction in hospital length of stay and antibiotic costs.

8. Bhagat H, Sikka MK, Sukerman ES, Makadia J, Lewis JS 2nd, Streifel AC: Evaluation of opportunities for oral antibiotic therapy in bone and joint infections. *Ann Pharmacother* 2023;57(2):156-162.

   Most patients treated with outpatient parenteral antimicrobial therapy for BJIs were candidates for oral antibiotics. A change in practice would result in cost savings to the US health care system.

9. McMeekin N, Geue C, Briggs A, et al: Cost-effectiveness of oral versus intravenous antibiotics (OVIVA) in patients with bone and joint infection: Evidence from a non-inferiority trial. *Wellcome Open Res* 2019;4:108.

   Treating patients with BJIs for the first 6 weeks of therapy with oral antibiotics is both less costly and does not result in detectable differences in quality of life compared with treatment with intravenous antibiotics.

10. Seaton RA, Ritchie ND, Robb F, Stewart L, White B, Vallance C: From 'OPAT' to 'COpAT': Implications of the

OVIVA study for ambulatory management of bone and joint infection. *J Antimicrob Chemother* 2019;74(8):2119-2121.

Ambulatory antibiotic therapy (whether intravenous or oral) in this patient group requires expert multidisciplinary management, monitoring, and follow-up and ideally should be undertaken within existing outpatient parenteral antimicrobial therapy or, more accurately, complex outpatient antibiotic therapy services.

11. Sclar DA, Tartaglione TA, Fine MJ: Overview of issues related to medical compliance with implications for the outpatient management of infectious diseases. *Infect Agents Dis* 1994;3(5):266-273.

12. Hamad Y, Dodda S, Frank A, et al: Perspectives of patients on outpatient parenteral antimicrobial therapy: Experiences and adherence. *Open Forum Infect Dis* 2020;7(6):ofaa205.

The purpose of this study is to determine the rate of nonadherence and factors associated with it. Less frequent antibiotic dosing and better social support were associated with improved adherence to outpatient parenteral antimicrobial therapy. In contrast, younger age, lower income, and lack of time were associated with nonadherence.

13. Kruse CC, Ekhtiari S, Oral I, et al: The use of rifampin in total joint arthroplasty: A systematic review and meta-analysis of comparative studies. *J Arthroplasty* 2022;37(8):1650-1657.

Rifampin appears to confer a protective effect against treatment failure following PJI and treatment effect is particularly pronounced in the context of exchange arthroplasty.

14. Spellberg B, Lipsky BA: Systemic antibiotic therapy for chronic osteomyelitis in adults. *Clin Infect Dis* 2012;54(3):393-407.

15. Wilson BM, Bessesen MT, Doros G, et al: Adjunctive rifampin therapy for diabetic foot osteomyelitis in the Veterans Health Administration. *JAMA Netw Open* 2019;2(11):e1916003.

Patients who were administered rifampin experienced lower rates of death and amputation than patients not treated with rifampin; these rates remained significant after adjustment for confounders.

16. Valour F, Trouillet-Assant S, Riffard N, et al: Antimicrobial activity against intraosteoblastic Staphylococcus aureus. *Antimicrob Agents Chemother* 2015;59(4):2029-2036.

17. Conlon BP, Rowe SE, Lewis K: Persister cells in biofilm associated infections. *Adv Exp Med Biol* 2015;831:1-9.

18. Beldman M, Lowik C, Soriano A, et al: If, when, and how to use rifampin in acute staphylococcal periprosthetic joint infections, a multicentre observational study. *Clin Infect Dis* 2021;73(9):1634-1641.

Data support the use of rifampin in acute staphylococcal PJIs treated with surgical débridement, particularly in knees. Immediate start of rifampin after surgical débridement should probably be discouraged, but requires further investigation.

19. Tornero E, Morata L, Martinez-Pastor JC, et al: Importance of selection and duration of antibiotic regimen in prosthetic joint infections treated with debridement and implant retention. *J Antimicrob Chemother* 2016;71(5):1395-1401.

20. Pushkin R, Iglesias-Ussel MD, Keedy K, et al: A randomized study evaluating oral fusidic acid (CEM-102) in combination with oral rifampin compared with standard-of-care antibiotics for treatment of prosthetic joint infections: A newly identified drug-drug interaction. *Clin Infect Dis* 2016;63(12):1599-1604.

21. Grosset J, Truffot-Pernot C, Lecoeur H, Guelpa-Lauras CC: Activity of rifampicin administered daily and intermittently on experimental tuberculosis in mice [Article in French]. *Pathol Biol (Paris)* 1983;31(5):446-450.

22. Kadurugamuwa JL, Sin LV, Yu J, Francis KP, Purchio TF, Contag PR: Noninvasive optical imaging method to evaluate postantibiotic effects on biofilm infection in vivo. *Antimicrob Agents Chemother* 2004;48(6):2283-2287.

23. Riedel DJ, Weekes E, Forrest GN: Addition of rifampin to standard therapy for treatment of native valve infective endocarditis caused by Staphylococcus aureus. *Antimicrob Agents Chemother* 2008;52(7):2463-2467.

24. Tuloup V, France M, Garreau R, et al: Model-based comparative analysis of rifampicin and rifabutin drug-drug interaction profile. *Antimicrob Agents Chemother* 2021;65(9):e0104321.

This study discusses a model-based approach showing that drug-drug interactions caused by low-dose rifampin were twice as potent as those caused by rifabutin. In contrast to rifampin, rifabutin appeared unlikely to cause severe drug-drug interactions.

25. Thill P, Robineau O, Roosen G, et al: Rifabutin versus rifampicin bactericidal and antibiofilm activities against clinical strains of Staphylococcus spp. isolated from bone and joint infections. *J Antimicrob Chemother* 2022;77(4):1036-1040.

Using the determination of minimum biofilm eradication concentration values, this study suggests that rifabutin is more effective than rifampicin against clinical strains of *Staphylococcus* spp. obtained from PJIs. Using minimum biofilm eradication concentrations instead of minimum inhibitory concentrations seems to be of interest when considering biofilms.

26. Metzler K, Hansen GM, Hedlin P, Harding E, Drlica K, Blondeau JM: Comparison of minimal inhibitory and mutant prevention drug concentrations of 4 fluoroquinolones against clinical isolates of methicillin-susceptible and -resistant Staphylococcus aureus. *Int J Antimicrob Agents* 2004;24(2):161-167.

27. Widmer AF: New developments in diagnosis and treatment of infection in orthopedic implants. *Clin Infect Dis* 2001;33(suppl 2):S94-S106.

28. Murillo O, Pachon ME, Euba G, et al: High doses of levofloxacin vs moxifloxacin against staphylococcal experimental foreign-body infection: The effect of higher MIC-related pharmacokinetic parameters on efficacy. *J Infect* 2009;58(3):220-226.

29. Shortridge D, Flamm RK: Comparative in vitro activities of new antibiotics for the treatment of skin infections. *Clin Infect Dis* 2019;68(suppl 3):S200-S205.

Delafloxacin is unique in being active against both gram-positive and gram-negative pathogens, including those resistant to other antimicrobial agents.

30. FDA In Brief: FDA warns that fluoroquinolone antibiotics can cause aortic aneurysm in certain patients, 2018. Available at: https://www.fda.gov/news-events/fda-brief/fda-brief-fda-warns-fluoroquinolone-antibiotics-can-cause-aortic-aneurysm-certain-patients. Accessed June 30, 2022.

    The FDA issued a Drug Safety Communication warning to health care professionals to avoid prescribing fluoroquinolone antibiotics to patients who have an aortic aneurysm or are at risk for an aortic aneurysm, such as patients with a history of blood vessel blockages or aneurysms, high blood pressure, and certain genetic conditions such as Marfan syndrome and Ehlers-Danlos syndrome and elderly patients.

31. Veve MP, Stuart M, Davis SL: Comparison of neutropenia associated with ceftaroline or ceftriaxone in patients receiving at least 7 days of therapy for severe infections. *Pharmacotherapy* 2019;39(8):809-815.

    The objective was to determine drug and patient factors associated with neutropenia in patients receiving ceftaroline or ceftriaxone for deep-seated infections. The data showed that prolonged ceftaroline use was an independent risk factor for developing mild neutropenia.

32. Haddad NA, Schreier DJ, Fugate JE, et al: Incidence and predictive factors associated with beta-lactam neurotoxicity in the critically Ill: A retrospective cohort study. *Neurocrit Care* 2022;37(1):73-80.

    This study sought to define the incidence of neurotoxicity, derive a prediction model for β-lactam neurotoxicity, and then validate the model in an independent cohort of critically ill adults. In this single-center cohort of critically ill patients, β-lactam neurotoxicity was demonstrated less frequently than previously reported and obesity was identified as a novel risk factor for the development of neurotoxicity.

33. Alvarez-Arango S, Ogunwole SM, Sequist TD, Burk CM, Blumenthal KG: Vancomycin infusion reaction – Moving beyond "red man syndrome". *N Engl J Med* 2021;384(14):1283-1286.

    Vancomycin is now the most commonly used antibiotic in US hospitals, and without a specific infusion protocol, as many as half of patients who receive it experience symptoms consistent with vancomycin infusion reaction.

34. Liu C, Bayer A, Cosgrove SE, et al: Clinical practice guidelines by the Infectious Diseases Society of America for the treatment of methicillin-resistant Staphylococcus aureus infections in adults and children. *Clin Infect Dis* 2011;52(3):e18-e55.

35. Rybak MJ, Le J, Lodise TP, et al: Therapeutic monitoring of vancomycin for serious methicillin-resistant Staphylococcus aureus infections: A revised consensus guideline and review by the American Society of Health-System Pharmacists, the Infectious Diseases Society of America, the Pediatric Infectious Diseases Society, and the Society of Infectious Diseases Pharmacists. *Am J Health Syst Pharm* 2020;77(11):835-864.

    The review evaluates the current scientific data and controversies associated with vancomycin dosing and serum concentration monitoring for serious MRSA infections (including but not limited to bacteremia, sepsis, infective endocarditis, pneumonia, osteomyelitis, and meningitis) and provides new recommendations based on recent available evidence.

36. Gyamlani G, Potukuchi PK, Thomas F, et al: Vancomycin-associated acute kidney injury in a large veteran population. *Am J Nephrol* 2019;49(2):133-142.

    The study evaluates the association of vancomycin with acute kidney injury in relation to its serum concentration value to examine the risk of acute kidney injury in patients treated with vancomycin when compared with a matched cohort of patients receiving nonglycopeptide antibiotics (linezolid/daptomycin). The results show that vancomycin use is associated with a higher risk of acute kidney injury when serum levels exceed 20 mg/L.

37. Matt M, Duran C, Courjon J, et al: Dalbavancin treatment for prosthetic joint infections in real-life: A national cohort study and literature review. *J Glob Antimicrob Resist* 2021;25:341-345.

    This study describes a cohort of patients treated for PJI with dalbavancin and reviews the literature regarding this condition. The results of the study and literature data suggest that use of dalbavancin in PJI could be considered, even as salvage therapy. Dalbavancin appears to be a safe and easy treatment for patients with staphylococcal PJIs.

38. Morata L, Cobo J, Fernandez-Sampedro M, et al: Safety and efficacy of prolonged use of dalbavancin in bone and joint infections. *Antimicrob Agents Chemother* 2019;63(5):e02280-18.

    This is a multicenter retrospective study of patients with an osteoarticular infection treated with at least one dose of dalbavancin between 2016 and 2017 in 30 institutions in Spain. The results showed that dalbavancin is a well-tolerated antibiotic, even when more than 2 doses are administered, and is associated with a high cure rate.

39. Rappo U, Puttagunta S, Shevchenko V, et al: Dalbavancin for the treatment of osteomyelitis in adult patients: A randomized clinical trial of efficacy and safety. *Open Forum Infect Dis* 2019;6(1):ofy331.

    This is a randomized clinic trial in adult patients with osteomyelitis or those who receive dalbavancin versus standard of care. The study concluded that a 2-dose regimen of weekly dalbavancin is effective and well tolerated for the treatment of osteomyelitis in adults.

40. Malizos K, Sarma J, Seaton RA, et al: Daptomycin for the treatment of osteomyelitis and orthopaedic device infections: Real-world clinical experience from a European registry. *Eur J Clin Microbiol Infect Dis* 2016;35(1):111-118.

41. Parra-Ruiz J, Vidaillac C, Rose WE, Rybak MJ: Activities of high-dose daptomycin, vancomycin, and moxifloxacin alone or in combination with clarithromycin or rifampin in a novel in vitro model of Staphylococcus aureus biofilm. *Antimicrob Agents Chemother* 2010;54(10):4329-4334.

42. Geriak M, Haddad F, Rizvi K, et al: Clinical data on daptomycin plus ceftaroline versus standard of care monotherapy in the treatment of methicillin-resistant Staphylococcus aureus bacteremia. *Antimicrob Agents Chemother* 2019;63(5):e02483-18.

This study evaluated 40 adult patients with MRSA bacteremia who were randomized to receive combination therapy with daptomycin and ceftaroline compared with vancomycin monotherapy or daptomycin monotherapy. Although the study was initially designed to examine bacteremia duration, an unanticipated in-hospital mortality difference of zero (0 of 17 patients) for combination therapy and 26% (6 of 23 patients) for monotherapy (P = 0.029) halted the study earlier than anticipated.

43. Ezad S, Cheema H, Collins N: Statin-induced rhabdomyolysis: A complication of a commonly overlooked drug interaction. *Oxf Med Case Reports* 2018;2018(3):omx104.

    This case report highlights the need for awareness of common drug interactions associated with statins. It also emphasizes the significance of commencing statins at a lower dose in new patients, and last, the importance of early recognition and management of rhabdomyolysis to prevent the development of complications.

44. Vercillo M, Patzakis MJ, Holtom P, Zalavras CG: Linezolid in the treatment of implant-related chronic osteomyelitis. *Clin Orthop Relat Res* 2007;461:40-43.

45. Wiener M, Guo Y, Patel G, Fries BC: Lactic acidosis after treatment with linezolid. *Infection* 2007;35(4):278-281.

46. Bishop E, Melvani S, Howden BP, Charles PG, Grayson ML: Good clinical outcomes but high rates of adverse reactions during linezolid therapy for serious infections: A proposed protocol for monitoring therapy in complex patients. *Antimicrob Agents Chemother* 2006;50(4):1599-1602.

47. Gerson SL, Kaplan SL, Bruss JB, et al: Hematologic effects of linezolid: Summary of clinical experience. *Antimicrob Agents Chemother* 2002;46(8):2723-2726.

48. Rucker JC, Hamilton SR, Bardenstein D, Isada CM, Lee MS: Linezolid-associated toxic optic neuropathy. *Neurology* 2006;66(4):595-598.

49. Prokocimer P, De Anda C, Fang E, Mehra P, Das A: Tedizolid phosphate vs linezolid for treatment of acute bacterial skin and skin structure infections: The ESTABLISH-1 randomized trial. *J Am Med Assoc* 2013;309(6):559-569.

50. Ruhe JJ, Monson T, Bradsher RW, Menon A: Use of long-acting tetracyclines for methicillin-resistant Staphylococcus aureus infections: Case series and review of the literature. *Clin Infect Dis* 2005;40(10):1429-1434.

51. Barza M, Brown RB, Shanks C, Gamble C, Weinstein L: Relation between lipophilicity and pharmacological behavior of minocycline, doxycycline, tetracycline, and oxytetracycline in dogs. *Antimicrob Agents Chemother* 1975;8(6):713-720.

52. Lebrun-Vignes B, Kreft-Jais C, Castot A, Chosidow O, French Network of Regional Centers of Pharmacovigilance: Comparative analysis of adverse drug reactions to tetracyclines: Results of a French national survey and review of the literature. *Br J Dermatol* 2012;166(6):1333-1341.

53. Hanada Y, Berbari EF, Steckelberg JM: Minocycline-induced cutaneous hyperpigmentation in an orthopedic patient population. *Open Forum Infect Dis* 2016;3(1):ofv107.

54. Nisar MS, Iyer K, Brodell RT, Lloyd JR, Shin TM, Ahmad A: Minocycline-induced hyperpigmentation: Comparison of 3 Q-switched lasers to reverse its effects. *Clin Cosmet Investig Dermatol* 2013;6:159-162.

55. Blakely KM, Drucker AM, Rosen CF: Drug-induced photosensitivity-an update: Culprit drugs, prevention and management. *Drug Saf* 2019;42(7):827-847.

    Amiodarone, chlorpromazine, doxycycline, hydrochlorothiazide, nalidixic acid, naproxen, piroxicam, tetracycline, thioridazine, vemurafenib, and voriconazole are among the most consistently implicated drugs and warrant the most precaution by both the physician and patient.

56. Karlowsky JA, Steenbergen J, Zhanel GG: Microbiology and preclinical review of omadacycline. *Clin Infect Dis* 2019;69(suppl 1):S6-S15.

    This review outlines the microbiology and preclinical studies of omadacycline, including its mechanism of action; spectrum of activity; protein binding; activity in the presence of surfactant, serum, normal, and pH-adjusted urine, or bacterial biofilms; postantibiotic effect; pharmacodynamic properties; and in vitro and in vivo efficacy.

57. Garau J, Bouza E, Chastre J, Gudiol F, Harbarth S: Management of methicillin-resistant Staphylococcus aureus infections. *Clin Microbiol Infect* 2009;15(2):125-136.

58. Smilack JD: Trimethoprim-sulfamethoxazole. *Mayo Clin Proc* 1999;74(7):730-734.

59. Masters PA, O'Bryan TA, Zurlo J, Miller DQ, Joshi N: Trimethoprim-sulfamethoxazole revisited. *Arch Intern Med* 2003;163(4):402-410.

60. Perazella MA, Mahnensmith RL: Trimethoprim-sulfamethoxazole: Hyperkalemia is an important complication regardless of dose. *Clin Nephrol* 1996;46(3):187-192.

61. Ho JM, Juurlink DN: Considerations when prescribing trimethoprim-sulfamethoxazole. *CMAJ* 2011;183(16):1851-1858.

62. Giles A, Foushee J, Lantz E, Gumina G: Sulfonamide allergies. *Pharmacy (Basel)* 2019;7(3):132.

    This article describes the incidence, manifestations, and risk factors associated with sulfonamide allergies. The potential for cross-reactivity of allergies to sulfonamide antimicrobials with nonantimicrobial sulfonamide medications is also reviewed.

CHAPTER 14

Long-Term Antibiotic Suppression

ALEXANDER M. TATARA, MD, PhD • SANDRA B. NELSON, MD

ABSTRACT

Orthopaedic surgeons and infectious diseases physicians are sometimes faced with infections for which source control is not feasible or contraindicated, thereby rendering the likelihood of cure low. In these cases, suppressive antibiotic therapy may be considered as an alternative to curative surgery, with the goal of infection control rather than cure. Contingent on microbial susceptibility, host tolerance, and bioavailability, antibiotics may be taken over an extended period with the goal of containing an infection to prevent further tissue destruction, hardware complication, or distant spread. However, there is limited evidence in the literature to guide decisions regarding optimal patient selection, antibiotic choice, duration of therapy, and the relative risks and harms associated with long-term antibiotic suppression. It is important to review available data specific to orthopaedic infection and considerations for the use of suppressive antimicrobial therapy.

Keywords: hardware-associated infection; long-term suppression; orthopaedic device infection; prosthetic infection; suppressive antibiotic therapy

---

Dr. Nelson or an immediate family member serves as a board member, owner, officer, or committee member of Musculoskeletal Infection Society. Neither Dr. Tatara nor any immediate family member has received anything of value from or has stock or stock options held in a commercial company or institution related directly or indirectly to the subject of this chapter.

INTRODUCTION

In the absence of implanted material, bacterial infections are generally curable with antibiotic treatment and source control. Infection of implanted orthopaedic devices, such as prosthetic joints and spinal hardware, typically lead to biofilm generation, which challenges the eradication of infection. Biofilm decreases bacterial susceptibility to antibiotics, inhibits penetration of antibiotics, and facilitates immune evasion.[1,2] Complete device removal with tissue débridement followed by antibiotic therapy is the mainstay of therapy to physically eliminate biofilm and promote bacterial clearance. However, there is a subset of patients in whom source control cannot be achieved, either because of surgical factors, the potential for limb loss, or medical frailty. In cases in which infected orthopaedic hardware cannot be removed, suppressive antibiotic therapy (SAT) may be considered. SAT has carried different definitions in different studies; for this chapter, SAT is defined as the long-term use of antibiotics for an infection in which source control cannot be achieved and the likelihood of short-term cure is relatively low. The goal of SAT is to suppress the growth of bacteria and thereby contain the infection to mitigate further tissue damage, prevent systemic dissemination, preserve function, and minimize pain. SAT indications, factors in antibiotic selection, efficacy, duration of therapy, potential adverse events, and future directions for the field are discussed.

INDICATIONS

For patients with infection in which source control cannot be achieved, SAT may be considered following a therapeutic course of intravenous or highly bioavailable oral antibiotics. In the field of orthopaedics, this most frequently occurs in the setting of prosthetic joint infection (PJI), spinal fixation infection, and infection associated with osteofixation for trauma,[3] although SAT has also been used for non–hardware-associated bone infections.[4] The decision to proceed with SAT and no longer pursue source control for cure may be based on both medical and surgical factors (**Table 1**). Patients with medical comorbidities that increase surgical risk and/or with limited life expectancy may be considered for SAT. Patients in whom there are no reliable reconstructive options after device explantation, those who undergo a noncurative procedure (eg, débridement with implant retention in a chronic prosthetic infection), those with higher risk organisms (such as *Staphylococcus aureus* or *Candida* species), those for whom source control might lead to spinal instability or long bone collapse in the setting of nonunited fracture, and in some cases asymptomatic patients who would lose function and/or experience significant pain in the setting of explantation may be considered for SAT. At the 2018 second International Consensus Meeting on Musculoskeletal Infection, 95% of expert attendees agreed that long-term SAT was recommended for PJI when patients are not candidates for surgery, when surgery is not expected to improve functional outcome, and when patients decline surgery.[5] There are currently no high-quality prospective studies to determine optimal candidacy for SAT. Therefore, conversations about SAT are often multidisciplinary and include shared decision-making between the orthopaedic surgeon, infectious diseases physician, and the patient and caregivers. These decisions are often nuanced and should not be made lightly (**Figure 1**).

Given additional comorbidities, geriatric patients may be more likely to have surgical and/or medical contraindications leading to consideration of SAT. In one multicenter study of 136 patients older than 75 years with PJI treated with SAT, the reason for suppression was surgical or anesthetic contraindication in 40% of cases, refusal of surgery by the patient or their family in 33% of cases, negative risk/benefit assessment by medical staff in 19% of cases, and history of prior surgical failure in 10% of cases.[6]

In some cases, long-term antibiotics may be prescribed as secondary prophylaxis for higher-risk patients in the absence of known infection, such as in patients with frequent recurrences of hematogenous infection or after a second-stage reimplantation in the setting of cured PJI. Although the antibiotic risks associated with long-term secondary prophylaxis may be similar to those in which antibiotics are used for suppression of established infection, the balance of risks and potential benefits are different when infection is absent. Indications for and efficacy of secondary prophylaxis will not be discussed further in this chapter.

ANTIBIOTIC SELECTION

The selection of antibiotic for SAT depends on many factors, including bacterial susceptibility profile, drug bioavailability, drug adverse event profile, patient tolerance, other host factors including allergy, potential for drug-drug interactions, ease of delivery, and cost to patient. When feasible, antimicrobials that target the organism being suppressed while minimizing the effect on host microbial flora (limited antimicrobial spectrum) are preferred. Given the complexity of antibiotic selection and monitoring, infectious diseases physicians often guide these decisions.

There are a variety of oral antimicrobials available for SAT, including penicillins, cephalosporins, sulfonamides, tetracyclines, fluoroquinolones, lincomycins, oxazolidinones, rifamycins, and azoles. These different antibiotics have advantages and disadvantages as well as different dosing schedules[7] (**Table 2**). There have been no head-to-head trials comparing the efficacy of different regimens in SAT. The most prevalent regimens among studies with the largest amount of patients include tetracyclines[3,8] and

Table 1

Medical and Surgical Factors for Which Suppressive Antibiotic Therapy May Be Favored

Medical and Host Factors	Surgical Factors
Medical comorbidities that increase surgical risk	No reliable reconstruction options after device explantation and/or need for amputation
Limited life expectancy	Noncurative procedure performed (eg, débridement with implant retention in a chronic prosthetic infection)
High-risk organism (such as *Staphylococcus aureus* or *Candida* species)	Anticipated structural instability with device explantation or other curative procedure (eg, spinal instability, long bone collapse, fracture nonunion)
Strong patient preference to avoid curative surgery	Loss of function with device explantation or other curative procedure
Inability to use optimal antibiotic therapy	Significant pain with device explantation or other curative procedure

Chapter 14: Long-Term Antibiotic Suppression

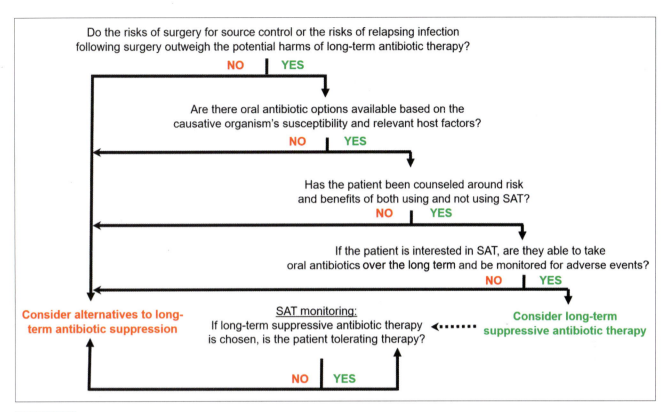

FIGURE 1 Proposed decision tree for consideration of suppressive antibiotic therapy and monitoring. SAT = suppressive antibiotic therapy

cephalosporins,[9,10] likely because of both antimicrobial spectrum and patient tolerance.

After deciding which regimens are feasible based on microbial susceptibility and host factors such as allergy and potential drug interactions, the relative toxicities specific to different antibiotics should be weighed. For example, trimethoprim/sulfamethoxazole may increase creatinine and can lead to hyperkalemia, especially in patients with borderline renal function[11] or on medications such as spironolactone. Fluoroquinolones are highly bioavailable but have a broad organism spectrum and have serious potential adverse effects including tendinitis and tendon rupture, aortic aneurysm and dissection, peripheral neuropathy, corrected QT interval (QTc) prolongation, and cardiac arrhythmia.[12] Linezolid is another example of a highly bioavailable potent antibiotic agent (effective against most gram-positive multidrug-resistant organisms), which also has a significant adverse effect profile with long-term usage, including thrombocytopenia, neuropathy, and dangerous drug-drug interactions that may lead to serotonin syndrome.[13] Therefore, fluoroquinolones and linezolid are rarely used for SAT and often only when there are no alternative options and after careful discussion of risks and benefits.

In addition to adverse events, certain antibiotic regimens may be impractical because of frequency; for example, the typical dosage for cephalexin is four times daily. Some practitioners decrease antibiotic frequency of four times daily or three times daily down to twice daily for the purposes of suppression,[7] although it is unknown whether dose reduction affects outcomes. Other regimens may not be accessible to some patients because of expense. Further prospective studies may clarify both the efficacy and adverse event profiles of different regimens for SAT.

Although SAT is almost always oral therapy, one exception may be in patients who undergo hemodialysis. Some intravenous antibiotics can be dosed during hemodialysis sessions and maintain meaningful concentrations between sessions.[14]

EFFICACY

Historically, the early literature studying SAT did not demonstrate efficacy. In studies from the late 1980s and early 1990s, patients treated with SAT for hardware infection had failure rates (defined as requiring prosthesis removal due to recurrent infection) as high as 77%,[15] adverse events requiring antibiotic changes in

Table 2

Antibiotics Commonly Used in Suppressive Antibiotic Therapy

Antimicrobial	Example[a]	Dosing for SAT[b]	Advantages	Disadvantages
Penicillins	Amoxicillin	500 mg bid-tid	Inexpensive; narrow spectrum; typically well tolerated	Relatively poor bioavailability
Cephalosporins	Cefadroxil Cephalexin	500 mg qd-bid 500 mg tid-qid	Typically well tolerated	Some may have poor bioavailability; some require frequent dosing. Second-generation and third-generation cephalosporins are broader spectrum
Sulfonamides	Trimethoprim-sulfamethoxazole	1 double strength bid	Inexpensive; good bioavailability; often active against MRSA	May cause nephrotoxicity, hepatotoxicity, and cytopenias; may lead to hyperkalemia; important drug-drug interactions (eg, methotrexate, spironolactone); can be associated with severe allergic reactions
Tetracyclines	Doxycycline Minocycline	100 mg bid 100 mg bid	Good bioavailability; generally safe and well tolerated	Bioavailability is limited with coadministration of cations; photosensitivity; hyperpigmentation with long-term use
Fluoroquinolones	Levofloxacin	500 mg qd	Good bioavailability	Associated with tendinopathy and tendon rupture; risk of neuropathy with long-term use; associated with aortic aneurysm rupture; may cause QTc prolongation. Broad spectrum; higher risk of *Clostridioides difficile* infection
Lincomycins	Clindamycin	300 mg tid-qid	Good bioavailability. Activity against gram-positive anaerobes	Increasing resistance among *Staphylococcus aureus* and streptococci; associated with *C difficile* infection. More frequent dosing sometimes required
Oxazolidinones	Linezolid	600 mg qd-bid	Good bioavailability. Activity against many multidrug-resistant gram-positive organisms	Drug-drug interactions associated with risk of serotonin syndrome; associated with thrombocytopenia and neuropathy. Requires CBC monitoring

Table 2
Antibiotics Commonly Used in Suppressive Antibiotic Therapy (Continued)

Antimicrobial	Example[a]	Dosing for SAT[b]	Advantages	Disadvantages
Rifamycins	Rifampin	600 mg qd	Good bioavailability. May have specific activity against biofilm-associated organisms	Never to be used as monotherapy because of rapid development of resistance; drug-drug interactions are common and may preclude use; risk of thrombocytopenia, nephrotoxicity, and hepatotoxicity; frequently associated with GI adverse effects
Azoles	Fluconazole	200 mg qd	Good bioavailability	Limited activity for invasive fungi outside of *Candida* species; drug-drug interactions are common and may preclude use; may cause QTc prolongation

bid = twice daily, CBC = complete blood count, GI = gastrointestinal, MRSA = methicillin-resistant *Staphylococcus aureus*, qd = daily, qid = four times daily, QTc = corrected QT interval, tid = three times daily
[a]This table is not intended to be fully comprehensive of all antimicrobials nor all advantages/disadvantages of any specific antimicrobial.
[b]Other factors such as renal function, weight, and dosing frequency may affect dose selection.[7]

38% of cases,[15] and resolution of symptoms in only 8% of cases.[16] However, recently reported outcomes have been more favorable, possibly because of factors such as antibiotics with improved bioavailability, improved débridement technique with hardware retention, and better understanding of appropriate patient selection for SAT. In a 2020 meta-analysis including seven studies and 437 patients with PJI who underwent débridement, antibiotics, and implant retention procedure followed by SAT for at least 1 year, 75% of patients had infection-free survival compared with historical rates without SAT of approximately 42% to 66%,[17] suggesting that SAT may improve outcomes in these cases. In a retrospective study of SAT in patients with predominantly infected spinal hardware, 47% of patients on SAT were infection free at 1 year and the use of SAT for at least 3 months was significantly associated with treatment success (defined as absence of surgery for persistent/recurrent inflammation, survival, and absence of prosthetic removal/amputation at 1 year) in comparison with patients who did not receive SAT.[3] Limited data are available on the efficacy of SAT in non–hardware-associated infections.

Factors predicting the success of SAT remain an area of interest, although the lack of standardized definitions for success and failure has limited this understanding. Considering surgical factors, several studies have suggested that SAT is more likely to fail (generally defined as requiring revision surgery after starting SAT, persistent fistula/drainage/pain, or patient death due to causes related to PJI) in treatment of infected total knee arthroplasty compared with total hip arthroplasty,[18,19] and a 2020 study found that upper limb PJI was more likely to fail with SAT than lower limb PJI.[8] In one retrospective study, patients with a megaprosthesis (most often due to tumor resection) were approximately three times more likely to fail SAT then those with a standard prosthesis, where failure was defined as persistent joint pain, additional need for surgical intervention to control infection, and/or death due to infection.[20] Host factors may also affect outcomes. Diabetes has been associated with recurrence of infection following cessation of SAT.[4] Despite increased comorbidities, retrospective studies in elderly populations on SAT for PJI demonstrated failure (with slightly different definitions depending on study) in only 6% to 16% and death related to infection in only 1.5% to 2.6% of patients.[6,21] Several studies suggest that younger patients have poorer outcomes regarding SAT.[8,9] However, this should be interpreted with caution as the indications for SAT may be different in younger patients, and these patients may also have more time available for infection to relapse.

The role of specific pathogens in the success or failure of SAT is also not fully understood. Retrospective studies of orthopaedic SAT have suggested that

S aureus is associated with increased SAT failure,[3,9,22,23] although one study suggested *S aureus* infection was associated with increased SAT success,[19] albeit with different definitions of success and failure between studies. One study also suggested that SAT is more likely to succeed (defined as absence of surgery for persistent/recurrent inflammation, survival, and absence of prosthetic removal/amputation at 1 year) in infected orthopaedic hardware cases caused by *Cutibacterium acnes* and fail in cases of gram-negative bacilli.[3] Culture-negative infection has been significantly associated with SAT success compared with culture-positive infection,[9] which authors speculated may be because of lower bacterial burden. Better quality data may shed more light on the effect of organism species on SAT success.

The effect of factors specific to antimicrobial usage on SAT success is likewise not fully understood. Although the optimal duration of antibiotic therapy for maximum efficacy is unknown, there is evidence that delay in initiating SAT following the initial antibiotic therapy results in poor outcomes. A 2019 retrospective study of SAT for total hip arthroplasty PJI showed that in 83% of patients who had an antibiotic-free period before the initiation of SAT, death related to PJI or new surgical intervention on the prosthesis occurred because of persistent or recurrent infection.[23] It is also unclear whether specific antibiotic selection is associated with success or failure of SAT. In one prospective study of SAT for PJI, regimens with trimethoprim/sulfamethoxazole or clindamycin had higher failure rates (defined as progressive pain, loosening of the implant, or drainage) than other regimens (including beta-lactams, fluoroquinolones, tetracyclines, and oxazolidinones) although patient number was too low for meaningful statistical comparisons.[22] In another small study of patients older than 80 years with PJI on SAT, two out of three patients treated with trimethoprim/sulfamethoxazole had treatment failure (one due to renal failure and one due to persistent infection with sinus tract).[21] These studies were not designed to evaluate the efficacy of individual regimens and likely should not contribute to decision-making until more robust data are available.

The literature suggests that in situ development of resistance is unlikely to be a major source of SAT failure. In one retrospective study of 134 patients treated for total knee arthroplasty with SAT, infection with recurrence of the original organism occurred in 19% of patients while on SAT; none of these isolates had resistance to the antibiotic used for suppression.[9] In a previously mentioned 2020 retrospective multicenter study featuring more than 300 patients on SAT for PJI, resistance developed in 15 patients (5%) and in situ development of resistance was thought to be responsible for only 12% of SAT failures.[8] This suggests that other factors, such as insurmountable biofilm burden or mechanical factors as a consequence of infection, may be contributing to failure.

DURATION OF SUPPRESSION

Suppressive antimicrobial therapy is intended for those infections in which cure is not likely to be achieved and therefore is often intended to be lifelong. However, adverse effects sometimes challenge the durability of suppression. In addition, a growing concern about the effect of long-term suppression on antimicrobial resistance may force patients and clinicians to reconsider the duration of SAT. The optimal duration for SAT remains unknown. Different groups have studied durations ranging from as short as 3 months to lifelong.[3,9,24] In one prospective observational study in total joint arthroplasty, increased duration of SAT appeared to correlate with increased time to relapse even beyond 2 years.[22] In a retrospective study of SAT for PJI after débridement, antibiotics, and implant retention procedure designed to study duration, the mean duration of SAT was 1.5 years. Patients were significantly more likely to experience failure (reinfection or revision) after SAT cessation rather than during SAT.[25] However, the duration of SAT before stopping did not appear to affect the likelihood of post-SAT infection and it was concluded that long-term antibiotic therapy may delay rather than prevent failure.

In a study of predominantly spinal hardware retention, patients were more than twice as likely to have treatment success at 1 year when SAT was used for at least 3 months; there was not a significant increased benefit seen at 6 and 12 months of SAT, although there were limited numbers of patients in those groups and indefinite suppression was not compared because success criteria were defined at 1-year follow-up.[3] Similarly, in a retrospective cohort study of SAT for knee PJI, it was concluded that there were diminishing returns in beneficial effect after 1 year.[19]

Radiographic or functional end points to determine SAT duration may be more meaningful than arbitrary time-based end points. For example, in one study of predominantly retained spinal hardware infection,[3] it was suggested that SAT be continued until spinal fusion is achieved in patients with early infection who have undergone successful débridement and treatment with parenteral antimicrobial agents. In long bone defects with infected hardware, radiographic union may be a reasonable SAT end point, assuming hardware could be safely removed in the setting of relapsing infection.

Because there are no high-quality data to guide decisions surrounding duration for SAT, the approach should be one of shared decision-making with the patient. If SAT is chosen, it is typically continued for at least 1 year.

Particularly for older patients, if antibiotics are well tolerated and relapse poses high morbidity, continued suppression with routine follow-up to both survey for adverse events as well as continue to revisit the risks and benefits of continuing SAT is recommended.

ADVERSE EVENTS

As with any medication, the use of antibiotics is not without risk. Long-term antimicrobial therapy may be complicated by allergic reactions (some of which may present in a delayed manner), direct toxicities (including hepatotoxicity, nephrotoxicity, and cytopenias), and harmful effect on host microbial flora. Perturbation of native flora may result in secondary infections (including cutaneous or mucosal candidiasis and *Clostridioides difficile* infection [CDI]) and may make incidental infections (such as urinary tract infections) more difficult to manage because of drug resistance. There are also some long-term harms associated with individual antibiotics, such as skin hyperpigmentation with minocycline[26] and neuropathy with linezolid.[13]

The most commonly reported adverse event during SAT is persistent diarrhea,[17] though most antimicrobial-associated diarrhea is not caused by *C difficile*. Rates of CDI in patients on long-term antibiotic therapy for osteoarticular infections (not necessarily hardware-related) are only 3.6%,[27] and in one retrospective study of 302 patients on SAT for PJI, CDI developed in only 1%.[8] In terms of adverse events resulting in antibiotic change, acute kidney injury was the most common in one study.[18] In elderly patients, renal failure was the most common adverse drug reaction in SAT.[6] Other more frequent adverse events related to SAT reported in the literature include drug-related rash, nausea, and dizziness.[10] In one study, beta-lactams used in SAT had significantly lower rates of adverse events than other classes of antibiotics[6] although more robust data are required to better understand differential adverse events between SAT regimens. Specific risks associated with commonly used antibiotic classes are outlined in **Table 2**.

With SAT, adverse events are important not only because they cause direct harm but also because they may result in changes to or cessation of the SAT regimen, thereby affecting the long-term success of SAT. In addition, regimen changes can be challenging, especially if the causative bacteria has drug resistance, and multiple antibiotic changes have been associated with increased SAT failure.[18] In a 2020 meta-analysis of seven studies of SAT for PJI including 437 patients, 15.4% had adverse effects, but only 4.3% required antibiotic discontinuation.[17] These numbers may be higher in specific populations. For example, in a study of SAT in elderly patients, 9% had antibiotic discontinuation (with rifampin being the most commonly discontinued agent) and an additional 9% required antibiotic change.[6] Interestingly, in one retrospective cohort study that compared patients treated with débridement, antibiotics, and implant retention procedure following PJI, there were no significant differences in adverse event rate between those who then had SAT versus those who did not have additional SAT.[10]

Development of antibiotic resistance is another known risk associated with long-term antimicrobial therapy. In one retrospective study of 211 patients receiving secondary prophylaxis following two-stage PJI treatment, patients who received prolonged oral antibiotic treatment were more likely to have resistant organisms on PJI recurrence although a prolonged course of oral antibiotics did not significantly affect recurrence rates.[28] In addition to potentially affecting resistance in organisms involved in the infected hardware, all patients on antimicrobial therapy have alterations in their native flora, although the long-term effect of this is not well understood. In some patients on long-term antibacterial therapy, cutaneous, oral, and/or vaginal candidiasis may develop and lead to significant discomfort. CDI is also a well-established risk of antimicrobial use, particularly in individuals receiving antimicrobial agents with greater effect on the gut microbiome. Antimicrobials such as trimethoprim-sulfamethoxazole and doxycycline may be safer for patients at higher risk of CDI. The use of long-term suppression may also promote drug-resistant urinary tract infection and contribute to colonization with organisms such as methicillin-resistant *S aureus* and vancomycin-resistant *Enterococcus*.

Discussing potential adverse events with patients before initiation of SAT is important. In one study of patients on life-long antibiotic therapy, 34% thought that they were not made aware of potential adverse effects.[24] Counseling patients on these potential adverse events better prepares them to self-assess for events so that they can be addressed earlier and allows for more nuanced decision-making in antibiotic selection as well as decision to pursue SAT.

FUTURE DIRECTIONS

Although recent retrospective data suggest that SAT may be successful in infection suppression for specific clinical scenarios, there are no randomized controlled trials demonstrating the efficacy of SAT. In general, SAT is guided by retrospective data and expert opinion. Understanding which patients benefit most from SAT will further enhance decisions around patient selection and reduce unnecessary exposure to long-term antimicrobial agents. Prospective studies evaluating efficacy and risks associated with specific antimicrobial agents and assessing the optimal duration of SAT are needed. There is also a lack of data regarding SAT in atypical infections, including mycobacterial and fungal hardware infection. With the increasing use of orthopaedic devices and the increasing medical complexity of the patient population receiving these devices, the field would benefit from high-quality data to guide decision-making in the use of SAT.

SUMMARY

SAT may be indicated in orthopaedic patients who otherwise are not candidates for a curative approach to their infections. SAT antibiotic selection is multifactorial and must consider the bacterial susceptibility profile, tolerance, bioavailability, and the ability of the patient to adhere to therapy. Adverse events are typically manageable, although changing antibiotics regimens multiple times is associated with failure of SAT. If SAT is pursued, it should be initiated immediately following the intensive treatment period for infection without an antimicrobial holiday. The optimal duration of SAT is unknown and has ranged from several months to lifelong. Although there are no high-quality studies on the efficacy of SAT, it is likely most successful in total hip arthroplasty PJI, compared with other arthroplasty infections, spinal hardware infection, and non–hardware-associated osteomyelitis. As the population ages and presents with increasingly complicated comorbidities, the group of patients with orthopaedic infection and contraindications for surgery may increase. There is currently a dearth of evidence to guide decision-making in SAT; well-designed studies to better understand the best management practices for these challenging cases are needed.

KEY STUDY POINTS

- SAT may be indicated for hardware-associated infections without source control in which surgery is contraindicated or refused and safe and tolerable oral antibiotic options are available.
- The choice of antibiotic for SAT is dictated by organism susceptibility, bioavailability, adverse event profile, and ease of administration including frequency and cost.
- Potential adverse events associated with SAT should be carefully considered in weighing risks/benefits, although less commonly result in the need to discontinue SAT entirely.
- There is limited high-quality evidence to support decision-making in the use of SAT, and this should be a priority area in clinical research for the field of orthopaedic hardware infection.

ANNOTATED REFERENCES

1. Arciola CR, Campoccia D, Montanaro L: Implant infections: Adhesion, biofilm formation and immune evasion. *Nat Rev Microbiol* 2018;16(7):397-409.

   In this review, the fundamental principles of implant infection microbiology are reviewed including the challenge of biofilm and other virulence mechanisms.

2. Shah SR, Tatara AM, D'Souza RN, Mikos AG, Kasper FK: Evolving strategies for preventing biofilm on implantable materials. *Mater Today* 2013;16:177-182.

3. Keller SC, Cosgrove SE, Higgins Y, Piggott DA, Osgood G, Auwaerter PG: Role of suppressive oral antibiotics in orthopedic hardware infections for those not undergoing two-stage replacement surgery. *Open Forum Infect Dis* 2016;3(4):ofw176.

4. Nowak MA, Winner JS, Beilke MA: Prolonged oral antibiotic suppression in osteomyelitis and associated outcomes in a Veterans population. *Am J Health Syst Pharm* 2015;72(23 suppl 3):S150-S155.

5. Calabrò F, Coen M, Franceschini M, et al: Hip and knee section, treatment, antimicrobial suppression: Proceedings of international consensus on orthopedic infections. *J Arthroplasty* 2019;34(2 suppl):S483-S485.

   In 2018, there was a consensus meeting for orthopaedic infections. There was discussion and debate on the use of SAT for chronic PJI in which 95% of attendees agreed that SAT may be considered for patients in whom surgery is not a reasonable option. The authors acknowledged that there were no specific studies on the profile of candidates for long-term SAT.

6. Prendki V, Ferry T, Sergent P, et al: Prolonged suppressive antibiotic therapy for prosthetic joint infection in the elderly: A national multicentre cohort study. *Eur J Clin Microbiol Infect Dis* 2017;36(9):1577-1585.

7. Osmon DR, Berbari EF, Berendt AR, et al: Diagnosis and management of prosthetic joint infection: Clinical practice guidelines by the Infectious Diseases Society of America. *Clin Infect Dis* 2013;56(1):e1-e25.

8. Escudero-Sanchez R, Senneville E, Digumber M, et al: Suppressive antibiotic therapy in prosthetic joint infections: A multicentre cohort study. *Clin Microbiol Infect* 2020;26(4):499-505.

   In this retrospective multicenter study, 302 patients with PJI treated with SAT were studied to determine success. SAT was successful in 58.6% of patients and tetracyclines were the most commonly used antibiotic agent. Failure was more frequent in patients younger than 70 years, infections with organisms other than gram-positive cocci, and in upper extremity prostheses. Level of evidence: III.

9. Weston JT, Watts CD, Mabry TM, Hanssen AD, Berry DJ, Abdel MP: Irrigation and debridement with chronic antibiotic suppression for the management of infected total knee arthroplasty: A contemporary analysis. *Bone Joint J* 2018;100-B(11):1471-1476.

In this retrospective single center study, 134 cases of total knee arthroplasties were treated with débridement, antibiotics, and implant retention followed by suppressive antibiotic therapy. Infection-free survival was at 5 years was 66%, and staphylococcal infection and increased age were associated with reinfection. Level of evidence: III.

10. Shah NB, Hersh BL, Kreger A, et al: Benefits and adverse events associated with extended antibiotic use in total knee arthroplasty periprosthetic joint infection. *Clin Infect Dis* 2020;70(4):559-565.

    In this retrospective multicenter cohort study, patients with total knee arthroplasty PJI were treated with débridement, antibiotics, and implant retention alone or débridement, antibiotics, and implant retention plus SAT. Patients who underwent SAT had statistically significantly higher infection-free survival and similar rates of adverse events. Level of evidence: III.

11. Fraser TN, Avellaneda AA, Graviss EA, Musher DM: Acute kidney injury associated with trimethoprim/sulfamethoxazole. *J Antimicrob Chemother* 2012;67(5):1271-1277.

12. Baggio D, Ananda-Rajah MR: Fluoroquinolone antibiotics and adverse events. *Aust Prescr* 2021;44(5):161-164.

    Although fluoroquinolones have good oral bioavailability and broad-spectrum antimicrobial activity, they are associated with rare but significant adverse events including tendon rupture, aortic aneurysm dissection, neuropathy, and cardiac arrhythmias as a result of QTc prolongation. This review describes the adverse events and their relative frequency associated with fluoroquinolones.

13. Beekmann SE, Gilbert DN, Polgreen PM, IDSA Emerging Infections Network: Toxicity of extended courses of linezolid: Results of an Infectious Diseases Society of America Emerging Infections Network survey. *Diagn Microbiol Infect Dis* 2008;62(4):407-410.

14. Vilay AM: Antibiotic dosing in chronic kidney disease and end-stage renal disease: A focus on contemporary challenges. *Adv Chronic Kidney Dis* 2019;26(1):61-71.

    Patients with renal failure have different requirements regarding antibiotic dosing to avoid toxicity as well as subtherapeutic concentrations. This review discusses the different challenges in this population.

15. Tsukayama DT, Wicklund B, Gustilo RB: Suppressive antibiotic therapy in chronic prosthetic joint infections. *Orthopedics* 1991;14(8):841-844.

16. Johnson DP, Bannister GC: The outcome of infected arthroplasty of the knee. *J Bone Joint Surg Br* 1986;68(2):289-291.

17. Malahias MA, Gu A, Harris EC, et al: The role of long-term antibiotic suppression in the management of peri-prosthetic joint infections treated with debridement, antibiotics, and implant retention: A systematic review. *J Arthroplasty* 2020;35(4):1154-1160.

    In this meta-analysis that defined suppression as at least 1 year of SAT, 437 patients were studied from 6 retrospective studies and 1 prospective study on PJI treated with débridement, antibiotics, and implant retention and SAT. Infection-free survival was 75% and *S aureus* was the most common organism. Adverse event rate was 15.4% and discontinuation rate was 4.3%. Level of evidence: II.

18. Burr RG, Eikani CK, Adams WH, Hopkinson WJ, Brown NM: Predictors of success with chronic antibiotic suppression for prosthetic joint infections. *J Arthroplasty* 2022;37(8 suppl):S983-S988.

    In this retrospective cohort study, 45 patients with PJI treated with SAT were studied to determine markers of success, defined as revision surgery or death due to PJI. With a median follow-up of 50 months, total hip arthroplasty PJI was more likely to succeed than total knee arthroplasty PJI and patients with gram-positive infections were more likely to succeed than gram-negative infections. Multiple SAT antibiotic regimen changes were associated with failure. Level of evidence: III.

19. Siqueira MB, Saleh A, Klika AK, et al: Chronic suppression of periprosthetic joint infections with oral antibiotics increases infection-free survivorship. *J Bone Joint Surg Am* 2015;97(15):1220-1232.

20. Wouthuyzen-Bakker M, Nijman JM, Kampinga GA, van Assen S, Jutte PC: Efficacy of antibiotic suppressive therapy in patients with a prosthetic joint infection. *J Bone Jt Infect* 2017;2:77-83.

21. Prendki V, Zeller V, Passeron D, et al: Outcome of patients over 80 years of age on prolonged suppressive antibiotic therapy for at least 6 months for prosthetic joint infection. *Int J Infect Dis* 2014;29:184-189.

22. Rao N, Crossett LS, Sinha RK, Le Frock JL: Long-term suppression of infection in total joint arthroplasty. *Clin Orthop Relat Res* 2003;414:55-60.

23. Leijtens B, Weerwag L, Schreurs BW, Kullberg BJ, Rijnen W: Clinical outcome of antibiotic suppressive therapy in patients with a prosthetic joint infection after hip replacement. *J Bone Jt Infect* 2019;4(6):268-276.

    In this retrospective study, 23 patients with total hip arthroplasty PJI were treated with SAT with success in preventing revision surgery or death due to PJI in 56.5% with a median follow-up of 33 months. *S aureus* was significantly associated with poor outcome and doxycycline was the most commonly used antibiotic. Patients with an antibiotic-free period before SAT did poorly. Level of evidence: IV.

24. Lau JSY, Bhatt S, Streitberg R, Bryant M, Korman TM, Woolley I: Surveillance of life-long antibiotics-A cross-sectional cohort study assessing patient attitudes and understanding of long-term antibiotic consumption. *Infect Dis Health* 2019;24(4):179-186.

    In this study, 29 patients on life-long antibiotic treatment (mostly for hardware-associated infection) were surveyed to better analyze their understanding of SAT. Nineteen patients consented to microbiologic screening for drug-resistant organisms and one patient was found to be colonized with bacteria resistant to their SAT antibiotic. Level of evidence: IV.

25. Byren I, Bejon P, Atkins BL, et al: One hundred and twelve infected arthroplasties treated with 'DAIR' (debridement, antibiotics and implant retention): Antibiotic duration and outcome. *J Antimicrob Chemother* 2009;63(6):1264-1271.

26. Hanada Y, Berbari EF, Steckelberg JM: Minocycline-induced cutaneous hyperpigmentation in an orthopedic patient population. *Open Forum Infect Dis* 2016;3(1):ofv107.

27. Schindler M, Bernard L, Belaieff W, et al: Epidemiology of adverse events and Clostridium difficile-associated diarrhea during long-term antibiotic therapy for osteoarticular infections. *J Infect* 2013;67(5):433-438.

28. Kelly MP, Gililland JM, Blackburn BE, Anderson LA, Pelt CE, Certain LK: Extended oral antibiotics increase bacterial resistance in patients who fail 2-stage exchange for periprosthetic joint infection. *J Arthroplasty* 2022;37(8 suppl):S989-S996.

In this retrospective study, 211 patients who underwent two-stage exchange for PJI were studied to determine if an extended course of oral antibiotics (at least 2 weeks following second implantation) affected the outcome. Extended oral antibiotics did not prevent PJI recurrence but was associated with increased resistance of organisms during recurrence. Level of evidence: III.

SECTION 4

Prosthetic Joint Infections

Section Editor:
Brian A. Klatt, MD, FAAOS

CHAPTER 15

Diagnosis of Prosthetic Joint Infection

SAAD TARABICHI, MD • JAVAD PARVIZI, MD, FAAOS, FRCS

ABSTRACT

Prosthetic joint infection (PJI) is a catastrophic complication following total joint arthroplasty. Recent estimates have placed the incidence of PJI between 1% and 2% after total joint arthroplasty. To date, no single test with the sufficient accuracy necessary to diagnose PJI has been identified. As a result, the diagnosis of PJI can be challenging. However, diagnostic criteria have been established that have helped significantly improve sensitivity and specificity in this setting. Further, efforts are underway to improve the diagnosis of infection and to better identify the infecting organisms.

Keywords: diagnosis; European Bone and Joint Infection Society; International Consensus Meeting; Musculoskeletal Infection Society; prosthetic joint infection; serologic tests; synovial biomarkers

---

Dr. Parvizi or an immediate family member has received royalties from Becton Dickenson and Corentec; serves as a paid consultant to or is an employee of Becton Dickenson, Cardinal Health, Corentec, Ethicon, KCI/3M (Acelity), MicroGenDx, Peptilogics, Tenor, and Zimmer Biomet; has stock or stock options held in Acumed, LLC, Alphaeon, Ceribell, Coracoid, Elute, Hip Innovation Technology, Illuminus, Intellijoint, Molecular Surface Technologies, Nanooxygenic, Osteal, Parvizi Surgical Innovations and Subsidiaries, Peptilogic, PRN-Veterinary, and Sonata; and has received research or institutional support from 3M, Aesculap, AO Spine, Biomet, Cempra, CeramTec, DePuy, Integra, Lima, Myoscience, National Institutes of Health (NIAMS & NICHD), NDRI, Novartis, OREF, Orthospace, Pfizer, Rotation Medical, Simplify Medical, Smith & Nephew, Stelkast, Stryker, Synthes, TissueGene, Tornier, and Zimmer Biomet. Neither Dr. Tarabichi nor any immediate family member has received anything of value from or has stock or stock options held in a commercial company or institution related directly or indirectly to the subject of this chapter.

INTRODUCTION

Diagnosis of prosthetic joint infection (PJI) following primary and revision total joint arthroplasty (TJA) can be challenging. To date, no single test has demonstrated absolute accuracy in the diagnosis of PJI. Physicians currently rely on a combination of clinical signs, serological tests, and synovial markers in order to workup patients with suspected PJI. This chapter will provide a concise review of the available literature examining the utility of different tests for the diagnosis of PJI.

PROSTHETIC JOINT INFECTION IN TOTAL JOINT ARTHROPLASTY

Total joint arthroplasty is rapidly becoming one of the most commonly performed elective procedures in the developed world.[1] Prosthetic joint infection (PJI) is a devastating complication and a well-documented cause of implant failure following arthroplasty procedures.[2-5] Despite concerted international efforts, studies of large arthroplasty registries have shown that the incidence of PJI is increasing.[6] Recent estimates have placed the incidence of PJI between 0.5% and 2% after total knee arthroplasty, 0.5% and 1% after total hip arthroplasty, and less than 1% after total shoulder arthroplasty.[2,7]

As of 2020, no single gold standard test has demonstrated absolute accuracy in the diagnosis of PJI;[8] hence, it can be challenging.[9] Physicians tend to rely on a combination of serologic tests, synovial markers, intraoperative findings, and clinical judgment in the workup of patients with a painful prosthesis.[10] Advancements in technology have provided the surgeons with newer diagnostic modalities that were developed to improve diagnostic confidence in this setting.[11,12] Although this led to the identification of promising tests that are substantially relied on,[13,14] it also introduced many tests that have neither been validated nor had their usefulness properly investigated. It is important to review the most recent literature on the utility of different modalities currently used for the diagnosis of PJI.

DIAGNOSIS OF PJI

Presentation in the Hip, Knee, and Shoulder

Because of the varying clinical presentations of PJI, the proper identification of an infected prosthesis is paramount. To ensure that a diagnosis of PJI is not missed, physicians must use a high index of suspicion in all patients presenting with a painful prosthetic joint. Regardless of the affected joint, the diagnosis of PJI typically involves two steps. First, patients undergo laboratory tests for analysis of serologic markers. If these markers are elevated, arthrocentesis is performed to obtain synovial fluid for biomarker evaluation. The second step in the diagnosis of PJI involves the identification of the infecting organism. In addition to biomarker testing, culture is routinely performed on synovial fluid obtained during arthrocentesis.[15] A randomized controlled trial from 2020 demonstrated that in cases of culture-positive PJI, the identification of a pathogen can help physicians administer targeted antimicrobial therapy, greatly improving chances of treatment success.[16]

Imaging

Plain Radiographs

Conventional plain radiographs are still the gold standard imaging modality used for the diagnosis of osteoarthritis. In addition, plain radiographs are also ordered routinely during the initial workup of any painful prosthetic joint.[17] However, their use in the diagnosis of PJI is limited. Several radiologic findings on conventional radiographs, such as loosening and periosteal bone formation, have been identified as indicative of infection.[18] Despite this, it is estimated that physicians fail to identify signs of infection on radiographs in up to 50% of confirmed PJI cases.[19] Further, plain radiographs of infected prostheses often appear normal, especially in the acute phase.[20]

Nuclear Imaging

The first step in a three-phase scintigraphic bone scan involves intravenous administration of bone-seeking agents, such as diphosphonates, that have technetium-99m attached.[21] Subsequently, images are obtained at 1 to 3 seconds, followed by another image obtained during what is referred to as the blood pool phase. Following a period of 2 to 3 hours after the initial injection, the third phase involves obtaining images of the entire lower half of the body. The utility of three-phase bone scans in the diagnosis of PJI remains a contentious issue. As a result, the use of bone scans in the routine workup of patients with suspected PJI has been largely discontinued. A 2021 study reported that, in general, bone scans rely on the hypothesis that increased uptake of intravenously administered radioactive tracers (technetium or indium) by bone exhibiting abnormally high levels of structural remodeling is suggestive of an ongoing infectious process.[22] However, increases in bone remodeling have also been shown to be a constitutional part of the pathophysiology of mechanical loosening, making the test nonspecific for PJI.[23] In addition, bone remodeling is also part of the normal physiologic response following TJA. Thus, bone scans can yield false-positive results for up to 2 years following surgery.[24] In a 2020 meta-analysis, three-phase bone scans had a pooled sensitivity and specificity of 64% and 97%, respectively.[25] In addition, the next step following a positive bone scan is supplementary nuclear imaging that may not only fail to definitively diagnose PJI but also incur substantial additional costs.[26]

CT Scan and Ultrasonography

In cases of suspected PJI, it is well-established that arthrocentesis of the affected joint can be a useful diagnostic tool. However, it was noted in 2020 that although most joint aspirations can be performed in the clinic, these procedures can be technically challenging and may require the use of CT or ultrasonographic guidance.[27] Furthermore, these techniques are particularly useful when attempting to determine the significance of periprosthetic fluid collections.[28]

MAGNETIC RESONANCE IMAGING

Despite its widespread availability, MRI has little value in the diagnosis of PJI.[18] Although MRI provides greater anatomic visualization, which, in theory, can be useful to help determine the extent of infection that may have spread to the periprosthetic tissues, the metal composition of most conventional implants generates considerable metallic artifact, making the interpretation of these images challenging.[29] In addition, there remains a paucity of data on the utility of this modality in this setting. As a result, MRI is by no means routinely performed in the workup of patients with suspected PJI.

Preoperative and Intraoperative Testing

Serologic Markers

C-reactive Protein Level and Erythrocyte Sedimentation Rate

Because of their accessibility, low cost, and high sensitivity, serologic markers, such as C-reactive protein (CRP) level and erythrocyte sedimentation rate (ESR), are commonly used to help rule out PJI in patients presenting with a painful prosthetic joint.[13] This widespread use culminated in the endorsement of both aforementioned markers in the 2018 publication of clinical practice guidelines on the diagnosis of PJI.[30] However, several studies in the literature have since demonstrated that CRP level and ESR have poor specificity and are often normal in patients with low-grade infection.[31] Currently, it appears that a CRP cutoff of 10 mg/L and an ESR cutoff of 30 mm/hr are the ideal thresholds for the diagnosis of PJI.

D-dimer
In 2021, D-dimer was noted as a marker for infection following reports in the literature on its ability to predict outcomes in patients with sepsis.[32] Subsequently, promising reports in the orthopaedic literature led to its inclusion in the most recent International Consensus Meeting (ICM) definition of PJI.[33,34] Further, a 2023 large prospective study found that D-dimer demonstrated higher sensitivity than CRP and ESR in the diagnosis of PJI caused by indolent organisms.[35] However, in 2020, widespread use of this marker was met with some resistance because of conflicting reports.[36] Because of its high sensitivity, a 2022 study reported that D-dimer may have a role in screening of patients with suspected PJI.[37] In 2020, it was noted that because of heterogeneity in the measurement of D-dimer levels, different threshold levels have been proposed for the use of D-dimer in the diagnosis of PJI.[38] However, a 2023 study reported that a D-dimer threshold of 664 ng/mL was found to have the best utility for the diagnosis of PJI.[35]

Interleukin 6 and Procalcitonin
Interleukin 6 (IL-6) is a cytokine commonly secreted by macrophages after tissue injury. Once it enters the systemic circulation, IL-6 primarily acts on the liver, resulting in the production of acute phase reactants that drive inflammation.[39] Procalcitonin, also a marker of nonspecific inflammation, is thought to be produced by derivatives of embryologic neural crest cells. Although the diagnostic utility of both markers has since been determined in the literature, a lack of consensus on an optimal cutoff, as well as limited availability, precludes them from widespread adoption in this setting.[40]

Synovial Fluid Analysis
White Blood Cell Count and Polymorphonuclear Leukocyte Percentage
Several studies throughout the literature have demonstrated the utility of synovial white blood cell (WBC) count and polymorphonuclear leukocyte percentage (PMN%) in the diagnosis of PJI.[41,42] As a result, both markers are commonly present in most validated criteria used in the diagnosis of PJI. In 2018, the second ICM on musculoskeletal infection proposed new threshold levels of 3,000 cells/µL and 80% for WBC count and PMN%, respectively.[34] A subsequent study found that using those levels, WBC count demonstrated a sensitivity and specificity of 86% and 83%, respectively, whereas PMN% exhibited a sensitivity and specificity of 86% and 81%, respectively.[10]

Leukocyte Esterase Strip Test
The leukocyte esterase strip test has shown significant utility in the diagnosis of PJI. One study found that the sensitivity and specificity of leukocyte esterase in the diagnosis of PJI was 80.6% and 100%, respectively. However, it is important to note that the test cannot be used in cases of bloody synovial fluid. Furthermore, the interpretation of a leukocyte esterase result is subjective and may therefore affect the accuracy of this test.[43,44] However, the leukocyte esterase test is limited by the subjective nature of its colorimetric response and as such is not yet universally adopted.

Synovial Biomarker Test
One infection panel was first introduced as a laboratory test in 2013. In addition to measuring levels of WBC count and PMN%, it also evaluates additional biomarkers such as synovial CRP, alpha-defensin, and human neutrophil elastase.[45] Although all synovial biomarkers generally have high accuracy for the diagnosis of PJI,[44] alpha-defensin was shown to outperform other markers in one study with a reported area under the curve of 0.950 and sensitivity and specificity of 100% and 98%, respectively.[46] The latter finding was disputed by two studies from 2021 that have shown little utility for routine measurement of alpha-defensin, as diagnostic accuracy of alpha-defensin was not found to be higher than synovial cell count and/or neutrophil percentage.[47,48] Another marker that is part of the Synovasure panel is synovial CRP. In a 2022 study, it was found that synovial CRP demonstrated an area under the curve of 0.951 with a sensitivity and specificity of 74.2% and 98.0%, respectively.[49]

Pathology
In 2018, neutrophil infiltration of periprosthetic tissues on histopathologic examination was shown to be highly suggestive of PJI.[50] Also, in 2018, the ICM on musculoskeletal infection identified a cutoff of five neutrophils per high-power field as having the best diagnostic utility for PJI.[34] In one study from 2018, histopathology demonstrated a sensitivity of 78% and specificity of 90% for the diagnosis of PJI.[51] However, interobserver reliability in this setting is still a primary concern. In addition, improvements in the accuracy of preoperative serologic and synovial biomarker testing have resulted in a sharp decline in the reliance on this previously popular technique.[30] Histopathologic examination is an important tool and can provide surgeons with valuable information, particularly when performed intraoperatively.

Microbial Identification
Culture
Even with the advent of newer technologies, culture testing remains the most common method for pathogen isolation in PJI.[9] In a 2019 meta-analysis, culture demonstrated a pooled sensitivity and specificity of 70% and 97%, respectively, in the diagnosis of PJI.[52] However, as reported in 2019, the rate of culture-negative infections is increasing and can be up to 45%.[53] To maximize the diagnostic yield of culture, the ICM on musculoskeletal infection recommends that at least 3 to 5 high-quality intraoperative samples be obtained

from patients undergoing revision TJA.[54] Further, a 2023 study demonstrated that holding cultures for 14 days was sufficient to capture most organisms.[55] However, although holding cultures for 14 days may help improve the detection of indolent organisms, this practice may also increase the potential for false-positive results. It is also important to note that the diagnostic accuracy of culture depends on the type of specimen being processed. In 2020, it was reported that, although preoperative joint aspiration presents the surgeon with the unique opportunity of culturing synovial fluid for pathogen identification, the risk of contamination in joint aspirations is high, making the accuracy of synovial fluid cultures questionable.[56] In one study, synovial fluid cultures were found to have a sensitivity and specificity of 55% and 100%, respectively, in the diagnosis of PJI.[57] However, because of the development of protocols focused on proper specimen collection and preparation, positive cultures of intraoperative tissue samples often correctly identify the actual infecting organism.[58] As a result, current recommendations advice that cultures of tissue be given priority over cultures of swabs and synovial fluid. Furthermore, reports in the literature on the concordance between preoperative aspiration cultures and intraoperative cultures have found varying results (44% to 85%).[59,60] More recently, sonication of the implant has garnered attention in this setting following promising reports in the literature. This technique disrupts sessile bacteria that are present in biofilm to help improve the overall yield of culture. Further, it has been suggested that sonication culture is not affected by the administration of antibiotics. One study found that implant sonication culture demonstrated a sensitivity and specificity of 97% and 90%, respectively, in the diagnosis of PJI.[57] A 2019 study noted that it is now evident that gram stain testing has little to no role in the diagnosis of PJI.[61]

Polymerase Chain Reaction and Next-Generation Sequencing

As the awareness of concepts such as viable but nonculturable bacteria increases, it is evident that culture is severely limited as a method of pathogen identification.[62] Therefore, the utilization of molecular techniques to identify pathogens in this setting is increasingly common, especially in cases of culture-negative infection.[63] Molecular techniques, such as multiplex polymerase chain reaction (PCR) testing and next-generation sequencing (NGS), can detect and identify bacterial and fungal DNA without the need for isolation on culture.[64] Hence, these techniques are highly sensitive and, per a report from 2019, can significantly increase the chances of pathogen identification, compared with traditional culture.[65] Multiplex PCR, via the use of primers, can detect both microbial DNA and resistance genes. However, its diagnostic capabilities are dependent on the availability of gene-specific primers that only exist for a selection of microbes.[66] Thus, it can fail to detect pathogens that are uncommon.[67] NGS is another molecular technique that has recently gained traction in this setting, following favorable reports in 2018.[68,69] In contrast to multiplex PCR, NGS targets two specific regions of the rRNA gene: (1) the 16S region to detect bacteria, and (2) the internal transcribed spacer region to identify fungi. This results in the production of sequence reads that are then referenced against the GenBank database from the National Institutes of Health. In a large multicenter study from 2022, NGS was capable of identifying a pathogen in 65.9% of culture-negative patients.[70] In addition to this, it is important to note that different laboratories establish different thresholds for the number of sequence reads necessary when reporting a positive result. However, because NGS targets microbial DNA, a perceived limitation of this technology is that it is not able to distinguish between organisms that are alive or dead.[71] Furthermore, NGS often identifies multiple organisms and can therefore lead to therapeutic challenges when determining appropriate antimicrobial therapy. Nevertheless, a 2018 study reported that, as molecular techniques become more readily available, their superior sensitivity and faster turnaround time may allow surgeons to administer more targeted antimicrobial therapy sooner, increasing the chances of treatment success in patients with PJI.[72]

Mass Spectrometry Analysis

Advancements in technology have resulted in the discovery of several techniques that have shown promise in the diagnosis of PJI.[11] Mass spectrometry is one such technique that is best known for its superior accuracy in the identification of different microbial species.[73] In 2021, a study reported that mass spectrometry has also demonstrated near-perfect accuracy in the diagnosis of PJI, with one study reporting an area under the curve of 0.975.[74] However, mass spectrometry machines are expensive and require highly trained laboratory personnel to perform analyses. As a result, spectrometric analysis is often inaccessible and is therefore not routinely performed in patients with suspected PJI.

Criteria

Musculoskeletal Infection Society Criteria

In 2011, the workgroup of the Musculoskeletal Infection Society (MSIS), based on the most up-to-date evidence at the time, put forward a new definition of PJI.[75] PJI was defined as either the presence of one of two major criteria or, in the absence of a single major criterion, the presence of at least four of six minor criteria. The two major criteria were as follows: (1) presence of a sinus tract that communicates with and extends down to the level of the prosthesis and (2) two positives cultures that isolate the same pathogen from two separate tissue or synovial fluid samples. The six minor criteria were as follows: (1) elevated serum CRP level (>1 mg/dL) and ESR (30 mm/hr), (2) elevated synovial WBC count, (3) elevated synovial PMN%, (4) intraoperative purulence, (5) a single positive culture from either tissue or synovial fluid, and (6) more than 5 neutrophils per high-power field on histologic examination (×400 magnification) of tissue. Although the MSIS criteria greatly improved diagnostic confidence in this setting, a notable limitation of these criteria is that it was constructed based on the expert consensus and has not been validated.

ICM Criteria

Although very similar to the original MSIS criteria, the 2013 ICM criteria were the first such criteria to propose diagnostic thresholds for different synovial tests.[76] In addition, following promising reports in the literature, it also endorsed the incorporation of a positive synovial leukocyte esterase strip test (++) as a minor criterion.[44] However, as is the case with the MSIS criteria, the diagnostic utility of the 2013 ICM criteria has never been validated. Subsequently, in 2018, the second ICM on musculoskeletal infection put forth the first evidence-based and validated criteria for the diagnosis of PJI[34] (**Figure 1**). To maximize clinical relevance, the diagnostic utility of the markers included in the 2018 ICM definition of infection was assessed in a stepwise manner. The first step involved the evaluation of serologic markers, followed by the examination of synovial markers, and finally, the evaluation of intraoperative findings. Random forest analyses were performed after each step to determine the weight and score of each of the variables studied. Following application of the criteria, patients are classified as infected (≥6), inconclusive (4 or 5), or aseptic (0 to 3). When assessing the diagnostic utility of different definitions of PJI proposed over the years, the 2018 ICM criteria (sensitivity 97.7%, specificity 99.5%) significantly outperformed the 2013 ICM criteria (sensitivity 86.9%, specificity 99.5%) and the MSIS criteria

Preoperative diagnosis

Major criteria (at least one of the following)	Decision
Two positive cultures of the same organism	Infected
Sinus tract with evidence of communication to the joint or visualization of the prosthesis	

	Minor criteria	Score	Decision
Serum	Elevated CRP *or* D-dimer	2	≥6 Infected
Serum	Elevated ESR	1	
Synovial	Elevated synovial *WBC count or LE*	3	2-5 Possibly infected [a]
Synovial	Positive alpha-defensin	3	
Synovial	Elevated synovial PMN (%)	2	0-1 Not infected
Synovial	Elevated synovial CRP	1	

Intraoperative diagnosis

Inconclusive preoperative *or* dry tap [a]	Score	Decision
Preoperative score	-	≥6 infected
Positive histology	3	4-5 Inconclusive [b]
Positive purulence	3	
Single positive culture	2	≤3 Not infected

FIGURE 1 2018 International Consensus Meeting definition for hip and knee prosthetic joint infection. CRP = C-reactive protein, ESR = erythrocyte sedimentation rate, LE = leukocyte esterase, PMN = polymorphonuclear leukocyte, WBC = white blood cell. (Reprinted from Parvizi J, Tan TL, Goswami K, et al: The 2018 definition of periprosthetic hip and knee infection: An evidence-based and validated criteria. *J Arthroplasty* 2018;33[5]:1309-1314.e2. Copyright 2018, with permission from Elsevier.)
[a] For patients with inconclusive minor criteria, operative criteria can also be used to fulfill definition for PJI.
[b] Consider further molecular diagnostics such as next-generation sequencing.

Section 4: Prosthetic Joint Infections

	Infection Unlikely (all findings negative)	**Infection Likely** (two positive findings)[a]	**Infection Confirmed** (any positive finding)
Clinical and blood workup			
Clinical features	Clear alternative reason for implant dysfunction (eg, fracture, implant breakage, malposition, tumor)	1) Radiologic signs of loosening within the first 5 years after implantation 2) Previous wound healing problems 3) History of recent fever or bacteremia 4) Purulence around the prosthesis[b]	Sinus tract with evidence of communication to the joint or visualization of the prosthesis
C-reactive protein		>10 mg/L (1 mg/dL)[c]	
Synovial fluid cytologic analysis[d]			
Leukocyte count[c] (cells/µL)	≤1,500	>1,500	>3,000
PMN (%)[c]	≤65%	>65%	>80%
Synovial fluid biomarkers			
Alpha-defensin[e]			Positive immunoassay or lateral flow assay[e]
Microbiology[f]			
Aspiration fluid		Positive culture	
Intraoperative (fluid and tissue)	All cultures negative	Single positive culture[g]	≥ two positive samples with the same microorganism
Sonication[h] (CFU/mL)	No growth	>1 CFU/mL of any organism[g]	>50 CFU/mL of any organism
Histology[c,i]			
High-power field (400× magnification)	Negative	Presence of ≥ five neutrophils in a single HPF	Presence of ≥ five neutrophils in ≥ five HPF
			Presence of visible microorganisms
Others			
Nuclear imaging	Negative three-phase isotope bone scan[c]	Positive WBC scintigraphy[j]	

Summary Key

a. Infection is only likely if there is a positive clinical feature or raised serum C-reactive protein, together with another positive test (synovial fluid, microbiology, histology, or nuclear imaging).

b. Except in adverse local tissue reaction (ALTR) and crystal arthropathy cases.

c. Should be interpreted with caution when other possible causes of inflammation are present: gout or other crystal arthropathy, metallosis, active inflammatory joint disease (eg, rheumatoid arthritis), periprosthetic fracture, or the early postoperative period.

d. These values are valid for hip and knee periprosthetic joint infection (PJI). Parameters are only valid when clear fluid is obtained and no lavage has been performed. Volume for the analysis should be >250 µL, ideally 1 mL, collected in an EDTA-containing tube and analyzed in <1 hour, preferentially using automated techniques. For viscous samples, pretreatment with hyaluronidase improves the accuracy of optical or automated techniques. In case of blood samples, the adjusted synovial WBC= synovial WBC $_{observed}$ − [WBC $_{blood}$ / RBC blood × RBC $_{synovial\ fluid}$] should be used.

e. Not valid in cases of ALTR, hematomas, or acute inflammatory arthritis or gout.

f. If antibiotic treatment has been given (not simple prophylaxis), the results of microbiologic analysis may be compromised. In these cases, molecular techniques may have a place. Results of culture may be obtained from preoperative synovial aspiration, preoperative synovial biopsies, or (preferred) intraoperative tissue samples.

g. Interpretation of a single positive culture (or <50 CFU/mL in sonication fluid) must be cautious and taken together with other evidence. If a preoperative aspiration identified the same microorganism, they should be considered as two positive confirmatory samples. Uncommon contaminants or virulent organisms (eg, *Staphylococcus aureus* or gram-negative rods) are more likely to represent infection than common contaminants (such as coagulase-negative staphylococci, micrococci, or *Cutibacterium acnes*).

h. If centrifugation is applied, then the suggested cutoff is 200 CFU/mL to confirm infection. If other variations to the protocol are used, the published cutoff for each protocol must be applied.

i. Histologic analysis may be from preoperative biopsy, intraoperative tissue samples with either paraffin, or frozen section preparation.

j. WBC scintigraphy is regarded as positive if the uptake is increased at the 20-hour scan, compared with the earlier scans (especially when combined with complementary bone marrow scan).

FIGURE 2 2021 European Bone and Joint Infection Society definition of prosthetic joint infection. CFU = colony-forming unit, EDTA = ethylenediaminetetraacetic acid, HPF = high-power field, PMN = polymorphonuclear leukocyte, RBC = red blood cell, WBC = white blood cell. (Reprinted with permission of British Editorial Society of Bone & Joint Surgery McNally M, Sousa R, Wouthuyzen-Bakker M, et al: The EBJIS definition of periprosthetic joint infection. *Bone Joint J* 2021;103-B[1]:18-25.)

(sensitivity 79.3%, specificity 99.5%).[34] However, it is important to note that the analysis of all criteria included as part of the 2018 ICM criteria is paramount to maximize diagnostic confidence.

European Bone and Joint Infection Society Criteria

The European Bone and Joint Infection Society criteria were first proposed in 2019[77] (**Figure 2**). These criteria, through the absence or presence of different markers for infection, classify patients into three groups: (1) infection unlikely, (2) infection likely, or (3) infection confirmed. However, a potential pitfall of these criteria is that they automatically classify patients as infected based on the positivity of single synovial biomarkers, not accounting for the inherent limitations of these tests.[48] In addition, its diagnostic utility has not been validated, significantly decreasing diagnostic confidence in its proposed criteria.

SUMMARY

A single gold standard test for the diagnosis of PJI has not been identified. Therefore, the diagnosis of PJI is extremely challenging. A concise review of the available literature examining the diagnostic utility of different synovial biomarkers, serologic tests, imaging techniques, and histopathologic tests currently available to aid in the diagnosis of this complex disease process is provided. In addition, the different proposed diagnostic criteria have not only significantly increased diagnostic confidence but also have helped standardize global research efforts.

KEY STUDY POINTS

- No single test has demonstrated absolute accuracy in the diagnosis of PJI.
- Several different serologic and synovial biomarkers have demonstrated excellent utility in the diagnosis of PJI.
- Molecular techniques are the future of pathogen identification in PJI.
- Criteria proposed by international orthopaedic societies have helped significantly improve diagnostic confidence.

ANNOTATED REFERENCES

1. Sloan M, Premkumar A, Sheth NP: Projected volume of primary total joint arthroplasty in the U.S., 2014 to 2030. *J Bone Joint Surg Am* 2018;100(17):1455-1460.

    The annual volume of primary and revision TJA is expected to reach an all-time high over the next 2 decades.

2. Namba RS, Inacio MCS, Paxton EW: Risk factors associated with deep surgical site infections after primary total knee arthroplasty: An analysis of 56,216 knees. *J Bone Joint Surg Am* 2013;95(9):775-782.

3. Tarabichi S, Chisari E, Van Nest DS, Krueger CA, Parvizi J: Surgical helmets used during total joint arthroplasty harbor common pathogens: A cautionary note. *J Arthroplasty* 2022;37(8):1636-1639.

    Surgical helmets are commonly contaminated by pathogens that are known to cause PJI and are a source of significant bioburden. Level of evidence: II.

4. Tarabichi S, Parvizi J: Prevention of surgical site infection: A ten-step approach. *Arthroplasty* 2023;5(1):21.

    Prevention of surgical site infection is multimodal and requires a multidisciplinary approach. This article highlights 10 important steps for the prevention of surgical site infection and PJI.

5. Tarabichi S, Parvizi J: Preventing the impact of hyperglycemia and diabetes on patients undergoing total joint arthroplasty. *Orthop Clin North Am* 2023;54(3):247-250.

    Hyperglycemia and diabetes continue to be a major cause of poor outcomes in patients undergoing TJA. Current standard-of-care glycemic indices possess little prognostic value.

6. Springer BD, Cahue S, Etkin CD, Lewallen DG, McGrory BJ: Infection burden in total hip and knee arthroplasties: An international registry-based perspective. *Arthroplast Today* 2017;3(2):137-140.

7. Edwards JR, Peterson KD, Mu Y, et al: National Healthcare Safety Network (NHSN) report: Data summary for 2006 through 2008, issued December 2009. *Am J Infect Control* 2009;37(10):783-805.

8. Wasterlain AS, Goswami K, Ghasemi SA, Parvizi J: Diagnosis of periprosthetic infection: Recent developments. *J Bone Joint Surg Am* 2020;102(15):1366-1375.

    Diagnosis of PJI remains challenging. Recently, several serum and synovial biomarkers that can help improve diagnostic confidence in this setting have been identified.

9. Kim SJ, Cho YJ: Current guideline for diagnosis of periprosthetic joint infection: A review article. *Hip Pelvis* 2021;33(1):11-17.

    Currently, there is no gold standard test for the diagnosis of PJI. Physicians rely on a combination of serologic and synovial tests to help guide surgical decision making.

10. Shahi A, Tan TL, Kheir MM, Tan DD, Parvizi J: Diagnosing periprosthetic joint infection: And the winner is? *J Arthroplasty* 2017;32(9 suppl):S232-S235.

11. Patel R, Alijanipour P, Parvizi J: Advancements in diagnosing periprosthetic joint infections after total hip and knee arthroplasty. *Open Orthop J* 2016;10:654-661.

12. Tarabichi S, Goh GS, Fernández-Rodríguez D, Baker CM, Lizcano JD, Parvizi J: Plasma D-dimer is a promising marker to guide timing of reimplantation: A prospective cohort study. *J Arthroplasty* 2023; May 11 [Epub ahead of print].

    When compared with conventional serologic markers, plasma D-dimer was found to demonstrate superior prognostic utility in identifying infection control before reimplantation. Level of evidence: II.

13. Alijanipour P, Bakhshi H, Parvizi J: Diagnosis of periprosthetic joint infection: The threshold for serological markers. *Clin Orthop Relat Res* 2013;471(10):3186-3195.

14. Tarabichi S, Chen AF, Higuera CA, Parvizi J, Polkowski GG: 2022 American Association of Hip and Knee Surgeons Symposium: Periprosthetic joint infection. *J Arthroplasty* 2023;38(7 suppl 2):S45-S49.

    This article reviews recent strategies in the prevention, diagnosis, and management of acute and chronic PJI of the hip and knee.

15. Parvizi J, Fassihi SC, Enayatollahi MA: Diagnosis of periprosthetic joint infection following hip and knee arthroplasty. *Orthop Clin North Am* 2016;47(3):505-515.

16. Yang J, Parvizi J, Hansen EN, et al: 2020 Mark Coventry Award: Microorganism-directed oral antibiotics reduce the rate of failure due to further infection after two-stage revision hip or knee arthroplasty for chronic infection – A multicentre randomized controlled trial at a minimum of two years. *Bone Joint J* 2020;102-B(6 suppl A):3-9.

    In this randomized controlled trial, targeted antimicrobial therapy was found to reduce failure rates following a two-stage exchange for chronic PJI. Level of evidence: II.

17. Lohmann CH, Rampal S, Lohrengel M, Singh G: Imaging in peri-prosthetic assessment: An orthopaedic perspective. *EFORT Open Rev* 2017;2(5):117-125.

18. Bauer TW, Bedair H, Creech JD, et al: Hip and knee section, diagnosis, laboratory tests: Proceedings of international consensus on orthopedic infections. *J Arthroplasty* 2019;34(2 suppl):S351-S359.

    This article is a summary of the hip and knee diagnostics section from the international consensus meeting on musculoskeletal infection.

19. Zajonz D, Wuthe L, Tiepolt S, et al: Diagnostic work-up strategy for periprosthetic joint infections after total hip and knee arthroplasty: A 12-year experience on 320 consecutive cases. *Patient Saf Surg* 2015;9:20.

20. Math KR, Zaidi SF, Petchprapa C, Harwin SF: Imaging of total knee arthroplasty. *Semin Musculoskelet Radiol* 2006;10(1):47-63.

21. Dinh T, McWhorter N: Triple phase bone scan, in *StatPearls*. StatPearls Publishing, 2022. Available at: http://www.ncbi.nlm.nih.gov/books/NBK535390/. Accessed March 2, 2023.

    Triple-phase bone scans use radioisotopes to determine areas of increased metabolic activity.

22. Pinski JM, Chen AF, Estok DM, Kavolus JJ: Nuclear medicine scans in total joint replacement. *J Bone Joint Surg Am* 2021;103(4):359-372.

    Because of the increasing availability of imaging technologies, nuclear medicine scans have been used increasingly to help identify infection following TJA.

23. Weiss PE, Mall JC, Hoffer PB, Murray WR, Rodrigo JJ, Genant HK: 99mTc-methylene diphosphonate bone imaging in the evaluation of total hip prostheses. *Radiology* 1979;133(3 pt 1):727-729.

24. Glaudemans AW, Galli F, Pacilio M, Signore A: Leukocyte and bacteria imaging in prosthetic joint infection. *Eur Cell Mater* 2013;25:61-77.

25. Figa R, Veloso M, Bernaus M, et al: Should scintigraphy be completely excluded from the diagnosis of periprosthetic joint infection? *Clin Radiol* 2020;75(10):797.e1-797.e7.

    In this study, scintigraphy was found to have limited diagnostic utility in the workup of patients with suspected PJI of the hip, knee, and shoulder.

26. Patton DD: Cost-effectiveness in nuclear medicine. *Semin Nucl Med* 1993;23(1):9-30.

27. Romanò CL, Petrosillo N, Argento G, et al: The role of imaging techniques to define a peri-prosthetic hip and knee joint infection: Multidisciplinary consensus statements. *J Clin Med* 2020;9(8):2548.

    Advanced imaging techniques should not be used as part of the routine workup of patients presenting with a painful prosthetic joint. Nonetheless, they have some diagnostic utility in patients with equivocal laboratory findings.

28. Signore A, Sconfienza LM, Borens O, et al: Consensus document for the diagnosis of prosthetic joint infections: A joint paper by the EANM, EBJIS, and ESR (with ESCMID endorsement). *Eur J Nucl Med Mol Imaging* 2019;46(4):971-988.

    This is a review on the utility and feasibility of radiological techniques in the diagnosis of periprosthetic joint infection.

29. Hayter CL, Gold SL, Koff M, et al: MRI findings in painful metal-on-metal hip arthroplasty. *AJR Am J Roentgenol* 2012;199(4):884-893.

30. Goswami K, Parvizi J, Maxwell Courtney P: Current recommendations for the diagnosis of acute and chronic PJI for hip and knee—Cell counts, alpha-defensin, leukocyte esterase, next-generation sequencing. *Curr Rev Musculoskelet Med* 2018;11(3):428-438.

    This study provided recommendations for the use of synovial tests for the diagnosis of acute and chronic periprosthetic joint infection.

31. Kanafani ZA, Sexton DJ, Pien BC, Varkey J, Basmania C, Kaye KS: Postoperative joint infections due to propionibacterium species: A case-control study. *Clin Infect Dis* 2009;49(7):1083-1085.

32. Han YQ, Yan L, Zhang L, et al: Performance of D-dimer for predicting sepsis mortality in the intensive care unit. *Biochem Med* 2021;31(2):020709.

    D-dimer was found to be an accurate predictor of mortality in patients who were admitted to the intensive care unit. Level of evidence: III.

33. Shahi A, Kheir MM, Tarabichi M, Hosseinzadeh HRS, Tan TL, Parvizi J: Serum D-dimer test is promising for the diagnosis of periprosthetic joint infection and timing of reimplantation. *J Bone Joint Surg Am* 2017;99(17):1419-1427.

34. Parvizi J, Tan TL, Goswami K, et al: The 2018 definition of periprosthetic hip and knee infection: An evidence-based and validated criteria. *J Arthroplasty* 2018;33(5):1309-1314.e2.

    Using random forest analyses, the authors of this study developed the first validated definition for chronic PJI. Level of evidence: III.

35. Tarabichi S, Goh GS, Baker CM, Chisari E, Shahi A, Parvizi J: Plasma D-dimer is noninferior to serum C-reactive protein in the diagnosis of periprosthetic joint infection. *J Bone Joint Surg Am* 2023;105(7):501-508.

Plasma D-dimer was found to have comparable diagnostic accuracy with conventional serologic markers. However, it demonstrated superior sensitivity in the detection of indolent organisms. Level of evidence: II.

36. Ackmann T, Möllenbeck B, Gosheger G, et al: Comparing the diagnostic value of serum D-dimer to CRP and IL-6 in the diagnosis of chronic prosthetic joint infection. *J Clin Med* 2020;9(9):2917.

    D-dimer was found to be inferior to serum CRP and IL-6 in the diagnosis of PJI. Level of evidence: III.

37. Muñoz-Mahamud E, Tornero E, Estrada JA, Fernández-Valencia JA, Martínez-Pastor JC, Soriano Á: Usefulness of serum D-dimer and platelet count to mean platelet volume ratio to rule out chronic periprosthetic joint infection. *J Bone Jt Infect* 2022;7(3):109-115.

    Serum D-dimer outperformed conventional serologic markers and had higher diagnostic utility for the detection of PJI. Level of evidence: III.

38. Pearson LN, Moser KA, Schmidt RL: D-dimer varies widely across instrument platforms and is not a reliable indicator of periprosthetic joint infections. *Arthroplast Today* 2020;6(4):686-688.

    D-dimer levels were found to differ significantly among different assays and laboratories.

39. Selberg O, Hecker H, Martin M, Klos A, Bautsch W, Köhl J: Discrimination of sepsis and systemic inflammatory response syndrome by determination of circulating plasma concentrations of procalcitonin, protein complement 3a, and interleukin 6. *Crit Care Med* 2000;28(8):2793-2798.

40. Yoon JR, Yang SH, Shin YS: Diagnostic accuracy of interleukin-6 and procalcitonin in patients with periprosthetic joint infection: A systematic review and meta-analysis. *Int Orthop* 2018;42(6):1213-1226.

    In this meta-analysis, IL-6 and procalcitonin were found to have moderate to good diagnostic utility for the detection of PJI.

41. Bedair H, Ting N, Jacovides C, et al: The Mark Coventry Award: Diagnosis of early postoperative TKA infection using synovial fluid analysis. *Clin Orthop Relat Res* 2011;469(1):34-40.

42. Dinneen A, Guyot A, Clements J, Bradley N: Synovial fluid white cell and differential count in the diagnosis or exclusion of prosthetic joint infection. *Bone Joint J* 2013;95-B(4):554-557.

43. Chisari E, Yacovelli S, Goswami K, Shohat N, Woloszyn P, Parvizi J: Leukocyte esterase versus ICM 2018 criteria in the diagnosis of periprosthetic joint infection. *J Arthroplasty* 2021;36(8):2942-2945.e1.

    Synovial leukocyte esterase demonstrated high diagnostic accuracy when compared with the 2018 ICM for PJI. Level of evidence: III.

44. Parvizi J, Jacovides C, Antoci V, Ghanem E: Diagnosis of periprosthetic joint infection: The utility of a simple yet unappreciated enzyme. *J Bone Joint Surg Am* 2011;93(24):2242-2248.

45. Commissioner of Food and Drug Administration: FDA permits marketing of first diagnostic test to aid in detecting prosthetic joint infections. FDA, 2020. Available at: https://www.fda.gov/news-events/press-announcements/fda-permits-marketing-first-diagnostic-test-aid-detecting-prosthetic-joint-infections. Accessed July 25, 2022.

    Alpha-defensin received FDA approval in early 2020.

46. Frangiamore SJ, Gajewski ND, Saleh A, Farias-Kovac M, Barsoum WK, Higuera CA: α-Defensin accuracy to diagnose periprosthetic joint infection-best available test? *J Arthroplasty* 2016;31(2):456-460.

47. Kleeman-Forsthuber LT, Johnson RM, Brady AC, Pollet AK, Dennis DA, Jennings JM: Alpha-defensin offers limited utility in routine workup of periprosthetic joint infection. *J Arthroplasty* 2021;36(5):1746-1752.

    Alpha-defensin demonstrated comparable diagnostic accuracy with conventional synovial markers. Thus, there is limited to no value in routine ordering of alpha-defensin in patients presenting with a painful prosthetic. Level of evidence: III.

48. Ivy MI, Sharma K, Greenwood-Quaintance KE, et al: Synovial fluid α defensin has comparable accuracy to synovial fluid white blood cell count and polymorphonuclear percentage for periprosthetic joint infection diagnosis. *Bone Joint J* 2021;103-B(6):1119-1126.

    Alpha defensin was found to demonstrate no additional benefit for the diagnosis of PJI, when compared to more readily available synovial markers such as synovial white blood cell count and differential. Level of evidence: III.

49. Baker CM, Goh GS, Tarabichi S, Shohat N, Parvizi J: Synovial C-reactive protein is a useful adjunct for diagnosis of periprosthetic joint infection. *J Arthroplasty* 2022;37(12):2437-2443.e1.

    Synovial CRP level was found to demonstrate high diagnostic accuracy and can therefore be used as an adjunct in the workup of patients with suspected PJI. Level of evidence: III.

50. Bori G, McNally MA, Athanasou N: Histopathology in periprosthetic joint infection: When will the morphomolecular diagnosis be a reality? *Biomed Res Int* 2018;2018:1412701.

    Morphomolecular diagnostic techniques in the diagnosis of PJI are experiencing a surge in popularity.

51. Bémer P, Léger J, Milin S, et al: Histopathological diagnosis of prosthetic joint infection: Does a threshold of 23 neutrophils do better than classification of the periprosthetic membrane in a prospective multicenter study? *J Clin Microbiol* 2018;56(9):e00536-18.

    A threshold of 23 neutrophils per high-power field was found to have high accuracy for the diagnosis of PJI.

52. Li C, Ojeda-Thies C, Trampuz A: Culture of periprosthetic tissue in blood culture bottles for diagnosing periprosthetic joint infection. *BMC Musculoskelet Disord* 2019;20(1):299.

    Blood culture bottles are a cost-effective method for sample incubation and have a rapid turnaround time.

53. Palan J, Nolan C, Sarantos K, Westerman R, King R, Foguet P: Culture-negative periprosthetic joint infections. *EFORT Open Rev* 2019;4(10):585-594.

    Instances of culture-negative PJI are increasing and expected to reach an all-time high of 40%.

54. Zmistowski B, Della Valle C, Bauer TW, et al: Diagnosis of periprosthetic joint infection. *J Arthroplasty* 2014;29(2 suppl):77-83.

55. Tarabichi S, Goh GS, Zanna L, et al: Time to positivity of cultures obtained for periprosthetic joint infection. *J Bone Joint Surg Am* 2023;105(2):107-112.

    Time to positivity of cultures obtained for PJI was found to vary by microbial species and specimen type. Level of evidence: III.

56. Declercq P, Neyt J, Depypere M, et al: Preoperative joint aspiration culture results and causative pathogens in total hip and knee prosthesis infections: Mind the gap. *Acta Clin Belg* 2020;75(4):284-292.

    There is poor agreement between preoperative aspiration cultures and intraoperative tissue cultures.

57. Rothenberg AC, Wilson AE, Hayes JP, O'Malley MJ, Klatt BA: Sonication of arthroplasty implants improves accuracy of periprosthetic joint infection cultures. *Clin Orthop Relat Res* 2017;475(7):1827-1836.

58. Peel TN, Spelman T, Dylla BL, et al: Optimal periprosthetic tissue specimen number for diagnosis of prosthetic joint infection. *J Clin Microbiol* 2017;55(1):234-243.

59. Li H, Xu C, Hao L, Chai W, Jun F, Chen J: The concordance between preoperative aspiration and intraoperative synovial fluid culture results: Intraoperative synovial fluid re-cultures are necessary whether the preoperative aspiration culture is positive or not. *BMC Infect Dis* 2021;21(1):1018.

    Preoperative synovial fluid cultures cannot be relied on in patients undergoing revision TJA. Level of evidence: III.

60. Zanna L, Sangaletti R, Akkaya M, et al: What is the concordance rate of preoperative synovial fluid aspiration and intraoperative biopsy in detecting periprosthetic joint infection of the shoulder? *J Shoulder Elbow Surg* 2023;32(3):492-499.

    Discordance between preoperative and intraoperative culture rates in patients undergoing revision shoulder arthroplasty was found to be greater than 40%. Level of evidence: III.

61. Wouthuyzen-Bakker M, Shohat N, Sebillotte M, Arvieux C, Parvizi J, Soriano A: Is Gram staining still useful in prosthetic joint infections? *J Bone Jt Infect* 2019;4(2):56-59.

    Gram staining has no role in pathogen identification in patients with PJI. Level of evidence: III.

62. Ramamurthy T, Ghosh A, Pazhani GP, Shinoda S: Current perspectives on viable but non-culturable (VBNC) pathogenic bacteria. *Front Public Health* 2014;2:103.

63. Weile J, Knabbe C: Current applications and future trends of molecular diagnostics in clinical bacteriology. *Anal Bioanal Chem* 2009;394(3):731-742.

64. Tsui CK, Woodhall J, Chen W, et al: Molecular techniques for pathogen identification and fungus detection in the environment. *IMA Fungus* 2011;2(2):177-189.

65. Sigmund IK, Holinka J, Sevelda F, et al: Performance of automated multiplex polymerase chain reaction (mPCR) using synovial fluid in the diagnosis of native joint septic arthritis in adults. *Bone Joint J* 2019;101-B(3):288-296.

    Multiplex PCR testing demonstrated good diagnostic utility in patients with native joint septic arthritis.

66. Fenollar F, Roux V, Stein A, Drancourt M, Raoult D: Analysis of 525 samples to determine the usefulness of PCR amplification and sequencing of the 16S rRNA gene for diagnosis of bone and joint infections. *J Clin Microbiol* 2006;44(3):1018-1028.

67. Cazanave C, Greenwood-Quaintance KE, Hanssen AD, et al: Rapid molecular microbiologic diagnosis of prosthetic joint infection. *J Clin Microbiol* 2013;51(7):2280-2287.

68. Tarabichi M, Alvand A, Shohat N, Goswami K, Parvizi J: Diagnosis of Streptococcus canis periprosthetic joint infection: The utility of next-generation sequencing. *Arthroplast Today* 2018;4(1):20-23.

    This case report demonstrates the utility of NGS in identifying *Streptococcus canis*. Level of evidence: II.

69. Tarabichi M, Shohat N, Goswami K, Parvizi J: Can next generation sequencing play a role in detecting pathogens in synovial fluid? *Bone Joint J* 2018;100-B(2):127-133.

    This prospective study examined the utility of next generation sequencing in identifying pathogens in the synovial fluid of infected patients. Level of evidence: II.

70. Goswami K, Clarkson S, Phillips CD, et al: An enhanced understanding of culture-negative periprosthetic joint infection with next-generation sequencing: A multicenter study. *J Bone Joint Surg Am* 2022;104(17):1523-1529.

    NGS was capable of identifying a pathogen in more than 60% of culture-negative cases of PJI. Level of evidence: II.

71. Canvin JM, Goutcher SC, Hagig M, Gemmell CG, Sturrock RD: Persistence of Staphylococcus aureus as detected by polymerase chain reaction in the synovial fluid of a patient with septic arthritis. *Br J Rheumatol* 1997;36(2):203-206.

72. Tarabichi M, Shohat N, Goswami K, et al: Diagnosis of periprosthetic joint infection: The potential of next-generation sequencing. *J Bone Joint Surg Am* 2018;100(2):147-154.

    NGS was found to identify more than 80% of cases of culture-negative PJI. Level of evidence: II.

73. Fox A: Mass spectrometry for species or strain identification after culture or without culture: Past, present, and future. *J Clin Microbiol* 2006;44(8):2677-2680.

74. Li R, Song L, Quan Q, et al: Detecting periprosthetic joint infection by using mass spectrometry. *J Bone Joint Surg Am* 2021;103(20):1917-1926.

    Mass spectrometry demonstrates near-perfect accuracy in the diagnosis of PJI. Level of evidence: II.

75. Parvizi J, Zmistowski B, Berbari EF, et al: New definition for periprosthetic joint infection: From the Workgroup of the Musculoskeletal Infection Society. *Clin Orthop Relat Res* 2011;469(11):2992-2994.

76. Parvizi J, Gehrke T, Chen AF: Proceedings of the international consensus on periprosthetic joint infection. *Bone Joint J* 2013;95-B(11):1450-1452.

77. McNally M, Sousa R, Wouthuyzen-Bakker M, et al: The EBJIS definition of periprosthetic joint infection. *Bone Joint J* 2021;103-B(1):18-25.

    This is the new definition of PJI as put forth by the European Bone and Joint Society. Level of evidence: III.

CHAPTER 16

Surgical Treatment of Hip and Knee Prosthetic Joint Infections

MARK A. HAIMES, MD, MS • MICHAEL J. O'MALLEY, MD, FAAOS

ABSTRACT

Prosthetic joint infection (PJI) is a devastating condition with high morbidity and mortality. With the increased number of hip and knee replacements being performed, the expected number of PJIs is likely to increase as well. Treatment is usually surgical; however, the choice of surgical procedure is not universally agreed on. The spectrum of surgical treatment includes débridement with exchange of modular components (débridement, antibiotics, and implant retention), revision of all components in either a single-stage or two-stage manner, or a salvage procedure. A two-stage revision of components is the standard treatment for chronic PJI in the United States; however, single-stage revision is becoming more common internationally and in some centers in the United States. Débridement, antibiotics, and implant retention is commonly used for the treatment of acute infections with less virulent organisms and when patients cannot tolerate a full revision of components. The 1.5-stage procedure has resulted, as some patients and surgeons have both decided to defer second-stage reimplantation because of their satisfaction with their temporary spacer. The surgical options should be weighed to consider the patient's symptoms, microbiology, medical comorbidities, prior surgeries/implants, and goals for quality of life. When all other options are most likely to fail, salvage procedures should be discussed with the patient.

Keywords: 1.5-stage revision; antibiotics, débridement, and implant retention; prosthetic joint infection; single-stage revision; two-stage revision

INTRODUCTION

Generally, the treatment of prosthetic joint infection (PJI) consists of both surgical débridement and antimicrobial therapy. The proper surgical and antimicrobial approach depends on the timing of symptoms, microbiology, stability of prosthesis, quality of soft-tissue envelope, and individual patient function. Surgical options include débridement with retention of prosthesis, resection arthroplasty with reimplantation at one or two stages, arthrodesis, resection arthroplasty alone, or amputation. There is no universal standard treatment and there are differences in practice based on the region of the world. However, there are general guidelines and strong evidence in certain cases that can help surgeons plan the appropriate surgical treatment of PJI of the hip or knee.

DÉBRIDEMENT, ANTIBIOTICS, AND IMPLANT RETENTION

Indications

A 2019 literature review discussed the traditional indications for a débridement, antibiotics, and implant retention (DAIR) procedure: patients with a PJI who have well-fixed components, absence of a sinus tract, less than 3 weeks of symptoms, less than 4 weeks since index surgery, or those for whom alternative surgical strategies are unacceptable.[1] DAIR has obvious appeal if successful in that the retention of well-fixed

---

Dr. O'Malley or an immediate family member serves as a paid consultant to or is an employee of Smith & Nephew and Stryker. Neither Dr. Haimes nor any immediate family member has received anything of value from or has stock or stock options held in a commercial company or institution related directly or indirectly to the subject of this chapter.

components avoids the patient morbidity associated with removing the implants and the subsequent more difficult recovery.

Surgical Technique
The least-invasive surgical treatment of PJI is the arthroscopic DAIR procedure. A 2020 study reported only a 15% to 20% success rate for arthroscopic DAIR; subsequently, the procedure has become less common because of the low likelihood of success.[2] These results are most likely due to the inability to exchange modular components. The exchange of modular components (polyethylene in total knee arthroplasty [TKA] or head and liner in total hip arthroplasty) allows for not only removal of foreign material with a potential biofilm but also better visualization and the ability to perform a more thorough débridement. Therefore, there is no current role for arthroscopic DAIR in hip and knee PJI.[2]

Appropriate DAIR procedures consist of an open arthrotomy, extensive débridement of the synovium, irrigation, and removal and exchange of modular components. A 2020 study supported the exchange of modular components when possible.[3] The procedure itself differs among surgeons in the extent of the débridement/synovectomy as well as the local delivery of antibiotics and irrigation solutions. The optimal extent of débridement or local adjunct treatment of antibiotics and irrigation is yet to be determined. However, at the second International Consensus Meeting (ICM) on Musculoskeletal Infection, there was strong group consensus recommending irrigation with 6 to 9 L of fluid.[4]

Postoperatively, patients are treated with intravenous antibiotics for 6 weeks, followed by oral antibiotic suppression for an extended period. A 2020 retrospective review supported giving 3 to 6 months of extended oral antibiotic treatment with one study advocating for 1 year.[5]

Outcomes
The overall success of a DAIR in the literature varies widely, from zero to 90%.[6,7] The likelihood of success depends the timing of symptoms, microbiology, laboratory study results, the ability to exchange modular components, and patient comorbidities.[6-11] With recent protocols, one study from 2019 found that 84% of patients who underwent DAIR for PJI were free of infection at 2 years.[12] Another study has less-promising results, reporting a 4-year failure of 57% and a 5-year mortality of 20%.[13]

The timing of symptoms is an important prognostic indicator. In a retrospective analysis of 99 patients who underwent DAIR for PJI, 88% of patients with less than 2 days of symptoms were successfully treated in contrast to 55% with more than 2 days of symptoms.[7]

In a 2019 study of 83 patients who underwent DAIR, the mean time from onset of symptoms to surgery was 6.2 days for successfully treated patients versus 10.7 days for those with treatment failure.[11] This shifts the urgency of the DAIR procedure, once indicated, to days rather than weeks.

The infectious organism also plays a significant role in predicting successful treatment with a DAIR procedure. *Staphylococcus aureus* PJIs have a higher failure rate when compared with *Staphylococcus epidermidis* or streptococcal species.[14] This finding has persisted throughout the literature with reports of 71% failure rate of *S aureus* PJI versus 30% failure rate of *S epidermidis* PJI.[8] Another study reported a success rate of 74% for streptococcal infections versus 50% for staphylococcal infection.[7] Reported outcomes with methicillin-resistant *S aureus* continue to show a high failure rate of DAIR, as high as 84%.[9] Finally, two studies from 2019 reported that polymicrobial, antibiotic-resistant species, and fungal infections also have been shown to have a significantly higher failure rate when performing DAIR.[15,16]

Several host factors have been associated with failed DAIR treatment. A 2019 retrospective review of 199 patients who underwent DAIR for PJI found treatment failure associated with multiple factors after multivariate analysis, including acute hematogenous infection, previous revision surgery, and increased Charlson Comorbidity Index.[15] Diabetes mellitus, chronic obstructive pulmonary disease, and history of malignancy were patient comorbidities associated with treatment failure.[15] Predictive algorithms have been developed to guide treatment decisions. The KLIC-score (kidney, liver, index surgery, cemented prosthesis, and C-reactive protein value) is shown to be predictive of early failure of DAIR.[17] The CRIME80 score (C-reactive protein greater than 150 mg/L, chronic obstructive pulmonary disease, rheumatoid arthritis, fracture as indication for the prosthesis, male sex, not exchanging the mobile components during débridement, and age older than 80 years [+2, +1, +3, +3, +1, +1, and +2, respectively]) can be useful in predicting treatment failure in late acute infections. A score of 3 or greater was associated with higher treatment failure and mortality with a DAIR procedure when compared with implant removal[10] (Table 1).

There is a concern that undergoing a DAIR procedure causes worse outcomes for a subsequent two-stage revision. A multicenter retrospective cohort study demonstrated 28 failures (34%) of 83 knees that underwent a two-stage revision TKA after previous DAIR.[18] The authors attribute this high failure rate for two-stage revision TKA to the initial DAIR procedure itself. This study has limitations because it lacks a comparative group of patients and no evidence that the DAIR procedure itself caused an increase in subsequent two-stage revision TKA

Table 1

CRIME80 Score Used to Predict Treatment Failure

Chronic obstructive pulmonary disease	+2
C-reactive protein >150 mg/L	+1
Rheumatoid arthritis	+3
Fracture as indication for the prosthesis	+3
Male sex	+1
Not exchanging the modular components	+1
Age older than 80 years	+2

A score of 3 or above is associated with higher treatment failure and mortality with a débridement, antibiotics, and implant retention procedure compared with implant removal.

failure. Other studies have questioned these findings and have not shown an increase in failure rate of subsequent two-stage treatment after a failed DAIR procedure.[19-22] A 2019 multicenter retrospective review of 291 patients with knee PJI included 63 patients who underwent two-stage revision TKA alone and 228 who underwent DAIR and had a mean follow-up of 6.2 years.[22] Seventy-five patients underwent DAIR, which was unsuccessful, and subsequent two-stage revision TKA. This study demonstrated 72% success in the failed DAIR group and 81% in the staged-only group. This difference was not significant, and considering the morbidity of a two-stage revision TKA, and it was concluded that DAIR is a reasonable treatment attempt.

There has been increased interest in attempting DAIR in the more complex cases of PJI. This includes patients who previously underwent a two-stage revision or in the case of extensive instrumentation for which complete explant of hardware would have very high morbidity. One study analyzed 60 patients (42 knees, 18 hips) whose two-stage revisions had failed who then underwent subsequent procedures.[23] A DAIR procedure was performed in 37 cases, resulting in failure in 21 patients (57%). Forty patients underwent a two-stage revision TKA (17 from the DAIR group). Outcomes also were poor in the two-stage revision group, with only 26 of 40 patients (65%) undergoing second-stage reimplantation and only 16 patients (40%) of those remained infection free at 2-year follow-up. The authors note that DAIR has a high failure rate, but the outcomes of a two-stage revision are also very poor, so there are limited options in this setting. Another group of patients with complex issues includes those with extensive instrumentation and PJI. Extensive instrumentation has been defined as long revision prostheses, fully cemented constructs, and those with ingrown cones or sleeves. In a group of 87 patients with PJI and extensive instrumentation who were retrospectively reviewed, 56 underwent DAIR procedure and 31 underwent two-stage revision.[6] There was no difference in outcomes for those who underwent DAIR versus two-stage revision in terms of revision surgery or mortality; however, more patients in the DAIR cohort were ambulatory (76.8% versus 54.8%) and maintained a functional bending knee joint (85.7% versus 45.2%). The decision to undergo DAIR versus a two-stage revision was made by the treating surgeon, introducing potential bias to the groups. However, 27% of the patients who underwent DAIR had symptoms for longer than 4 weeks and 25% had a draining sinus. These previously considered contraindications for a DAIR procedure seem to still allow for reasonable results in these difficult situations. It is important to note that antibiotics were continued indefinitely in the DAIR population in this study.

DAIR can be a successful treatment option if the indications are appropriate. The timing of surgery is critical and, if possible, patients should undergo surgery within days of diagnosis. Patients with streptococcal or *S epidermidis* infection have better results than those with *S aureus* infection, antimicrobial-resistant organism infection, polymicrobial infections, or fungal infections. Extended oral antibiotics after 6 weeks of intravenous antibiotics increase the rate of successful DAIR. DAIR procedure failed in patients with an acute hematogenous infection, bacteremia, elevated erythrocyte sedimentation rate, diabetes, chronic obstructive pulmonary disease, or previous revision surgery. However, in the appropriate setting, patients with extensive hardware may benefit from an attempted DAIR procedure and chronic suppressive antibiotics rather than the morbidity associated with a two-stage revision. Future studies are needed to find the ideal irrigation solutions that have the highest yield for infection control, what antibiotic regimen and duration is most appropriate, and which local antibiotic delivery modality is best. Genomic sequencing may play a role in the future to improve pathogen identification and tailor appropriate treatment.

TWO-STAGE REVISION ARTHROPLASTY

The most commonly used treatment for hip and knee PJI in North America is a two-stage revision of components. First described in 1983, the components are removed during the first procedure, along with extensive débridement and irrigation.[24] Commonly, a temporary spacer is placed to maintain the joint space and deliver antibiotics locally. The patient is placed on parenteral antibiotics for a period of 6 to 12 weeks and a second surgery is performed with repeat débridement and irrigation followed by reimplantation of new components. Outside of chronic PJI, other indications include conditions in which DAIR or a single-stage procedure is more likely to fail such as PJI with active sepsis or virulent/resistant pathogens.

Stage One and Antibiotic Spacers

The first stage involves the removal of implants, extensive débridement, and usually, the insertion of an antibiotic spacer. Implant removal can be extremely complex and time consuming if the implants are well-fixed. The goal with any implant removal is to perform an extensive synovectomy and preserve as much bone as possible. Techniques to remove implants are beyond the scope of this chapter but are integral to master when performing revisions for infection.

Inserting a spacer during the interval between the first and second stage of a two-stage revision serves several purposes. It maintains the joint space and often can be a functional joint, providing patients comfort and making reimplantation easier. In addition, spacers are used to deliver antibiotics locally, which may aid in infection control. Spacers can be defined as static (nonarticulating) or dynamic (articulating). Dynamic spacers can be made entirely of cement or composed of normal arthroplasty components with a metal-on-polyethylene articulation, commonly referred to as a low-friction spacer.

Knee

A 2019 study reported on the use of static spacers as a temporary arthrodesis with antibiotic-loaded cement between the femur and tibia, usually with an intramedullary device extending into the diaphysis of the femur and tibia.[25] These serve to maintain the joint space and provide increased stability of the knee. These are generally indicated for severe bone loss, collateral ligament insufficiency (**Figure 1**), periarticular fracture, or extensor mechanism disruption.[26,27] Articulating cement spacers can be prefabricated or made intraoperatively. The benefit of the prefabricated spacers (**Figure 2**) is time saved in the operating room. However, the antibiotic agent present in the prosthesis cannot be tailored to the sensitivities of the pathogen. Limitations of these spacers include patient discomfort, as they often report a grinding sensation with joint movement. In addition, these spacers can dislodge or fracture (**Figure 3**). Low-friction spacers are gaining popularity because the joint feels more normal to patients (**Figure 4**). Concerns regarding the use of metal and polyethylene in an infected joint are expected, but a 2020 study reported no increase in failure or subsequent reinfection with these spacers.[28] Some surgeons place antibiotic dowels in the medullary canal to help stabilize the implant and to deliver additional antibiotics. A 2019 study evaluating their use reported no increase in infection eradication.[29]

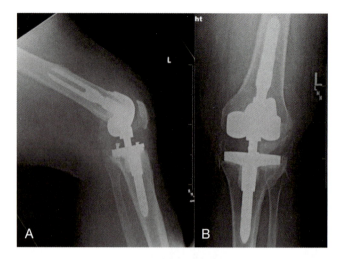

FIGURE 1 **A** and **B**, Lateral and AP radiographs showing previous hinged total knee arthroplasty with collateral ligament insufficiency. **C** and **D**, AP and Lateral radiographs show the same knee with subsequent prosthetic joint infection treated with static spacer rather than an articulating spacer because of collateral ligament insufficiency.

Hip

Nonarticulating (Girdlestone) spacers in the hip are usually composed of packed antibiotic-laden cement in the acetabulum and in the open femoral canal (**Figure 5**). Antibiotic beads can also be used. The primary indication for nonarticulating hip spacers is inadequate bone stock to support a dynamic spacer. Similar to the knee, dynamic spacers in the hip vary in design and composition. Hip spacers can be prefabricated with antibiotic cement or can be sized and molded intraoperatively. Real-component, low-friction spacers have gained popularity in the hip as well (**Figure 6**). The benefit of articulating spacers is that the patient obtains a functioning hip during the interval between stages. Complications however have been described, including fracture, bone erosion, and dislocation.

Chapter 16: Surgical Treatment of Hip and Knee Prosthetic Joint Infections

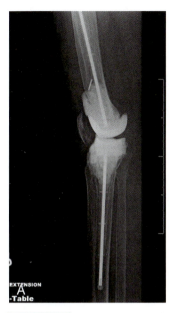
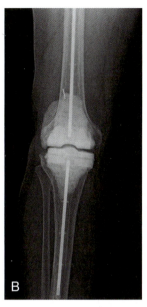

FIGURE 2 **A** and **B**, Plain lateral and AP radiographs show a total knee arthroplasty prosthetic knee infection treated with a prefabricated cement spacer.

The antibiotics used in the spacer should be tailored to the infectious organism, as well as bactericidal, water soluble, and thermodynamically stable. These include most commonly tobramycin, gentamycin, and vancomycin. Spacers have varying antibiotic compositions with no randomized controlled trials to compare them.[28] However, there is evidence to support the use of more than 2 g of vancomycin per 40-g bag of cement in the spacer construct, as a decrease in treatment failure has been reported.[20]

Two randomized controlled trials comparing static and articulating spacers, one published in 2020 for knees[30] and the other published in 2021 for hips,[31] demonstrate favorable outcomes with articulating spacers. Sixty-eight patients undergoing two-stage exchange for knee PJI were randomized to either static spacer or articulating spacer made intraoperatively with the use of silicone molds. The static spacer group had a longer hospital stay (6.1 versus 5.1 days), decreased arc of motion at follow-up (100° versus 113°), and lower Knee Society Score (69.8 versus 79.4). Although not statistically significant, there was also a greater need for extensile exposure at the time of reimplantation (16.7% versus 4.0%) and a higher reoperation rate (25.0% versus 8.0%) in the static spacer group.[30] Fifty-two patients undergoing two-stage exchange for hip PJI were randomized to either static spacer or articulating spacer made intraoperatively with the use of silicone molds. There was no difference in surgical time at second-stage reimplantation (143 minutes static versus 145 articulating). Hospital stay was longer in the static cohort after stage one (8.6 versus 5.4 days) and stage two (6.3 versus 3.6 days). Although it did not reach statistical significance, the static cohort was more often discharged to an extended care facility after stage one (65% versus 30%, $P = 0.056$).[31]

The optimal spacer construct has yet to be determined. In a systematic meta-analysis of 34 articles containing

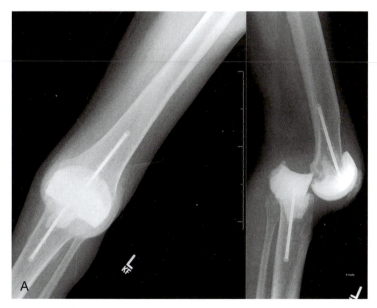
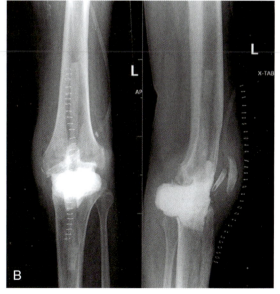

FIGURE 3 **A**, AP and Lateral radiographs showing an articulating spacer dislocation. **B**, Revision spacer exchange to a static spacer created with antibiotic cement and intramedullary placement of an external fixator bar.

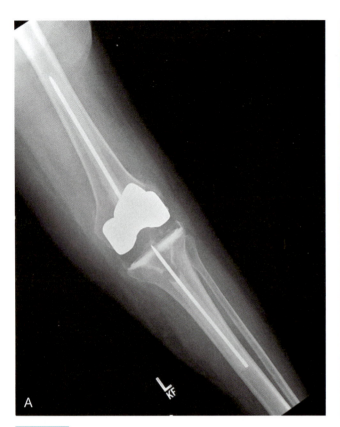

FIGURE 4 **A** and **B**, AP and Lateral radiographs of a low-friction articulating knee spacer created with primary total knee arthroplasty components, including a metal femur and an all-polyethylene tibia. This spacer has intramedullary dowels secured using Steinmann pins.

1,016 spacers, metal-on-polyethylene spacers had an increased range of motion, fewer spacer-specific complications, and no spacer fractures compared with the four other spacer types. There was no difference in terms of reinfection rates or difficulty with reimplantation between spacers.[32] Another systematic review of 48 reports comparing 962 articulating and 707 static spacers with mean follow-up of 4 years found both groups had similar Knee Society Scores, reinfection rates, complication rates, or reoperation rates.[33] However, the articulating spacer group had improved range of motion.

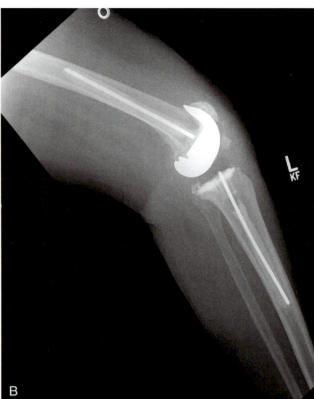

FIGURE 5 Radiograph from a patient who underwent revision to a nonarticulating Girdlestone spacer because of persistent infection with an articulating spacer.

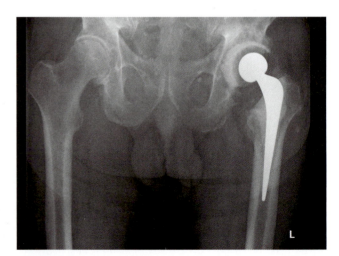

FIGURE 6 Radiograph of a low-friction spacer made with primary total hip arthroplasty components and high antibiotic-laden cement.

Spacer complications do occur. A 2019 study reported that, in a group of patients with varying types of hip spacers, 48 of 185 patients (26%) were reported to have spacer complications.[34] Dislocation occurred in 17 patients (9%) and was associated with reduced femoral offset of greater than 5 mm and increased bone loss. Spacer fracture occurred in 14 of 185 patients (8%), 12% (12 of 97 patients) of molded versus 8% (2 of 23 patients) of handmade spacers. Periprosthetic fracture was associated with the use of an extended trochanteric osteotomy and increased offset greater than 5 mm.

Stage Two

Most patients receive 4 to 6 weeks of intravenous antibiotics after resection of the infected prosthesis. Reimplantation is delayed until the soft tissues have healed and the infection is treated. As of 2019, there was no consensus on the timing of reimplantation,[35] with some surgeons opting for a 2- to 6-week antibiotics holiday. The rationale for this is to allow for the emergence of persistent infection before reimplantation. The 2018 ICM guidelines report limited evidence to support the use of an antibiotic holiday before reimplantation.[36]

Although the Musculoskeletal Infection Society (MSIS) guidelines are very helpful in diagnosing PJI, they are not useful in the determination of persistent infection before reimplantation.[37] Serum erythrocyte sedimentation rate and C-reactive protein level are commonly assessed; however, they have a low sensitivity in this setting.[38] Declining serum erythrocyte sedimentation rate and C-reactive protein level are inferred to indicate appropriate response to treatment of the infection,[36] although this no association was shown with risk for reinfection.[39,40] Therefore, surgeons do not need to wait for these markers to normalize before reimplantation.[36] Synovial fluid analysis, reported in 2022, has also varying results, with white blood cell count and polymorphonuclear leukocyte percentage demonstrating high specificity (95%) and poor sensitivity (21%) in predicting persistent infection.[41] The synovial biomarker alpha-defensin has also shown poor sensitivity (7%) and poor overall accuracy (73%; area under the curve = 0.5) in detecting infection control with spacers.[42,43] Frozen section and leukocyte esterase are two intraoperative metrics that are available. The utility of frozen section during the second-stage surgery has been debated. Original studies demonstrated that frozen section correlated with standard histology and had sensitivity, specificity, positive predictive value, and negative predictive values of 25%, 98%, 50%, and 95%, respectively.[44,45] Another analysis demonstrated the five neutrophils per high-power field method to have a high specificity (98%) and positive predictive value but a low sensitivity (28%).[46] Therefore, the test has limited benefit in this setting. Leukocyte esterase is an appealing test as it is both quickly attainable intraoperatively and inexpensive. This test showed promising results in 2022, with a sensitivity, specificity, positive predictive value, and negative predictive value of 82%, 99%, 90%, and 97%, respectively.[47]

Outcomes Following Two-Stage Revision

Outcomes following two-stage revision arthroplasty as treatment for chronic PJI can be very successful. Several studies report 90% treatment success at 2-year follow-up and 80% to 90% at 5- to 10-year follow-up.[48] However, reports are highly variable and need to be taken in the context of the individual treatment protocols and definition of success.[49] A 2019 publication from the MSIS workgroup details tiers of outcomes to better differentiate in the literature: (1) infection control with no continued antibiotics, (2) infection control with continued antibiotics, (3) need for revision surgery (with subgroups based on the type of surgical procedure), and (4) death (due to infection or not).[50]

Many preoperative factors are associated with treatment failure. A review of 108 two-stage revision TKAs for infection with 16 treatment failures analyzed 31 risk factors to identify associations with treatment failure.[48] Overall treatment success was 91% at 2 years, and multivariate analysis revealed four potential risk factors that may predict treatment failure: body mass index of 30 kg/m² or greater, surgical time greater than 4 hours, gout, and the presence of *Enterococcus* species during resection arthroplasty. Other studies demonstrated that body mass index greater than 40 kg/m² is associated with three- to fivefold increase in reinfection, revision, and reoperation rates.[51,52] Similar to all PJI treatment strategies, a two-stage revision also has a higher failure rate when infection with antibiotic-resistant organisms occurs. In 37 patients with PJI due to resistant organisms, 9 (24%) experienced reinfection, but only 4 (14%) were infected with the original organism.[53]

One relative indication for two-stage revision for PJI is a previous failed surgery for infection, and this continues to be researched. In a retrospective review of 45 patients who have undergone two or more two-stage revision TKA for PJI, failure rates were compared using a PJI grading system[54] that accounts for host grade and extremity compromising factors.[55] Uncompromised hosts (MSIS type A) with an acceptable wound (MSIS type 1 or 2) had treatment success with 7 of 10 hosts, whereas type B2 hosts had success with 10 of 20, and type C3 had no treatment success with 2 hosts. This illustrates the importance of host factors in the treatment of PJI, and salvage strategies should be considered for those more compromised hosts that have a high likelihood for failure. Another study reported poor outcomes following a second attempt at two-stage treatment for recurrent PJI.

Of the 40 patients in this study who underwent intended two-stage treatment, only 26 (65%) patients underwent the second stage for reimplantation and only 62% of these patients had treatment success.[23]

During the two-stage protocol, there is a high attrition and a high mortality rate following the first stage. One study of 616 patients found that 111 patients (18%) did not receive reimplantation.[49] Of the 111 patients, 29 (26.1%) did well with their retained spacer, 23 (20.7%) underwent salvage procedures, and 59 (53.2%) were medically unfit, with 34 of the patients dying within 1 year of spacer insertion. In a smaller 2020 study of 89 patients,[56] 28 (31%) did not undergo reimplantation. Of 61 patients whose reimplantation was completed, 9 (14.8%) had a reimplantation that failed with a repeat or recurrent PJI, and the mortality rate was 23.6% (21 of 89 patients) at a mean follow-up of 4.5 years.[56] With the high attrition rate in the interim between the first and second stage, there are emerging arguments to expand the indications for treatment strategies with one surgical procedure such as DAIR, single-stage, or 1.5-stage procedures.

Two-stage revision remains the standard treatment for a chronic PJI. Articulating spacers have improved patient function during treatment without sacrificing infection control. Further studies are required to improve treatment outcomes. The timing of stages, surgical protocols including ideal irrigation solutions used, and the duration and route of antibiotics remain areas of needed research.

REVISION ARTHROPLASTY IN 1.5 STAGES

A 1.5-stage revision arthroplasty as treatment for knee PJI is a novel technique that is gaining popularity at some centers. It is defined as a functional articulating antibiotic spacer implanted with the intention of being left in for an extended period, if not permanently. As with a single-stage procedure, many surgeons incorporate two surgical setups including a wound closure, reprepping, redraping, and reopening the incision into their protocol to simulate two separate surgical procedures. In addition, surgeons will properly balance the joint and use third-generation cementation technique with the goal of leaving the spacer as their functional joint. The rationale behind the technique is that patients are often very satisfied with their knee, as it can function as a normal knee replacement. Some patients choose to keep this knee and not undergo another surgical procedure. Some patients are deemed too high risk to undergo a revision and keep their spacer by default. The reasoning for a 1.5-stage instead of a true single-stage procedure is the potential for reinfection. If a patient becomes reinfected during a 1.5-stage construct, it is less morbid to remove the spacer than to perform a full revision that may have fully cemented stems with ingrown sleeves or cones.

A 2019 study reviewed 57 patients who underwent a 1.5-stage revision with a low-friction articulating spacer and 137 patients who underwent a traditional two-stage revision with an all-cement articulating spacer.[57] Although no comparisons were statistically significant, at 2-year follow-up, the 1.5-stage group had a higher treatment success rate (78.9% versus 70.8%) and greater range of motion (105.8° versus 101.8°), with lower rates of reinfection (14.0% versus 24.1%) and revision surgery (19.3% versus 27.7%). Another study in 2022 compared 114 patients who underwent a 1.5-stage revision with low-friction articulating spacers and 48 patients who underwent a two-stage revision.[58] This showed a survival rate free of infection in the 1.5-stage group that was higher, but not significant. The Knee Injury and Osteoarthritis Outcome Score, Joint Replacement and postoperative complications were better in the 1.5-stage group as well, but this was biased because the population undergoing two-stage procedures was evaluated 5 years before the population undergoing 1.5-stage procedures, and not all of the two-stage spacers were the articulating type. In a 2021 study of 31 patients who planned to undergo a two-stage revision TKA, but were satisfied with their low-friction articulating spacer (28 patients) or medically unfit to undergo the reimplantation (3 patients), 25 of 31 initial spacers (81%) were in situ at a mean follow-up of 2.7 years.[59]

Overall, a 1.5-stage revision is a reasonable option for patients who either choose not to have or are medically unfit to undergo a second-stage surgical procedure. Infection control and patient functional outcomes appear comparable with those of two-stage revision. Literature is limited at this time and protocols differ significantly.

SINGLE-STAGE REVISION ARTHROPLASTY

One-stage, also referred to as single-stage, revision for the treatment of PJI is highly used in Europe and is becoming more common at some centers in the United States. As with any treatment for PJI, the goal of a single-stage revision is infection control. There are several purported benefits to single-stage revision, including less morbidity, reduced time in treatment for the patient, and less cost to the hospital system.

Technique

Several high-volume centers in Europe have published their protocol for single-stage treatment of PJI. One example from the United Kingdom is published[60] and another from the Endo-Klinik, Germany.[61] These protocols emphasize radical débridement with removal of all nonbleeding tissue and bone, including collateral ligaments, if necessary, followed by irrigation with minimum of 12 L of solution that includes continued mechanical débridement with brushes and pulse lavage. Antiseptic solutions such as 1% povidone-iodine solution and 3% hydrogen peroxide are then applied, followed by a second normal saline wash. Povidone-iodine or polymeric biguanide-hydrochloride (polyhexanide)–soaked swabs are placed in the wound and the incision is closed and dressed. The entire surgical team rescrubs, the patient is reprepped and draped, and all new surgical instruments are used. The wound is reincised, irrigated with normal saline, and the final revision implant is placed.[60,61]

Indications

The ICM on PJI considers single-stage revision arthroplasty to be a reasonable treatment for PJI when the patient is a good host and not septic, there is no sinus tract or severe soft-tissue involvement, and the organism is identified and not drug resistant.[62] In 2022, a systematic review reported on updated indications for single-stage revision, which include the absence of severe immunocompromise, significant soft-tissue or bony compromise, and concurrent acute sepsis.[63] It was concluded that a two-stage approach should be used for multidrug-resistant or atypical organisms such as fungus. Overall success rates reported in this systematic review of the single-stage approach were 82% to 100% at 2 years. There are efforts to make single-stage treatment more common at centers in the United States. However, one tertiary referral center reported in 2020 that of 91 patients who underwent two-stage treatment, only 19% would qualify for single-stage treatment based on the ICM criteria.[64]

Outcomes

A 2019 retrospective review of 111 patients who underwent single-stage revision with noncemented reconstruction for total hip arthroplasty PJI found that 99 of 111 patients (89.2%) were free of infection at a mean of 6 years.[65] A 2019 retrospective case review demonstrated favorable long-term results of single-stage revision for total hip arthroplasty PJI with a 10-year infection-free survival rate of 94% and a surgery-free survival rate of 75.9%, with the most common indication for revision being instability in 10 of 20 patients.[66] This study of 230 one-stage exchanges did have significant loss to follow-up during the study time frame (only 85 [37%] were available for final follow-up), but follow-up was relatively long term at 10 years. A 2019 study created a Monte Carlo simulation for the hypothetic situation of knee PJI with all pathogens and one for difficult-to-treat pathogens.[67] This expected value decision tree was constructed to estimate the change in quality of life and costs associated with single-stage versus two-stage revision. Single-stage revision was the dominant strategy for patients in approximately 85% and 69% of the trials, respectively. Single-stage revision is more cost effective for hospital centers, with a savings of approximately $20,000 per patient.[68] However, as of 2019, the physician reimbursement for a single-stage revision is approximately one-third the hourly rate of a primary procedure.[69] Despite the challenges, the use of single-stage revision is likely to increase in the United States.

SALVAGE PROCEDURES

Unfortunately, some patients are unable to remain infection free. In patients whose procedures result in repeated failure, severe soft-tissue damage, significant host compromise, and those unable to tolerate multiple surgeries, salvage procedures such as knee arthrodesis, resection arthroplasty, or amputation/disarticulation should be considered. Although rare, knee resection arthroplasty was described in 2020 as an alternative to amputation with an infection control rate of 84%.[70] One study of patients who underwent knee resection arthroplasty found that 45% were community ambulators, 35% were household ambulators, and 20% were only able to transfer. All patients require a knee-ankle-foot orthosis and walking aid, and 15% of patients were on chronic narcotic medications. Regarding knee arthrodesis, it can be performed with multiple fixation options including an Ilizarov frame, intramedullary fusion nail, intramedullary arthrodesis system that obtains biologic fixation, or plate fixation (**Figures 7** and **8**). There is a paucity of literature on the specific implants available and outcomes. A 2021 retrospective review of 20 patients who underwent transfemoral amputation and 23 patients who underwent knee arthrodesis demonstrated a similar

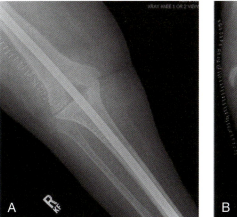

FIGURE 7 **A**, AP and **B**, lateral radiographs showing knee arthrodesis with a reamed, statically locked, intramedullary nail from the proximal femur to the distal tibia.

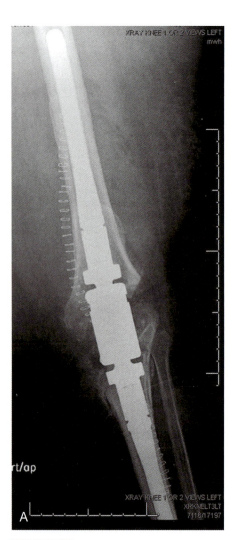 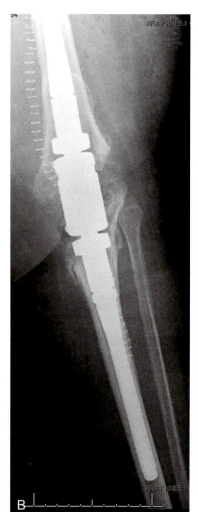 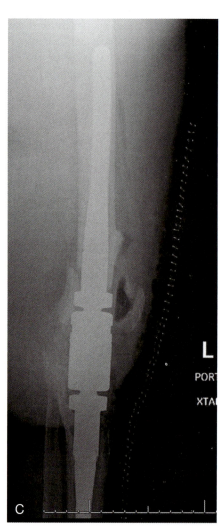

FIGURE 8 **A**, AP knee, **B**, AP tibia, and **C**, lateral radiographs. The radiographic series show knee arthrodesis with an intramedullary fusion device including an intercalary segment. This can be used in severe bone loss to prevent significant limb shortening with other arthrodesis instrumentation.

rate of recurrent infection.[71] Follow-up was significantly longer for the arthrodesis group: 9.7 versus 4.2 years. The number of previous revisions and time between the primary arthroplasty and the follow-up surgical procedure was greater in the transfemoral amputation group. Functional scores (visual analog scale pain, DN4, Parker and Palmer, and 36-Item Short Form scores) were all better in the transfemoral amputation group. Patients who underwent transfemoral amputation had less pain, more autonomy, and higher quality of life than those who underwent arthrodesis.[71,72] Patients who underwent a Girdlestone resection arthroplasty have significantly lower health status and quality-of-life scores than those who did not. A 2018 study reported that patients undergoing Girdlestone resection had health scores even lower than patients who underwent lower limb amputation or who experienced myocardial infarction.[73]

Overall, salvage procedures have worse outcomes than other procedures for hip and knee PJI; however, their use may become necessary when the likelihood of success is so low with other joint revision procedures.

SUMMARY

The diagnosis and treatment for hip and knee PJI continues to evolve because of thoughtful and innovative work of musculoskeletal physicians worldwide. Currently, two-stage revision is the standard in the United States. However, there are often strong indications and successful outcomes with DAIR and 1.5-stage and single-stage revisions. DAIR is a reasonable option for patients who have acute symptoms or those with implants or medical/social factors that contraindicate exchange procedures that are more invasive and have higher morbidity. The

1.5-stage procedures for PJI are becoming more common and likely are the natural progression for some surgeons to move toward single-stage revisions. Single-stage revisions are popular outside of North America but have become more prevalent at some centers within the United States. For the appropriately indicated patient (good host, known nonresistant organism, healthy soft-tissue envelope), these procedures are successful and more cost effective. Finally, salvage procedures should always remain an option in poor hosts, for which repeated surgeries add morbidity, with limited potential for success.

KEY STUDY POINTS

- Treatment for hip and knee PJI is usually surgical, with varying options available.
- DAIR is the least-invasive surgical option with the greatest risk for infection recurrence, but is a good option in patients with an acute infection, a nonresistant organism, and a good host.
- Two-stage revision is still the standard treatment for PJI that has the highest rate of infection control.
- Single-stage and 1.5-stage revisions are becoming more common and can have better outcomes and cost as the techniques and patient selection processes are refined.

ANNOTATED REFERENCES

1. Chotanaphuti T, Courtney PM, Fram B, et al: Hip and knee section, treatment, algorithm: Proceedings of international consensus on orthopedic infections. *J Arthroplasty* 2019;34(2 suppl):S393-S397.

    This is an article on the proceedings of the ICM, with literature review.

2. Johns BP, Loewenthal MR, Davis JS, Dewar DC: Open debridement is superior to arthroscopic debridement for the infected total knee arthroplasty. *J Arthroplasty* 2020;35(12):3716-3723.

    This retrospective cohort study evaluated open DAIR procedures in 96 patients and arthroscopic DAIR procedures in 45 patients and found that the success rates were 45% and 16%, respectively. Level of evidence: IV.

3. Shohat N, Goswami K, Tan TL, et al: 2020 Frank Stinchfield Award: Identifying who will fail following irrigation and debridement for prosthetic joint infection. *Bone Joint J* 2020;102-B(7 suppl B):11-19.

    A machine learning algorithm analyzed 1,174 patients retrospectively to predict failure of a DAIR procedure. Variables associated with failure were serum C-reactive protein levels, positive blood cultures, an indication for index arthroplasty other than osteoarthritis, not exchanging the modular components, the use of immunosuppressive medication, late acute (hematogenous) infections, methicillin-resistant *S aureus* infection, overlying skin infection, polymicrobial infection, and older age. Level of evidence: IV.

4. Argenson JN, Arndt M, Babis G, et al: Hip and knee section, treatment, debridement and retention of implant: Proceedings of international consensus on orthopedic infections. *J Arthroplasty* 2019;34(2 suppl):S399-S419.

    This is an article on the proceedings of the ICM, with literature review.

5. Shah NB, Hersh BL, Kreger A, et al: Benefits and adverse events associated with extended antibiotic use in total knee arthroplasty periprosthetic joint infection. *Clin Infect Dis* 2020;70(4):559-565.

    A retrospective review of 108 patients who underwent treatment for PJI. Fifty-one of the 108 patients received an extended course of antibiotics treatment. A multivariate analysis determined that extended antibiotic therapy for longer than 6 weeks was an independent predictor of success. Level of evidence: IV.

6. Barry JJ, Geary MB, Riesgo AM, Odum SM, Fehring TK, Springer BD: Irrigation and debridement with chronic antibiotic suppression is as effective as 2-stage exchange in revision total knee arthroplasty with extensive instrumentation. *J Bone Joint Surg Am* 2021;103(1):53-63.

    In this study, 56 patients who underwent a DAIR procedure were compared with 31 patients who underwent a two-stage revision. The DAIR cohort had better patient function with no difference in reinfection. Surgical treatment was determined by the surgeon, and the DAIR cohort was on lifetime antibiotic suppression. Level of evidence: III.

7. Klare CM, Fortney TA, Kahng PW, Cox AP, Keeney BJ, Moschetti WE: Prognostic factors for success after irrigation and debridement with modular component exchange for infected total knee arthroplasty. *J Arthroplasty* 2018;33(7):2240-2245.

    Retrospective cohort study reporting the outcome of 99 patients after irrigation and débridement with modular component exchange. They report at 35% reoperation rate at average 2.6 year follow up. Level of evidence: IV.

8. Gardner J, Gioe TJ, Tatman P: Can this prosthesis be saved?: Implant salvage attempts in infected primary TKA. *Clin Orthop Relat Res* 2011;469(4):970-976.

9. Bradbury T, Fehring TK, Taunton M, et al: The fate of acute methicillin-resistant Staphylococcus aureus periprosthetic knee infections treated by open debridement and retention of components. *J Arthroplasty* 2009;24(6 suppl):101-104.

10. Wouthuyzen-Bakker M, Sebillotte M, Lomas J, et al: Timing of implant-removal in late acute periprosthetic joint infection: A multicenter observational study. *J Infect* 2019;79(3):199-205.

    In this multicenter retrospective review of 445 patients, 340 of those who underwent DAIR demonstrated that a CRIME80 score greater than 3 is associated with DAIR treatment failure. Level of evidence: IV.

11. Chung AS, Niesen MC, Graber TJ, et al: Two-stage debridement with prosthesis retention for acute periprosthetic joint infections. *J Arthroplasty* 2019;34(6):1207-1213.

    This retrospective study evaluated the success of infection prevention at 1 year after a two-stage débridement with implant retention: 83% of patients who underwent total hip arthroplasty and 90% of patients who underwent TKA remained infection free at 1 year. Level of evidence: IV.

12. Ottesen CS, Troelsen A, Sandholdt H, Jacobsen S, Husted H, Gromov K: Acceptable success rate in patients with periprosthetic knee joint infection treated with debridement, antibiotics, and implant retention. *J Arthroplasty* 2019;34(2):365-368.

    Fifty-eight patients with acute PJI were reviewed. DAIR was successful in 43 of 48 of patients (90%) who underwent the procedure within 90 days of their index procedure regardless of antibiotic organism. Level of evidence: IV.

13. Urish KL, Bullock AG, Kreger AM, et al: A multicenter study of irrigation and debridement in total knee arthroplasty periprosthetic joint infection: Treatment failure is high. *J Arthroplasty* 2018;33(4):1154-1159.

    A multicenter, observational cohort study of 216 patients that underwent irrigation and débridement with implant retention. The authors report a failure rate of 57.4% at 4 years. Level of evidence: III.

14. Deirmengian C, Greenbaum J, Lotke PA, Booth RE Jr, Lonner JH: Limited success with open debridement and retention of components in the treatment of acute Staphylococcus aureus infections after total knee arthroplasty. *J Arthroplasty* 2003;18(7 suppl 1):22-26.

15. Shohat N, Goswami K, Tan TL, Fillingham Y, Parvizi J: Increased failure after irrigation and debridement for acute hematogenous periprosthetic joint infection. *J Bone Joint Surg Am* 2019;101(8):696-703.

    This analysis of 199 patients with PJI treated with DAIR demonstrated a failure rate of 56% for those with acute hematogenous infections versus 31% for those with acute postsurgical infections. Level of evidence: I.

16. Nace J, Siddiqi A, Talmo CT, Chen AF: Diagnosis and management of fungal periprosthetic joint infections. *J Am Acad Orthop Surg* 2019;27(18):e804-e818.

    This review focuses on fungal PJIs. Level of evidence: IV.

17. Tornero E, Morata L, Martínez-Pastor J, et al: KLIC-score for predicting early failure in prosthetic joint infections treated with debridement, implant retention and antibiotics. *Clin Microbiol Infect* 2015;21(8):786.e9-786.e17.

18. Sherrell JC, Fehring TK, Odum S, et al: The Chitranjan Ranawat Award: Fate of two-stage reimplantation after failed irrigation and débridement for periprosthetic knee infection. *Clin Orthop Relat Res* 2011;469(1):18-25.

19. Brimmo O, Ramanathan D, Schiltz NK, Pillai AL, Klika AK, Barsoum WK: Irrigation and debridement before a 2-stage revision total knee arthroplasty does not increase risk of failure. *J Arthroplasty* 2016;31(2):461-464.

20. Nodzo SR, Boyle KK, Nocon AA, Henry MW, Mayman DJ, Westrich GH: The influence of a failed irrigation and debridement on the outcomes of a subsequent 2-stage revision knee arthroplasty. *J Arthroplasty* 2017;32(8):2508-2512.

21. Rajgopal A, Panda I, Rao A, Dahiya V, Gupta H: Does prior failed debridement compromise the outcome of subsequent two-stage revision done for periprosthetic joint infection following total knee arthroplasty? *J Arthroplasty* 2018;33(8):2588-2594.

    An observational cohort study of 184 knees that underwent a two-stage exchange for PJI. The authors reported that those patients who previously failed an attempt at irrigation and débridement with implant retention had inferior outcomes and higher failure rates after subsequent two-stage exchange. Level of evidence: IV.

22. Kim K, Zhu M, Cavadino A, Munro JT, Young SW: Failed debridement and implant retention does not compromise the success of subsequent staged revision in infected total knee arthroplasty. *J Arthroplasty* 2019;34(6):1214-1220.e1.

    This multicenter retrospective review analyzed 291 patients: 228 underwent DAIR and 63 underwent a staged revision. In the DAIR group, 75 patients experienced treatment failure. At a mean follow-up of 6.2 years, the success rates were 72% for the failed DAIR group and 81% in the staged revision group. Multivariate analysis suggested that previously failed DAIR does not significantly compromise success of a staged revision. Level of evidence: I.

23. Kheir MM, Tan TL, Gomez MM, Chen AF, Parvizi J: Patients with failed prior two-stage exchange have poor outcomes after further surgical intervention. *J Arthroplasty* 2017;32(4):1262-1265.

24. Insall JN, Thompson FM, Brause BD: Two-stage reimplantation for the salvage of infected total knee arthroplasty. *J Bone Joint Surg Am* 1983;65(8):1087-1098.

25. Hipfl C, Winkler T, Janz V, Perka C, Müller M: Management of chronically infected total knee arthroplasty with severe bone loss using static spacers with intramedullary rods. *J Arthroplasty* 2019;34(7):1462-1469.

    This study used sonication results to determine if intramedullary rods caused reinfection when used with a static spacer. Sonication results were positive in 2% of cases and none of those failed. Most reinfections grew different organisms than the initial infection. Level of evidence: IV.

26. Lichstein P, Su S, Hedlund H, et al: Treatment of periprosthetic knee infection with a two-stage protocol using static spacers. *Clin Orthop Relat Res* 2016;474(1):120-125.

27. Röhner E, Pfitzner T, Preininger B, Zippelius T, Perka C: Temporary arthrodesis using fixator rods in two-stage revision of septic knee prothesis with severe bone and tissue defects. *Knee Surg Sports Traumatol Arthrosc* 2016;24(1):84-88.

28. Lachiewicz PF, Wellman SS, Peterson JR: Antibiotic cement spacers for infected total knee arthroplasties. *J Am Acad Orthop Surg* 2020;28(5):180-188.

    This review focuses on spacers used in two-stage exchanged for PJI. Level of evidence: I.

29. Zielinski MR, Ziemba-Davis M, Warth LC, Keyes BJ, Meneghini RM: Do antibiotic intramedullary dowels assist

in eradicating infection in two-stage resection for septic total knee arthroplasty? *J Arthroplasty* 2019;34(10):2461-2465.

This study analyzed spacers with and without intramedullary dowels and found that those with dowels did not have lower infection rates. Treatment was successful in 85.7% of articulating spacers with intramedullary dowels, 89.8% of articulating spacers without intramedullary dowels, and 68.2% of static spacers with intramedullary dowels (P = 0.074). Level of evidence: IV.

30. Nahhas CR, Chalmers PN, Parvizi J, et al: A randomized trial of static and articulating spacers for the treatment of infection following total knee arthroplasty. *J Bone Joint Surg Am* 2020;102(9):778-787.

This randomized controlled trial of 68 patients found articulating knee spacers resulted in decreased length of stay, greater range of motion, and higher Knee Society Scores. Articulating spacers also required less extensile exposure and had a lower reoperation rate, but these results were not statistically significant (P = 0.189 and P = 0.138, respectively). Level of evidence: I.

31. Nahhas CR, Chalmers PN, Parvizi J, et al: Randomized trial of static and articulating spacers for treatment of the infected total hip arthroplasty. *J Arthroplasty* 2021;36(6):2171-2177.

This randomized controlled trial of 52 patients found articulating hip spacers with decreased length of stay and no difference in surgical time. Approximately twice as many patients with static spacers were discharged to an extended care facility as were those with articulating spacers (P = 0.056). Level of evidence: I.

32. Spivey JC, Guild GN 3rd, Scuderi GR: Use of articulating spacer technique in revision total knee arthroplasty complicated by sepsis: A systematic meta-analysis. *Orthopedics* 2017;40(4):212-220.

33. Pivec R, Naziri Q, Issa K, Banerjee S, Mont MA: Systematic review comparing static and articulating spacers used for revision of infected total knee arthroplasty. *J Arthroplasty* 2014;29(3):553-557.e1.

34. Jones CW, Selemon N, Nocon A, Bostrom M, Westrich G, Sculco PK: The influence of spacer design on the rate of complications in two-stage revision hip arthroplasty. *J Arthroplasty* 2019;34(6):1201-1206.

This retrospective study of hip spacers found complications in 48 of 185 patients (26%). Dislocations occurred in 17 (9%), and these were associated with reduced femoral offset greater than 5 mm and increased bone loss. Spacer fracture occurred in 14 (8%), and these were associated with molded spacers rather than handmade ones. Periprosthetic fracture was associated with increased offset greater than 5 mm and extended trochanteric osteotomy. Level of evidence: IV.

35. de Beaubien B, Belden K, Bell K, et al: Hip and knee section, treatment, antimicrobials: Proceedings of international consensus on orthopedic infections. *J Arthroplasty* 2019;34(2 suppl):S477-S482.

This is an article on the proceedings of the ICM, with literature review.

36. Aalirezaie A, Bauer TW, Fayaz H, et al: Hip and knee section, diagnosis, reimplantation: Proceedings of international consensus on orthopedic infections. *J Arthroplasty* 2019;34(2 suppl):S369-S379.

This is an article on the proceedings of the ICM, with literature review.

37. Frangiamore SJ, Siqueira MB, Saleh A, Daly T, Higuera CA, Barsoum WK: Synovial cytokines and the MSIS criteria are not useful for determining infection resolution after periprosthetic joint infection explantation. *Clin Orthop Relat Res* 2016;474(7):1630-1639.

38. Kusuma SK, Ward J, Jacofsky M, Sporer SM, Della Valle CJ: What is the role of serological testing between stages of two-stage reconstruction of the infected prosthetic knee? *Clin Orthop Relat Res* 2011;469(4):1002-1008.

39. Stambough JB, Curtin BM, Odum SM, Cross MB, Martin JR, Fehring TK: Does change in ESR and CRP guide the timing of two-stage arthroplasty reimplantation? *Clin Orthop Relat Res* 2019;477(2):364-371.

This retrospective review of 300 patients found that the percent change in serum erythrocyte sedimentation rate and C-reactive protein inflammatory markers before and after two-stage reimplantation for PJI was not associated with reinfection risk. Level of evidence: III.

40. Ghanem E, Azzam K, Seeley M, Joshi A, Parvizi J: Staged revision for knee arthroplasty infection: What is the role of serologic tests before reimplantation? *Clin Orthop Relat Res* 2009;467(7):1699-1705.

41. Pannu TS, Villa JM, Corces A, Riesgo AM, Higuera CA: Synovial white blood cell count and differential to predict successful infection management in a two-stage revision. *J Arthroplasty* 2022;37(6):1159-1164.

This retrospective study attempts to define thresholds for synovial white blood cell and polymorphonuclear leukocyte percentage to determine reimplantation survival, with a proposed white blood cell count of 2,733/μL and polymorphonuclear leukocyte percentage of 62%. In general, these tests had higher negative predictive values of approximately 75%. These tests had high specificity, but not very high overall accuracy. Level of evidence: IV.

42. Samuel LT, Sultan AA, Kheir M, et al: Positive alpha-defensin at reimplantation of a two-stage revision arthroplasty is not associated with infection at 1 year. *Clin Orthop Relat Res* 2019;477(7):1615-1621.

This multicenter retrospective analysis of 69 patients showed poor correlation with positive alpha-defensin and infection at 1 year. Level of evidence: IV.

43. Owens JM, Dennis DA, Abila PM, Johnson RM, Jennings JM: Alpha-defensin offers limited utility in work-up prior to reimplantation in chronic periprosthetic joint infection in total joint arthroplasty patients. *J Arthroplasty* 2022;37(12):2431-2436.

This retrospectively study reviewed 87 patients and found 4 categorized as infected and 68 were categorized as possibly infected, none of which had a positive result for alpha-

44. Feldman DS, Lonner JH, Desai P, Zuckerman JD: The role of intraoperative frozen sections in revision total joint arthroplasty. *J Bone Joint Surg Am* 1995;77(12):1807-1813.

45. Della Valle CJ, Bogner E, Desai P, et al: Analysis of frozen sections of intraoperative specimens obtained at the time of reoperation after hip or knee resection arthroplasty for the treatment of infection. *J Bone Joint Surg Am* 1999;81(5):684-689.

46. Bori G, Soriano A, García S, Mallofré C, Riba J, Mensa J: Usefulness of histological analysis for predicting the presence of microorganisms at the time of reimplantation after hip resection arthroplasty for the treatment of infection. *J Bone Joint Surg Am* 2007;89(6):1232-1237.

47. Logoluso N, Pellegrini A, Suardi V, et al: Can the leukocyte esterase strip test predict persistence of periprosthetic joint infection at second-stage reimplantation? *J Arthroplasty* 2022;37(3):565-573.

    This study showed promising results for leukocyte esterase strips in predicting persistence of PJI at reimplantation in 76 patients. The retrospective study demonstrated that sensitivity, specificity, positive predictive value, and negative predictive value of the leukocyte esterase assay were 82%, 99%, 90%, and 97%, respectively. Level of evidence: IV.

48. Ma CY, Lu YD, Bell KL, et al: Predictors of treatment failure after 2-stage reimplantation for infected total knee arthroplasty: A 2-to 10-year follow-up. *J Arthroplasty* 2018;33(7):2234-2239.

    Retrospective review of 108 knees that underwent two-stage exchange for infection. Authors report obesity, >4 hour OR time, gout, and Enterococcus species as risk factors for failure of two stage treatment. Level of evidence: IV.

49. Wang Q, Goswami K, Kuo FC, Xu C, Tan TL, Parvizi J: Two-stage exchange arthroplasty for periprosthetic joint infection: The rate and reason for the attrition after the first stage. *J Arthroplasty* 2019;34(11):2749-2756.

    This study analyzed 111 patients who never went on to reimplantation: 29 patients (26%) did well with their spacer, 23 (21%) underwent salvage procedure, and 59 (53%) were medically unfit. Level of evidence: IV.

50. Fillingham YA, Della Valle CJ, Suleiman LI, et al: Definition of successful infection management and guidelines for reporting of outcomes after surgical treatment of periprosthetic joint infection: From the Workgroup of the Musculoskeletal Infection Society (MSIS). *J Bone Joint Surg Am* 2019;101(14):e69.

    This is a workgroup consensus on defining outcomes for consistent reporting after PJI. Level of evidence: V.

51. Houdek MT, Wagner ER, Watts CD, et al: Morbid obesity: A significant risk factor for failure of two-stage revision total hip arthroplasty for infection. *J Bone Joint Surg Am* 2015;97(4):326-332.

52. Watts CD, Wagner ER, Houdek MT, et al: Morbid obesity: A significant risk factor for failure of two-stage revision total knee arthroplasty for infection. *J Bone Joint Surg Am* 2014;96(18):e154.

53. Mittal Y, Fehring TK, Hanssen A, Marculescu C, Odum SM, Osmon D: Two-stage reimplantation for periprosthetic knee infection involving resistant organisms. *J Bone Joint Surg Am* 2007;89(6):1227-1231.

54. McPherson EJ, Woodson C, Holtom P, Roidis N, Shufelt C, Patzakis M: Periprosthetic total hip infection: Outcomes using a staging system. *Clin Orthop Relat Res* 2002;403:8-15.

55. Fehring KA, Abdel MP, Ollivier M, Mabry TM, Hanssen AD: Repeat two-stage exchange arthroplasty for periprosthetic knee infection is dependent on host grade. *J Bone Joint Surg Am* 2017;99(1):19-24.

56. Barton CB, Wang DL, An Q, Brown TS, Callaghan JJ, Otero JE: Two-stage exchange arthroplasty for periprosthetic joint infection following total hip or knee arthroplasty is associated with high attrition rate and mortality. *J Arthroplasty* 2020;35(5):1384-1389.

    This retrospective study analyzed 89 patients who underwent resection arthroplasty with a planned second stage. Only 61 patients (69%) underwent reimplantation; of those, 9 (15%) had repeat infection. The mortality rate was 23.6% (21 of 89 patients). Level of evidence: IV.

57. Siddiqi A, Nace J, George NE, et al: Primary total knee arthroplasty implants as functional prosthetic spacers for definitive management of periprosthetic joint infection: A multicenter study. *J Arthroplasty* 2019;34(12):3040-3047.

    This study reviewed 137 patients with all-cement dynamic spacers and 57 patients with low-friction spacers and found no significant differences. However, low-friction spacers resulted in decreased rates of infection (14.0% versus 24.1%) and revision surgery (19.3% versus 27.7%), and increased range of motion (106° versus 102°) and improved success rates (78.9% versus 70.8%; $P > 0.05$ for all). Level of evidence: IV.

58. Nabet A, Sax OC, Shanoada R, et al: Survival and outcomes of 1.5-stage vs 2-stage exchange total knee arthroplasty following prosthetic joint infection. *J Arthroplasty* 2022;37(5):936-941.

    This study compared 114 patients who underwent a revision with a low-friction articulating spacer and 48 who underwent a two-stage revision with a traditional spacer. Outcomes were improved in the articulating group; however, the study was biased because not all two-stage spacers were articulating and the two-stage population was evaluated long before the low-friction spacer population was. Level of evidence: IV.

59. Hernandez NM, Buchanan MW, Seyler TM, Wellman SS, Seidelman J, Jiranek WA: 1.5-stage exchange arthroplasty for total knee arthroplasty periprosthetic joint infections. *J Arthroplasty* 2021;36(3):1114-1119.

    This study of 31 patients concluded that 1.5-stage exchange arthroplasty may be reasonable, with 25 patients (81%) having retained spacers at 2.7 years. Level of evidence: IV.

60. George DA, Haddad FS: One-stage exchange arthroplasty: A surgical technique update. *J Arthroplasty* 2017;32(9 suppl):S59-S62.

61. Gehrke T, Zahar A, Kendoff D: One-stage exchange: It all began here. *Bone Joint J* 2013;95-B(11 suppl A):77-83.

62. Parvizi J, Gehrke T, Chen A: Proceedings of the international consensus on periprosthetic joint infection. *Bone Joint J* 2013;95-B(11):1450-1452.

63. Thakrar R, Horriat S, Kayani B, Haddad F: Indications for a single-stage exchange arthroplasty for chronic prosthetic joint infection: A systematic review. *Bone Joint J* 2019; 101-B(1 suppl A):19-24.

    This systematic review included 962 patients to determine factors that would predict treatment failure in a single-stage revision for PJI. It was concluded that the indications are the absence of severe immunocompromise, significant soft-tissue or bony compromise, and concurrent sepsis. A two-stage revision should be used in patients with multidrug-resistant or atypical organisms causing their PJI. Level of evidence: III.

64. Dombrowski M, Wilson A, Wawrose R, O'Malley M, Urish K, Klatt B: A low percentage of patients satisfy typical indications for single-stage exchange arthroplasty for chronic periprosthetic joint infection. *Clin Orthop Relat Res* 2020;478(8):1780-1786.

    This study analyzed the patient population and determined that only 19% (20 of 108 patients) would actually meet the ICM criteria for a single-stage exchange. Level of evidence: III.

65. Ji B, Wahafu T, Li G, et al: Single-stage treatment of chronically infected total hip arthroplasty with cementless reconstruction: Results in 126 patients with broad inclusion criteria. *Bone Joint J* 2019;101-B(4):396-402.

    This study of 126 patients with broad inclusion criteria who underwent a single-stage revision reported that 99 of 111 patients (89%) were free of infection at mean follow-up of 58 months. Level of evidence: IV.

66. Zahar A, Klaber I, Gerken AM, et al: Ten-year results following one-stage septic hip exchange in the management of periprosthetic joint infection. *J Arthroplasty* 2019;34(6):1221-1226.

    This group's specific protocol for single-stage hip exchange had excellent 10-year infection-free survival rate of 94% and a surgery-free survival rate of 75.9% in patients who were followed up. Level of evidence: IV.

67. Srivastava K, Bozic KJ, Silverton C, Nelson AJ, Makhni EC, Davis JJ: Reconsidering strategies for managing chronic periprosthetic joint infection in total knee arthroplasty: Using decision analytics to find the optimal strategy between one-stage and two-stage total knee revision. *J Bone Joint Surg Am* 2019;101(1):14-24.

    A Monte Carlo simulation favored single-stage revision for quality-adjusted life-years and cost outcomes at 85% and 69%, respectively. Level of evidence: IV.

68. Bori G, Navarro G, Morata L, Fernández-Valencia JA, Soriano A, Gallart X: Preliminary results after changing from two-stage to one-stage revision arthroplasty protocol using cementless arthroplasty for chronic infected hip replacements. *J Arthroplasty* 2018;33(2):527-532.

    Prospective cohort study of 19 patients that underwent single-stage exchange for chronic PJI. The authors report successful treatment in 18 patients with significant cost savings as compared to two stage treatment. Level of evidence: IV.

69. Fehring KA, Curtin BM, Springer BD, Fehring TK: One-stage periprosthetic joint infection reimbursement—Is it worth the effort? *J Arthroplasty* 2019;34(9):2072-2074.

    Cost analysis of reimbursement divided by the intraoperative time demonstrated approximately one-third of the hourly rate for a physician performing a single-stage procedure. Level of evidence: III.

70. Goldman AH, Clark NJ, Taunton MJ, Lewallen DG, Berry DJ, Abdel MP: Definitive resection arthroplasty of the knee: A surprisingly viable treatment to manage intractable infection in selected patients. *J Arthroplasty* 2020;35(3):855-858.

    This study demonstrates very poor outcomes for a rare procedure of resection arthroplasty of the knee. Level of evidence: IV.

71. Trouillez T, Faure PA, Martinot P, et al: Above-the-knee amputation versus knee arthrodesis for revision of infected total knee arthroplasty: Recurrent infection rates and functional outcomes of 43 patients at a mean follow-up of 6.7 years. *Orthop Traumatol Surg Res* 2021;107(4):102914.

    This study reviewed 20 patients who underwent a transfemoral amputation and 23 patients who underwent knee arthrodesis. The patients who underwent transfemoral amputation had less pain and improved quality of life. Level of evidence: IV.

72. Hungerer S, Kiechle M, von Rüden C, Militz M, Beitzel K, Morgenstern M: Knee arthrodesis versus above-the-knee amputation after septic failure of revision total knee arthroplasty: Comparison of functional outcome and complication rates. *BMC Musculoskelet Disord* 2017;18:443-447.

73. Vincenten CM, Den Oudsten BL, Bos PK, Bolder SB, Gosens T: Quality of life and health status after Girdlestone resection arthroplasty in patients with an infected total hip prosthesis. *J Bone Jt Infect* 2019;4(1):10-15.

    Sixty-three patients who underwent a Girdlestone resection arthroplasty at a median follow-up of 48 months demonstrated poor outcomes. Quality-of-life measures were worse than in those with amputations or those patients with myocardial infarctions. Level of evidence: IV.

CHAPTER 17

Surgical Management of Prosthetic Joint Infection of the Shoulder

NOAH J. QUINLAN, MD • JASON E. HSU, MD, FAAOS

ABSTRACT

Prosthetic joint infection is a potentially devastating complication of shoulder arthroplasty. The most common bacterium involved is *Cutibacterium acnes*, which is a common commensal of the skin and can live in the sebaceous glands under the skin surface. These bacteria can evade normal surgical prophylaxis and cause pathologic changes after inoculating the deep wound and implants at the time of index arthroplasty. Given the lower virulence of *C acnes*, the presentation of prosthetic joint infection of the shoulder often lacks the classic signs and symptoms of infection and more commonly presents with less obvious vague complaints of pain, stiffness, and component loosening, sometimes years after initial arthroplasty. Workup and diagnosis can be challenging given the low sensitivity of diagnostic testing. Often, the treating surgeon does not have definitive knowledge of the presence of bacteria until after revision arthroplasty is complete. Treatment strategies range from débridement with implant retention to one-stage or two-stage revision to resection arthroplasty in persistently recalcitrant cases. Rates of infection control are reassuring, though functional outcomes vary. Antibiotic therapy can be started after revision surgery before cultures are finalized to cover potential low-virulence organisms.

Keywords: *Cutibacterium acnes*; prosthetic joint infection; revision arthroplasty; shoulder arthroplasty

INTRODUCTION

Prosthetic joint infection (PJI) of the shoulder is a potentially devastating complication after shoulder arthroplasty and is most commonly associated with *Cutibacterium acnes*, formerly known as *Propionibacterium acnes*. The prevention, diagnosis, and management of shoulder PJI differ from that of PJI of other joints, such as the hip and the knee, because of the unique microbiome of the shoulder. *C acnes* can exist both on the surface of the skin and in the subcutaneous sebaceous glands below the skin surface. Skin surface antiseptics often are unable to reach the bacteria in the sebaceous glands, allowing them to inoculate the deeper tissues at the time of shoulder arthroplasty. Because of the low virulence of most strains of *C acnes*, the presentation of shoulder PJI often is less obvious without any clinically apparent signs, symptoms, or laboratory tests indicative of infection. Often, diagnosis requires obtaining multiple tissue specimens at the time of revision arthroplasty. Surgical treatment and antibiotic therapy often are challenging given that results of intraoperative cultures are not known until days after the surgical procedure.

INCIDENCE AND EPIDEMIOLOGY

The incidence of PJI after primary shoulder arthroplasty has been reported from 1% to 5%.[1-6] Most shoulder PJI cases are attributed to *Cutibacterium*, followed by

---

Dr. Hsu or an immediate family member has received royalties from DJ Orthopaedics; serves as a paid consultant to or is an employee of DJ Orthopaedics; and serves as a board member, owner, officer, or committee member of American Shoulder and Elbow Surgeons. Dr. Quinlan or an immediate family member is a member of a speakers' bureau or has made paid presentations on behalf of DJ Orthopedics.

coagulase-negative staphylococci, accounting for 39% and 29% of cases, respectively.[7] This discrepancy in organisms compared with that of total knee and hip PJI can be attributed to the specific skin microbiome of the shoulder. The shoulder epidermal layer harbors different types of bacteria, whereas the dermis contains a much higher proportion of *C acnes*. The oily skin type around the shoulder, neck, and chest is concentrated with sebaceous glands where *C acnes* can reside[8] (**Figure 1**). Unlike other bacteria, *C acnes* can thrive in these glands under the skin surface, and as a result, it can escape normal prophylactic measures such as topical chlorhexidine skin preparation solutions.[9,10] Once incision is made at the time of surgical intervention, these bacteria in the dermal glands are released and can inoculate into the deeper structures at the time of surgery.[11] This is the mechanism by which is it postulated that *C acnes* biofilm and infections are established.

SURGICAL PROPHYLAXIS

Because of the evidence demonstrating the lack of efficacy of standard chlorhexidine gluconate surgical preparation, alternative means of surgical prophylaxis have been studied. Understanding the specific organisms of shoulder PJI has led to targeted efforts for prevention, including perioperative antibiotic and cleansing regimens such as benzoyl peroxide (BPO) and hydrogen peroxide.[12,13] Studies on use of BPO gel in comparison with chlorhexidine gluconate suggest a statistically significant reduction in, but not elimination of *C acnes* bioburden on the skin. A meta-analysis reported the rates of positive skin cultures after home prophylaxis regimens of BPO and chlorhexidine to be 17% and 37%, respectively.[14] BPO soap, as opposed to gel, has not been shown to be effective in reduction of bioburden.[15] Hydrogen peroxide has also been investigated as an adjunct to chlorhexidine to increase reduction of *C acnes* burden as a skin preparation solution used before skin incision. Several studies have evaluated this adjunctive measure with mixed results—recent studies demonstrated a reduction in positivity of deep tissue cultures,[12,16] but a 2021 study demonstrated no difference.[17] It is important to note that there have not been any studies on clinical efficacy in terms of reduction of shoulder PJI with use of BPO when compared with chlorhexidine.

Cefazolin is considered the gold standard for preincision antibiotic prophylaxis. Patients with a reported penicillin allergy can typically still receive cefazolin unless they have a history of anaphylaxis or severe reactions such as Stevens-Johnson syndrome, toxic epidermal necrosis, hepatitis, pneumonitis, or hematologic reactions to a beta-lactam antibiotic.[18] For patients with a verified anaphylactic or severe reaction to cephalosporins, an alternative should be considered. Weight-based vancomycin can be used in these scenarios but is inferior to cefazolin in PJI prevention.[19-22] Addition of preoperative doxycycline has not shown to be effective in decreasing bacterial load either when administered intravenously in addition to cefazolin or if given orally for 7 days before surgery.[23,24] Any patient with a reported history of methicillin-resistant *Staphylococcus aureus* should receive, in addition to cefazolin, a full dose of weight-based vancomycin administered before surgical incision.[20]

PRESENTATION

Clinical presentation of shoulder PJI varies markedly depending on the virulence of the involved organism. Regarding timing, shoulder PJI can be considered acute (<3 months), subacute (3 to 12 months), or chronic (>12 months), depending on when symptoms develop postoperatively.[25] However, in terms of management strategies, it is important to understand that the presentation may be on a wide spectrum from clinically obvious infection to stealth infections.[26]

Obvious PJI often presents in a manner consistent with classic musculoskeletal infections. These symptoms may include wound erythema with drainage, formation of a sinus tract (**Figure 2**), or frank intra-articular pus.[27] Systemic symptoms such as fevers, chills, or malaise may also be present. These obvious infections are more commonly associated with virulent organisms such as *Staphylococcus*. Although often considered a commensal

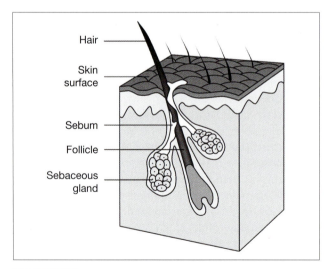

FIGURE 1 Illustration of the normal pilosebaceous unit. *Cutibacterium acnes* can reside in the sebaceous glands deep to the skin surface and away from normal skin surface antiseptic agents. (Reproduced from the National Institute of Arthritis and Musculoskeletal and Skin Diseases, US National Institutes of Health.)

Chapter 17: Surgical Management of Prosthetic Joint Infection of the Shoulder

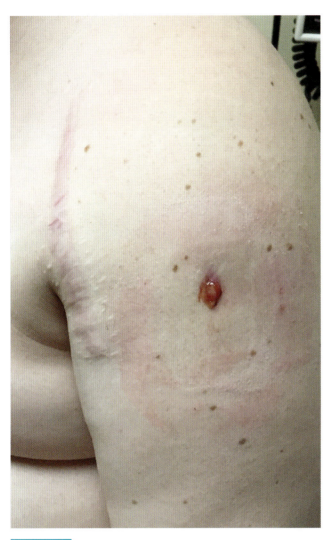

FIGURE 2 Photograph showing lateral shoulder sinus tract as an obvious sign in a patient with chronic prosthetic joint infection of the shoulder.

or low-virulence organism, *C acnes* can also present in this manner if associated with a virulent strain.

Stealth infections can be more challenging to recognize because of vague symptoms that may be overshadowed by presumably mechanical causes. Patients may present with pain, stiffness, and component loosening without any other obvious infectious symptoms. Therefore, infection should be part of the differential diagnosis for a patient who is unsatisfied with their shoulder arthroplasty. In contrast to obvious infections, stealth infections are more commonly attributed to less virulent organisms such as *C acnes*.

Stealth infection can be difficult to diagnose because positive cultures at revision arthroplasty may provide the only definitive guidance to defining infection. Further complicating the matter is that these results often are known only days to weeks after surgical intervention. Therefore, understanding the clinical presentation and risk factors for stealth infections is essential to guide appropriate treatment, although it is important to differentiate risk factors for the presence of *C acnes* as opposed to PJI (**Table 1**). PJI has been associated with prior surgery, younger age, male sex, index procedure for osteoarthritis, early aseptic revision, testosterone supplement use, lower American Society of Anesthesiologists score, diabetes mellitus, weight loss/nutritional deficiency, drug abuse, anemia from blood loss, iron deficiency, high loads of *C acnes* on the unprepared skin, and intraoperative finding of synovitis.[2-7,28-30] In contrast, a systematic review reported older age and higher body mass index to be associated with PJI.[7] Regarding the presence of *C acnes*, on the unprepared epidermis it is seen more commonly in males and those with higher serum testosterone levels.[8,9,31] In the dermal or subdermal layer after incision, *C acnes* has been associated with male sex, younger age, American Society of Anesthesiologists class 1, use of testosterone supplements, prior shoulder surgery, high *C acnes* load on the unprepared skin, and serum testosterone.[8,9,31] Finally, regarding deep cultures, *C acnes* has been associated with male sex, positive unprepared skin cultures, positive dermal cultures, glenoid erosions/wear, glenoid osteolysis, glenoid loosening, humeral loosening, humeral osteolysis, membrane formation, and cloudy fluid.[8,26,32] In a series of patients undergoing an open shoulder procedure without concern for infection, two or more preoperative corticosteroid injections was also associated with a positive deep culture.[33]

WORKUP

Evaluation for PJI begins with obtaining a comprehensive history focused on the timeline of any symptoms. Patients with stealth infections often can have a honeymoon period of good comfort and function after arthroplasty followed by unexplained pain or decline in function. History of any prior superficial or deep infection involving the ipsilateral extremity or recent systemic infections are important to document. Use of exogenous testosterone is associated with higher *Cutibacterium* skin loads and may be a potential risk factor for infection.[31] Physical examination may reveal the presence of a sinus tract, wound erythema, or drainage, but absence of these signs does not rule out potential infection.

Serum laboratory workup includes standard infection entities such as erythrocyte sedimentation rate, C-reactive protein level, and white blood cell count. These may be elevated in obvious infection, but these laboratory values are known to have low sensitivity in ruling out potential low-grade infection. A 2018 national database study noted a combination of elevated erythrocyte sedimentation rate (>25 mm/hr), C-reactive protein (>10 mg/L), and white blood cell (11,000 cells/mL) had

Table 1

Risk Factors Associated With Prosthetic Joint Infection and Positive *Cutibacterium acnes* Culture of Skin, After Incision (Dermal/Subdermal Layer), and Deep

Risk Factors			
Prosthetic Joint Infection	***C acnes* Skin**	***C acnes* Dermal/Subdermal**	***C acnes* Deep**
Prior surgery	Male	Prior surgery	Male
Younger age	Higher serum testosterone	Younger age	Positive skin cultures
Male		Male	Positive dermal cultures
Index procedure for arthritis		Testosterone supplement use	Glenoid erosions/wear
Early aseptic revision		Higher serum testosterone	Glenoid osteolysis
Testosterone supplement use		ASA class 1	Glenoid loosening
Lower ASA score		Higher *C acnes* load on skin	Humeral loosening
Diabetes			Humeral osteolysis
Weight loss/nutritional deficiency			Membrane formation
Drug abuse			Cloudy fluid
Anemia from blood loss			
Iron deficiency			
Higher *C acnes* load on skin			
Intraoperative synovitis			

ASA = American Society of Anesthesiologists

---

the highest specificity (92%) for PJI but that sensitivity remained low (7% to 42%).[34] Therefore, elevated inflammatory markers can be helpful in confirming infection, but normal values do not definitively rule out shoulder PJI. Additional serum inflammatory markers, such as interleukin (IL)-6 and D-dimer, have not been found to be helpful for diagnosis of shoulder PJI.[27,35]

Plain radiographs should be scrutinized for evidence of loosening or osteolysis, and in particular, humeral loosening or subsidence is a concerning sign for infection (**Figure 3**). Comparison of interval radiographs may be helpful. Advanced imaging such as CT or MRI may be helpful for purposes of planning for surgical revision with regard to cuff integrity, bone loss, or deformity. Lymphadenopathy, joint effusion, and synovitis on advanced metal artifact reduction sequence MRI have been reported to have high diagnostic accuracy, but confirmatory studies are necessary.[36] Nuclear imaging has been investigated though appropriate use has yet to be delineated and not routinely recommended.[27]

Further workup can include aspiration and surgical biopsy before revision.[27] Although aspiration is a critical step for evaluation of knee or hip PJI, dry taps are not uncommon in the shoulder, and even when an adequate sample is obtained, the results can be difficult to interpret given the lack of established cell count and percent polymorphonuclear leukocyte threshold values for shoulder PJI. Although some studies report a high specificity of aspiration in shoulder PJI, others note significant concern regarding the false-positive rate of air and swab negative controls. Additionally, *Cutibacterium* may primarily exist in biofilms in a nonplanktonic state and may not be adequately identified in synovial fluid.

A number of synovial markers have been proposed to improve diagnostic utility of an aspirate. The following cytokines have been found to be elevated in synovial samples of PJI: IL-6, granulocyte-macrophage colony–stimulating factor, interferon gamma, IL-1β, IL-2, IL-8, and IL-10. Although requiring further validation, these markers when considered independently or in combination show promise of more reliably predicting PJI.[37] Synovial alpha-defensin may have some utility with a sensitivity and specificity of 63% and 95%, respectively.[38] Synovial leukocyte esterase testing has a limited role in detecting shoulder PJI.[39] Alternative strategies such as next-generation sequencing are under investigation; to date, there is minimal evidence to support its use and bacterial species with questionable clinical significance may be detected.[27,40]

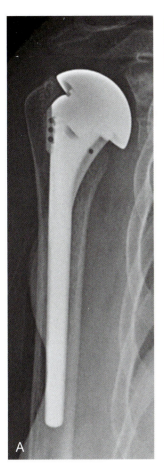
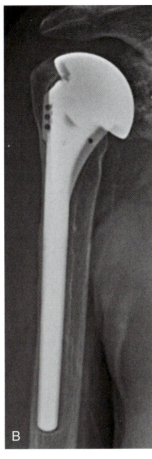

FIGURE 3 **A** and **B**, Humeral loosening and subsidence evident on interval AP radiographs, suggestive of low-grade infection.

The utility of intraoperative frozen section and histology has been studied. Similar to other diagnostic studies, this method has been shown to be less reliable than in the hip and knee literature, likely because of the lower virulence of *C acnes*.[27] An evaluation of intraoperative frozen histology using historical guidelines for PJI of five or more polymorphonuclear leukocytes per high-power field in each of three or more fields found the sensitivity and specificity for PJI related to *C acnes* to be 50% and 100%, respectively. Even when optimizing the cutoff to 10 polymorphonuclear leukocytes per five high-powered fields, the sensitivity for *C acnes* PJI was only 72%.[41] As a result, intraoperative histology has not been widely adopted.

Prerevision arthroscopic or open tissue biopsy for culture has been suggested as an alternative to increase sensitivity of diagnosis in comparison with serum or synovial samples. One study reported on 19 patients who underwent revision arthroplasty following aspiration and arthroscopic biopsy. Although both diagnostic methods demonstrated 100% specificity, biopsy was 100% sensitive compared with 17% with aspiration.[42] Another study noted that staged biopsy and revision due to concern for infection resulted in a sensitivity of 90% and specificity of 86% for PJI.[43] Prerevision biopsy may have most value when the surgeon would consider more extensive surgery (eg, removal of a well-fixed or cemented humeral stem) if bacteria were identified preoperatively.

At the time of revision surgery, multiple tissue or explant samples can be sent for culture to identify any bacteria present. The 2018 International Consensus Meeting guidelines recommend that if cultures are taken, particularly at the time of revision surgery, five tissue samples from a variety of sites around the shoulder should be sampled, specifically targeting any areas of necrotic or infected-appearing tissue.[27] Specimens should be sent for aerobic and anaerobic culture but do not routinely need to be sent for atypical culture, such as fungal or acid-fast organisms, as these are rare and add considerable cost. The suggested length of hold for cultures ranges anywhere from 7 to 21 days because of the slower growth of *C acnes*.[8,27] Time to obtain positive culture results can be considered as a potential indicator of clinical relevance. In one study, time to positive results in cases with probable true positive cultures was a mean 5 days compared with 9 days in probable contaminant cases. True positive cases were identified as those with more than one positive intraoperative culture or one positive intraoperative culture with additional signs/symptoms of infection. Probable contaminant cases were identified as those with one positive intraoperative culture, but no other indication of infection. No probable true-positive cases resulted after 11 days as opposed to 44% of probable contaminants.[44] In a 2022 study of negative and positive control samples by the American Shoulder and Elbow Surgeons (ASES) PJI Multicenter Group, it was found that time to positivity was significantly lower and strength of positivity was significantly higher in true-positive results when compared with false-positive results.[45] Sonication of implants has been studied to a limited extent without clear evidence that it improves culture yield over tissue specimen.[27]

Whether to obtain cultures in all revision shoulder arthroplasty cases is controversial. In a number of studies in which cultures were obtained in consecutive revisions, the rate of culture positivity was relatively high, but the clinical effect of these positive cultures is uncertain.[28,32,46] Positive cultures are most strongly associated with male sex.[29] The clinical significance of positive cultures can sometimes be difficult to interpret because of multiple studies on the substantial proportion of negative control cultures that grow *Cutibacterium*[33] and the knowledge that deep cultures can only be procured after cutting through the subcutaneous tissues in which the bacteria often reside.[11] In clinical follow-up studies, 107 revision arthroplasties with positive cultures were studied and it was noted that persistent infection was found in 10% and that in 25% of cases, the positive cultures had no clinical relevance.[29] Similarly, in another study, 17 patients who underwent single-stage revision ended up with positive cultures and recurrence of infection was found in only 6%.[46] Ultimately, it remains difficult to interpret whether positive cultures are associated with true infection or whether the bacteria can be considered a contaminant that is not contributing to the reason for undergoing revision arthroplasty.[27] Whether to obtain cultures during an aseptic revision remains the preference of the surgeon, with arguments to support both sides.

DIAGNOSTIC CRITERIA

Although workup has been well described, because of the vastly different presentations and findings associated with shoulder PJI, there has been inconsistency in the literature regarding diagnostic criteria. According to a systematic review, 27% of studies did not define what constituted shoulder PJI, whereas 14% used classification systems specific to the hip and knee.[47]

In 2018, a consensus definition of shoulder PJI from the 2018 International Consensus Meeting was published[48] (Table 2). Definite PJI was defined as: presence of a sinus tract from prosthesis to skin, frank intra-articular pus, or two positive tissue cultures of identical organisms. The study authors then report a scoring system for a number of minor criteria. A score of 6 or higher with an identified organism represents probable infection, and a score of 6 or higher without an organism represents possible infection. With a score of 6 or lower, if there is a single culture for virulent organism or two cultures of a less virulent organism, then PJI is possible. If cultures are negative and score is lower than 6, PJI is unlikely. Outside of the International Consensus Meeting criteria for definite infection (sinus tract, intra-articular pus, two or more positive cultures with virulent bacteria), multiple positive intraoperative cultures are often necessary to appropriately categorize a shoulder as having probable, possible, or unlikely PJI. Management often is particularly difficult given that the diagnosis of PJI often cannot be made until after surgical revision. The objectives of these guidelines are to help surgeons diagnose and manage shoulder PJI as well as establish a consistent definition to be used in research efforts going forward.

SURGICAL MANAGEMENT

Surgical management of shoulder PJI is dependent on signs, symptoms, and chronicity. In the case of obvious infection (eg, sinus tract, erythema, pus), the choice of management may be straightforward. However, diagnosis of shoulder PJI before surgery is often difficult because of the low sensitivity of available tests, and so often the surgeon is pursuing revision surgery without a definitive diagnosis of shoulder PJI. Often, the diagnosis is not made until after culture results are finalized, and treatment decisions at the time of revision surgery are often not clear.

In the case of obvious infection in which there are definite signs (eg, sinus tract, intra-articular pus) or test results (elevated erythrocyte sedimentation rate/C-reactive protein, positive preoperative aspiration) consistent

Table 2

Diagnostic Criteria for Prosthetic Shoulder Infections

Major Criteria

Presence of a sinus tract from the skin to the prosthesis
Gross intra-articular pus
Two positive tissue cultures with phenotypically identical virulent organisms

Minor Criteria	Score
Unexpected wound drainage	4
Single positive tissue culture with virulent organism	3
Second positive tissue culture (identical low-virulence organism)	
Humeral loosening	
Positive frozen section (5 PMNs in >5 high-power fields)	
Positive preoperative aspirate culture (low or high virulence)	
Elevated synovial neutrophil percentage (>80%)	2
Elevated synovial WBC (>3,000 cells/µL)	
Elevated ESR (>30 mm/hr)	
Elevated CRP (>10 mg/L)	
Elevated synovial alpha-defensin level	
Cloudy fluid	
Single positive tissue culture with low-virulence organism	1

CRP = C-reactive protein, ESR = erythrocyte sedimentation rate, PJI = prosthetic joint infection, PMN = polymorphonuclear leukocyte, WBC = white blood cell

Definite PJI is defined as the presence of any of the major criteria. Regarding the minor criteria, a score of 6 or more with an identified organism represents probable infection, and a score of 6 or higher without an organism represents possible infection. With a score lower than 6, if there is a single culture for virulent organism or two cultures of a less virulent organism, then PJI is possible. If cultures are negative and score is lower than 6, PJI is unlikely.

Adapted with permission from Garrigues GE, Zmistowski B, Cooper AM, Green A: Proceedings from the 2018 International Consensus Meeting on Orthopedic Infections: The definition of periprosthetic shoulder infection. *J Shoulder Elbow Surg* 2019;28(6 suppl):S8-S12. Copyright 2019, Journal of Shoulder and Elbow Surgery Board of Trustees.

with shoulder PJI with virulent bacteria, treatment often is based on chronicity. In the case of an acute obvious infection, early irrigation and débridement may be considered. Implants are retained, though all modular components should be exchanged. If infection is cleared with this approach, morbidity may be minimized by avoiding aggressive resection and reconstruction procedures. If considered subacute or chronic, typically a two-stage exchange is considered in shoulder PJI associated with virulent bacteria. This requires explant of all implants, insertion of an antibiotic spacer, antibiotic treatment typically for 6 weeks followed by a 6-week antibiotic holiday, and then insertion of the final implant if serum inflammatory markers are at normal levels (**Figure 4**). Joint aspiration before the second-stage procedure also can be considered to rule out infection before reimplantation. Typically, a reverse shoulder arthroplasty is performed if the bone stock and soft-tissue balance are adequate.

In contrast, shoulder PJI without obvious preoperative or intraoperative signs, symptoms, or test results is more challenging because the presence of bacteria is often not known until the revision surgery is complete. Often, a single-stage exchange can be considered if there is suspicion that a nonvirulent bacterial species will grow from tissue specimens obtained at the time of revision surgery (**Figure 5**). It typically is recommended that a complete single-stage exchange with thorough débridement is performed rather than a partial single-stage exchange in which implants are retained. In some cases, however, a cemented stem or one with heavy ingrowth can lead to significant morbidity and loss of critical bone stock. In these cases, preoperative aspiration and arthroscopic or open biopsy could be considered if the surgeon wants to confidently rule out potential PJI before retaining the stem. However, it should be noted that no prerevision test or procedure has reliably demonstrated good sensitivity in prediction of positive cultures.

Alternatively, a two-stage procedure as described previously can be considered if there is any suspicion for infection. In this scenario, the surgeon can determine whether PJI is present at the first stage and can more confidently treat any potential infection with antibiotics before insertion of the final prosthesis. The downside to this approach is the potential morbidity associated with two surgical procedures with regard to anesthesia, bone loss, and soft-tissue scarring/contracture from additional surgery.

POSTOPERATIVE ANTIBIOTICS

The decision to administer postoperative antibiotics after revision arthroplasty for PJI presents a challenge for surgeons given that culture results often are not obtained until days after the procedure. However, a delay in antibiotic administration theoretically may leave the

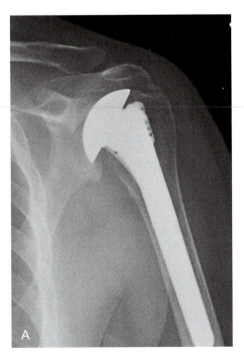 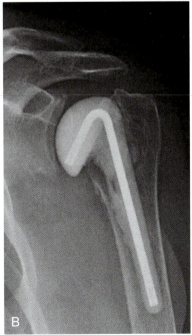 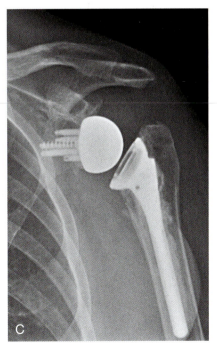

FIGURE 4 **A** through **C**, AP radiographs demonstrating two-stage reconstruction with revision to antibiotic spacer followed by reverse shoulder arthroplasty in a patient with obvious signs of gross intra-articular pus and cultures positive for methicillin-resistant *Staphylococcus aureus*.

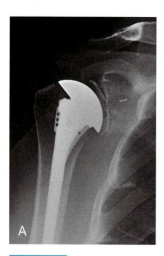 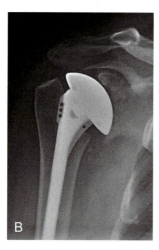

FIGURE 5 **A** and **B**, AP radiographs showing a complete single-stage exchange performed for a patient with a loose glenoid component without any obvious signs of infection. Multiple samples from revision surgery grew *Cutibacterium acnes*.

patient vulnerable to recurrence if bacteria are found to be present. Additionally, if antibiotics are administered, the decision on whether to administer antibiotics orally or intravenously is controversial.

One approach to antibiotic administration is based on the surgeon's suspicion of infection based on patient characteristics, signs and symptoms, and preoperative and intraoperative testing. Prior studies have suggested that younger, healthier, male patients with a history of prior infection, prior surgery, or exogenous testosterone use are at risk for positive cultures.[28] If suspicion for infection is high, the surgeon may consider administration of intravenous antibiotics until cultures are finalized, whereas if the suspicion for infection is low, the administration of oral antibiotics may be considered. If two or more cultures of the same bacterial species are positive, then the patient is treated with intravenous antibiotics for 6 weeks total followed by 3 to 6 months of oral antibiotics, whereas if cultures are negative, antibiotic therapy is discontinued. A 2022 study reported on initial antibiotic management in 92 patients undergoing revision shoulder arthroplasties. Because of high index of suspicion for PJI, 37 patients immediately began an intravenous antibiotic regimen, whereas the rest received oral antibiotics postoperatively. Further antibiotic management was directed by culture results. At a mean 4.1-year follow-up, there was no difference in revision or recurrent infection rates with comparable function and satisfaction.[49] Although intravenous antibiotics may be necessary, they should be used judiciously because intravenous antibiotics as well as a longer course of treatment have been associated with adverse effects.[50]

Alternatively, a more conservative approach to oral-only antibiotic therapy can be considered based on more recent evidence that oral antibiotic administration may be noninferior to intravenous antibiotic administration for bone and joint infections.[51] With this approach, all patients are given oral antibiotics (typically doxycycline or amoxicillin/clavulanate) after revision surgery until cultures are finalized at 14 days. If cultures are positive for two or more bacteria of the same species, then antibiotics are continued for another 3 to 6 months. If cultures are negative, then antibiotic therapy can be discontinued.

With any revision shoulder arthroplasty procedure for which infection is suspected, consultation with a musculoskeletal infectious disease specialist may be beneficial to ensure that the type of antibiotic is appropriate for the suspected or confirmed bacterial species.

OUTCOMES

Few studies report on irrigation and débridement with retention of implants because this is less commonly indicated for shoulder PJI. Regarding staged procedures, results are mixed. One study reported on 19 patients with PJI who underwent implant removal and antibiotic spacer followed by 6 weeks of directed antibiotic therapy, open biopsy, and revision if cultures were negative. At the time of open biopsy, 22% demonstrated persistent infection requiring repeat irrigation and débridement before proceeding with reimplantation. Ultimately, reimplantation was performed in all patients with no evidence of recurrent infection at minimum 1-year follow-up and average ASES score of 71.[52] One study reported on experience with two-stage revision for PJI with mean 63-month follow-up, demonstrating a rate of recurrence of infection of 26%. Average ASES score was 69 and forward flexion improved postoperatively to 119° from 58°.[53] Similarly, another study on two-stage reimplantation for PJI noted infection control in 85% of patients studied. However, 39% had an unsatisfactory result in terms of shoulder pain, function, or need for subsequent surgery.[54] A 2019 study reported on a three-stage protocol that entailed (1) explant with spacer and antibiotics followed by (2) open débridement and biopsy, and then (3) final reimplantation. In 28 patients, there were no instances of recurrence at a mean follow-up of 32 months. Patients in this study who underwent revision surgery had outcomes similar to those of a cohort of patients who underwent aseptic revision to reverse total shoulder arthroplasty.[55] However, it should be noted that the use of spacers is not without consequences. One study followed 53 patients who had a total of 60 spacers placed for two-stage treatment of shoulder infection. Although there were no issues at initial spacer implantation, among those who proceeded to second-stage revision there were 18 complications including glenoid erosion (6), spacer fracture (4) humeral shaft erosion (2), spacer rotation (3), and humerus fracture (3). In those who retained the spacer, there were four complications: humeral shaft erosion (3) and humerus fracture (1).[56]

A few studies have evaluated one-stage revisions. One study compared results of one-stage revision arthroplasty in patients who had positive *C acnes* cultures with those in patients in whom cultures were negative, noting comparable functional outcomes and subsequent procedures. These results support the efficacy of single-stage revision in select cases and that the presence of *C acnes* PJI does not necessarily impart a worse outcome compared with other indications for revision.[57] Similarly, in a report on a series of patients undergoing revision arthroplasty without suspicion of infection, 24% had an unexpected positive culture (UPC) though they demonstrated no difference in subsequent revision surgery rate compared with those in whom cultures were negative.[58] A 2022 study reviewed patients treated with single-stage revision and intravenous antibiotics for suspected infection. Failure of treatment was associated with higher *C acnes* load on skin and deep cultures at the time of revision.[30] In cases where revision reconstruction is not an option, a 2022 meta-analysis compared permanent antibiotic spacer with resection arthroplasty. Although similar infection control rates ranging from 72% to 90% were demonstrated, permanent spacers helped patients achieve improved function in terms of forward flexion and American Shoulder and Elbow Surgeons score.[59]

A number of systematic reviews and meta-analyses have been performed to compare results of these treatment strategies. A systematic review covered a range of treatments for shoulder PJI with their associated success rate of infection control: antibiotic therapy alone (50%), irrigation and débridement with implant retention (69%), resection arthroplasty (93%), definitive antibiotic spacer (90%), one-stage revision (90% if UPC, 92% without UPC), and two-stage revision (94%). On further analysis, there was no difference in success between single-stage, two-stage, or resection arthroplasty. One-stage revision had the highest Constant-Murley score whereas permanent spacer had the lowest.[7] Similarly, a meta-analysis of one-stage versus two-stage revision for PJI found no significant difference in infection control rate at 6% and 10%, respectively.[60] This is in contrast to another systematic review reporting improved infection control with one-stage revision compared with two-stage revision, though better function with two-stage revision. The study authors note the decision to proceed with one-stage revision versus two-stage revision is biased by several patient and surgeon factors that also likely affect outcome.[61] Although each of these treatment strategies may be effective in the right setting, management should be determined on a case-by-case basis accounting for severity/acuity of infection, patient factors, implant stability, and patient goals.

SUMMARY

PJI of the shoulder is driven primarily by the unique microbiome of the skin surrounding the shoulder. Most shoulder PJI is associated with *C acnes*. Prevention is difficult given that *C acnes* often can survive under the skin surface in the sebaceous glands, and skin surface preparations often fail to eliminate subsurface bacteria. Because of the nonvirulent nature of these bacteria, the clinical significance of positive tissue cultures is controversial, and definitive diagnosis of shoulder PJI is made difficult by the lack of usual signs and symptoms of infection. Surgical management often consists of single-stage or two-stage reconstruction, with two-stage reconstruction performed for more obvious infection. However, surgeons often need to make decisions without definitive knowledge about the presence or absence of bacteria around an implant. In these cases, a complete single-stage exchange can be considered. Similarly, postoperative antibiotic therapy is often selected before intraoperative culture results are finalized. Often, treatment with oral or intravenous antibiotics is considered until cultures are finalized. Although understanding of shoulder PJI and treatment strategies have drastically improved in recent years, further research in the field is needed to assist surgeons in clinical decision making and to optimize patient outcomes.

KEY STUDY POINTS

- The incidence of PJI after shoulder arthroplasty ranges from 1% to 5% and is most commonly due to an abundance of *C acnes* in sebaceous glands about the shoulder.
- Although obvious PJI may be clinically apparent, stealth infections should be considered in any patient who underwent shoulder arthroplasty with persistent pain or functional concerns.
- Workup for shoulder PJI is unique compared with that for other joints, and diagnostic criteria specific to the shoulder have recently been established. Because of low sensitivity of preoperative testing, negative testing results do not rule out the potential presence of shoulder PJI.
- Whether cultures should be obtained in all patients undergoing revision shoulder arthroplasty and the significance of UPCs remain poorly understood.
- Treatment ranges widely, including antibiotics only, débridement with implant retention, single-stage revision, two-stage revision, permanent antibiotic spacer, and resection arthroplasty. Infection control rates are reassuring; however, functional outcomes with revision arthroplasty for infection are not as reliable as primary arthroplasty.

ANNOTATED REFERENCES

1. Bohsali KI, Bois AJ, Wirth MA: Complications of shoulder arthroplasty. *J Bone Joint Surg Am* 2017;99(3):256-269.

2. Florschütz AV, Lane PD, Crosby LA: Infection after primary anatomic versus primary reverse total shoulder arthroplasty. *J Shoulder Elbow Surg* 2015;24(8):1296-1301.

3. Morris BJ, O'Connor DP, Torres D, Elkousy HA, Gartsman GM, Edwards TB: Risk factors for periprosthetic infection after reverse shoulder arthroplasty. *J Shoulder Elbow Surg* 2015;24(2):161-166.

4. Padegimas EM, Maltenfort M, Ramsey ML, Williams GR, Parvizi J, Namdari S: Periprosthetic shoulder infection in the United States: Incidence and economic burden. *J Shoulder Elbow Surg* 2015;24(5):741-746.

5. Singh JA, Sperling JW, Schleck C, Harmsen WS, Cofield RH: Periprosthetic infections after total shoulder arthroplasty: A 33-year perspective. *J Shoulder Elbow Surg* 2012;21(11):1534-1541.

6. Werthel JD, Hatta T, Schoch B, Cofield R, Sperling JW, Elhassan BT: Is previous nonarthroplasty surgery a risk factor for periprosthetic infection in primary shoulder arthroplasty? *J Shoulder Elbow Surg* 2017;26(4):635-640.

7. Nelson GN, Davis DE, Namdari S: Outcomes in the treatment of periprosthetic joint infection after shoulder arthroplasty: A systematic review. *J Shoulder Elbow Surg* 2016;25(8):1337-1345.

8. Matsen FA 3rd, Butler-Wu S, Carofino BC, Jette JL, Bertelsen A, Bumgarner R: Origin of propionibacterium in surgical wounds and evidence-based approach for culturing propionibacterium from surgical sites. *J Bone Joint Surg Am* 2013;95(23):e1811-e1817.

9. MacNiven I, Hsu JE, Neradilek MB, Matsen FA 3rd: Preoperative skin-surface cultures can help to predict the presence of propionibacterium in shoulder arthroplasty wounds. *JB JS Open Access* 2018;3(1):e0052.

   Preoperative skin cultures in 66 patients undergoing primary shoulder arthroplasty correlated with cultures of the freshly incised dermis. Level of evidence: III.

10. Lee MJ, Pottinger PS, Butler-Wu S, Bumgarner RE, Russ SM, Matsen FA 3rd: Propionibacterium persists in the skin despite standard surgical preparation. *J Bone Joint Surg Am* 2014;96(17):1447-1450.

11. Falconer TM, Baba M, Kruse LM, et al: Contamination of the surgical field with propionibacterium acnes in primary shoulder arthroplasty. *J Bone Joint Surg Am* 2016;98(20):1722-1728.

12. Chalmers PN, Beck L, Stertz I, Tashjian RZ: Hydrogen peroxide skin preparation reduces Cutibacterium acnes in shoulder arthroplasty: A prospective, blinded, controlled trial. *J Shoulder Elbow Surg* 2019;28(8):1554-1561.

    A prospective, controlled, parallel/noncrossover, nonrandomized, single-blind trial in 61 patients undergoing primary shoulder arthroplasty compared standard skin preparation with standard skin preparation plus hydrogen peroxide. There were significantly fewer triple-positive cultures (skin, dermis, and joint) and positive joint cultures in the hydrogen peroxide group, indicating it may be an effective measure to reduce contamination. Level of evidence: II.

13. Sabetta JR, Rana VP, Vadasdi KB, et al: Efficacy of topical benzoyl peroxide on the reduction of Propionibacterium acnes during shoulder surgery. *J Shoulder Elbow Surg* 2015;24(7):995-1004.

14. Nhan DT, Woodhead BM, Gilotra MN, Matsen FA 3rd, Hsu JE: Efficacy of home prophylactic benzoyl peroxide and chlorhexidine in shoulder surgery: A systematic review and meta-analysis. *JBJS Rev* 2020;8(8):e2000023.

    A meta-analysis of eight studies demonstrated BPO is a more effective home skin-disinfection regimen than chlorhexidine in reduction of *C acnes* on the skin. Level of evidence: III.

15. Hsu JE, Whitson AJ, Woodhead BM, Napierala MA, Gong D, Matsen FA 3rd: Randomized controlled trial of chlorhexidine wash versus benzoyl peroxide soap for home surgical preparation: Neither is effective in removing Cutibacterium from the skin of shoulder arthroplasty patients. *Int Orthop* 2020;44(7):1325-1329.

    A randomized controlled trial of 50 male patients undergoing shoulder arthroplasty treated preoperatively with 4% chlorhexidine solution or 10% BPO soap demonstrated neither preparation was effective in reducing *C acnes* skin load. Level of evidence: II.

16. Stull JD, Nicholson TA, Davis DE, Namdari S: Addition of 3% hydrogen peroxide to standard skin preparation reduces Cutibacterium acnes-positive culture rate in shoulder surgery: A prospective randomized controlled trial. *J Shoulder Elbow Surg* 2020;29(2):212-216.

    In a prospective randomized controlled trial, 70 male patients undergoing shoulder arthroplasty were treated with standard skin preparation either with or without the addition of 3% hydrogen peroxide. Those treated with the addition of hydrogen peroxide had a lower rate of positive C acnes culture. Level of evidence: I.

17. Grewal G, Polisetty T, Boltuch A, Colley R, Tapia R, Levy JC: Does application of hydrogen peroxide to the dermis reduce incidence of Cutibacterium acnes during shoulder arthroplasty: A randomized controlled trial. *J Shoulder Elbow Surg* 2021;30(8):1827-1833.

    A prospective, randomized controlled trial of 60 patients undergoing primary shoulder arthroplasty demonstrated no difference in the rate of positive cultures among those assigned to standard skin preparation and antibiotic prophylaxis either with or without addition of hydrogen peroxide following incision. Level of evidence: I.

18. Khan DA, Banerji A, Blumenthal KG, et al: Drug allergy: A 2022 practice parameter update. *J Allergy Clin Immunol* 2022;150(6):1333-1393.

    Practice parameters and recommendations regarding drug reactions established by a workgroup after literature review. Level of evidence: V.

19. Marigi EM, Bartels DW, Yoon JH, Sperling JW, Sanchez-Sotelo J: Antibiotic prophylaxis with cefazolin is associated with lower shoulder periprosthetic joint infection rates than non-cefazolin alternatives. *J Bone Joint Surg Am* 2022;104(10):872-880.

    This is a retrospective review of 7,713 patients who underwent primary shoulder arthroplasty, with minimum 2-year follow-up. Those receiving perioperative cefazolin had significantly lower rates of PJI compared with those receiving noncefazolin antibiotics. Level of evidence: III.

20. Garrigues GE, Zmistowski B, Cooper AM, Green A, ICM Shoulder Group: Proceedings from the 2018 International Consensus Meeting on Orthopedic Infections: Prevention of periprosthetic shoulder infection. *J Shoulder Elbow Surg* 2019;28(6 suppl):S13-S31.

    Second International Consensus Meeting on Orthopedic Infections in July 2018 included a shoulder workgroup that provided consensus recommendations on 16 questions related to prevention of PJI of the shoulder. Level of evidence: V.

21. Yian EH, Chan PH, Burfeind W, Navarro RA, Singh A, Dillon MT: Perioperative clindamycin use in penicillin allergic patients is associated with a higher risk of infection after shoulder arthroplasty. *J Am Acad Orthop Surg* 2020;28(6):e270-e276.

    A retrospective study of 7,140 primary shoulder arthroplasties demonstrated no difference in the rate of deep infection in those treated with perioperative cefazolin compared with vancomycin. However, there was a higher rate of infection in those treated with clindamycin. Level of evidence: III.

22. Oprica C, Nord CE, ESCMID Study Group on Antimicrobial Resistance in Anaerobic Bacteria: European surveillance study on the antibiotic susceptibility of Propionibacterium acnes. *Clin Microbiol Infect* 2005;11(3):204-213.

23. Rao AJ, Chalmers PN, Cvetanovich GL, et al: Preoperative doxycycline does not reduce Propionibacterium acnes in shoulder arthroplasty. *J Bone Joint Surg Am* 2018;100(11):958-964.

    Randomized controlled trial of 56 patients undergoing shoulder arthroplasty received either perioperative cefazolin or a combination of cefazolin and doxycycline. There was no significant difference in operative skin or deep culture results. Patients with positive cultures were younger, male, and had a lower Charlson Comorbidity Index. Level of evidence: I.

24. Namdari S, Nicholson T, Parvizi J, Ramsey M: Preoperative doxycycline does not decolonize Propionibacterium acnes from the skin of the shoulder: A randomized controlled trial. *J Shoulder Elbow Surg* 2017;26(9):1495-1499.

25. Strickland JP, Sperling JW, Cofield RH: The results of two-stage re-implantation for infected shoulder replacement. *J Bone Joint Surg Br* 2008;90(4):460-465.

26. Hsu JE, Neradilek MB, Russ SM, Matsen FA 3rd: Preoperative skin cultures are predictive of Propionibacterium load in deep cultures obtained at revision shoulder arthroplasty. *J Shoulder Elbow Surg* 2018;27(5):765-770.

    Preoperative skin cultures in 60 patients undergoing revision shoulder arthroplasty without clinical concern for infection correlated with deep tissue and explant cultures *C acnes* load. Level of evidence: I.

27. Garrigues GE, Zmistowski B, Cooper AM, Green A, ICM Shoulder Group: Proceedings from the 2018 International Consensus Meeting on Orthopedic Infections: Evaluation of periprosthetic shoulder infection. *J Shoulder Elbow Surg* 2019;28(6 suppl):S32-S66.

    Second International Consensus Meeting on Orthopedic Infections in July of 2018 which included a shoulder workgroup that provided consensus recommendations on 27 questions related to shoulder periprosthetic joint infection evaluation. Level of evidence: V.

28. Matsen FA 3rd, Whitson A, Neradilek MB, Pottinger PS, Bertelsen A, Hsu JE: Factors predictive of Cutibacterium periprosthetic shoulder infections: A retrospective study of 342 prosthetic revisions. *J Shoulder Elbow Surg* 2020;29(6):1177-1187.

    A retrospective reviews of 342 patients undergoing revision shoulder arthroplasty demonstrated that younger age, male sex, index procedure for osteoarthritis, testosterone supplement use, lower American Society of Anesthesiologists score, lower body mass index, higher preoperative skin *C acnes* load, and intraoperative synovitis were associated with *C acnes* periprosthetic infection. Level of evidence: IV.

29. Foruria AM, Fox TJ, Sperling JW, Cofield RH: Clinical meaning of unexpected positive cultures (UPC) in revision shoulder arthroplasty. *J Shoulder Elbow Surg* 2013;22(5):620-627.

30. Schiffman CJ, Mills ZD, Hsu JE, Whitson AJ, Matsen Iii FA: Factors associated with failure of surgical revision and IV antibiotics to resolve Cutibacterium periprosthetic infection of the shoulder. *Int Orthop* 2022;46(3):555-562.

    Review of 35 patients treated with single-stage revision shoulder arthroplasty followed by intravenous antibiotics for suspected *C acnes* periprosthetic joint infection. Those with ≥2 positive cultures at time of revision were more likely to be male, have had ream and run procedures, and have higher *C acnes* loads on their skin. Failure of this treatment protocol was associated with higher skin and deep *C acnes* loads.

31. Schiffman CJ, Hsu JE, Khoo KJ, et al: Association between serum testosterone levels and Cutibacterium skin load in patients undergoing elective shoulder arthroplasty: A cohort study. *JB JS Open Access* 2021;6(4):e21.00030.

    Preoperative serum testosterone levels in 51 patients undergoing shoulder arthroplasty were obtained and a correlation with *C acnes* levels on the skin and surgical wound was demonstrated. Level of evidence: II.

32. Pottinger P, Butler-Wu S, Neradilek MB, et al: Prognostic factors for bacterial cultures positive for Propionibacterium acnes and other organisms in a large series of revision shoulder arthroplasties performed for stiffness, pain, or loosening. *J Bone Joint Surg Am* 2012;94(22):2075-2083.

33. Mook WR, Klement MR, Green CL, Hazen KC, Garrigues GE: The incidence of Propionibacterium acnes in open shoulder surgery: A controlled diagnostic study. *J Bone Joint Surg Am* 2015;97(12):957-963.

34. Chalmers PN, Sumner S, Romeo AA, Tashjian RZ: Do elevated inflammatory markers associate with infection in revision shoulder arthroplasty? *J Shoulder Elbow Arthroplasty* 2018;2:2471549217750465.

    National database study of 1,392 patients undergoing revision shoulder arthroplasty to assess laboratory data most associated with infection within 1 year post-operatively. A combination of CRP, ESR, and WBC was the most specific (92%) though had limited sensitivity (7% to 42%). Level of evidence: III.

35. Villacis D, Merriman JA, Yalamanchili R, Omid R, Itamura J, Rick Hatch GF 3rd: Serum interleukin-6 as a marker of periprosthetic shoulder infection. *J Bone Joint Surg Am* 2014;96(1):41-45.

36. Fritz J, Meshram P, Stern SE, Fritz B, Srikumaran U, McFarland EG: Diagnostic performance of advanced metal artifact reduction MRI for periprosthetic shoulder infection. *J Bone Joint Surg Am* 2022;104(15):1352-1361.

    Review of 89 patients with suspected PJI who underwent MARS-MRI demonstrating good interreader and intrareader reliability of imaging findings in diagnosing shoulder PJI. Level of evidence: III.

37. Frangiamore SJ, Saleh A, Grosso MJ, et al: Neer Award 2015: Analysis of cytokine profiles in the diagnosis of periprosthetic joint infections of the shoulder. *J Shoulder Elbow Surg* 2017;26(2):186-196.

38. Frangiamore SJ, Saleh A, Grosso MJ, et al: α-Defensin as a predictor of periprosthetic shoulder infection. *J Shoulder Elbow Surg* 2015;24(7):1021-1027.

39. Nelson GN, Paxton ES, Narzikul A, Williams G, Lazarus MD, Abboud JA: Leukocyte esterase in the diagnosis of shoulder periprosthetic joint infection. *J Shoulder Elbow Surg* 2015;24(9):1421-1426.

40. Namdari S, Nicholson T, Abboud J, et al: Comparative study of cultures and next-generation sequencing in the diagnosis of shoulder prosthetic joint infections. *J Shoulder Elbow Surg* 2019;28(1):1-8.

    Review of culture and next-generation sequencing data in 44 patients undergoing revision shoulder arthroplasty in which *C acnes* was the most commonly cultured and identified on next-generations sequencing in cases of definite and probable infection. Concordance between diagnostic criteria for infection using culture or sequencing was only fair, with more probable contaminant cases using culture. Level of evidence: II.

41. Grosso MJ, Frangiamore SJ, Ricchetti ET, Bauer TW, Iannotti JP: Sensitivity of frozen section histology for identifying Propionibacterium acnes infections in revision shoulder arthroplasty. *J Bone Joint Surg Am* 2014;96(6):442-447.

42. Dilisio MF, Miller LR, Warner JJ, Higgins LD: Arthroscopic tissue culture for the evaluation of periprosthetic shoulder infection. *J Bone Joint Surg Am* 2014;96(23):1952-1958.

43. Tashjian RZ, Granger EK, Zhang Y: Utility of prerevision tissue biopsy sample to predict revision shoulder arthroplasty culture results in at-risk patients. *J Shoulder Elbow Surg* 2017;26(2):197-203.

44. Frangiamore SJ, Saleh A, Grosso MJ, et al: Early versus late culture growth of Propionibacterium acnes in revision shoulder arthroplasty. *J Bone Joint Surg Am* 2015;97(14):1149-1158.

45. American Shoulder and Elbow Surgeons ASES Periprosthetic Joint Infection PJI Multicenter Group, Hsu JE, Bumgarner RE, et al: What do positive and negative Cutibacterium culture results in periprosthetic shoulder infection mean? A multi-institutional control study. *J Shoulder Elbow Surg* 2022;31(8):1713-1720.

    Laboratory evaluation at 11 institutions of 12 blinded samples with different concentrations of *C acnes* from a failed total shoulder arthroplasty with probable infection. True-positive cultures had significantly shorter time to positivity and higher strength of positivity. All of the specimens at the 4 highest concentrations were positive for *C acnes*, while 14% of the negative controls were positive for *C acnes*. Level of evidence: IV.

46. Grosso MJ, Sabesan VJ, Ho JC, Ricchetti ET, Iannotti JP: Reinfection rates after 1-stage revision shoulder arthroplasty for patients with unexpected positive intraoperative cultures. *J Shoulder Elbow Surg* 2012;21(6):754-758.

47. Hsu JE, Somerson JS, Vo KV, Matsen FA 3rd: What is a "periprosthetic shoulder infection"? A systematic review of two decades of publications. *Int Orthop* 2017;41(4):813-822.

48. Garrigues GE, Zmistowski B, Cooper AM, Green A, ICM Shoulder Group: Proceedings from the 2018 International Consensus Meeting on Orthopedic Infections: The definition of periprosthetic shoulder infection. *J Shoulder Elbow Surg* 2019;28(6 suppl):S8-S12.

    Second International Consensus Meeting on Orthopedic Infections in July of 2018 which included the committee provided consensus on the definition of periprosthetic shoulder infection. Level of evidence: V.

49. Yao JJ, Jurgensmeier K, Whitson AJ, Pottinger PS, Matsen FA 3rd, Hsu JE: Oral and IV antibiotic administration after single-stage revision shoulder arthroplasty: Study of survivorship and patient-reported outcomes in patients without clear preoperative or intraoperative infection. *J Bone Joint Surg Am* 2022;104(5):421-429.

    This is a review of 92 patients undergoing revision shoulder arthroplasty treated initially with either intravenous or oral antibiotics based on surgeon index of suspicion and tailored following culture results. Subsequent re-revision was required in 18% of patients, with no difference between those initially on intravenous or oral antibiotics at mean 4.1 years follow-up. Level of evidence: IV.

50. Yao JJ, Jurgensmeier K, Woodhead BM, et al: The use and adverse effects of oral and intravenous antibiotic administration for suspected infection after revision shoulder arthroplasty. *J Bone Joint Surg Am* 2020;102(11):961-970.

    This is a review of 175 patients undergoing revision shoulder arthroplasty treated with either intravenous or oral antibiotics based on surgeon index of suspicion for infection and subsequently tailored based on culture results. Surgeons correctly anticipated culture results in 75% of cases with male sex, history of infection, and membrane formation as predictors of initiating intravenous antibiotics based on multivariate analysis. Complications were significantly lower in those treated with oral antibiotics and a shorter course. Level of evidence: IV.

51. Li HK, Rombach I, Zambellas R, et al: Oral versus intravenous antibiotics for bone and joint infection. *N Engl J Med* 2019;380(5):425-436.

    In this randomized trial, 1,054 patients with bone or joint infection treated with or without surgery were assigned to an initial 6-week treatment course of intravenous or oral antibiotic therapy and followed up to 1 year. The failure rate was similar in the intravenous group compared with oral group (15% versus 13%), and noninferiority of oral antibiotics was demonstrated. Level of evidence: I.

52. Zhang AL, Feeley BT, Schwartz BS, Chung TT, Ma CB: Management of deep postoperative shoulder infections: Is there a role for open biopsy during staged treatment? *J Shoulder Elbow Surg* 2015;24(1):e15-e20.

53. Buchalter DB, Mahure SA, Mollon B, Yu S, Kwon YW, Zuckerman JD: Two-stage revision for infected shoulder arthroplasty. *J Shoulder Elbow Surg* 2017;26(6):939-947.

54. Assenmacher AT, Alentorn-Geli E, Dennison T, et al: Two-stage reimplantation for the treatment of deep infection after shoulder arthroplasty. *J Shoulder Elbow Surg* 2017;26(11):1978-1983.

55. Tseng WJ, Lansdown DA, Grace T, et al: Outcomes of revision arthroplasty for shoulder periprosthetic joint infection: A three-stage revision protocol. *J Shoulder Elbow Surg* 2019;28(2):268-275.

    Retrospective review of 28 cases treated with a 3-stage protocol for shoulder prosthetic joint infection with no recurrences of infection. Those revised to reverse total shoulder arthroplasty had no significant functional differences compared to a cohort of patients revised to reverse total shoulder arthroplasty for non-infectious causes. Level of evidence: III.

56. McFarland EG, Rojas J, Smalley J, Borade AU, Joseph J: Complications of antibiotic cement spacers used for shoulder infections. *J Shoulder Elbow Surg* 2018;27(11):1996-2005.

    A retrospective review of 60 commercially available antibiotic cement spacers placed for shoulder infection as part of 2-stage treatment demonstrated no complications at spacer placement. Second stage was completed at average 6 months with 18 complications of which two required revision surgeries. Of the 10 patients who retained the spacer, 4 complications were noted. Level of evidence: IV.

57. Hsu JE, Gorbaty JD, Whitney IJ, Matsen FA 3rd: Single-stage revision is effective for failed shoulder arthroplasty with positive cultures for propionibacterium. *J Bone Joint Surg Am* 2016;98(24):2047-2051.

58. Padegimas EM, Lawrence C, Narzikul AC, et al: Future surgery after revision shoulder arthroplasty: The impact of unexpected positive cultures. *J Shoulder Elbow Surg* 2017;26(6):975-981.

59. Xiao M, Money AJ, Pullen WM, Cheung EV, Abrams GD, Freehill MT: Outcomes after resection arthroplasty versus permanent antibiotic spacer for salvage treatment of shoulder periprosthetic joint infections: A systematic review and meta-analysis. *J Shoulder Elbow Surg* 2022;31(3):668-679.

    Meta-analysis of 23 studies comparing outcomes of resection arthroplasty to permanent antibiotic spacer for shoulder periprosthetic joint infection. These procedures demonstrated similar eradication rates (82% versus 85%, respectively) and visual analog scale pain (3.7 versus 3.4, respectively), though the permanent spacer group had significantly better forward flexion and American Shoulder and Elbow Surgeons Score. Level of evidence: IV.

60. Belay ES, Danilkowicz R, Bullock G, Wall K, Garrigues GE: Single-stage versus two-stage revision for shoulder periprosthetic joint infection: A systematic review and meta-analysis. *J Shoulder Elbow Surg* 2020;29(12):2476-2486.

    A meta-analysis of 13 studies on single-stage revision and 30 studies on two-stage revision noted that in the setting of positive cultures *C acnes* were observed in 48% and 34% of cases, respectively. There was no significant difference in reinfection rate (6% versus 10%, respectively), though this may be biased by less virulent infections more frequently being treated with single-stage procedures. Level of evidence: IV.

61. Ruditsky A, McBeth Z, Curry EJ, Cusano A, Galvin JW, Li X: One versus 2-stage revision for shoulder arthroplasty infections: A systematic review and analysis of treatment selection bias. *JBJS Rev* 2021;9(9):e20.00219.

    A systematic review of 26 studies compared one-stage and two-stage revision for periprosthetic shoulder infection. Although one-stage revisions had higher infection clearance rates, two-stage procedures had greater functional improvement; however, these results may be biased based on reasoning for each approach. Level of evidence: III.

CHAPTER 18

Antibiotic Treatment of Prosthetic Joint Infections

LAURA CERTAIN, MD, PhD • JAKRAPUN PUPAIBOOL, MD, MS

ABSTRACT

After surgical management of prosthetic joint infection, patients receive prolonged courses of antimicrobial therapy, ideally under the direction of an infectious disease specialist. Although the data regarding the optimal duration of antimicrobial therapy are inconclusive, a minimum of 6 weeks is likely necessary, and much longer courses are used in patients treated with débridement and implant retention. Although serum markers of inflammation can provide some suggestions regarding which patients are more likely to have persistent infection, they do not have enough predictive value to be the deciding factor in whether to continue or stop antibiotic therapy.

Keywords: antibiotics; medical therapy; prosthetic joint infection

INTRODUCTION

The successful treatment of prosthetic joint infections (PJIs) requires a combination of surgery and antibiotics. In general, patients with PJI receive prolonged courses of antibiotics: anything from 6 weeks to 1 year or longer is typical. The perfect duration of antibiotics remains unknown. There also remain many active questions regarding the best choice of antibiotics to use: intravenous or oral, adding rifampin or not, and others. The best option varies from patient to patient, but it is important to outline general principles and recent clinical trial data.

PREOPERATIVE ANTIBIOTIC MANAGEMENT

Ideally, each patient with a PJI should be cotreated by an orthopaedic surgeon and an infectious disease specialist, with the infectious disease specialist directing and monitoring the antibiotic therapy, as reported in 2019.[1] In most cases, antibiotics should be held before surgical management of PJI.[2] Although a preoperative joint aspirate often reveals the pathogen, gathering additional tissue cultures intraoperatively, before starting antibiotics, can be necessary to identify the culprit organism or organisms. Similarly, starting antibiotics before diagnosis of PJI is ill advised. If a patient presents with examination findings concerning for possible PJI (joint warmth, erythema, swelling, drainage, etc), the best course of action is *not* to try an empiric course of antibiotics. Rather, the patient should be evaluated for PJI.

Once the diagnosis has been made, the patient is in the operating room, and tissue cultures have been collected, starting empiric antibiotics while awaiting culture data is standard. If the pathogen is known or suspected based on a preoperative synovial fluid culture, then targeted antibiotic therapy can be started instead of empiric therapy. In patients who present with sepsis from a PJI, blood cultures should be drawn before starting empiric antibiotics and the patient taken to the operating room as soon as possible for source control of the infection. One dose of preoperative antibiotics likely does not significantly affect culture yield.[3,4]

Dr. Certain or an immediate family member serves as a board member, owner, officer, or committee member of Musculoskeletal Infection Society. Neither Dr. Pupaibool nor any immediate family member has received anything of value from or has stock or stock options held in a commercial company or institution related directly or indirectly to the subject of this chapter.

EMPIRIC TREATMENT REGIMENS AND CULTURE-NEGATIVE PJI

When the pathogen is not known preoperatively, postoperative antibiotics should be directed toward the most common pathogens. Because most PJIs are caused by gram-positive bacteria, an antibiotic with broad gram-positive activity, such as vancomycin or daptomycin, should be used. Most clinicians will also include a third- or fourth-generation cephalosporin in the empiric regimen, as a small but nontrivial proportion of infections are gram-negative or polymicrobial.[5,6] Ideally, within a few days of surgery, the intraoperative cultures will identify the culprit organism, and antibiotics can be tailored to that organism, as outlined in the next section.

If all cultures remain negative, as is the case in approximately 25% of PJIs,[7-9] then the empiric regimen can be continued for the entire duration of therapy. Alternatively, one might choose to replace the cephalosporin with a fluoroquinolone, to cover atypical pathogens that might not grow easily on routine culture. For cases in which sequence-based diagnostics have been used clinically to identify a pathogen in culture-negative PJI, *Mycoplasma*[10,11] and *Ureaplasma*[12] have been found. There are many reasons contributing to negative cultures, such as antimicrobial therapy before obtaining specimens for cultures, difficult-to-grow organisms, and nonbacterial pathogens. Antimicrobial regimens covering both gram-positive and gram-negative bacteria are generally recommended. Consultation with an infectious disease specialist is particularly important in cases of culture-negative PJI to determine if the patient should be evaluated and/or empirically treated for rare pathogens, such as fungi, mycobacteria, *Coxiella*, *Brucella*, and others.

TARGETED TREATMENT REGIMENS

Staphylococcus aureus

S aureus is the most common organism causing early-onset and acute late-onset PJI.[13-15] For methicillin-susceptible *S aureus*, cefazolin is the antimicrobial of choice, whereas vancomycin is the first-line antimicrobial agent for methicillin-resistant *S aureus*.

Coagulase-Negative *Staphylococcus* Species

Coagulase-negative staphylococci (CoNS) are part of human skin flora. *Staphylococcus epidermidis* is the most commonly occurring species of this group causing PJI. CoNS are the most common organisms of delayed late-onset PJI, as reported in 2019.[13,15] Most of the CoNS are resistant to oxacillin, except *Staphylococcus lugdunensis*. Vancomycin is recommended for empiric treatment of CoNS infection.

Streptococcus Species

Streptococci mainly cause acute late-onset PJI.[13,15] *Streptococcus agalactiae* (group B streptococci) is the most frequently identified species of this group. Beta-hemolytic streptococci (groups A, B, C, and G) are generally susceptible to penicillin, whereas viridans group streptococci and *Streptococcus pneumoniae* can be penicillin resistant.

Cutibacterium (*Propionibacterium*) Species

Cutibacteria are part of human skin flora and are low-virulence organisms. A 2021 study reported that *Cutibacterium acnes* is the most common *Cutibacterium* species causing PJI, particularly of the shoulder, followed by *Cutibacterium avidum* and *Cutibacterium granulosum*.[16] PJIs caused by cutibacteria typically have indolent clinical presentations. Cutibacteria are susceptible to most antimicrobial agents used in bone and joint infections, such as beta-lactams, fluoroquinolones, doxycycline, vancomycin, and clindamycin.

Gram-Negative Bacilli

Gram-negative bacilli infection occurs somewhat commonly in early-onset PJI, especially PJI of the hip. The most frequent species of this group identified in most studies to be a causative organism of PJI is *Escherichia coli*, followed by *Pseudomonas aeruginosa*.[17-19] The empiric antimicrobial agent of choice depends on local antibiogram data. Ceftriaxone (or cefepime if pseudomonal coverage is needed) is generally the appropriate empiric therapy while awaiting species identification and antimicrobial susceptibility report. Antimicrobial therapy for each organism is summarized in **Table 1**.

ORAL ANTIMICROBIAL THERAPY FOR PJI

To date, there have been no randomized controlled trials (RCTs) evaluating the efficacy of oral antibiotic therapy exclusively for PJI. In 2019, the Oral versus Intravenous Antibiotics for Bone and Joint Infection (OVIVA) trial[20] investigated whether early switch (within 7 days of an index surgery) to oral antibiotic therapy was noninferior to standard parenteral antibiotic therapy at 1-year follow-up for the treatment of bone and joint infections. In the OVIVA trial, which included 20% to 30% patients with PJI, a correctly chosen oral antibiotic regimen was as effective as intravenous antibiotics for treating orthopaedic infections, including PJI. The duration of antibiotic therapy was longer than 6 weeks, with a median of 71 and 78 days in the oral antibiotic and intravenous antibiotic groups, respectively. In the sensitivity analysis, better outcomes were found both in patients in the

Table 1

Antimicrobial Therapy for Prosthetic Joint Infection

Organisms	Preferred Regimen or Regimens	Alternative Regimens
Oxacillin-susceptible *Staphylococcus* species	Cefazolin 2 g IV q 8 hours	Nafcillin 2 g IV q 6 hours Ceftriaxone 2 g IV q 24 hours Vancomycin 15 mg/kg IV q 12 hours (dose adjustment per serum level)
Oxacillin-resistant *Staphylococcus* species	Vancomycin 15 mg/kg IV q 12 hours (dose adjustment per serum level)	Daptomycin 6 to 8 mg/kg IV q 24 hours Linezolid 600 mg PO/IV q 12 hours
Streptococcus species	Penicillin G 18 to 20 million units IV q 24 hours (continuous infusion or in six divided doses)	Cefazolin 2 g IV q 8 hours Ceftriaxone 2 g IV q 24 hours Vancomycin 15 mg/kg IV q 12 hours (dose adjustment per serum level)
Ampicillin-susceptible *Enterococcus* species	Ampicillin 2 g IV q 4 hours	Penicillin G 20 to 24 MU IV q 24 hours (continuous infusion or in six divided doses) Vancomycin 15 mg/kg IV q 12 hours (dose adjustment per serum level) Daptomycin 8 to 10 mg/kg IV q 24 hours Linezolid 600 mg PO/IV q 12 hours
Ampicillin-resistant *Enterococcus* species	Vancomycin 15 mg/kg IV q 12 hours (dose adjustment per serum level)	Daptomycin 8 to 10 mg/kg IV q 24 hours Linezolid 600 mg PO/IV q 12 hours
Cutibacterium species	Penicillin G 20 to 24 mU IV q 24 hours (continuous infusion or in 6 divided doses)	Ceftriaxone 2 g IV q 24 hours Vancomycin 15 mg/kg IV q 12 hours Clindamycin 300 to 450 mg PO q 6 hours or 600 to 900 mg IV q 8 hours
Pseudomonas aeruginosa	Cefepime 2 g IV q 8 to 12 hours or 4 to 6 g IV continuous infusion q 24 hours Ceftazidime 2 g IV q 8 hours or 6 g IV continuous infusion q 24 hours Levofloxacin 750 mg PO q 24 hours Ciprofloxacin 750 mg PO q 12 hours	Piperacillin-tazobactam 4.5 g IV q 6 hours or 18 g IV continuous infusion q 24 hours Meropenem 500 mg IV q 6 hours or 1 g IV q 8 hours
Enterobacter species, *Citrobacter* species, *Serratia* species	Cefepime 2 g IV q 8 to 12 hours or 4 to 6 g IV continuous infusion q 24 hours Levofloxacin 750 mg PO q 24 hours Ciprofloxacin 750 mg PO q 12 hours	Ertapenem 1 g IV q 24 hours Meropenem 500 mg IV q 6 hours or 1 g IV q 8 hours
Escherichia coli and other Enterobacteriaceae	Ceftriaxone 2 g IV q 24 hours Levofloxacin 750 mg PO q 24 hours Ciprofloxacin 750 mg PO q 12 hours	Based on in-vitro susceptibilities
Culture-negative prosthetic joint infection	Vancomycin 15 mg/kg IV q 12 hours (dose adjustment per serum level) + Ceftriaxone 2 g IV q 24 hours or Levofloxacin 750 mg PO q 24 hours or Ciprofloxacin 750 mg PO q 12 hours	Daptomycin 6 to 8 mg/kg IV q 24 hours or linezolid 600 mg PO/IV q 12 hours + Ceftriaxone 2 g IV q 24 hours or Levofloxacin 750 mg PO q 24 hours or Ciprofloxacin 750 mg PO q 12 hours

IV = intravenous, PO = oral, q = daily

intravenous antibiotic group who underwent débridement, antibiotics, and implant retention (DAIR) or single-stage revisions and in patients in the oral antibiotic group who underwent removal of prosthetic joint or fracture fixation device for infection.

Although intravenous antibiotics are still commonly used after spacer placement, they are likely not necessary and the antibiotic regimen should be tailored to the individual patient, accounting for the infecting organism, drug-drug interactions, allergy profile, ability to adhere to an oral antibiotic regimen, and ability to manage a peripherally inserted central catheter. In theory, as long as an adequate antibiotic level in bone and surrounding soft tissue is achieved, the route of antibiotic administration should be of no consequence. Further studies are needed to confirm the findings of the OVIVA trial for PJI specifically, and the subsequent clinical trials could address doses of oral antibiotics and/or the individualized surgical procedures for PJI.

RIFAMPIN COMBINATION THERAPY

Rifampin is a broad-spectrum antimicrobial agent that is commonly used in combination with other antimicrobial agents to treat a variety of infections. It prevents protein synthesis by inhibiting DNA-dependent RNA polymerase and has activity against many bacteria, not just the staphylococci that are the focus of its use in orthopaedic infections. There are abundant in vitro and animal studies demonstrating its biofilm penetration ability against staphylococci. This led to recommendations to include rifampin in the three-drug regimen for treatment of staphylococcal prosthetic valve endocarditis.[21] In addition, it has been adopted to use for treatment of orthopaedic implant-associated infections.[22,23] However, clinical studies show conflicting benefits of rifampin in implant-associated infections.

Rifampin for *Staphylococcus* Species

Rifampin has been investigated in various clinical studies, most of which are retrospective studies in DAIR. The evidence for its use in the context of single-stage and two-stage revision arthroplasty is extremely limited. The retrospective studies in general showed at least modest benefit of rifampin for treatment of staphylococcal PJI after DAIR.[23-26] There have been three RCTs investigating the use of rifampin in staphylococcal PJI therapy[27-29] (**Table 2**), although two of the studies are small.[27,28] A 2020 RCT enrolled 99 patients with staphylococcal PJI treated with DAIR; 48 patients were included in the final analyses.[29] At 2-year follow-up, no significant difference of success rates of eradiation of PJI (17 of 23 patients [74%] versus 18 of 25 patients [72%]) were found between the two treatment groups (95% confidence interval, 0.73 to 1.45; $P = 0.88$). However, the study is underpowered because of a high dropout rate. In addition, antimicrobial agents with high oral bioavailability and bone penetration such as fluoroquinolones, trimethoprim-sulfamethoxazole, and doxycycline were not used in this study. The study used high-dose rifampin (900 mg/d) in combination with oral cloxacillin for the treatment of methicillin-susceptible *S aureus* infection and intravenous vancomycin for the treatment of methicillin-resistant *S aureus* infection.

Rifampin for *Streptococcus* Species

Biofilm formation is also a virulence factor of streptococci; therefore, rifampin might have a role in combination antimicrobial therapy regimens for treatment of streptococcal PJI. Four retrospective studies reported results that trended toward better outcomes when rifampin was used to treat streptococcal PJI, but statistical significance was achieved in only one.[30-33] It is unclear whether adding rifampin to the antimicrobial regimen is needed for streptococcal PJI.

Rifampin for *Cutibacterium* (*Propionibacterium*) Species

Although the evidence is limited, it was reported in 2018 that *Cutibacterium* species do have biofilm formation capability.[34] The results of two retrospective studies showed similar results regarding the success rates of rifampin combination treatment of *Cutibacterium*-associated PJI of the shoulder, hip, and knee.[16,35] These two studies observed a potentially beneficial effect of adding rifampin to the antimicrobial regimen. More evidence is required to support whether the addition of rifampin should be recommended for treatment of PJI caused by *Cutibacterium* species.

Because of the limitations of the existing clinical evidence and the absence of good-quality RCTs, the role

Table 2

Randomized Controlled Trials of Investigating Rifampin in Staphylococcal Prosthetic Joint Infection

First Author	Year of Publication	Types of Arthroplasty Revision	Sample Size	Cure Rate (Rifampin Versus Control)
Zimmerli	1998	DAIR	33	100% versus 58%
Pushkin	2016	Two-Stage exchange, DAIR	14	57% versus 57%
Karlsen	2020	DAIR	99	74% versus 72%

DAIR = débridement, antibiotics, and implant retention

of rifampin as an adjunctive therapy for PJI caused by gram-positive bacteria is still debatable. However, a 2019 report showed that there are abundant in vitro and experimental implant-associated infections in animal studies demonstrating strong evidence of the benefit of rifampin in terms of biofilm penetration.[36] Of note, because bacteria treated with rifampin monotherapy can readily develop resistance, rifampin should always be used in combination with at least one other antibiotic agent when used to treat PJI.

DURATION OF ANTIBIOTIC TREATMENT

The optimal duration of antibiotics for PJI is still being investigated, but depends, in general, on the surgical approach used to treat the PJI, the goals of the patient, and the feasibility of further surgeries if the patient experiences recurrent PJI. Total antibiotic treatment duration varies widely, from a minimum of 6 weeks to indefinite chronic suppression in some cases. In contrast to most other infections, where studies show that shorter courses of antibiotics are as effective as longer courses,[37] PJI remains an instance in which prolonged courses of antibiotics are necessary An RCT published in 2021 compared 6 and 12 weeks of antibiotic use for the treatment of PJI (the DAPTIPO [Duration of Antibiotic Treatment in Prosthetic Joint Infection] trial).[38] Notably, the trial included patients treated with any surgical strategy: one-stage exchange, two-stage exchange, or DAIR. Patients were randomized to receive either 6 or 12 weeks of antibiotics after their surgery and then were monitored for infection recurrence for 2 years. The study was designed as a noninferiority trial and found that 6 weeks was NOT noninferior to 12 weeks. Overall, 17% of patients treated with 6 weeks of antibiotics had a recurrent infection compared with 8% of patients treated with 12 weeks.[38] Although the effect was most pronounced for patients treated with DAIR (30% versus 15% recurrence), the trend toward better outcomes with the longer treatment option was present in all surgical subgroups. However, most clinicians still treat differently, depending on the specific surgical history.

Duration of Antibiotics After Two-Stage Exchange

One of the most common approaches to treating PJI is a two-stage exchange. This approach involves an initial surgery to remove the infected prosthesis and place an antibiotic spacer (stage one), treatment with a prolonged course of antibiotics, and then another surgery to implant a new prosthetic joint (stage two). Traditional management of these cases was to provide 6 weeks of intravenous antibiotics after spacer placement, then stop and observe the patient off antibiotics, then place a new joint if the infection appeared to be cured.[22] Although that is still the standard approach, the Duration of Antibiotic Treatment in Prosthetic Joint Infection (DATIPO) trial indicates that treating for 12 weeks after spacer placement may be preferred. However, that increased duration of antibiotics must be balanced against any increased harm to the patient by delaying surgery, for example, by needing to maintain non–weight-bearing status. In addition, a smaller unblinded randomized trial from 2019 indicated that 4 weeks of antibiotic therapy could be acceptable.[39]

An area of active debate is when the reimplantation surgery should be performed. As discussed further later, patients are typically monitored while on therapy, and then after completing antibiotic therapy, in an effort to reassure the patient and the surgeon that the infection is eradicated before implanting a new joint. Because the best test of cure is the absence of signs of infection after stopping antibiotics, traditionally patients have an antibiotic holiday before reimplantation. However, it is not clear that this approach improves outcomes compared with continuing antibiotics through the reimplantation surgery without a break, according to a 2019 report.[40]

The duration of antibiotics after the second stage of the reimplantation surgery is another area of active research. The Infectious Diseases Society of America guidelines from 2012 did not recommend any further antibiotic treatment after stage two. However, the relatively high rate of PJI recurrence after stage two (approximately 20%)[41,42] has led some surgeons to treat patients with prophylactic oral antibiotics after stage two. An RCT demonstrated that giving patients 3 months of oral antibiotics after stage two reduces the rate of recurrent PJI.[43,44] However, a 2022 report shows that this benefit must be weighed against the risk of selecting for resistant organisms in any recurrent PJI.[45] A 2018 report noted that another relatively common practice is to start oral antibiotics after stage two, but then stop after 2 to 3 weeks if the incision is healing well and the intraoperative cultures obtained at the time of reimplantation were negative, similar to high-risk primary arthroplasty patients.[46]

Duration of Antibiotics After Single-Stage Exchange or Destination Spacer

There are fewer data to inform the duration of antibiotics after single-stage exchange. The 2012 Infectious Diseases Society of America guidelines recommend 6 to 12 weeks, with consideration of indefinite suppression thereafter.[22] Based on the results of the DATIPO trial, which included 150 patients treated with a single-stage exchange, 12 weeks is reasonable.[38] Other, smaller studies have suggested that 6 weeks may be adequate, including one from 2020.[47] In addition to planned single-stage exchanges, more patients are receiving semipermanent spacers without any immediate plans for stage two reimplantation surgery. A 2019 study reported that it is reasonable to treat these patients similar to those undergoing a single-stage exchange, with a 6- to 12-week course of antibiotics.[48]

Duration of Antibiotics After Débridement With Implant Retention

For patients treated with DAIR, all should receive a minimum of 12 weeks of antibiotics.[38] Whether and how long to continue antibiotics beyond 12 weeks remains an area of debate. Most studies do show a lower risk of recurrent PJI in patients maintained on so-called suppressive antibiotics.[49,50] However, it is worth remembering that the rate of recurrent PJI for patients treated with 12 weeks of antibiotics in the DATIPO trial was only 15%, which is at least as good a success rate as seen in large cohort studies of patients on prolonged oral antibiotics.[49,51,52] Therefore, although at least 12 weeks is indicated, and there may be some benefits in extending antibiotics up to 1 year after DAIR, the benefit of indefinite suppression remains unproven. In general, lifelong suppression should be reserved for those patients for whom a recurrent PJI would result in amputation or who are too frail to undergo any further surgeries.

Duration of Antibiotics After Amputation or Arthrodesis

In unfortunate cases, salvaging a functional joint from a PJI is not possible, and the patient is treated with amputation or arthrodesis. In these cases, when no foreign material (orthopaedic hardware) remains, the duration of therapy after surgery depends on whether there is any residual infected bone (osteomyelitis). If all infected bone is removed surgically, then only a short course of antibiotics is indicated, generally less than 7 days, to treat any residual soft-tissue infection. If there is concern for retained infected bone, then 6 weeks of antibiotics after resection is typical.

MONITORING DURING TREATMENT

The prolonged duration of antimicrobial therapy for PJI can cause serious adverse reactions. Serial laboratory testing, in addition to clinical monitoring, should be obtained to monitor for those adverse reactions while receiving antimicrobial therapy. There are no generalized recommendations on frequency of laboratory testing because it depends on various factors including age of patients, underlying comorbidities, antimicrobial tolerability, and type of antimicrobial agents. However, weekly complete blood counts and blood chemistry analyses are standard while receiving outpatient parenteral antimicrobial therapy.[53] For outpatient oral antimicrobial therapy, laboratory testing can be less frequent, although certain antibiotics (linezolid, high-dose trimethoprim-sulfamethoxazole) require close monitoring. The chemistry monitoring for most antimicrobial agents includes electrolytes and renal and hepatic functions. Additional laboratory testing is needed for certain antimicrobial agents: for example, creatinine kinase for daptomycin, vancomycin level for vancomycin, and electrocardiogram for fluoroquinolones.

Monitoring serum inflammatory markers such as serum erythrocyte sedimentation rate (ESR) and C-reactive protein (CRP) is common practice, although how best to use the information remains unclear. Many clinicians will check ESR and CRP level at the beginning and end of therapy, to look for a response to treatment. Obtaining serum ESR and CRP during treatment is reasonable when clinical findings are suspicious of treatment failure or recurrent infection. However, concrete evidence for using ESR and CRP to determine success and/or failure of PJI treatment is limited. A 2023 retrospective study demonstrated that elevations in both serum ESR and CRP level before reimplantation of total knee arthroplasty (second-stage revision) was associated with reinfection compared with elevated either ESR or CRP level alone.[54] Another 2020 retrospective study showed that the ESR:CRP ratio performed better than either serum ESR or CRP level alone in predicting failure after DAIR for chronic PJI, but had poor prognostic capability for failure after DAIR for acute PJI.[55] Results of other retrospective studies showed similar results and supported the utility of serum ESR and CRP as indicators of the resolution of PJI.[56,57]

However, other studies have had different results. A retrospective study published in 2022 showed that only elevated serum CRP level was strongly associated with failure of two-stage reimplantation, whereas elevated serum ESR had trends toward reinfection but was not significant.[58] Furthermore, a few published studies showed no significant associations of ESR and/or CRP with reinfection in DAIR or two-stage revision for hip or knee PJI.[59,60] A retrospective study published in 2022 demonstrated that serum ESR, CRP level, and the ratio of ESR:CRP did not predict failure of reimplantation in patients treated with two-stage exchange for hip or knee PJI.[61] Overall, ESR and CRP may be additional data points and may cause the clinician more or less worry about a patient, but they are not predictive enough to dictate care.

Frequently, ESR and CRP level do not return to normal by the end of antimicrobial therapy. Decisions to determine success and timing for reimplantation must consider multiple factors, not just serum inflammatory markers. Preimplantation joint aspiration is another (unproven) strategy that can be used to determine treatment failure or persistent infection. Other serum markers, such as D-dimer, plasma fibrinogen, fibrin degradation products, and thromboelastography, have also been studied in an attempt to improve monitoring and assist on timing of reimplantation. However, so far, the best monitoring strategy for treatment of PJI remains unknown.

FUTURE DIRECTIONS

Although many studies have been published on the treatment of PJI, there remain many clinical questions. As outlined previously, the optimal duration of antibiotic therapy after the various surgical approaches remains unknown. In addition, although the OVIVA trial demonstrated that oral antibiotics can be as effective as intravenous antibiotics for managing orthopaedic infection, there is no clear guidance on which specific oral antimicrobials are best for which pathogens or for which patients. Investigating how and when to use oral antimicrobials instead of intravenous antimicrobials is ongoing. Other areas of research interest include better diagnostics for identifying the culprit pathogen, local antibiotic delivery, and phage therapy. Phages are viruses that can infect bacterial cells and cause bacterial cell lysis during the lytic phase of the viral replication life cycle. Phage therapy could potentially be an alternative treatment modality for PJI management, adjunct to antimicrobial therapy, or for PJI prevention. However, current clinical data on PJI are still limited.[62]

SUMMARY

A multidisciplinary team approach is mandatory for the successful management of PJI, as both skilled surgical débridement and appropriate antimicrobial therapy are key. Empiric antibiotic therapy should be withheld until after tissue samples and/or synovial fluid are obtained, except for those patients with unstable vital signs or with sepsis. The empiric therapy should provide adequate coverage against gram-positive organisms, and some cases may need empiric therapy for aerobic gram-negative bacilli, such as early-onset PJI and immunocompromised hosts. PJI should be treated with systemic antimicrobials for at least 6 weeks, and in many cases at least 12 weeks; however, the duration of treatment should be tailored to each patient and their surgical procedures. Chronic suppressive antimicrobial therapy is often used in patients with retained hardware for whom another surgery is not possible. Oral antimicrobial therapy is appropriate in certain patients with the guidance of an infectious disease specialist, but more research is needed to clarify best regimens. Rifampin is often included in the antimicrobial regimen for staphylococcal PJI after DAIR or single-stage revision, given excellent activity against biofilms in in vitro and animal studies. There are few RCTs on antimicrobial therapy for PJI, monitoring while on therapy, and treatment outcomes. These data are mostly from small RCTs, retrospective studies, and case series.

KEY STUDY POINTS

- Successful management of PJI requires a combination of surgery and prolonged antimicrobial therapy.
- When possible, the antimicrobial therapy for PJI should be directed at the culprit pathogen and managed by an infectious disease specialist.
- There is no test of cure for PJI and the most effective duration of antibiotics for any individual patient remains unknown. Chronic suppressive therapy can be a reasonable option in some cases.

ANNOTATED REFERENCES

1. Vasoo S, Chan M, Sendi P, Berbari E: The value of ortho-ID teams in treating bone and joint infections. *J Bone Jt Infect* 2019;4(6):295-299.

   This editorial describes the value of orthopaedic infectious disease specialists and multidisciplinary teams.

2. Shahi A, Deirmengian C, Higuera C, et al: Premature therapeutic antimicrobial treatments can compromise the diagnosis of late periprosthetic joint infection. *Clin Orthop Relat Res* 2015;473(7):2244-2249.

3. Burnett RS, Aggarwal A, Givens SA, McClure JT, Morgan PM, Barrack RL: Prophylactic antibiotics do not affect cultures in the treatment of an infected TKA: A prospective trial. *Clin Orthop Relat Res* 2010;468(1):127-134.

4. Anagnostopoulos A, Bossard DA, Ledergerber B, et al: Perioperative antibiotic prophylaxis has no effect on time to positivity and proportion of positive samples: A cohort study of 64 Cutibacterium acnes bone and joint infections. *J Clin Microbiol* 2018;56(2):e01576-17.

   This is a single-center cohort study looking at the effect of perioperative antibiotics on the rate of positive intra-operative cultures, looking specifically at cultures positive for *C acnes*.

5. Moran E, Masters S, Berendt AR, McLardy-Smith P, Byren I, Atkins BL: Guiding empirical antibiotic therapy in orthopaedics: The microbiology of prosthetic joint infection managed by debridement, irrigation and prosthesis retention. *J Infect* 2007;55(1):1-7.

6. Rosteius T, Jansen O, Fehmer T, et al: Evaluating the microbial pattern of periprosthetic joint infections of the hip and knee. *J Med Microbiol* 2018;67(11):1608-1613.

   This single-center cohort study describes the causative pathogens of hip and knee PJI in cases from 2003 to 2011.

7. Nelson SB, Certain LK: Microbes and antibiotics, in Rubash HE, ed: *The Adult Knee*, ed 2. Lippincott Williams & Wilkins, 2020.

   This text book chapter covers the microbiology and antibiotic treatment of knee infections.

8. Palan J, Nolan C, Sarantos K, Westerman R, King R, Foguet P: Culture-negative periprosthetic joint infections. *EFORT Open Rev* 2019;4(10):585-594.

   This is a review article about culture-negative PJI and available diagnostic methods.

9. Tan TL, Kheir MM, Shohat N, et al: Culture-negative periprosthetic joint infection: An update on what to expect. *JBJS Open Access* 2018;3(3):e0060.

   This single-center cohort study reported on patients with culture-negative PJI in cases from 2000 to 2014.

10. Thoendel M, Jeraldo P, Greenwood-Quaintance KE, et al: A novel prosthetic joint infection pathogen, Mycoplasma salivarium, identified by metagenomic shotgun sequencing. *Clin Infect Dis* 2017;65(2):332-335.

11. Wang C, Huang Z, Li W, Fang X, Zhang W: Can metagenomic next-generation sequencing identify the pathogens responsible for culture-negative prosthetic joint infection? *BMC Infect Dis* 2020;20(1):253.

    This single-center study of 27 patients with culture-negative PJI compared patients treated with empiric antibiotics with those treated with antibiotics targeting organisms identified by next-generation sequencing methods. The study was too small to be conclusive.

12. Whiting Z, Doerre T: Diagnosis of culture-negative septic arthritis with polymerase chain reaction in an immunosuppressed patient: A case report. *JBJS Case Connect* 2020;10(3):e20.00057.

    This is a case report of native joint culture-negative septic arthritis caused by *Ureaplasma*, identified by polymerase chain reaction.

13. Benito N, Mur I, Ribera A, et al: The different microbial etiology of prosthetic joint infections according to route of acquisition and time after prosthesis implantation, including the role of multidrug-resistant organisms. *J Clin Med* 2019;8(5):673.

    This multicenter study from Spain describes the microbiology of PJI in cases from 2003 to 2012.

14. Tande AJ, Patel R: Prosthetic joint infection. *Clin Microbiol Rev* 2014;27(2):302-345.

15. Triffault-Fillit C, Ferry T, Laurent F, et al: Microbiologic epidemiology depending on time to occurrence of prosthetic joint infection: A prospective cohort study. *Clin Microbiol Infect* 2019;25(3):353-358.

    This single-center study from France describes the microbiology of PJI in cases from 2011 to 2016.

16. Kusejko K, Auñón Á, Jost B, et al: The impact of surgical strategy and rifampin on treatment outcome in Cutibacterium periprosthetic joint infections. *Clin Infect Dis* 2021;72(12):e1064-e1073.

    This multicenter retrospective study reported on 187 patients with *Cutibacterium* PJI. There was a significant trend toward improved outcomes with rifampin.

17. Aboltins CA, Dowsey MM, Buising KL, et al: Gram-negative prosthetic joint infection treated with debridement, prosthesis retention and antibiotic regimens including a fluoroquinolone. *Clin Microbiol Infect* 2011;17(6):862-867.

18. Rodríguez-Pardo D, Pigrau C, Lora-Tamayo J, et al: Gram-negative prosthetic joint infection: Outcome of a debridement, antibiotics and implant retention approach. A large multicentre study. *Clin Microbiol Infect* 2014;20(11):O911-O919.

19. Zmistowski B, Fedorka CJ, Sheehan E, Deirmengian G, Austin MS, Parvizi J: Prosthetic joint infection caused by gram-negative organisms. *J Arthroplasty* 2011;26(6 suppl):104-108.

20. Li HK, Rombach I, Zambellas R, et al: Oral versus intravenous antibiotics for bone and joint infection. *N Engl J Med* 2019;380(5):425-436.

    This large randomized clinical trial in the United Kingdom compared oral with intravenous antibiotics for bone and joint infections. There was no difference in rate of treatment failure between the two groups, indicating that oral antibiotics can be as effective as intravenous antibiotics for the treatment of orthopaedic infections.

21. Baddour LM, Wilson WR, Bayer AS, et al: Infective endocarditis in adults: Diagnosis, antimicrobial therapy, and management of complications – A scientific statement for healthcare professionals from the American Heart Association. *Circulation* 2015;132(15):1435-1486.

22. Osmon DR, Berbari EF, Berendt AR, et al: Diagnosis and management of prosthetic joint infection: Clinical practice guidelines by the Infectious Diseases Society of America. *Clin Infect Dis* 2013;56(1):1-25.

23. Beldman M, Löwik C, Soriano A, et al: If, when, and how to use rifampin in acute staphylococcal periprosthetic joint infections, a multicentre observational study. *Clin Infect Dis* 2021;73(9):1634-1641.

    This is a retrospective multicenter study looking at the effect of rifampin use on outcomes for patients with staphylococcal PJI treated with débridement and implant retention. Patients treated with rifampin had lower rates of treatment failure.

24. Becker A, Kreitmann L, Triffaut-Fillit C, et al: Duration of rifampin therapy is a key determinant of improved outcomes in early-onset acute prosthetic joint infection due to Staphylococcus treated with a debridement, antibiotics and implant retention (DAIR): A retrospective multicenter study in France. *J Bone Jt Infect* 2020;5(1):28-34.

    This is a retrospective multicenter study looking at the effect of rifampin use on outcomes for patients with staphylococcal PJI treated with débridement and implant retention. Patients treated with rifampin had lower rates of treatment failure.

25. El Helou OC, Berbari EF, Lahr BD, et al: Efficacy and safety of rifampin containing regimen for staphylococcal prosthetic joint infections treated with debridement and retention. *Eur J Clin Microbiol Infect Dis* 2010;29(8):961-967.

26. Holmberg A, Thórhallsdóttir VG, Robertsson O, W-Dahl A, Stefánsdóttir A: 75% success rate after open debridement, exchange of tibial insert, and antibiotics in knee prosthetic joint infections. *Acta Orthop* 2015;86(4):457-462.

27. Pushkin R, Iglesias-Ussel MD, Keedy K, et al: A randomized study evaluating oral fusidic acid (CEM-102) in combination with oral rifampin compared with standard-of-care antibiotics for treatment of prosthetic joint infections: A newly identified drug-drug interaction. *Clin Infect Dis* 2016;63(12):1599-1604.

28. Zimmerli W, Widmer AF, Blatter M, Frei R, Ochsner PE: Role of rifampin for treatment of orthopedic implant-related staphylococcal infections: A randomized controlled trial. Foreign-Body Infection (FBI) Study Group. *J Am Med Assoc* 1998;279(19):1537-1541.

29. Karlsen ØE, Borgen P, Bragnes B, et al: Rifampin combination therapy in staphylococcal prosthetic joint infections: A randomized controlled trial. *J Orthop Surg Res* 2020;15(1):365.

   This RCT studied the use of adjunctive rifampin for patients with early staphylococcal PJI treated with débridement and implant retention. There was no benefit to rifampin; however, the study only included one-half (48 of 99) of enrolled patients in the final analysis.

30. Fiaux E, Titecat M, Robineau O, et al: Outcome of patients with streptococcal prosthetic joint infections with special reference to rifampicin combinations. *BMC Infect Dis* 2016;16(1):568.

31. Andronic O, Achermann Y, Jentzsch T, et al: Factors affecting outcome in the treatment of streptococcal periprosthetic joint infections: Results from a single-centre retrospective cohort study. *Int Orthop* 2021;45(1):57-63.

   In this single-center retrospective cohort study of streptococcal PJI cases from 2011 to 2019, no benefit of rifampin was seen.

32. Mahieu R, Dubée V, Seegers V, et al: The prognosis of streptococcal prosthetic bone and joint infections depends on surgical management – A multicenter retrospective study. *Int J Infect Dis* 2019;85:175-181.

   In this multicenter retrospective cohort study of streptococcal PJI of cases from 2010 to 2012, no benefit of rifampin was seen.

33. Wouthuyzen-Bakker M, Sebillotte M, Lomas J, et al: Clinical outcome and risk factors for failure in late acute prosthetic joint infections treated with debridement and implant retention. *J Infect* 2019;78(1):40-47.

   An international multicenter retrospective study showed an overall failure rate of 45% of DAIR in acute late-onset PJI. Risk factors of the failure were fracture as indication for the prosthesis, rheumatoid arthritis, age older than 80 years, male sex, and CRP level greater than 150 mg/L. The rifampin combination therapy group had a significantly lower failure rate in staphylococcal PJI, but not in streptococcal PJI.

34. Kuehnast T, Cakar F, Weinhäupl T, et al: Comparative analyses of biofilm formation among different Cutibacterium acnes isolates. *Int J Med Microbiol* 2018;308(8):1027-1035.

   This basic science article describes the biofilm-forming properties of various strains of *C acnes*.

35. Jacobs AM, Van Hooff ML, Meis JF, Vos F, Goosen JH: Treatment of prosthetic joint infections due to Propionibacterium. Similar results in 60 patients treated with and without rifampicin. *Acta Orthop* 2016;87(1):60-66.

36. Zimmerli W, Sendi P: Role of rifampin against staphylococcal biofilm infections *in vitro*, in animal models, and in orthopedic-device-related infections. *Antimicrob Agents Chemother* 2019;63(2):e01746-18.

   This literature review of rifampin in orthopaedic device–related infection revealed good efficacy against in vitro biofilms and animal models under favorable conditions, which were low bacterial inoculum, young biofilm, and prolonged treatment duration, as well as in small human studies treated with DAIR.

37. Spellberg B, Rice LB: Duration of antibiotic therapy: Shorter is better. *Ann Intern Med* 2019;171(3):210-211.

   This is a commentary on the increasing volume of literature indicating that, for many infections, shorter courses of antibiotics are as effective as longer courses.

38. Bernard L, Arvieux C, Brunschweiler B, et al: Antibiotic therapy for 6 or 12 weeks for prosthetic joint infection. *N Engl J Med* 2021;384(21):1991-2001.

   The DATIPO trial was an open-label, randomized controlled, noninferiority study that demonstrated that 6 weeks of antibiotic therapy was *not* noninferior to 12 weeks of treatment in patients with microbiologically confirmed PJI at 104 weeks after completion of antibiotic therapy.

39. Benkabouche M, Racloz G, Spechbach H, Lipsky BA, Gaspoz J, Uçkay I: Four versus six weeks of antibiotic therapy for osteoarticular infections after implant removal: A randomized trial. *J Antimicrob Chemother* 2019;74(8):2394-2399.

   This single-center, unblinded, randomized trial found no significant difference in recurrence of clinical infection between patients treated with 4 or 6 weeks of antibiotic therapy for orthopaedic implant infection after implant removal.

40. Ascione T, Balato G, Mariconda M, Rotondo R, Baldini A, Pagliano P: Continuous antibiotic therapy can reduce recurrence of prosthetic joint infection in patients undergoing 2-stage exchange. *J Arthroplasty* 2019;34(4):704-709.

   This observational study of two orthopaedic practices (with different approaches to PJI management) showed a favorable cure rate at 96-week follow-up in patients with PJI who underwent stage two reimplantation surgery without an antibiotic holiday (the approach of practice A) compared with patients who were off antibiotics for 2 weeks pre-reimplantation (the approach of practice B).

41. Mortazavi SM, Vegari D, Ho A, Zmistowski B, Parvizi J: Two-stage exchange arthroplasty for infected total knee arthroplasty: Predictors of failure. *Clin Orthop Relat Res* 2011;469(11):3049-3054.

42. Ascione T, Pagliano P, Balato G, Mariconda M, Rotondo R, Esposito S: Oral therapy, microbiological findings, and comorbidity influence the outcome of prosthetic joint infections undergoing 2-stage exchange. *J Arthroplasty* 2017;32(7):2239-2243.

43. Frank JM, Kayupov E, Moric M, et al: The Mark Coventry, MD, Award: Oral antibiotics reduce reinfection after two-stage exchange – A multicenter, randomized controlled trial. *Clin Orthop Relat Res* 2017;475(1):56-61.

44. Yang JW, Parvizi J, Hansen EN, et al: 2020 Mark Coventry Award: Microorganism-directed oral antibiotics reduce the rate of failure due to further infection after two-stage revision hip or knee arthroplasty for chronic infection – A multicentre randomized controlled trial at a minimum of two years. *Bone Joint J* 2020;102-B(6 suppl A):3-9.

    This multicenter RCT showed that patients with PJI treated with microorganism-directed oral antibiotic agent for 3 months following reimplantation had significantly lower rate of repeat infection compared with patients with no antibiotic agent following reimplantation at 2-year follow-up.

45. Kelly MP, Gililland JM, Blackburn BE, Anderson LA, Pelt CE, Certain LK: Extended oral antibiotics increase bacterial resistance in patients who fail 2-stage exchange for periprosthetic joint infection. *J Arthroplasty* 2022;37(8 suppl):S989-S996.

    This retrospective study showed that prolonged oral antibiotic therapy following reimplantation increased the rate of subsequent PJI from antibiotic-resistant organisms significantly.

46. Inabathula A, Dilley JE, Ziemba-Davis M, et al: Extended oral antibiotic prophylaxis in high-risk patients substantially reduces primary total hip and knee arthroplasty 90-day infection rate. *J Bone Jt Surg* 2018;100(24):2103-2109.

    This retrospective study showed that a 7-day course of antibiotic prophylaxis following primary total knee or hip arthroplasty reduced the infection rates in the 90-day postoperative period in patients with high risk of postoperative infection, especially in patients with body mass index greater than 40 kg/m^2 and with diabetes mellitus.

47. Chieffo G, Corsia S, Rougereau G, et al: Six-week antibiotic therapy after one-stage replacement arthroplasty for hip and knee periprosthetic joint infection. *Med Mal Infect* 2020;50(7):567-574.

    This retrospective study showed an overall remission rate of 90% with a 6-week course of antibiotic therapy for knee and hip PJI in patients who underwent single-stage exchange.

48. Valencia JCB, Abdel MP, Virk A, Osmon DR, Razonable RR: Destination joint spacers, reinfection, and antimicrobial suppression. *Clin Infect Dis* 2019;69(6):1056-1059.

    This retrospective study showed that chronic antibiotic suppression therapy did not prevent recurrent infection following destination joint spacer surgery for PJI, especially in patients with preoperative sinus drainage.

49. Shah NB, Hersh BL, Kreger A, et al: Benefits and adverse events associated with extended antibiotic use in total knee arthroplasty periprosthetic joint infection. *Clin Infect Dis* 2020;70(4):559-565.

    This multicenter retrospective study demonstrated that patients with knee PJI who underwent DAIR treated with an extended course of oral antibiotics had a significantly lower failure rate compared with those who received a standard course of intravenous antibiotics. However, the benefit of antibiotic after 1 year was not observed.

50. Barry JJ, Geary MB, Riesgo AM, Odum SM, Fehring TK, Springer BD: Irrigation and debridement with chronic antibiotic suppression is as effective as 2-stage exchange in revision total knee arthroplasty with extensive instrumentation. *J Bone Joint Surg Am* 2021;103(1):53-63.

    This retrospective study evaluating infections following TKA revision showed that DAIR with chronic antibiotic suppressive therapy had a similar rate of recurrent infection compared with two-stage exchange.

51. Siqueira MB, Saleh A, Klika AK, et al: Chronic suppression of periprosthetic joint infections with oral antibiotics increases infection-free survivorship. *J Bone Joint Surg Am* 2015;97(15):1220-1232.

52. Byren I, Bejon P, Atkins BL, et al: One hundred and twelve infected arthroplasties treated with "DAIR" (debridement, antibiotics and implant retention): Antibiotic duration and outcome. *J Antimicrob Chemother* 2009;63(6):1264-1271.

53. Norris AH, Shrestha NK, Allison GM, et al: 2018 Infectious Diseases Society of America clinical practice guideline for the management of outpatient parenteral antimicrobial therapy. *Clin Infect Dis* 2019;68:1-35.

    These are the practice guidelines for the management of patients on prolonged courses of intravenous antibiotics.

54. Klemt C, Padmanabha A, Esposito JG, Laurencin S, Smith EJ, Kwon YM: Elevated ESR and CRP prior to second-stage reimplantation knee revision surgery for periprosthetic joint infection are associated with increased reinfection rates. *J Knee Surg* 2023;36(4):354-361.

    This retrospective study showed that in patients with chronic PJI, both elevated serum ESR and CRP level before reimplantation were associated with reinfection after surgery compared with those with elevated ESR or CRP level alone.

55. Maier SP, Klemt C, Tirumala V, Oganesyan R, van den Kieboom J, Kwon YM: Elevated ESR/CRP ratio is associated with reinfection after debridement, antibiotics, and implant retention in chronic periprosthetic joint infections. *J Arthroplasty* 2020;35(11):3254-3260.

    This retrospective cohort study of 179 patients examined ESR:CRP ratio as a predictor of failure after DAIR.

56. Lindsay CP, Olcott CW, Del Gaizo DJ: ESR and CRP are useful between stages of 2-stage revision for periprosthetic joint infection. *Arthroplast Today* 2017;3(3):183-186.

57. Tikhilov R, Bozhkova S, Denisov A, et al: Risk factors and a prognostic model of hip periprosthetic infection recurrence after surgical treatment using articulating and non-articulating spacers. *Int Orthop* 2016;40(7):1381-1387.

58. Hartman CW, Daubach EC, Richard BT, et al: Predictors of reinfection in prosthetic joint infections following two-stage reimplantation. *J Arthroplasty* 2022;37(7 suppl):S674-S677.

    This retrospective study showed that elevated serum CRP level before reimplantation was associated with reinfection in patients with PJI treated with two-stage exchange.

59. Fu J, Ni M, Li H, et al: The proper timing of second-stage revision in treating periprosthetic knee infection: Reliable indicators and risk factors. *J Orthop Surg Res* 2018;13(1):214.

    This retrospective study evaluating indicators and proper timing for reimplantation in patients with PJI showed that intraoperative frozen section was beneficial, whereas serum ESR and CRP level were poor predictors of reinfection.

60. Stambough JB, Curtin BM, Odum SM, Cross MB, Martin JR, Fehring TK: Does change in ESR and CRP guide the timing of two-stage arthroplasty reimplantation? *Clin Orthop Relat Res* 2019;477(2):364-371.

    This multicenter retrospective study demonstrated poor association of serum ESR and CRP level with reinfection after reimplantation in patients with hip and knee PJI.

61. Johnson NR, Rowe TM, Valenzeula MM, Scarola GT, Fehring TK: Do pre-reimplantation erythrocyte sedimentation rate/C-reactive protein cutoffs guide decision-making in prosthetic joint infection? Are we flying blind? *J Arthroplasty* 2022;37(2):347-352.

    This retrospective study showed no significant association of serum ESR, serum CRP level, and ESR:CRP ratio with reinfection in patients with chronic PJI after second-stage exchange.

62. Cano EJ, Caflisch KM, Bollyky PL, et al: Phage therapy for limb-threatening prosthetic knee Klebsiella pneumoniae infection: Case report and in vitro characterization of anti-biofilm activity. *Clin Infect Dis* 2021;73(1):e144-e151.

    This case report describes successful treatment of a refractory drug-resistant PJI using phage therapy.

SECTION 5

Fracture-Related Infections

Section Editor:
Charalampos G. Zalavras, MD, PhD, FAAOS, FACS

CHAPTER 19

Definition, Diagnosis, and Socioeconomic Effect of Fracture-Related Infections

WILLEM-JAN METSEMAKERS, MD, PhD
WILLIAM T. OBREMSKEY, MD, MPH, MMHC, FAAOS

ABSTRACT

Fracture-related infection (FRI) remains one of the most challenging musculoskeletal complications in orthopaedic trauma surgery. Its diagnosis is a multistage process that is based on various diagnostic pillars. The recently validated FRI consensus definition offers clinicians the opportunity to standardize clinical reports and improve the quality of published literature. The consensus definition is based on diagnostic criteria, which are considered either confirmatory (infection definitely present) or suggestive (infection possibly present). The presence of at least one clinical or microbiologic confirmatory sign is associated with a high diagnostic performance and is pathognomonic for the presence of an FRI. Very rarely patients will demonstrate suggestive signs only, and these cases should be discussed within a multidisciplinary team. A standardized clinical approach toward the diagnostic workup of patients with suspected FRI should facilitate early diagnosis and treatment and improve the outcome of patients with FRI. This is important, as FRI negatively affects a patients' quality of life, the ability to return to work, and overall health care costs.

Keywords: definition; diagnosis; fracture-related infection; microbiology; serum inflammatory markers

---

Dr. Obremskey or an immediate family member serves as a board member, owner, officer, or committee member of Southeastern Fracture Consortium. Neither Dr. Metsemakers nor any immediate family member has received anything of value from or has stock or stock options held in a commercial company or institution related directly or indirectly to the subject of this chapter.

INTRODUCTION

Fracture-related infection (FRI) is a serious complication following orthopaedic trauma. Over the past decades, heterogeneous bone-related infections, including infections related to fractures, were grouped together under the singular term osteomyelitis, which has prompted efforts to differentiate some of these infections into discrete disease entities such as prosthetic joint infection (PJI), diabetic foot infection, and native osteomyelitis. However, until recently, this was not the case for FRI. The first purpose of this chapter is to summarize the available evidence related to the diagnosis of FRI, to discuss the diagnostic criteria included in the FRI consensus definition, and to provide specific recommendations on microbiology specimen sampling and laboratory procedures. The second purpose is to provide an overview of the socioeconomic effect of FRI.

INCIDENCE OF FRI

With an estimated 180 million new fractures occurring worldwide every year and infection rates ranging between 1% and 30%, the incidence of this complication cannot be underestimated.[1-3] Although infections related to skeletal fractures have been known for centuries, accurately estimating the incidence and outcome of this complication has been hampered by the lack of a clear terminology.[4] Historically, studies focusing on FRI either provided no definition, developed their own, or used the definition for surgical site infection, issued by the Centers for Disease Control and Prevention. However, the practical applicability of these Centers for Disease Control and Prevention criteria published in 2021 for FRI is limited as they do not include nonsurgically treated patients with FRI (often seen in low-income countries), certain anatomic areas, as well as infections occurring after 90 days.[5]

An FRI is an infection that involves a healed or unhealed bone fracture, whereby pathogenic microorganisms may be present at any part of the fracture site. The first essential step in the management of FRI is an adequate diagnosis.[6] Because of the previous lack of standardized guidelines regarding the diagnosis of FRI, an international group of experts (the FRI Consensus Group) created a consensus definition based on diagnostic criteria, which are considered either confirmatory (infection definitely present) or suggestive (infection possibly present).[4,6] The criteria proposed by the FRI consensus group are provided in **Table 1**.

In a 2022 study, 637 patients who were treated for suspicion of infection were retrospectively evaluated and the confirmatory criteria for FRI validated.[7] Because of a previous lack of a diagnostic gold standard for FRI, intention to treat as recommended by the multidisciplinary team was used as a reference standard to subdivide patients into the FRI group and the control group. The presence of at least one clinical or microbiologic confirmatory sign was associated with a sensitivity of 97.5% and a specificity of 100%. The study showed that orthopaedic trauma patients very rarely demonstrate only one or more suggestive signs, and it is highly recommended that these cases are discussed within a multidisciplinary team.

This recently validated FRI consensus definition offers clinicians the opportunity to standardize clinical reports and improve the quality of published literature.

Table 1

Diagnostic Criteria Based on the Consensus Definition for Fracture-Related Infection

	Confirmatory Criteria	Suggestive Criteria

Clinical	Fistula, sinus, or wound breakdown (with communication with the bone or implant)
	Purulent drainage from the wound or presence of pus during surgery
		Local clinical signs of inflammation:
		  Local redness
		  Pain (without weight bearing, increasing over time, new onset)
		  Local swelling
		  Local warmth
		Systemic clinical signs:
		  Fever (single oral temperature measurement ≥38.3°C [101°F])
		Other clinical signs:
		  New-onset joint effusion
		  Persistent, increasing, or new-onset wound drainage, beyond the first few days postoperatively, without solid alternative explanation

Microbiology	Phenotypically indistinguishable microorganisms isolated from at least two separate deep-tissue or implant specimens	Pathogenic organism identified by culture from a single deep-tissue or implant specimen
Histopathology	Presence of microorganisms in deep-tissue specimens confirmed by histopathology For chronic or late-onset cases: The presence of at least five polymorphonuclear neutrophils per high-power field	—
Radiology	—	Radiologic signs on conventional radiography, CT, and/or MRI
Nuclear imaging	—	Nuclear imaging signs on WBC scan and/or ^{18}F FDG-PET
Laboratory	—	Elevated serum inflammatory markers (WBC count, CRP level, and/or ESR)

CRP = C-reactive protein, ESR = erythrocyte sedimentation rate, FDG-PET = fluorodeoxyglucose positron emission tomography, WBC = white blood cell

DIAGNOSTIC CRITERIA

Clinical Criteria

Patients with FRI can present with a large variety of clinical symptoms, depending on the healing state of the fracture, the virulence of the organism, the anatomic localization, and the mode of infection.[6,8] The clinical symptoms were evaluated by two systematic reviews that analyzed the diagnostic criteria related to FRI.[9,10] Purulent drainage and wound dehiscence or wound breakdown were found as the only two clinical symptoms that are pathognomonic for FRI.[9,10] The presence of a fistula (**Figure 1**), sinus or wound breakdown (with communication to the bone or implant) (**Figures 2** and **3**), and/or (intraoperative) purulent drainage are indeed included as clinical confirmatory criteria in the consensus definition for FRI[4,6] (**Table 1**).

Symptoms such as local warmth, redness, swelling, pain, fever (≥38.3°C; 101°F), and new-onset or persisting wound drainage are signs of general infection, and therefore, not specific for FRI.[4,6] For example, pain can be caused by several conditions, and in trauma patients, pain may be related to the fracture or the soft-tissue injury. These general infection symptoms are therefore

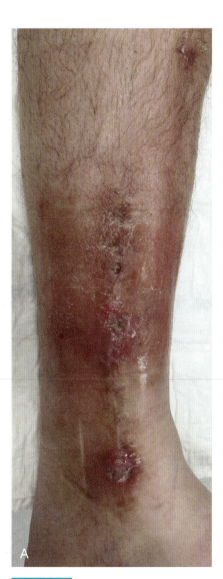
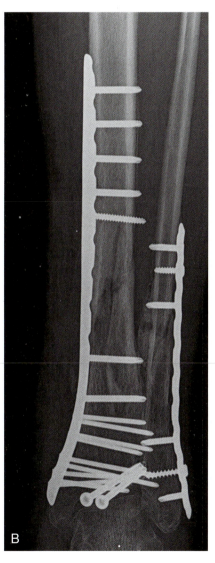
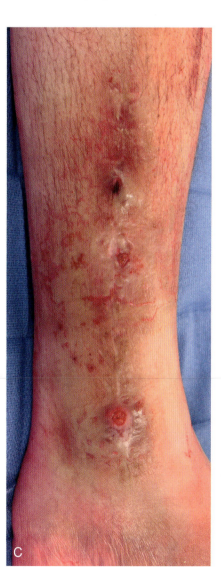

FIGURE 1 Images of a monomicrobial fracture-related infection (FRI) in a 39-year-old man obtained 7 months following a closed distal tibia and fibula fracture managed with plate-and-screw osteosynthesis. **A**, Clinical photograph shows redness, swelling, and fistulae at presentation. **B**, AP radiograph of the left lower leg shows the tibial and fibular fractures stabilized with plate-and-screw osteosynthesis. **C**, Intraoperative photograph shows the two fistulae in more detail. The presence of at least one clinical confirmatory sign (in this case, a fistula) is pathognomonic for FRI. During revision surgery the plate and screws were removed. Multiple tissue cultures were obtained and the implant was sent for sonication. Culture results showed multiple positive cultures with *Staphylococcus aureus*.

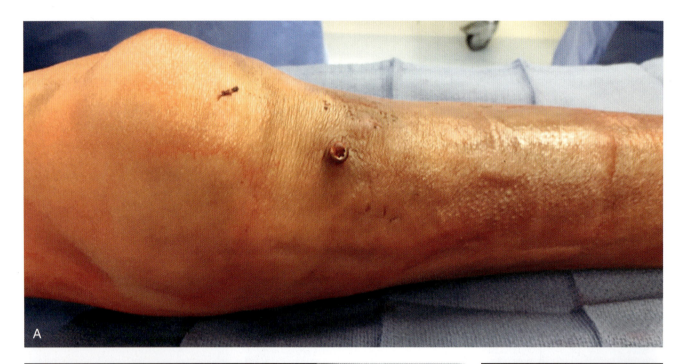

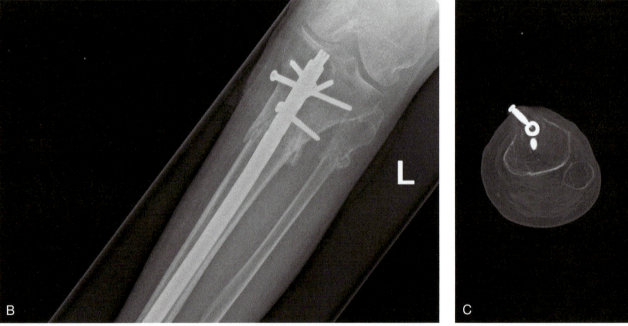

FIGURE 2 Images of a polymicrobial fracture-related infection (FRI) in a 64-year-old man obtained 3 months following intramedullary nailing of a tibial fracture. **A**, Clinical photograph of the left leg with wound breakdown caused by implant loosening at the level of one of the proximal locking screws. AP radiograph (**B**) and transaxial CT image (**C**) of the left lower leg show the tibial fracture treated with an intramedullary nail. Both imaging studies revealed loosening of one of the proximal locking screws. The presence of a clinical (wound breakdown) confirmatory sign is pathognomonic for FRI. The nail was removed and the intramedullary canal débrided. Multiple tissue cultures were obtained and the implant was sent for sonication. Culture results showed multiple positive cultures with *Staphylococcus epidermidis*, *Staphylococcus capitis*, and *Streptococcus mitis*.

included in the consensus definition as suggestive criteria.[4,6] A 2022 validation study found specificities exceeding 80% for the presence of any local clinical sign (ie, local warmth, redness, swelling, wound drainage), excluding pain, in patients in whom a clinical confirmatory sign was not present. This implies that if these signs are present when a patient returns to a clinic or urgent/urgent care center, the presence of an FRI should be

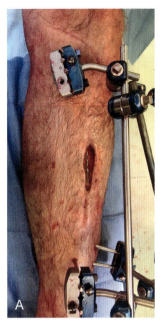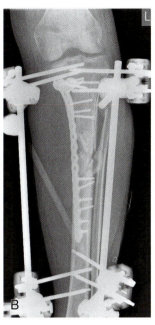

FIGURE 3 Images of a polymicrobial fracture-related infection (FRI) in a 35-year-old man obtained 3 months following a type IIIA open tibial fracture treated with a combination of plate osteosynthesis and external fixation. **A**, Clinical photograph of the left leg with wound breakdown with visualization of the plate osteosynthesis. **B**, AP radiograph of the left lower leg shows the tibial fracture stabilized with a combination of plate osteosynthesis and external fixation. The presence of at least one clinical confirmatory sign (in this case, wound breakdown) is pathognomonic for FRI. The plate and external fixation were removed, and the intramedullary canal débrided. Multiple tissue cultures were obtained and the plate was sent for sonication. Culture results showed multiple positive cultures with *Staphylococcus aureus* and *Staphylococcus capitis*.

strongly considered.[7] Attributing these signs to a superficial incisional infection, as defined by the Centers for Disease Control and Prevention criteria for surgical site infection, should be performed with caution and the patient should be followed closely to ensure that symptoms have completely resolved. Attributing persistent suggestive signs to a superficial incisional infection will delay the diagnosis of FRI. A 2021 study reported that a delay in diagnosis and treatment may be associated with a worse outcome.[11] Although, in rare cases (eg, elderly patients with comorbidities) suppressive antibiotics can be considered, prescribing antimicrobial therapy without performing adequate surgical débridement with tissue sampling should be discouraged.[7]

Serologic Evaluation

Laboratory findings that can be related to infection include the elevation of serum inflammatory markers such as white blood cell (WBC) count, C-reactive protein (CRP) level, and erythrocyte sedimentation rate (ESR).[6,12,13] In 2018, it was reported that in trauma patients, these markers are considered to be suggestive of infection in case of a consistent elevation over a longer period or in case of a secondary rise after an initial decrease.[14] The evidence for the use of serum inflammatory markers in the diagnostic workup for FRI is scarce, as these biomarkers typically also increase in the acute phase after trauma and in many inflammatory conditions.[14] For example, in patients with a fracture, CRP levels increase to a maximal level on the second day and return to normal after 2 weeks.[15] Most studies that investigated the diagnostic performance of serum inflammatory markers are therefore limited to chronic or late-onset FRI, in which the infection is typically less prominent and more difficult to diagnose.[7] Depending on the specific inflammatory marker (WBC count, CRP level, or ESR), these studies have reported sensitivities ranging between 17.0% and 100%, and specificities ranging between 34.3% and 95.0%.[14,16] The limited amount of data that are available on both acute/early-onset and chronic/late-onset FRIs show similar results.[7]

Other biomarkers such as interleukin 6 (IL-6), D-dimer, procalcitonin, and fibrinogen are used in the diagnosis of PJI or sepsis, but their use in the diagnosis of FRI currently lacks support and may even be inferior to more commonly used biomarkers such as CRP.[17-20]

The diagnosis of FRI should not solely be based on the presence of elevated serum inflammatory markers as they appear to be only suggestive of infection.

Microbiology

Biofilm formation on implants or necrotic bone is one of the major challenges in the diagnosis and management of FRI. A 2020 review reported that bacteria residing in biofilms have a low metabolic activity and are therefore difficult to culture.[21] As the surgical approach is chosen in tandem with targeted antimicrobial treatment,[21,22] it is important that sampling and culture techniques are performed meticulously.[6,22]

In both 2019[23] and 2020,[6] standardized protocols for intraoperative sampling with respect to FRI were published. If possible, antibiotic treatment should be stopped at least 2 weeks before the surgery.[6,23] In 2019, a study noted that, to avoid false-positive results due to cross-contamination, surgical samples should be obtained separately, each with a clean instrument and without touching the patient's skin.[23] The specimens should be transferred rapidly to the laboratory.[6] The culture yield can be optimized by increasing the number of intraoperative deep-tissue samples.[22,24] Current recommendations state that preferably a minimum of five deep-tissue samples should be obtained intraoperatively, from sites surrounding the fracture and the implant.[21,22,24] A systematic literature review reported that swab cultures should not be used because of their low sensitivity and high risk of contamination.[25] The same applies to superficial, skin, or sinus tract samples as they are not predictive of the causative pathogen and may be colonized with surface bacteria. Bone needle aspiration, used in pediatric and vertebral osteomyelitis, and image-guided closed bone needle biopsies are not used in the diagnosis of FRI because of a poor yield.[26,27] Compared with PJI, aspiration in the case of FRI is only rarely indicated (eg, joint effusion, deep abscess formation [pelvis]). In certain cases, it can even be contraindicated, as the implant can be very close to the skin (eg, ankle fractures), thereby increasing the risk of infection.[6,21]

The use of sonication fluid samples as an adjunct to standard deep-tissue cultures has been validated for the diagnosis of PJI, especially for patients who received antimicrobial therapy before sampling.[28,29] When the implant is removed, it is submerged into sterile fluid and subjected to low-intensity ultrasound waves, thereby dislodging the biofilm from the implant. This technique does not affect bacterial viability so that the sonicaed fluid can be cultured.[29] FRI studies evaluating the diagnostic performance of sonication fluid sampling are scarce, and often apply different methodologies, which makes it difficult to compare results.[25,30,31] Based on the available studies, sonication fluid cultures are not superior to standard deep-tissue cultures, but they may have a complementary value in the diagnostic pathway of FRI. Within the FRI consensus definition, a positive sonication fluid culture is evaluated as a single culture result.[21]

Positive cultures of two phenotypically indistinguishable pathogens of at least two separate deep-tissue/implant samples are considered a confirmatory microbiologic criterion of FRI. A pathogenic microorganism identified from a single deep-tissue/implant specimen is only suggestive for FRI. However, one positive sample with a highly virulent pathogen (arbitrarily defined as gram-negative bacilli, *Staphylococcus aureus*, enterococci, beta-hemolytic streptococci, milleri group streptococci, *Streptococcus pneumonia*, and *Candida* spp.) should raise a high suspicion of infection.[7]

Medical Imaging

Diagnostic imaging may be indicated if more certainty is required regarding the presence of FRI, to visualize the anatomic details of the disease and/or to evaluate the degree of fracture consolidation and implant stability. The choice of diagnostic imaging modality depends on local preference and availability.[6]

Conventional methods such as standard radiography and CT can detect secondary signs of infection such as impaired fracture healing, bone lysis, and implant loosening. However, because these signs can also occur in aseptic cases, standard radiography and CT have a low diagnostic performance for FRI.[32,33] MRI has a better resolution to distinguish infection or inflammation signs in the soft tissues (such as a fistula). However, a 2020 systematic literature review reported that the presence of fracture fixation devices may cause artifact and MRI does not differentiate well between infection and aseptic inflammation.[33]

Nuclear imaging techniques have progressed rapidly over the past decades. Regarding FRI, nuclear imaging generally involves three-phase scintigraphic bone scan, WBC scintigraphy, and/or fluorodeoxyglucose positron emission tomography (FDG-PET). Although a bone scan has a high sensitivity, it is not recommended in the workup of FRI because of its low specificity.[6,32] This is because a variety of reasons that can cause increased tracer (technetium-99m–labeled phosphorous complexes) uptake, such as fracture healing and implant loosening.[32] WBC scintigraphy has a high diagnostic performance, as it is not affected by recent surgery and can distinguish between infection and inflammation. However, it is a more laborious and time-consuming technique. Because of high uptake of WBC in the liver, spleen, and bone marrow, WBC scintigraphy is less suited for the diagnostic workup of the axial skeleton.[6,32,34] ^{18}F FDG-PET relies on the increased uptake of glucose by activated leukocytes, monocytes, lymphocytes, macrophages, and giant cells at the infected site.[6] It provides an increased spatial resolution and is time efficient. However, this technique cannot distinguish between an inflammatory reaction caused by the presence of a fracture and infection.[32,33] FDG-PET is therefore not suitable in acute/early-onset cases (ie, less than 1 month after surgical fracture treatment).[6] Hybrid camera systems such as PET/CT, PET/MRI, and WBC scintigraphy with single photon emission CT/CT have gained interest as they combine both anatomic and physiologic information, which may result in higher spatial resolution and better quantification possibilities.[32] Although recent studies show promising results for the use of nuclear imaging in the diagnostic workup of FRI, evidence is lacking to suggest that one imaging technique is superior to another.[7] Until more evidence becomes available, radiologic and nuclear imaging can be used for surgical planning and estimating the degree of fracture healing, but can only be seen as a suggestive sign in the diagnostic pathway for FRI.

Molecular Diagnostics

The evidence regarding molecular diagnostics remains scarce in the field of FRI. Polymerase chain reaction (PCR) testing and next-generation sequencing (NGS) have been investigated in the diagnosis of PJI, where they can serve as adjunctive tests, especially in case of culture-negative infections.[35,36] These techniques have the advantage that they can be fully automated and have the potential to detect bacteria despite antibiotic therapy.[37] The development of real-time PCR, compared with the earlier gel-based PCR, has contributed to a higher speed and lower susceptibility to cross-contamination because it is performed in a closed system.[6] Regarding the diagnosis of FRI, PCR performed on tissue or sonication fluid samples can be complementary to standard deep-tissue cultures.[25,38] However, results obtained with PCR testing should be interpreted with caution, as scientific evidence in the field of FRI is scarce and false-positive results from contaminants may be obtained because of high resolution and sensitivity.[21] Other disadvantages of the technique are the high equipment costs, the inability to distinguish live from dead bacteria, the inability to provide broad information about the susceptibility of the bacteria to antibiotics, and the difficulty in picking up polymicrobial infections.

NGS is another molecular technique with an even higher resolution than PCR testing. However, the role of this molecular method in the diagnosis of orthopaedic device–related infections is still unclear. A 2022 prospective cohort study suggested that NGS should not substitute for or complement conventional tissue culture in cases with low suspicion of FRI.[39] In contrast, in culture-negative PJI, NGS has been proven useful in the identification of causative organisms.[21,40,41] NGS can sequence all DNA present in a given sample, resulting in a more complete picture of the microbial genomes present.[21,42] Current applications of NGS show high specificities, a low turnaround time, and even the potential to characterize antimicrobial resistance.[42-44] Although NGS appears to be a promising addition to conventional sampling methods, the use of this molecular method for the diagnosis of FRI needs to be investigated further.[21,45]

Histopathology

Histopathologic assessment of bone encompasses the full scope of inflammatory infiltrates, ranging from inflammatory exudate composed of fibrin, polymorphonuclear leucocytes and macrophages, to a predominant plasma cell infiltration accompanied by bone marrow fibrosis.[46,47] The direct presence of microorganisms, typically colonizing necrotic bone and spreading within lacunae and canaliculi, can also be visualized using specific staining techniques for bacteria and fungi.[46,48,49]

For many years, the evidence for the use of histopathology in the diagnosis of FRI remained scarce and contradictory.[25,50,51] This can be attributed to the fact that polymorphonuclear leucocytes not only play a part in infection but they are also involved in the early phases of fracture healing, which makes this diagnostic technique theoretically less useful in acute cases. Three to 4 weeks after the fracture, the number of acute inflammatory cells related to the occurrence of a fracture decreases and higher counts may be more confidently associated with infection.[25]

Therefore, a 2018 study solely focused on surgically managed chronic/late-onset FRIs (ie, nonunions).[51] The histopathologic inflammatory response was assessed by mean polymorphonuclear neutrophil (PMN) count per high-power field (HPF) and compared with the established diagnosis. The use of a bimodal cutoff was found to have a high diagnostic value: the presence of more than five PMNs/HPF had a sensitivity of 80% and a specificity of 100%. To diagnose aseptic nonunion, a cutoff of 0 PMNs/HPF had a sensitivity of 85% and a specificity of 98%.[51] Based on this study, the histopathologic criterion of more than five PMNs/HPF was included in the consensus criteria, as a confirmatory sign of FRI.[6,52] Furthermore, the presence of microorganisms, as demonstrated by using specific staining techniques for bacteria (eg, Gram stain, Ziehl-Neelsen stain) or fungi (eg, Grocott methenamine silver stain), is considered to be pathognomonic for FRI and is therefore also included as a confirmatory criterion in the consensus definition of FRI[4,6] (Table 1).

SOCIOECONOMIC EFFECT

FRI has an important effect on patients and health care systems. Compared with surgical site infection in general, studies that solely focus on the socioeconomic effect of FRI are limited. Although a few studies investigated the socioeconomic consequences of infections related to fractures, most of them included heterogeneous patient cohorts, evaluated country-specific data, and primarily focused on direct hospital-related health care costs.[53-57] Nevertheless, studies suggest that FRI places a high burden on total health care expenditure, with length of stay as an important cost driver. Indirect costs arise as a secondary consequence of FRI treatment and are a relevant cost item, as health problems tend to have a negative effect on people's ability to work.[58]

Although earlier studies published that FRI results in a two- to fourfold increase in health care costs,[53,55] more recent data suggest a significantly higher cost.[54,58] A 2021 study compared direct hospital-related costs of infected and uninfected long bone fractures and found that FRI was correlated with an eightfold higher direct cost compared with uninfected long bone fractures.[58] In this study, the total health care costs were mainly driven by hospitalization costs, where FRI was associated with prolonged length of stay. Moreover, this study showed that FRI has an important negative effect on workplace absence and both short-term and long-term disability.

The indirect costs were approximately fourfold higher than that of noninfected patients.[58]

Although a negative effect on the patient's quality of life is obvious, published literature evaluating whether and to what extent FRI is associated with a decrement in this aspect is also limited.[55] Two studies from 2021 evaluated the effect of FRI on quality of life.[58,59] Regardless of the measurement instrument used (36-Item Short-Form, EuroQol 5-Dimension questionnaire, or Patient-Reported Outcome Measurement Information System physical function and pain interference scales), significantly poorer outcomes were obtained for patients who sustained FRI, even after a mean follow-up of up to 4.2 years.[58,59]

SUMMARY

The presence of at least one clinical or microbiologic confirmatory sign is associated with a high diagnostic performance and is pathognomonic for the presence of an FRI. Very rarely patients will present with only suggestive signs, and these cases should be discussed within a multidisciplinary team. If certain clinical signs are present such as wound drainage, local warmth, and redness, it is highly likely that an FRI is present, even in the absence of clinical confirmatory criteria. Treating physicians should avoid misdiagnosing these as superficial infections and should consider surgical débridement to attain adequate cultures for establishing the diagnosis and guiding antimicrobial treatment. Because FRI negatively affects a patients' quality of life, the ability to return to work, and overall health care costs, early diagnosis and adequate treatment are important.

KEY STUDY POINTS

- The presence of at least one clinical or microbiologic confirmatory sign is pathognomonic for an FRI.
- When patients present with redness, swelling, and wound drainage, the presence of an FRI should be strongly considered.
- Because targeted antimicrobial treatment is an important factor in the treatment of FRI, adequate sampling and culture techniques are important.
- Although radiologic and nuclear imaging techniques can be used for surgical planning and estimating the degree of fracture healing, they can only be seen as a suggestive sign of FRI.
- Because FRI has serious socioeconomic consequences, early diagnosis and adequate treatment are important.

ANNOTATED REFERENCES

1. GBD 2019 Fracture Collaborators, Wu AM, Bisignano C, et al: Global, regional, and national burden of bone fractures in 204 countries and territories, 1990-2019: A systematic analysis from the Global Burden of Disease Study 2019. *Lancet Healthy Longev* 2021;2(9):e580-e592.

   This study used the framework of the Global Burden of Diseases, Injuries, and Risk Factors Study (GBD) 2019 to assess the global incidence of fractures across the 21 GBD regions from 1990 to 2019. In 2019, an estimated 180 million new fractures have occurred worldwide.

2. Jennison T, Brinsden M: Fracture admission trends in England over a ten-year period. *Ann R Coll Surg Engl* 2019;101(3):208-214.

   This study analyzed fracture admissions in England over a 10-year period between 2004 and 2014. The risk of admission for fracture was 47.84 per 10,000 population; hip fractures accounted for 58% of hospital bed days, ankle fractures for 10% and femur fractures for 10%. Level of evidence: III.

3. Papakostidis C, Kanakaris NK, Pretel J, Faour O, Morell DJ, Giannoudis PV: Prevalence of complications of open tibial shaft fractures stratified as per the Gustilo-Anderson classification. *Injury* 2011;42(12):1408-1415.

4. Metsemakers WJ, Morgenstern M, McNally MA, et al: Fracture-related infection: A consensus on definition from an international expert group. *Injury* 2018;49(3):505-510.

   To enable the standardization and comparison of studies of FRI, an expert group developed a consensus definition for FRI. Two levels of certainty are defined for diagnostic criteria: confirmatory and suggestive. Level of evidence: V.

5. Sliepen J, Onsea J, Zalavras CG, et al: What is the diagnostic value of the Centers for Disease Control and Prevention criteria for surgical site infection in fracture-related infection? *Injury* 2021;52(10):2879-2885.

   This retrospective cohort study showed that, compared with the Centers for Disease Control and Prevention criteria for organ/space surgical site infection, most patients with suspected FRI can correctly be classified when applying the FRI consensus definition. Level of evidence: III.

6. Govaert GAM, Kuehl R, Atkins BL, et al: Diagnosing fracture-related infection: Current concepts and recommendations. *J Orthop Trauma* 2020;34(1):8-17.

   In this study, the available evidence is summarized and recommendations for the diagnosis of FRI are provided. An update to the initial FRI consensus definition is provided. Level of evidence: V.

7. Onsea J, Van Lieshout EMM, Zalavras C, et al: Validation of the diagnostic criteria of the consensus definition of fracture-related infection. *Injury* 2022;53(6):1867-1879.

   In this multicenter, retrospective cohort study, the diagnostic criteria of the consensus definition for FRI are validated. The presence of any confirmatory criterion can identify the most patients (97.5%) with an FRI. The presence of a single positive deep-tissue culture with a virulent pathogen should raise suspicion that an FRI may be present. Level of evidence: III.

8. Fang C, Wong TM, Lau TW, To KK, Wong SS, Leung F: Infection after fracture osteosynthesis – Part I. *J Orthop Surg (Hong Kong)* 2017;25(1):2309499017692712.

9. Bezstarosti H, Van Lieshout EMM, Voskamp LW, et al: Insights into treatment and outcome of fracture-related infection: A systematic literature review. *Arch Orthop Trauma Surg* 2019;139(1):61-72.

   In this systematic literature study, an overview of available diagnostic criteria, classifications, treatment protocols, and outcome measures for surgically treated patients with FRI is provided. Purulent drainage and wound dehiscence or wound breakdown are pathognomonic clinical signs for FRI.

10. Metsemakers WJ, Kortram K, Morgenstern M, et al: Definition of infection after fracture fixation: A systematic review of randomized controlled trials to evaluate current practice. *Injury* 2018;49(3):497-504.

    In this systematic literature study, different definitions, based on diagnostic criteria, used in scientific literature to describe infectious complications after fracture fixation are summarized. Purulent drainage and wound dehiscence or wound breakdown are pathognomonic clinical signs for FRI.

11. Morgenstern M, Kuehl R, Zalavras CG, et al: The influence of duration of infection on outcome of debridement and implant retention in fracture-related infection. *Bone Joint J* 2021;103-B(2):213-221.

    This systematic literature study shows that acute/early FRI, with a short duration of infection, can successfully be treated with implant retention. The limited available data suggest that chronic/late onset FRI treated with implant retention may be associated with a higher rate of recurrence. Successful outcome is dependent on managing all aspects of the infection. Thus, time from fracture fixation is not the only factor that should be considered in treatment planning of FRI

12. Brinker MR, Macek J, Laughlin M, Dunn WR: Utility of common biomarkers for diagnosing infection in nonunion. *J Orthop Trauma* 2021;35(3):121-127.

    In this cohort study of patients with nonunion, it was shown that common biomarkers such as WBC count, ESR, and CRP level were not significant predictors of infection. Level of evidence: II.

13. Stucken C, Olszewski DC, Creevy WR, Murakami AM, Tornetta P: Preoperative diagnosis of infection in patients with nonunions. *J Bone Joint Surg Am* 2013;95(15):1409-1412.

14. van den Kieboom J, Bosch P, Plate JDJ, et al: Diagnostic accuracy of serum inflammatory markers in late fracture-related infection: A systematic review and meta-analysis. *Bone Joint J* 2018;100-B(12):1542-1550.

    In this systematic literature review, the diagnostic value of CRP level, WBC count, and ESR in late FRI was evaluated. Based on the available evidence, and because these parameters also respond to conditions other than FRI, it seemed that CRP level, WBC count, and ESR are insufficiently accurate to diagnose late FRI. They may be used as suggestive signs in the diagnostic pathway of FRI. The sensitivity of CRP level ranged from 60% to 100% and the specificity from 34.3% to 85.7%. For WBC count, the sensitivity ranged between 22.9% and 72.6% and the specificity from 73.5% to 85.7%.

15. Neumaier M, Scherer MA: C-reactive protein levels for early detection of postoperative infection after fracture surgery in 787 patients. *Acta Orthop* 2008;79(3):428-432.

16. Sigmund IK, Dudareva M, Watts D, Morgenstern M, Athanasou NA, McNally MA: Limited diagnostic value of serum inflammatory biomarkers in the diagnosis of fracture-related infections. *Bone Joint J* 2020;102-B(7):904-911.

    In this cohort study of patients who underwent surgery for suspected septic nonunion after failed fracture fixation, the diagnostic value of preoperative CRP level and WBC count was evaluated. The sensitivity and specificity of CRP were 67% and 61%, respectively. For WBC count, a sensitivity of 17% and a specificity of 95% were found. Level of evidence: III.

17. Aichmair A, Frank BJ, Simon S, et al: Postoperative IL-6 levels cannot predict early onset periprosthetic hip/knee infections: An analysis of 7,661 patients at a single institution. *Eur Cell Mater* 2022;43:293-298.

    In this study comparing patients with and without early-onset PJI following total hip arthroplasty and total knee arthroplasty, there was no statistically significant difference in serum IL-6 levels on postoperative day 3. Level of evidence: III.

18. Sigmund IK, Puchner SE, Windhager R: Serum inflammatory biomarkers in the diagnosis of periprosthetic joint infections. *Biomedicines* 2021;9:1128.

    This study reviews the diagnostic value of established (serum CRP level, ESR, WBC count) and novel serum inflammatory markers (eg, fibrinogen, D-dimer, IL-6, procalcitonin, neutrophil percentage) for the preoperative diagnosis of PJI. Serum parameters in general have insufficient accuracy for diagnosing PJI because of a lack of specificity.

19. Stevenson MC, Slater JC, Sagi HC, Palacio Bedoya F, Powers-Fletcher MV: Diagnosing fracture-related infections: Where are we now? *J Clin Microbiol* 2022;60(2):e0280720.

    This review summarizes available evidence regarding diagnostic tests for FRI. There currently is no support for the use of IL-6, D-dimer, procalcitonin, or fibrinogen in the diagnosis of FRI, and in some cases, such as for IL-6, these biomarkers are inferior to common biomarkers such as CRP level.

20. Wang S, Yin P, Quan C, et al: Evaluating the use of serum inflammatory markers for preoperative diagnosis of infection in patients with nonunions. *Biomed Res Int* 2017;2017:9146317.

21. Depypere M, Morgenstern M, Kuehl R, et al: Pathogenesis and management of fracture-related infection. *Clin Microbiol Infect* 2020;26(5):572-578.

    This review summarizes the evidence regarding the pathogenesis of FRI and provides current practice guidelines for the management of FRI. To optimize targeted antimicrobial treatment, sampling and culture techniques should be performed meticulously.

22. Dudareva M, Barrett L, Figtree M, et al: Sonication versus tissue sampling for diagnosis of prosthetic joint and other orthopedic device-related infections. *J Clin Microbiol* 2018;56(12):e00688-18.

   This study compares the performance of paired tissue and sonication cultures. Tissue culture was more sensitive than sonication for both PJI and FRI (69% versus 57%). The combined sensitivity of tissue and sonication fluid culture was 76% and increased with the number of tissue specimens obtained, indicating that sonication fluid samples can be used as an adjunct to standard deep-tissue cultures. A minimum of five deep-tissue cultures should be obtained. Level of evidence: III.

23. Hellebrekers P, Rentenaar RJ, McNally MA, et al: Getting it right first time: The importance of a structured tissue sampling protocol for diagnosing fracture-related infections. *Injury* 2019;50(10):1649-1655.

   This study shows that the use of a structured sampling protocol is superior to an ad hoc approach, resulting in more microbiologically confirmed infections and more certainty regarding the causative pathogens. The protocol included the cessation of antibiotic therapy at least 2 weeks before sampling, the use of clean instruments to obtain tissue samples, and the retrieval of at least five deep-tissue cultures.

24. Dudareva M, Barrett LK, Morgenstern M, Atkins BL, Brent AJ, McNally MA: Providing an evidence base for tissue sampling and culture interpretation in suspected fracture-related infection. *J Bone Joint Surg Am* 2021;103(11):977-983.

   This study evaluated the accuracy of different numbers of specimens and diagnostic cutoffs for microbiologic testing of deep-tissue specimens in patients undergoing surgical treatment for suspected FRI. The culture yield can be optimized by increasing the number of samples. It is recommended to analyze at least five deep-tissue samples in patients with suspected FRI. Level of evidence: III.

25. Onsea J, Depypere M, Govaert G, et al: Accuracy of tissue and sonication fluid sampling for the diagnosis of fracture-related infection: A systematic review and critical appraisal. *J Bone Jt Infect* 2018;3(4):173-181.

   This systematic literature review reports the evidence regarding the use of different diagnostic tests, including tissue and sonication fluid culture, molecular diagnostics, and histopathology. Swab cultures are contraindicated for the diagnosis of FRI because of their low sensitivity and high risk of contamination.

26. Schlung JE, Bastrom TP, Roocroft JH, Newton PO, Mubarak SJ, Upasani VV: Femoral neck aspiration aids in the diagnosis of osteomyelitis in children with septic hip. *J Pediatr Orthop* 2018;38(10):532-536.

   This retrospective study showed that femoral aspiration can aid in the diagnosis of osteomyelitis in children in whom septic arthritis was already diagnosed. This was especially the case in patients with false-negative MRI findings for osteomyelitis. Level of evidence: III.

27. Pupaibool J, Vasoo S, Erwin PJ, Murad MH, Berbari EF: The utility of image-guided percutaneous needle aspiration biopsy for the diagnosis of spontaneous vertebral osteomyelitis: A systematic review and meta-analysis. *Spine J* 2015;15(1):122-131.

28. Rothenberg AC, Wilson AE, Hayes JP, O'Malley MJ, Klatt BA: Sonication of arthroplasty implants improves accuracy of periprosthetic joint infection cultures. *Clin Orthop Relat Res* 2017;475(7):1827-1836.

29. Trampuz A, Piper KE, Jacobson MJ, et al: Sonication of removed hip and knee prostheses for diagnosis of infection. *N Engl J Med* 2007;357(7):654-663.

30. Bellova P, Knop-Hammad V, Konigshausen M, Schildhauer TA, Gessmann J, Baecker H: Sonication in the diagnosis of fracture-related infections (FRI)-a retrospective study on 230 retrieved implants. *J Orthop Surg Res* 2021;16(1):310.

   This study assessed the diagnostic performance of the inoculation of sonication fluid into blood culture bottles. This technique increases sensitivity but does not allow colony-forming unit counting in contrast to standard sonication fluid culture. Level of evidence: III.

31. Finelli CA, da Silva CB, Murca MA, et al: Microbiological diagnosis of intramedullary nailing infection: Comparison of bacterial growth between tissue sampling and sonication fluid cultures. *Int Orthop* 2021;45(3):565-573.

   This study evaluated the accuracy of sonication fluid cultures in patients suspected with FRI after intramedullary nailing. The results of this study suggest that sonication fluid cultures offer no additional benefit over tissue cultures for the microbiologic diagnosis of FRI after intramedullary nailing. Level of evidence: II.

32. Zhang Q, Dong J, Shen Y, Yun C, Zhou D, Liu F: Comparative diagnostic accuracy of respective nuclear imaging for suspected fracture-related infection: A systematic review and Bayesian network meta-analysis. *Arch Orthop Trauma Surg* 2021;141(7):1115-1130.

   This systematic literature review compares the accuracy of available nuclear imaging modalities in the diagnosis of FRI. WBC scintigraphy, FDG-PET/CT, and PET nuclear imaging all present good satisfactory accuracy for the diagnosis of FRI.

33. Bosch P, Glaudemans AWJM, de Vries JPPM, et al: Nuclear imaging for diagnosing fracture-related infection. *Clin Transl Imaging* 2020;8:289-298.

   This systematic literature review outlines the evidence for the use of nuclear imaging techniques to diagnose FRI. Findings were based on retrospective studies. FDG-PET/CT was associated with an accuracy of 0.83 and WBC scintigraphy with single photon emission CT/CT with an accuracy of 0.92.

34. Govaert GAM, Bosch P, IJpma FFA, et al: High diagnostic accuracy of white blood cell scintigraphy for fracture related infections: Results of a large retrospective single-center study. *Injury* 2018;49(6):1085-1090.

   The accuracy of WBC scintigraphy was evaluated in this retrospective cohort study. A sensitivity and specificity of 79% and 97% were found, respectively. A diagnostic accuracy of

0.92 was found for detecting FRIs in the peripheral skeleton. Level of evidence: III.

35. Saeed K, Ahmad-Saeed N: The impact of PCR in the management of prosthetic joint infections. *Expert Rev Mol Diagn* 2015;15(7):957-964.

36. Qu X, Zhai Z, Li H, et al: PCR-based diagnosis of prosthetic joint infection. *J Clin Microbiol* 2013;51(8):2742-2746.

37. Hischebeth GT, Randau TM, Buhr JK, et al: Unyvero i60 implant and tissue infection (ITI) multiplex PCR system in diagnosing periprosthetic joint infection. *J Microbiol Methods* 2016;121:27-32.

38. Morgenstern M, Kühl R, Eckardt H, et al: Diagnostic challenges and future perspectives in fracture-related infection. *Injury* 2018;49(suppl 1):S83-S90.

    This review describes the current diagnostic modalities and an interdisciplinary diagnostic algorithm based on the publication of the consensus definition for FRI in 2018. Future diagnostic techniques, including PCR and NGS, are also discussed.

39. Natoli RM, Marinos DP, Montalvo RN, et al: Poor agreement between next-generation DNA sequencing and bacterial cultures in orthopaedic trauma procedures. *J Bone Joint Surg Am* 2022;104(6):497-503.

    This prospective cohort study investigated the potential use of NGS in the diagnosis of FRI. In this study, NGS identified bacterial presence more frequently than culture, but only with slight agreement between both modalities. Based on these results, the authors conclude that NGS should not substitute for or complement conventional cultures in patients with a low suspicion for FRI. Level of evidence: II.

40. Street TL, Sanderson ND, Atkins BL, et al: Molecular diagnosis of orthopedic-device-related infection directly from sonication fluid by metagenomic sequencing. *J Clin Microbiol* 2017;55(8):2334-2347.

41. Tarabichi M, Shohat N, Goswami K, et al: Diagnosis of periprosthetic joint infection: The potential of next-generation sequencing. *J Bone Joint Surg Am* 2018;100(2):147-154.

    The findings from this prospective study suggest that some cases of monomicrobial PJI may have additional organisms escaping detection when culture is used. In these cases, NGS may be a useful adjunct. Level of evidence: I.

42. Indelli PF, Ghirardelli S, Violante B, Amanatullah DF: Next generation sequencing for pathogen detection in periprosthetic joint infections. *EFORT Open Rev* 2021;6(4):236-244.

    This review summarizes current evidence for the use of NGS techniques for the diagnosis of PJI. Because NGS can sequence all DNA present in a sample, a more complete picture of the microbial genomes present is obtained. Current applications show high specificities, low turnaround times, and even the potential to detect antimicrobial resistance.

43. Petersen LM, Martin IW, Moschetti WE, Kershaw CM, Tsongalis GJ: Third-generation sequencing in the clinical laboratory: Exploring the advantages and challenges of nanopore sequencing. *J Clin Microbiol* 2019;58(1):e01315-19.

    This review highlights the general challenges of pathogen detection in clinical samples by metagenomic sequences, the properties of the Oxford Nanopore Technologies platform, and how research supports the potential future use of nanopore sequencing in the diagnosis of infectious diseases.

44. Wang C, Huang Z, Li W, Fang X, Zhang W: Can metagenomic next-generation sequencing identify the pathogens responsible for culture-negative prosthetic joint infection? *BMC Infect Dis* 2020;20(1):253.

    This study found that metagenomic NGS is a reliable tool for the identification of pathogens related to culture-negative PJI, which can therefore also attribute to the treatment of culture-negative PJI by adjusting antibiotic treatment to the NGS results. Level of evidence: III.

45. Goswami K, Tipton C, Clarkson S, et al: Fracture-associated microbiome and persistent nonunion: Next-generation sequencing reveals new findings. *J Orthop Trauma* 2022;36(suppl 2):S40-S46.

    In this prospective, multicenter study, the application of NGS pathogen detection to diagnose infected nonunion was investigated. It is suggested that the fracture-associated microbiome may be a significant risk factor for persistent nonunion. Level of evidence: II.

46. Bruder E, Jundt G, Eyrich G: Pathology of osteomyelitis, in Baltensperger MM, Eyrich GKH, eds: *Osteomyelitis of the Jaws*. Springer, 2009, pp 121-133.

47. Tiemann A, Hofmann GO, Krukemeyer MG, Krenn V, Langwald S: Histopathological Osteomyelitis Evaluation Score (HOES) – An innovative approach to histopathological diagnostics and scoring of osteomyelitis. *GMS Interdiscip Plast Reconstr Surg DGPW* 2014;3:Doc08.

48. de Mesy Bentley KL, MacDonald A, Schwarz EM, Oh I: Chronic osteomyelitis with Staphylococcus aureus deformation in submicron canaliculi of osteocytes: A case report. *JBJS Case Connect* 2018;8(1):e8.

    This study presents a case report of a patient with an infected diagnostic foot ulcer and *S aureus* chronic osteomyelitis. Using transmission electron microscopy, the deformation of *S aureus* in the submicron osteocytic-canalicular networks of amputated bone tissue was demonstrated. The invasion of the osteocytic-canalicular system in human bone is a new mechanism of infection persistence in chronic osteomyelitis. Level of evidence: IV.

49. de Mesy Bentley KL, Trombetta R, Nishitani K, et al: Evidence of Staphylococcus aureus deformation, proliferation, and migration in canaliculi of live cortical bone in murine models of osteomyelitis. *J Bone Miner Res* 2017;32(5):985-990.

50. Egol KA, Karunakar MA, Marroum MC, Sims SH, Kellam JF, Bosse MJ: Detection of indolent infection at the time of revision fracture surgery. *J Trauma* 2002;52(6):1198-1201.

51. Morgenstern M, Athanasou NA, Ferguson JY, Metsemakers WJ, Atkins BL, McNally MA: The value of quantitative histology in the diagnosis of fracture-related infection. *Bone Joint J* 2018;100-B(7):966-972.

The role of quantitative histopathologic analysis in the diagnosis of FRI was evaluated in a prospective study including 156 surgically treated nonunions. A bimodal cutoff was presented for the histopathologic diagnosis of FRI. The presence of more than five PMNs is confirmatory for FRI (positive predictive value of 100%), whereas the complete absence of PMNs is almost always indicative of aseptic nonunion (positive predictive value of 98%). Level of evidence: III.

52. McNally M, Govaert G, Dudareva M, et al: Definition and diagnosis of fracture-related infection. *EFORT Open Rev* 2020;5:614-619.

The advances that have been made in recent years toward establishing good diagnostic pathways with validated investigations including histopathology, microbiology, and imaging techniques are summarized in this literature review.

53. Thakore RV, Greenberg SE, Shi H, et al: Surgical site infection in orthopedic trauma: A case-control study evaluating risk factors and cost. *J Clin Orthop Trauma* 2015;6(4):220-226.

54. Metsemakers WJ, Smeets B, Nijs S, Hoekstra H: Infection after fracture fixation of the tibia: Analysis of healthcare utilization and related costs. *Injury* 2017;48(6):1204-1210.

55. Parker B, Petrou S, Masters JPM, Achana F, Costa ML: Economic outcomes associated with deep surgical site infection in patients with an open fracture of the lower limb. *Bone Joint J* 2018;100-B(11):1506-1510.

This study aimed at identifying economic outcomes associated with infectious complications after open fractures of the lower limb. Significantly impaired health-related quality of life and increased economic costs are associated with infectious complications after an open fracture of the lower limb. Level of evidence: III.

56. Ziegler P, Schlemer D, Flesch I, et al: Quality of life and clinical-radiological long-term results after implant-associated infections in patients with ankle fracture: A retrospective matched-pair study. *J Orthop Surg Res* 2017;12(1):114.

57. Hoekstra H, Smeets B, Metsemakers WJ, Spitz AC, Nijs S: Economics of open tibial fractures: The pivotal role of length-of-stay and infection. *Health Econ Rev* 2017;7(1):32.

58. Iliaens J, Onsea J, Hoekstra H, Nijs S, Peetermans WE, Metsemakers WJ: Fracture-related infection in long bone fractures: A comprehensive analysis of the economic impact and influence on quality of life. *Injury* 2021;52(11):3344-3349.

Direct and indirect health care costs related to long bone fractures in patients with and without FRI were compared as well as the effect of FRI on the patient's quality of life. Direct health care costs are eight times that of non-FRI long bone fractures. FRI is also significantly associated with poorer outcomes on physical function and pain interference Patient-Reported Outcome Measurement Information System scales. Level of evidence: III.

59. Walter N, Rupp M, Hierl K, et al: Long-term patient-related quality of life after fracture-related infections of the long bones. *Bone Joint Res* 2021;10(5):321-327.

The long-term effect of FRI on patients' physical health and psychologic well-being was assessed in patients who were successfully treated for long bone FRI using EuroQol 5-Dimension questionnaire and 36-Item Short-Form 36 outcome measurements. Even after a mean follow-up of 4.2 years after eradication of infection, patients report significantly lower quality of life compared with patients in whom this complication did not develop. Level of evidence: III.

CHAPTER 20

Prevention of Infection in Open Fractures

MICHAEL J. PATZAKIS, MD, FAAOS
CHARALAMPOS G. ZALAVRAS, MD, PHD, FAAOS, FACS

ABSTRACT

Patients with open fractures should be evaluated for associated potentially life-threatening, injuries. Systemic antibiotic therapy should be initiated on patient presentation and local antibiotic delivery added in severe injuries. The extent of contamination, soft-tissue damage, and bone injury should be determined intraoperatively to classify the open fracture correctly. Thorough débridement with removal of all devitalized tissue and foreign bodies is essential for prevention of infection. Definitive or provisional stable fixation of the open fracture should be achieved. The timing and technique of fixation depend on bone, soft-tissue, and patient characteristics, and on surgeon's expertise. Primary wound closure is an option for less-severe injuries if only healthy, viable tissue is present in the wound after thorough débridement. Delayed closure with a second-look débridement after 48 hours is recommended for more severe injuries. At that time, the wound can be closed if possible. In extensive soft-tissue injuries, reconstruction with a local or free flap may be necessary. Principle-based management of open fractures will help achieve the goals of infection prevention, fracture union, and restoration of function of the injured extremity.

Keywords: antibiotics; débridement; infection; open fracture

Neither of the following authors nor any immediate family member has received anything of value from or has stock or stock options held in a commercial company or institution related directly or indirectly to the subject of this chapter: Dr. Patzakis and Dr. Zalavras.

INTRODUCTION

Open fractures are especially problematic because of exposure of the fracture site to the outside environment. The healing potential and the host response to contaminating microorganisms are compromised because of the soft-tissue and bone injury. Therefore, open fractures are associated with an increased risk for infection and nonunion, are a challenging problem to both patient and treating physician, and require a principle-based approach to improve prognosis.

The principles of management of open fracture consist of detailed patient and injury evaluation, early administration of systemic antibiotics that can be supplemented by local delivery, thorough débridement and irrigation, fracture stabilization, and wound management that may require flap coverage in severe injuries. Management based on these principles will help achieve the goals of infection prevention, fracture union, and restoration of function.

ASSESSMENT

Patient and Injury Evaluation

Open fractures are defined by the presence of an associated soft-tissue injury that results in communication of the fracture site with the outside environment and contamination of the fracture site[1] and are often the result of high-energy trauma, especially in younger men.[2] Therefore, thorough assessment of every patient with an open fracture should be undertaken to identify other associated injuries (eg, thoracic or abdominal) that may even be life threatening. Evaluation of the injured extremity should include a careful neurovascular examination and assessment of the size, location, and contamination of the wound. Compartment syndrome may still complicate an open fracture, especially in crush injuries, despite the presence of the wound. Fracture characteristics, such as articular involvement and comminution, should be evaluated by radiographs and other imaging studies, as appropriate, to plan fracture fixation.

Open Fracture Classification

Depending on the mechanism of injury, great variability exists on the severity of open fractures, which has implications for both management and prognosis. The Gustilo-Anderson classification system,[3] subsequently modified 1 decade later,[4] has been extensively used and is detailed in **Table 1**.

The severity of the open fracture, as determined by using the Gustilo-Anderson classification, is associated with the risk of infection. In a series of more than 1,100 patients, the infection rate was 1.4% (7 of 497 patients) in type I, 3.6% (25 of 695 patients) in type II, and 22.7% (45 of 198 patients) in type III open fractures.[5]

The reliability of the Gustilo-Anderson classification may be suboptimal, with 60% mean agreement among surgeons asked to classify open fractures of the tibia on the basis of videotaped case presentations.[6] The Orthopaedic Trauma Association classification system evaluates skin, muscle, and arterial injury; bone loss; and contamination to determine the severity of open fractures.[7] The mean interobserver agreement was 86% overall, but interobserver reliability on muscle injury and contamination was moderate.[8] It is important to remember that optimal assessment of the extent and severity of injury and degree of contamination can only be performed in the operating room after wound exploration and débridement.

INITIAL MANAGEMENT

On presentation to the emergency department, the patient should be appropriately resuscitated and other serious or even life-threatening injuries should be managed as necessary according to advanced trauma life support protocols.

Patient, extremity, wound, and fracture assessment are undertaken as outlined previously. The wound is irrigated, gross contamination is removed, and a sterile dressing is applied. The fractured extremity should be grossly realigned and immobilized with a splint. Intravenous antibiotic therapy should be started and tetanus prophylaxis should be given depending on the patient's immunization status.

ANTIBIOTICS

Systemic Antibiotic Administration

Antibiotic administration should be started as soon as is feasible on patient presentation in the emergency department.[5,9]

The necessity of antibiotic administration in patients with open fractures was established. In a landmark study that was the first in the world to use cephalosporin in the management of open fractures.[10] This study reported a significantly decreased infection rate of 2.3% (2 of 84 fractures) when cephalothin, a first-generation cephalosporin, was administered compared with 13.9% (11 of 79 fractures) in the group not receiving antibiotics and 9.7% (9 of 92 fractures) in the group receiving penicillin and streptomycin.[10] A first-generation cephalosporin (cefazolin) is still the mainstay of antibiotic recommendations in open fractures.

A combination of gram-positive coverage (eg, a first-generation cephalosporin, such as cefazolin) and gram-negative coverage (eg, an aminoglycoside, such as gentamicin) is widely accepted for severe (type III) open fractures,[11-14] whereas gram-positive coverage only has been recommended for less severe (type I and II) open fractures.[12-14] However, a type IIIA open fracture with a small wound may be misclassified in the emergency department as type I or II open fracture and broad-spectrum coverage may not be initiated until much later.

Table 1

Gustilo-Anderson Classification System of Open Fractures

Type	Description
Type I	Wound of 1 cm or less, with minimal contamination or muscle crushing
Type II	Wound more than 1 cm long with moderate soft-tissue damage and crushing. Bone coverage is adequate and comminution is minimal.
Type IIIA	Extensive soft-tissue damage, often due to a high-energy injury with a crushing component. Massively contaminated wounds and severely comminuted or segmental fractures are included in this subtype. Bone coverage is adequate.
Type IIIB	Extensive soft-tissue damage with periosteal stripping and bone exposure, usually with severe contamination and bone comminution. Flap coverage is required.
Type IIIC	Arterial injury requiring repair

Data from Gustilo RB, Anderson JT: Prevention of infection in the treatment of one thousand and twenty-five open fractures of long bones: Retrospective and prospective analyses. *J Bone Joint Surg Am* 1976;58(4):453-458 and Gustilo RB, Mendoza RM, Williams DN: Problems in the management of type III (severe) open fractures: A new classification of type III open fractures. *J Trauma* 1984;24(8):742-746.

Systemic administration of vancomycin has not been recommended based on the potential for emergence of glycopeptide-resistant organisms.[14] A randomized controlled trial compared administration of a combination of vancomycin and cefazolin with administration of only cefazolin and reported no difference in the infection rates of methicillin-resistant *Staphylococcus aureus* between the two groups.[15] Anaerobic coverage (eg, penicillin, clindamycin, or metronidazole) is recommended in severe injuries with extensive contamination or potential contamination with clostridial organisms (eg, agricultural injuries).[11,14,16]

Open wound cultures are not useful in selecting the optimal antibiotic regimen. These culture results are obtained with a delay of days, and in most cases, fail to identify the pathogen causing a subsequent infection because such infections are often caused by nosocomial organisms.[17]

The recommended duration of antibiotic therapy is 72 hours, which in type I and II open fractures can be shortened to 24 hours after wound closure.[12] Prolonged duration of antibiotic therapy beyond 72 hours does not appear to be beneficial in the prevention of infection[18,19] and may even increase the infection rate, especially in mildly contaminated fractures.[18,20] However, an analysis from 2020 reported that severely contaminated fractures may benefit from antibiotic duration beyond 72 hours.[20]

A systematic review from 2022 reported that the evidence on antibiotic selection and duration is limited and further studies are needed to determine the optimal regimen.[19] Such studies should have a follow-up period longer than 90 days: a retrospective study from 2022 reported that a follow-up period of less than 90 days captures only 64% of fracture-related infections in open fractures.[21] However, it is critical to remember that even optimal antibiotic therapy is not a substitute for thorough surgical débridement.

Local Antibiotic Delivery

Local antibiotic administration via antibiotic-impregnated delivery vehicles has been used in addition to systemic antibiotic administration. Polymethyl methacrylate (PMMA) cement is a widely used delivery vehicle that can be molded to create beads of 5- to 10-mm diameter or spacer blocks of larger size. Antibiotics that are heat stable and available in powder form, such as aminoglycosides and vancomycin, can be incorporated into PMMA cement for local delivery.[22]

Elution, which is the process of release of antibiotics from the delivery vehicle to the surrounding tissues, is determined by the antibiotic concentration gradient between the antibiotic delivery system and its environment. A fluid medium is necessary for elution. Following insertion of antibiotic-impregnated PMMA beads, the open fracture wound should be sealed by a semipermeable barrier, to maintain the eluted antibiotics at the wound site and achieve a high local concentration. The antibiotic bead pouch technique achieves a high local concentration of antibiotics without a high systemic concentration, thereby maximizing efficacy at the injury site and minimizing toxicity.[23] Sealing of the wound from the external environment by the semipermeable barrier also prevents secondary contamination by nosocomial pathogens and establishes an aerobic wound environment.

The antibiotic bead pouch technique has been shown to reduce the infection rate when used in addition to systemic antibiotics for management of severe open fractures.[24,25] A retrospective study of 1,085 open fractures compared the use of systemic antibiotics with combined treatment with the use of both systemic antibiotics and the bead pouch technique and reported a significant reduction of infection from 20.6% (21 of 102) to 6.5% (22 of 340) in type III open fractures when the bead pouch technique was used.[24] A systematic review from 2018 showed a significantly lower infection rate when local antibiotics were used in addition to standard systemic antibiotics (4.6% [91 of 1986] versus 16.5% [124 of 752]).[25]

Alternatives to antibiotic-impregnated PMMA beads include bioabsorbable delivery vehicles such as calcium sulfate[26] and intrawound antibiotic powder.[27] A 2021 randomized controlled trial examined the effect of intrawound vancomycin powder in 980 patients with tibial plateau or pilon fractures at high risk for infection. In 191 patients with open fractures, the deep infection rate was 12.7% in the treatment group and 19.3% in the control group ($P = 0.23$).[27] Further research on intrawound antibiotics is warranted to clarify their effect on infection, especially when gram-negative coverage is provided.

DÉBRIDEMENT AND IRRIGATION

Technique

Débridement consists of the removal of foreign bodies and nonviable bone and soft tissues from the open fracture wound. Thorough surgical débridement is critical in the management of open fractures because devitalized tissue and foreign material promote the growth of microorganisms and development of biofilm.

When the open fracture wound is insufficient for detailed evaluation of the injury, surgical extension of the wound is required and should be performed in a way that respects the vascularity of soft tissues and facilitates fracture fixation and any anticipated reconstruction procedures. A retrospective study from 2018 reported that if the location of a small traumatic wound is such that an incision incorporating the wound would not facilitate subsequent procedures, a surgical approach to the fracture can be established without incorporating the traumatic wound and the open fracture can be débrided through this approach.[28] Débridement should be performed in a systematic and atraumatic manner while protecting adjacent neurovascular structures. Bone fragments should be left in place only if they have soft-tissue attachments, indicating vascularity of the fragments. Free fragments are avascular and should be removed, with the exception of articular fragments that are large enough to be useful in reconstruction of the involved joint.

Irrigation of the open fracture wound following débridement may further mechanically remove small foreign bodies and reduce bacterial concentration. A randomized controlled trial compared the effects of different irrigation solutions (castile soap versus normal saline) and irrigation pressures (high-pressure versus low-pressure versus very-low-pressure pulsatile lavage) on the reoperation rate in patients with open fractures.[29] The rates of reoperation were similar regardless of irrigation pressure, indicating that very low pressure is an acceptable, low-cost alternative for open fractures irrigation. The reoperation rate was lower in the saline group compared with the soap group.[29]

Timing

Concerns that delays in surgical management beyond 6 hours would lead to increased infection rates have not been substantiated in most of the literature.[5,30-32] In 307 patients with severe open lower extremity fractures, the infection rates were 28%, 29%, and 26% in patients who underwent débridement earlier than 5 hours, at 5 to 10 hours, and at more than 10 hours after injury, respectively.[30] A secondary analysis from 2021 of 2,286 patients with open fractures enrolled in a randomized controlled trial found that, when accounting for other variables, débridement and irrigation performed beyond 6 hours after injury did not independently increase the risk of revision surgery.[32] However, a 2021 meta-analysis reported a progressive increase in the risk of infection in type III open fractures with increased time, especially with delays of more than 24 hours.[33] Although bacterial populations in an untreated contaminated wound increase over time, it appears that early antibiotic administration and thorough surgical débridement can effectively reduce the contamination present. As a result, small delays in surgical treatment do not appear to translate to increased infection rates and may allow for stabilization and resuscitation of the patient, as well as for treatment of the patient by experienced surgical teams with all necessary equipment available.

FRACTURE FIXATION

Stabilization of the open fracture with restoration of length, alignment, and rotation is an important part of management. Stability at the fracture site prevents further injury to the soft tissues, enhances the host response to contaminating organisms, facilitates wound and patient care, and allows early motion of the extremity. Fracture stabilization can be definitive or provisional and can be accomplished with intramedullary nailing, plate-and-screw fixation, or external fixation. Selection among these options depends on careful evaluation of fracture, soft-tissue, and patient characteristics. More than one method may be applicable to a specific injury and surgeon expertise and implant availability should also be accounted for.

Intramedullary nailing is an effective method of stabilization of diaphyseal fractures of the lower extremity.[34,35] Statically interlocked intramedullary nailing maintains length and alignment of the fracture bone, is biomechanically superior to other methods, and does not interfere with soft-tissue management. An animal study demonstrated an adverse effect of reaming on endosteal perfusion; however, callus perfusion and early strength of union were similar following intramedullary nailing with or without reaming.[36]

Plate-and-screw fixation is useful for open diaphyseal fractures of the upper extremity and for periarticular fractures to allow anatomic reduction and restoration of joint congruency.

External fixation can be applied in a technically easy and expedient way with minimal blood loss and is beneficial in situations of damage control, such as with type IIIC open fractures and unstable polytrauma patients.[37] External fixation is also useful as a provisional joint-spanning fixation in open periarticular fractures to be followed by definitive fixation at a second stage.[38]

SOFT-TISSUE MANAGEMENT

Primary Wound Closure

Primary wound closure had not been advocated for open fractures because it had been associated with wound infections, including the catastrophic complication of gas gangrene. However, clinical studies comparing primary with delayed closure have not shown increased infection rates following primary closure.[5,39]

Primary closure of carefully selected open fracture wounds may prevent secondary contamination and reduce surgical morbidity and is a viable option if: (1) there is no severe soft-tissue injury and contamination,

(2) early administration of antibiotics has occurred, (3) a thorough débridement has been performed, and (4) the wound edges can be approximated without tension. If there is any doubt about the viability of the tissues or the adequacy of the débridement, the open fracture wound should not be closed primarily and a second-look débridement should be performed. The surgical extension of the wound created to facilitate débridement can be closed primarily, leaving only the injury wound open.

Delayed Wound Closure

Delayed wound closure prevents an anaerobic environment in the wound and allows viable but compromised tissues to declare themselves and, if found to be nonviable, to be débrided at a subsequent procedure (second-look débridement). However, this additional procedure results in increased hospital stay and cost. Delayed wound closure is preferable in severe injuries with extensive soft-tissue damage and contamination, in patients presenting with a considerable delay, and in wounds that cannot be closed without tension.

When the planned treatment of an open fracture wound is delayed closure, or when closure is not possible and flap coverage is required, the wound should not be left exposed to the outside environment. Instead, the antibiotic bead pouch technique[22,24] or negative pressure wound therapy (NPWT)[40] should be used to seal the wound and avoid contamination with nosocomial pathogens.

The literature does not show a clear association of NPWT with specific outcomes in patients with open fractures. A randomized controlled trial reported a significant reduction in infection rates in patients with severe open fractures of the tibia when NPWT was used instead of wet-to-dry dressings (5.4% versus 28%).[40] Similarly, a systematic review from 2020 reported that NPWT decreased the likelihood of deep infection compared with conventional dressings.[41] However, a randomized controlled trial from 2018 found no difference in patient disability, quality of life, surgical site infections, or other complications at any point in the 12 months after surgery when NPWT was used.[42] Further, a secondary analysis of data from the Fluid Lavage of Open Wounds randomized controlled trial reported in 2022 that NPWT increased the likelihood of deep infection by 4.5 times.[43] These conflicting results may be because of several reasons: confounding patient and injury factors that were unaccounted for, variability in the dressing used in the control groups, and variability in the duration of NPWT. It should be emphasized that in severe injuries, NPWT is only a temporizing measure that will not eliminate the need for flap coverage when bone and/or implants are exposed.

Soft-Tissue Reconstruction

Soft-tissue reconstruction is required when extensive soft-tissue injury precludes delayed wound closure and adequate bone coverage (type IIIB open fractures). A well-vascularized soft-tissue envelope enhances fracture healing, facilitates antibiotic delivery, and by covering the exposed anatomic structures prevents secondary contamination. Soft-tissue reconstruction is usually achieved with local or free flaps depending on the location and size of the soft-tissue defect.[44,45] A microvascular surgeon is an essential member of the multidisciplinary team treating a patient with an open fracture with extensive soft-tissue damage.

Soft-tissue reconstruction should be performed as early as is feasible, preferably within the first 5 to 7 days from injury because delays in soft-tissue coverage have been associated with increased rates of infection and flap complications.[9,46] However, delay to coverage in published studies may have been a result of a greater degree of soft-tissue injury and contamination (requiring further débridement procedures and increasing the infection risk) or because of the critical condition of the patient, therefore outside the control of the treating surgeon.[9]

SUMMARY

Open fractures are associated with increased risk for infection, which can be reduced by following the principles of detailed patient assessment and resuscitation as needed, careful extremity evaluation and classification of the open fracture, systemic antibiotic therapy that may be supplemented with local antibiotic delivery, thorough débridement with removal of all foreign material and devitalized tissue, stabilization of the open fracture, and finally, wound management to achieve fracture coverage with viable soft tissue.

KEY STUDY POINTS

- Open fractures are associated with increased risk for infection, which can be reduced by using principle-based management.
- Open fractures should be classified intraoperatively and not in the emergency department.
- Early administration of antibiotics reduces the infection rate.
- Thorough débridement is critical to treatment.
- The open fracture wound may be closed primarily in the absence of severe contamination and soft-tissue damage. If the wound is not closed primarily, it should be sealed with the bead pouch technique or NPWT dressing.

ANNOTATED REFERENCES

1. Zalavras CG, Patzakis MJ: Open fractures: Evaluation and management. *J Am Acad Orthop Surg* 2003;11(3):212-219.

2. Court-Brown CM, Bugler KE, Clement ND, Duckworth AD, McQueen MM: The epidemiology of open fractures in adults. A 15-year review. *Injury* 2012;43(6):891-897.

3. Gustilo RB, Anderson JT: Prevention of infection in the treatment of one thousand and twenty-five open fractures of long bones: Retrospective and prospective analyses. *J Bone Joint Surg Am* 1976;58(4):453-458.

4. Gustilo RB, Mendoza RM, Williams DN: Problems in the management of type III (severe) open fractures: A new classification of type III open fractures. *J Trauma* 1984;24(8):742-746.

5. Patzakis MJ, Wilkins J: Factors influencing infection rate in open fracture wounds. *Clin Orthop Relat Res* 1989;243:36-40.

6. Brumback RJ, Jones AL: Interobserver agreement in the classification of open fractures of the tibia. The results of a survey of two hundred and forty-five orthopaedic surgeons. *J Bone Joint Surg Am* 1994;76(8):1162-1166.

7. Orthopaedic Trauma Association: Open Fracture Study Group: A new classification scheme for open fractures. *J Orthop Trauma* 2010;24(8):457-464.

8. Agel J, Evans AR, Marsh JL, et al: The OTA open fracture classification: A study of reliability and agreement. *J Orthop Trauma* 2013;27(7):379-384.

9. Lack WD, Karunakar MA, Angerame MR, et al: Type III open tibia fractures: Immediate antibiotic prophylaxis minimizes infection. *J Orthop Trauma* 2015;29(1):1-6.

10. Patzakis MJ, Harvey JP Jr, Ivler D: The role of antibiotics in the management of open fractures. *J Bone Joint Surg Am* 1974;56(3):532-541.

11. Zalavras CG, Marcus RE, Levin LS, Patzakis MJ: Management of open fractures and subsequent complications. *J Bone Joint Surg Am* 2007;89(4):884-895.

12. Hoff WS, Bonadies JA, Cachecho R, Dorlac WC: East Practice Management Guidelines Work Group: Update to practice management guidelines for prophylactic antibiotic use in open fractures. *J Trauma* 2011;70(3):751-754.

13. Obremskey WT, Metsemakers WJ, Schlatterer DR, et al: Musculoskeletal infection in orthopaedic trauma: Assessment of the 2018 International Consensus Meeting on Musculoskeletal Infection. *J Bone Joint Surg Am* 2020;102(10):e44.

    This article summarizes the recommendations for diagnosis and management of fracture-related infections from the International Consensus Meeting in Philadelphia in July, 2018. Level of evidence: V.

14. Sagi HC, Patzakis MJ: Evolution in the acute management of open fracture treatment? Part 1. *J Orthop Trauma* 2021;35(9):449-456.

    This article discusses the evolution in antibiotic administration in the acute management of open fractures. Level of evidence: V.

15. Saveli CC, Morgan SJ, Belknap RW, et al: Prophylactic antibiotics in open fractures: A pilot randomized clinical safety study. *J Orthop Trauma* 2013;27(10):552-557.

16. Wynn M, Kesler K, Morellato J, et al: Agricultural trauma causing open fractures: Is antibiotic coverage against anaerobic organisms indicated? *J Orthop Trauma* 2022;36(2):e51-e55.

    This retrospective review found that open lower extremity fractures caused by agriculture-related trauma have higher rates of anaerobic infection and infection overall compared with open fractures due to nonagricultural trauma. Level of evidence: III.

17. Lee J: Efficacy of cultures in the management of open fractures. *Clin Orthop Relat Res* 1997;339:71-75.

18. Declercq P, Zalavras C, Nijssen A, et al: Impact of duration of perioperative antibiotic prophylaxis on development of fracture-related infection in open fractures. *Arch Orthop Trauma Surg* 2021;141(2):235-243.

    This retrospective study evaluated 502 patients with 559 long bone open fractures and 24-month follow-up and found that administration of prophylactic antibiotics beyond 72 hours is not warranted. Analyses adjusted for known confounding factors even revealed a higher risk for infection with longer antibiotic administration. Level of evidence: III.

19. Vanvelk N, Chen B, Van Lieshout EMM, et al: Duration of perioperative antibiotic prophylaxis in open fractures: A systematic review and critical appraisal. *Antibiotics (Basel)* 2022;11(3):293.

    This systematic review demonstrated that prolonged antibiotic administration does not appear to be beneficial in prevention of infection in open fractures. However, it was noted that existing studies investigating the effect of antibiotic duration on fracture-related infection have limitations. Level of evidence: III.

20. Stennett CA, O'Hara NN, Sprague S, et al: Effect of extended prophylactic antibiotic duration in the treatment of open fracture wounds differs by level of contamination. *J Orthop Trauma* 2020;34(3):113-120.

    This is a secondary analysis of 2,400 patients with open extremity fractures who participated in the Fluid Lavage of Open Wounds randomized controlled trial. The study found that antibiotic use for more than 72 hours after definitive wound closure was protective against deep infection in patients with severe contamination. Level of evidence: III.

21. Zalavras CG, Aerden L, Declercq P, Belmans A, Metsemakers WJ: Ninety-day follow-up is inadequate for diagnosis of fracture-related infections in patients with open fractures. *Clin Orthop Relat Res* 2022;480(1):139-146.

    This retrospective study found that follow-up of 90 days captured only 64% of fracture-related infections in patients with open fractures, whereas follow-up of 1 year captured 89% of infections overall and 95% of infections in the presence of an already healed fracture. Level of evidence: III.

22. Zalavras CG, Patzakis MJ, Holtom P: Local antibiotic therapy in the treatment of open fractures and osteomyelitis. *Clin Orthop Relat Res* 2004;427:86-93.

23. Adams K, Couch L, Cierny G, Calhoun J, Mader JT: In vitro and in vivo evaluation of antibiotic diffusion from antibiotic-impregnated polymethylmethacrylate beads. *Clin Orthop Relat Res* 1992;278:244-252.

24. Ostermann PA, Seligson D, Henry SL: Local antibiotic therapy for severe open fractures. A review of 1085 consecutive cases. *J Bone Joint Surg Br* 1995;77(1):93-97.

25. Morgenstern M, Vallejo A, McNally MA, et al: The effect of local antibiotic prophylaxis when treating open limb fractures: A systematic review and meta-analysis. *Bone Joint Res* 2018;7(7):447-456.

    This meta-analysis showed a significantly lower infection rate (4.6%) when local antibiotics were used compared with a control group receiving systemic antibiotic prophylaxis alone (16.5%). Level of evidence: III.

26. McKee MD, Wild LM, Schemitsch EH, Waddell JP: The use of an antibiotic-impregnated, osteoconductive, bioabsorbable bone substitute in the treatment of infected long bone defects: Early results of a prospective trial. *J Orthop Trauma* 2002;16(9):622-627.

27. Major Extremity Trauma Research Consortium (METRC), O'Toole RV, Joshi M, et al: Effect of intrawound vancomycin powder in operatively treated high-risk tibia fractures: A randomized clinical trial. *JAMA Surg* 2021;156(5):e207259.

    This randomized controlled trial examined the effect of intrawound vancomycin powder in 980 patients with tibial plateau or pilon fractures at high risk for infection; 191 of these patients had open fractures. The deep infection rate in patients with open tibial plateau or pilon fractures was reduced in the intrawound vancomycin powder group compared with the control group, but the difference was not significant with the numbers available (12.7% versus 19.3%, $P = 0.23$). Level of evidence: I.

28. Marecek GS, Nicholson LT, Auran RT, Lee J: Use of a defined surgical approach for the debridement of open tibia fractures. *J Orthop Trauma* 2018;32(1):e1-e4.

    This retrospective study found that the use of a defined surgical approach rather than direct extension of the traumatic wound for open diaphyseal tibial fractures is safe and may result in fewer revision surgeries. Level of evidence: III.

29. FLOW Investigators, Bhandari M, Jeray KJ, et al: A trial of wound irrigation in the initial management of open fracture wounds. *N Engl J Med* 2015;373(27):2629-2641.

30. Pollak AN, Jones AL, Castillo RC, Bosse MJ, MacKenzie EJ, LEAP Study Group: The relationship between time to surgical debridement and incidence of infection after open high-energy lower extremity trauma. *J Bone Joint Surg Am* 2010;92(1):7-15.

31. Schenker ML, Yannascoli SY, Baldwin KD, Ahn J, Mehta S: Does timing to operative debridement affect infectious complications in open long-bone fractures? A systematic review. *J Bone Joint Surg Am* 2012;94(12):1057-1064.

32. Johal H, Axelrod D, Sprague S, et al: The effect of time to irrigation and debridement on the rate of reoperation in open fractures: A propensity score-based analysis of the Fluid Lavage of Open Wounds (FLOW) study. *Bone Joint J* 2021;103-B(6):1055-1062.

    This is a secondary analysis of 2,286 patients with open extremity fractures who participated in the Fluid Lavage of Open Wounds randomized controlled trial. After controlling for confounding factors, irrigation and débridement performed within 6 hours of injury versus beyond 6 hours was not associated with subsequent revision surgery for infection or healing complications. Level of evidence: III.

33. Foote CJ, Tornetta P 3rd, Reito A, et al: A reevaluation of the risk of infection based on time to debridement in open fractures: Results of the GOLIATH meta-analysis of observational studies and limited trial data. *J Bone Joint Surg Am* 2021;103(3):265-273.

    This meta-analysis reported a progressive increase in risk of infection with progressive delay to débridement. Débridement later than 24 hours from the time of injury in type III open fractures was associated with a significant twofold increase in the likelihood of infection. Level of evidence: IV.

34. Brumback RJ, Ellison PS Jr, Poka A, Lakatos R, Bathon GH, Burgess AR: Intramedullary nailing of open fractures of the femoral shaft. *J Bone Joint Surg Am* 1989;71(9):1324-1331.

35. Study to Prospectively Evaluate Reamed Intramedullary Nails in Patients with Tibial Fractures Investigators, Bhandari M, Guyatt G, et al: Randomized trial of reamed and unreamed intramedullary nailing of tibial shaft fractures. *J Bone Joint Surg Am* 2008;90(12):2567-2578.

36. Schemitsch EH, Kowalski MJ, Swiontkowski MF, Harrington RM: Comparison of the effect of reamed and unreamed locked intramedullary nailing on blood flow in the callus and strength of union following fracture of the sheep tibia. *J Orthop Res* 1995;13(3):382-389.

37. Pape HC, Tornetta P 3rd, Tarkin I, Tzioupis C, Sabeson V, Olson SA: Timing of fracture fixation in multitrauma patients: The role of early total care and damage control surgery. *J Am Acad Orthop Surg* 2009;17(9):541-549.

38. Sirkin M, Sanders R, DiPasquale T, Herscovici D Jr: A staged protocol for soft tissue management in the treatment of complex pilon fractures. *J Orthop Trauma* 1999;13(2):78-84.

39. Jenkinson RJ, Kiss A, Johnson S, Stephen DJ, Kreder HJ: Delayed wound closure increases deep-infection rate associated with lower-grade open fractures: A propensity-matched cohort study. *J Bone Joint Surg Am* 2014;96(5):380-386.

40. Stannard JP, Volgas DA, Stewart R, McGwin G Jr, Alonso JE: Negative pressure wound therapy after severe open fractures: A prospective randomized study. *J Orthop Trauma* 2009;23(8):552-557.

41. Grant-Freemantle MC, Ryan EJ, Flynn SO, et al: The effectiveness of negative pressure wound therapy versus conventional dressing in the treatment of open fractures: A systematic review and meta-analysis. *J Orthop Trauma* 2020;34(5):223-230.

    This systematic review reported that NPWT was associated with decreased likelihood of deep infection and flap failure compared with conventional dressings in the management of open fractures not directly amenable to early closure. Level of evidence: I.

42. Costa ML, Achten J, Bruce J, et al: Negative-pressure wound therapy versus standard dressings for adults with an open lower limb fracture: The WOLLF RCT. *Health Technol Assess* 2018;22(73):1-162.

    This randomized controlled trial of 460 patients with severe lower extremity open fractures compared NPWT with standard dressings. There was no evidence of a difference between groups in patient disability, quality of life, surgical site infections, or other complications in the 12 months postoperatively. Level of evidence: I.

43. Atwan Y, Sprague S, Slobogean GP, et al: Does negative pressure wound therapy reduce the odds of infection and improve health-related quality of life in patients with open fractures? *Bone Jt Open* 2022;3(3):189-195.

    This is a secondary analysis of 1,322 patients with Gustilo-Anderson type II or III open fractures who participated in the Fluid Lavage of Open Wounds randomized controlled trial. After controlling for confounding factors, the odds of a deep infection requiring surgical management being developed within 12 months of initial injury was 4.5 times higher in patients who received NPWT compared with those who did not, but residual confounding factors may have been present. Level of evidence: III.

44. Gopal S, Majumder S, Batchelor AG, Knight SL, De Boer P, Smith RM: Fix and flap: The radical orthopaedic and plastic treatment of severe open fractures of the tibia. *J Bone Joint Surg Br* 2000;82(7):959-966.

45. Pollak AN, McCarthy ML, Burgess AR: Short-term wound complications after application of flaps for coverage of traumatic soft-tissue defects about the tibia. The Lower Extremity Assessment Project (LEAP) Study Group. *J Bone Joint Surg Am* 2000;82(12):1681-1691.

46. Cierny G 3rd, Byrd HS, Jones RE: Primary versus delayed soft tissue coverage for severe open tibial fractures. A comparison of results. *Clin Orthop Relat Res* 1983;178:54-63.

CHAPTER 21

Management of Fracture-Related Infections

CHARALAMPOS G. ZALAVRAS, MD, PhD, FAAOS, FACS • PAUL D. HOLTOM, MD
JOHN SONTICH, MD, FAAOS • RANDALL MARCUS, MD, FAAOS

ABSTRACT

The management principles of fracture-related infection include host optimization, surgical débridement, systemic and local antibiotic administration, fracture stabilization, soft-tissue coverage, and promotion of healing and/or bone defect reconstruction. Implementation of these principles will help achieve the goals of infection control, fracture healing, and restoration of function to the extent possible.

Keywords: antibiotics; fracture; fracture-related infection; nonunion; osteomyelitis

INTRODUCTION

Fracture-related infections (FRIs) are challenging to treat and are associated with considerable morbidity and socioeconomic effect. FRI management should be undertaken by a multidisciplinary team with the goals of infection control, fracture healing, and restoration of function. However, patient comorbidities, associated injuries, and bone/soft-tissue loss from previous trauma or surgical débridement may make these goals challenging to achieve. The management principles of FRIs include host optimization, aggressive surgical débridement, appropriate antibiotic administration, fracture stabilization, soft-tissue coverage (if needed), and promotion of healing and/or bone defect reconstruction, if needed.

MANAGEMENT OVERVIEW

Treatment of the patient with FRI may vary considerably in complexity and outcome depending on the health status and current function of the patient, the status of bone healing, the condition of the soft-tissue envelope, and the presence of bone and/or soft-tissue defects. A 2021 comprehensive analysis showed they reduce patient quality of life and increase hospitalization and health care costs.[1] Therefore, a detailed assessment of all previously mentioned factors is needed to assess the benefits and risks of various treatment options and determine, together with the patient, the optimal management plan.

The principles of management include detailed assessment of patient and FRI, host optimization, surgical débridement, antimicrobial therapy, fracture stabilization, soft-tissue coverage, and promotion of healing and/or bone defect reconstruction, if needed.[2-5] Management is optimized by the presence of a multidisciplinary team consisting at least of an orthopaedic surgeon, an infectious disease specialist, and a microvascular surgeon. Clinical pharmacists, musculoskeletal imaging specialists, nutritionists, physical therapists, occupational therapists, and specialized nurses are useful additions to the team.

Dr. Sontich or an immediate family member has received royalties from Stryker; is a member of a speakers' bureau or has made paid presentations on behalf of Stryker; and serves as a paid consultant to or is an employee of Stryker. Dr. Marcus or an immediate family member has received nonincome support (such as equipment or services), commercially derived honoraria, or other non–research-related funding (such as paid travel) from Blue Cross Blue Shield Association Pharmacy & Medical Policy Committee and Blue Cross Blue Shield Medical Advisory Panel. Neither of the following authors nor any immediate family member has received anything of value from or has stock or stock options held in a commercial company or institution related directly or indirectly to the subject of this chapter: Dr. Zalavras and Dr. Holtom.

Section 5: Fracture-Related Infections

ASSESSMENT

Each patient with an FRI presents a unique clinical scenario and the treating team often has to manage not only the infection but also other complications, such as compromised healing, bone loss, deformity, a poor soft-tissue envelope, joint stiffness, and limited function of the involved extremity. It is essential to perform a detailed assessment of all factors related to the involved bone and its status of healing, the existing implants, the pathogens, the soft-tissue envelope, the function of the involved extremity, and the status of the patient. Based on this assessment, an individualized treatment plan can be developed.[2-5]

The status of bone healing is very important because it determines the existing mechanical stability present at the fracture site and the need for fixation implants. FRIs are broadly classified into three categories: infections in healed fractures, infected nonunion, and infections in healing fractures; the relevant differences in management will be outlined later. It should be kept in mind that assessment of fracture healing, currently based on clinical and imaging findings, may not always be accurate, and for this reason, a 2021 review reinforced that there has been considerable variation in the definition of nonunion.[6] The presence of bone defects should be noted and their management should be incorporated in the plan. Existing implants should be identified by careful evaluation of radiographs and by obtaining previous medical records, so that specific extraction tools are available in the operating room.

Assessment of the pathogen or pathogens and their sensitivities, so as to optimize antimicrobial treatment, is ideally based on intraoperative cultures. However, useful information that may be available preoperatively may include blood culture results in febrile patients, joint aspiration results in intra-articular FRIs, or previous intraoperative culture results in recurrent cases.

In the presence of soft-tissue defects or poor vascularity of the soft-tissue envelope, early consultation with a microvascular surgeon is necessary so that soft-tissue coverage can be incorporated into the treatment plan. Previous incisions should be noted and used again, if possible. The presence of sinus tracts and soft-tissue abscesses should be noted to ensure adequate débridement.

The neurovascular status of the involved extremity should be carefully assessed and documented. Previous vascular injury or disease may compromise blood supply to the fracture/nonunion site and limit available soft-tissue coverage options. Functional deficits resulting from previous neurologic injury or disease, missed compartment syndrome, or stiffness of adjacent joints may compromise final outcome and prevent restoration of function after control of infection and bone healing.

The health status and functional needs of the patient should be carefully assessed. The presence of comorbidities compromises the patient's capacity for fracture healing and to mount an immune response to infection and patient comorbidities also increase the risk of surgery. Therefore, patient comorbidities must be assessed and corrected to the extent possible. The importance of the health status of the patient was recognized in a landmark study and patients were classified as type A (normal healthy host), type B (systemically and/or locally compromised host), or type C (host who is not a good surgical candidate) hosts.[7]

The functional needs and expectations of a patient and the willingness of a patient to undergo a potentially prolonged treatment plan that includes multiple hospitalizations and surgeries should also be carefully assessed to determine the management plan that offers the optimal risk-benefit ratio to the patient. In most patients, the goals of treatment are infection control, fracture healing, and restoration of function. However, other treatment options may be viable, or even preferable, in select patients. For example, nonsurgical treatment with the use of suppressive antibiotics may be an option for patients with chronic low-grade infections, who are not sick and have severe comorbidities and high surgical risk. Amputation of the involved extremity may be indicated in patients with uncontrolled sepsis and patients with severe comorbidities in whom reconstruction is complex and/or in whom poor functional outcomes are anticipated after reconstruction.

HOST OPTIMIZATION

Systemic health issues, such as diabetes mellitus, anemia, malnutrition, vitamin D deficiency, other metabolic and endocrine abnormalities, smoking, and use of certain medications, compromise bone healing, the response to infection, or both. Therefore, these issues should be optimized preoperatively to improve infection control and fracture healing. Early consultation with the appropriate specialist, such as an endocrinologist, a nutritionist, or others, may be extremely helpful.

Diabetes mellitus is associated with impaired fracture healing.[8] A 2019 review noted that blood glucose control in patients with diabetes mellitus improves fracture healing and decreases complications from perioperative infections.[9] Management of anemia is important for the optimization of a patient with an FRI. A 33% increase in nonunion rate has been reported in anemic animals, most likely as a result of a reduction in oxygen transport, which is associated with poor callus formation.[10]

Optimizing patient nutrition is important when treating patients with FRI. Protein deficiencies are associated with decreased callus strength and fracture healing can be enhanced via anabolic dietary supplementation.[11] Calcium and vitamin D homeostasis is also important for fracture healing. A large percentage of patients in developed countries have disturbances in calcium and vitamin D homeostasis.[12,13] Surgeons must ensure adequate calcium intake, a 25-hydroxyvitamin D serum level greater than 30 µg/L, and sufficient gastric acidification to enable calcium absorption in patients with FRI. Studies have shown that correction of these metabolic and endocrine abnormalities, even in patients with a presumed nonunion, can lead to fracture union without surgical intervention.[14,15]

Nicotine has a vasoconstriction effect and is directly toxic to osteoblasts. The use of nicotine products places the patient at risk for infection and nonunion.[16,17] Cessation of smoking, including vaping, should be strongly encouraged in the patient with FRI. Because of the difficulty in designing studies to determine how the duration of abstinence from the use of nicotine products affects wound and bone healing, it is difficult to provide an exact time for patients to stop the use of these products before surgical treatment.[18] However, even brief periods of abstinence from nicotine products preoperatively may be beneficial. It has been shown that concentrations of nicotine in the body decrease significantly within 12 hours of smoking cessation.[19] Furthermore, another study revealed that smoking cessation for 1 week before surgery produced a threefold decrease in wound complications requiring further surgical intervention.[20] At least a 1- to 3-week abstinence from nicotine use before surgery, which can be verified by obtaining patient nicotine levels preoperatively, is recommended.

Certain medications may adversely affect bone formation, infection control, or both. Corticosteroids inhibit the differentiation of mesenchymal cells, decrease bone healing, and increase infection risk.[21] NSAIDs, including cyclooxygenase-2 inhibitors, also have been reported to interfere with fracture healing, but the evidence is inconclusive.[21] Antibiotics, such as ciprofloxacin, may interfere with bone formation.[21] The treating surgeon should review the patient's current medications and consult the appropriate specialists to determine if relevant pharmacologic factors can be modified either in the perioperative period or, if possible, until infection control and fracture union have been achieved.

SURGICAL DÉBRIDEMENT

Débridement consists of removal of all nonviable tissue (including skin, soft tissues, and bone) and foreign bodies that are present at the fracture site.[22] Nonviable tissue and foreign bodies (such as fixation implants) promote biofilm development on their surface, which is a key pathogenetic mechanism of musculoskeletal infections.[23,24]

A biofilm is a highly structured multicellular community of microorganisms that adhere to an inert or living surface and are embedded within a self-produced polymeric matrix mainly composed by polysaccharides. Biofilm microorganisms demonstrate decreased susceptibility to antibiotics and host immune responses compared with individual (planktonic) organisms. As a result, formation of biofilm leads to persistence of infection.[23,24] Therefore, nonviable tissues and any foreign bodies, including existing implants, must be removed to achieve control of infection.

As a result, when infection occurs in the presence of internal fixation, the implants are a nidus for biofilm formation and implant retention will not allow infection control; however, a 2021 review reported that the stability provided by the implants is beneficial for fracture healing.[25] Animal studies have assessed the role of biomechanical stability on fracture healing in the presence of infection and a recent review of these studies showed that fracture healing can be achieved in the presence of infection when a stable implant is present.[25] Stability at the fracture site is also an important factor for infection control.[25] Therefore, the status of bone healing (healed fractures, infected nonunion, healing fractures) and the stability present are important factors in deciding whether to remove or retain the implants.[2,4]

In healed fractures, stability has been achieved and the implants are no longer needed; therefore, they have to be removed so that the associated biofilm that has formed on their surface is also removed and to maximize the probability of infection control.

In infected nonunion, the existing implants have to be removed as well. Even if they appear to be intact, they have failed to help the fracture achieve union, they have sustained fatigue and are susceptible to failure, and they are harboring biofilm that prevents infection control. An alternative fixation construct will be necessary after implant removal to achieve stability at the nonunion site.

In healing fractures with unstable fixation and/or unacceptable reduction, the fixation implants have to be removed and the fracture restabilized with new implants to achieve stability at the fracture site.

However, in healing fractures with intact fixation implants that provide stability and maintain an acceptable reduction, there are two options. The implants may be retained, in which case, the goal is not control but suppression of infection until the fracture heals; the implants will then be removed after fracture union.[26-28] An alternative approach would be to remove the existing implants, even if stable, and insert new ones to restabilize the healing fracture; this would be beneficial for infection control but revised fixation may not achieve adequate stability, especially in periarticular fractures and/or osteoporotic bone. Therefore, the decision to retain or remove the implants is not straightforward. Instead, it is a balancing act between the risk of infection recurrence if the implants are retained and the risk of not achieving the same degree of stability if the implants are removed and the fracture is restabilized. Clinical studies, in conjunction with animal studies, have shown that fracture healing can be achieved with implant retention.

A retrospective review of patients with 123 FRIs, which were diagnosed within 6 weeks after fracture fixation and treated with débridement, antibiotics, and implant retention (DAIR), reported that fracture healing was achieved in 71% of FRIs (87 of 123).[26] Inability to achieve healing with implant retention was significantly associated with open fractures and the presence of an intramedullary nail.[26] Infection recurred in 30% of the fractures (26 of 87) that were united with implant retention, which may appear high, but all recurrent infections resolved after implant removal and further antibiotic therapy.[26] As mentioned earlier, the goal is suppression of infection until the fracture heals. However, in FRIs of very short duration (up to 3 weeks after fixation), the infection may be successfully controlled with DAIR. A systematic literature review reported in 2021 that implant retention was associated with infection control rates of 86% to 100%.[27]

During débridement, multiple specimens of purulent fluid, soft tissue, and bone from the involved area are sent for aerobic and anaerobic cultures.[2,4] Mycobacterial and fungal cultures may be helpful in immunocompromised hosts or chronic infections. Histopathology may help confirm the diagnosis of FRI and identify atypical organisms.[4] In fractures stabilized with an intramedullary nail, reaming and irrigation of the intramedullary canal should be undertaken if the nail is removed.[28,29]

SYSTEMIC ANTIMICROBIAL THERAPY

Choice of Antimicrobial Agents

When patients are identified as having FRIs, information on the specific causative organism is usually not available, so treatment must be empiric based on likely organisms.

In most cases, the cause of infection is either *Staphylococcus aureus* or a *Streptococcus* species, although in patients with implanted hardware, coagulase-negative staphylococci are frequent. Methicillin-resistant *S aureus* (MRSA) is always a concern. The beta-lactam antibiotics remain the drugs of choice for these organisms (**Tables 1** and **2**). For the streptococci, penicillin or a penicillin derivative is the drug of choice. For methicillin-susceptible *S aureus*, cefazolin or nafcillin/oxacillin is superior to other drugs such as vancomycin. Because cefazolin has fewer adverse effects and no difference in outcomes compared with oxacillin or nafcillin, it has become the preferred agent. For MRSA, vancomycin remains the drug of choice. Although there have been many newer agents released with MRSA activity, none of these have been shown to be superior to vancomycin. Of the newer agents, linezolid has the advantage of excellent oral absorption and can be used as an oral alternative in patients who do not need continued hospitalization. Several older oral drugs may be effective against MRSA, such as clindamycin and trimethoprim/sulfamethoxazole, although resistance against these agents has been increasing.

Depending on the type of fracture and the extent of contamination, gram-negative bacilli (primarily the *Enterobacterales*) and anaerobes might need to be covered empirically. The drug of choice for gram-negative bacilli coverage is a third-generation cephalosporin such as ceftriaxone. The aminoglycosides have been used in the past, but because of their potential renal and ototoxicity, they have been generally replaced by cephalosporin. Metronidazole could be considered if anaerobic infection is considered likely. Antibiotic agent recommendations are summarized in **Tables 1** and **2**.

Route of Administration

The dogma that an intravenous route is necessary came from uncontrolled case series in the 1940s and 1950s. However, the oral antibiotics available at that time had limited bioavailability. Modern pharmacologic studies have demonstrated that numerous oral antimicrobial agents achieve levels in bone with standard oral dosing well above minimum inhibitory concentrations of susceptible pathogens.

There are no controlled investigations that show that intravenous-only therapy is superior to oral therapy with appropriate antimicrobial agents. Many observational studies have demonstrated that oral administration of antibiotics resulted in treatment success rates for osteomyelitis similar to those historically experienced with intravenous therapy. A 2019 large randomized controlled trial (RCT) from the United Kingdom compared oral versus intravenous antibiotic therapy for completion of the first 6 weeks of therapy in 1,054 adults with a diagnosis of bone, joint, or orthopaedic implant–associated infection who would receive at least 6 weeks of antibiotics and who had received 7 days or less of intravenous therapy from definitive surgery.[30] End point data were available for 1,015 participants (96.3%). Treatment failure (recurrence of infection within 12 months) occurred in 14.6% (74 of 506) and 13.2% (67 of 509) of participants randomized to intravenous and oral therapy, respectively, showing that oral therapy was noninferior to intravenous therapy. Oral therapy was associated with significantly fewer intravenous catheter complications (0.96%, 5 of 523) compared with intravenous therapy (9.37%, 49 of 523) and with cost savings of £2,740 per patient without

Chapter 21: Management of Fracture-Related Infections

Table 1
Common Antimicrobial Agents

Antimicrobial Agent	Spectrum of Activity	Route of Administration (IV, PO)	Complications	Comments
Cefazolin	MSSA, streptococci, limited gram-negative bacilli	IV	Anaphylaxis	Very low cross-reactivity with penicillin allergy
Oxacillin/nafcillin	MSSA	IV	Anaphylaxis, Toxic hepatitis	Cefazolin is preferred
Ceftriaxone	MSSA, streptococci, *Enterobacterales*	IV	Anaphylaxis	Very low cross-reactivity with penicillin allergy
Piperacillin/tazobactam	MSSA, streptococci, *Enterobacterales*, *Pseudomonas*, anaerobes	IV	Anaphylaxis	Used if there is concern for *Pseudomonas aeruginosa* in postoperative infections
Aminoglycosides (gentamicin, tobramycin)	*Enterobacterales*, *Pseudomonas*	IV	Nephrotoxicity, Ototoxicity	—
Ciprofloxacin	*Enterobacterales*, *Pseudomonas*	IV, PO	Tendinitis, QT prolongation	Poor coverage for MSSA, streptococci
Levofloxacin	MSSA, streptococci, *Enterobacterales*, *Pseudomonas*	IV, PO	Tendinitis, QT prolongation	—
Linezolid	MSSA, streptococci	IV, PO	Bone marrow suppression, neuropathy, interaction with other medications	—
Clindamycin	MSSA, streptococci, anaerobes	IV, PO	GI upset, diarrhea	—
Trimethoprim/sulfamethoxazole	MSSA, streptococci, Some *Enterobacterales*	IV, PO	Rash, Nausea	—
Rifampin	Synergy for MSSA	PO (IV available)	Orange urine, Cholestatic jaundice	Not for use as a single agent because resistance develops quickly

GI = gastrointestinal, IV = intravenous, MSSA = methicillin-susceptible *Staphylococcus aureus*, PO = per os (oral)

any significant difference in quality-adjusted life-years between the two arms of the trial.[30] Most trials have used oral fluoroquinolones, with or without rifampin, although other combinations of drugs (including trimethoprim/sulfamethoxazole plus rifampin) have been used in other studies.

Duration of Therapy

Current recommendations for duration of therapy are 4 to 6 weeks or even longer for chronic osteomyelitis. These treatment durations are based primarily on tradition and were originally recommended before the 1960s, when available antibiotics and surgical techniques were very different than those currently used.

There are no RCTs comparing lengths of therapy in FRIs. Two RCTs compared 6 weeks with 12 weeks of therapy, one in 351 patients with pyogenic vertebral osteomyelitis and one in 40 patients with nonsurgically treated diabetic foot osteomyelitis, and found no difference in infection remission with a longer duration of therapy.[31,32] Infection remission of pyogenic vertebral osteomyelitis at 12 months was 90.9% in both the 6-week and the 12-week group.[31] Infection remission of nonsurgically treated diabetic foot osteomyelitis at 12 months was 60% (12 of 20 patients) in the 6-week group and 70% (14 of 20 patients) in the 12-week group, which was not significant with the numbers available.[32] One RCT in 2019 compared 4 to 6 weeks of antibiotic

Table 2

Antimicrobial Agents for Specific Organisms

Organism	Preferred Antibiotic	Alternative Antibiotics
Staphylococcus aureus Methicillin-susceptible *S aureus*	Cefazolin	Clindamycin Vancomycin (in truly allergic patients)
S aureus Methicillin-resistant *S aureus*	Vancomycin	Clindamycin Linezolid Daptomycin
Streptococcus pyogenes	Penicillin	Clindamycin Vancomycin (in truly allergic patients)
Streptococcus pneumoniae	Ceftriaxone (if susceptible)	Vancomycin
Neisseria gonorrhoeae	Ceftriaxone	Must be guided by antimicrobial susceptibility testing
Enterobacteriaceae (not ESBL)	Ceftriaxone	Fluoroquinolone (if susceptible)
ESBL-producing gram negatives	Meropenem	Must be guided by antimicrobial susceptibility testing
Pseudomonas aeruginosa	Cefepime, ceftazidime, or meropenem	Must be guided by antimicrobial susceptibility testing
Candida albicans	Fluconazole	—

ESBL = extended spectrum beta-lactamase

therapy in 123 patients with osteoarticular infections treated with implant removal and found no statistically significant difference in the rates of infection recurrence between the 4-week group (6%, 4 of 62 patients) and the 6-week group (5%, 3 of 61 patients).[33]

In FRIs in healing fractures with stable implants that are retained with an aim to take the fracture to healing, the usual practice is to treat the infection with 6 weeks of directed antibiotics and then continue suppressive antibiotics until the implant can be removed. Lifelong suppression may be required in patients with severe comorbidities where surgical extirpation of the infection cannot be performed.

LOCAL ANTIMICROBIAL THERAPY

Local antibiotic administration via antibiotic-impregnated delivery vehicles is used, in addition to systemic administration, to achieve dead space management, high local concentration of antibiotics, minimal systemic toxicity, and prevention of secondary contamination.[34,35]

Polymethyl methacrylate (PMMA) cement is a widely used delivery vehicle. Antibiotics that are heat stable and available in powder form, such as aminoglycosides and vancomycin, can be incorporated into PMMA cement for local delivery. Following insertion of antibiotic-impregnated PMMA beads or spacers, the wound should be sealed by using a semipermeable barrier to maintain the eluted antibiotic agents at the wound, achieve a high local concentration, and prevent secondary contamination by nosocomial pathogens.

FRACTURE STABILIZATION

Stability at the infected fracture or nonunion site is necessary for both healing and infection control.[25] As mentioned earlier, implant retention is an option in healing fractures with stable fixation implants, but implant removal and restabilization are necessary in infected nonunion and healing fractures with unstable fixation.

Restabilization of the nonunion site usually is performed in a staged manner,[2,5] even though single-stage restabilization is an option.[36] Provisional fixation is achieved with a temporary external fixator or an antibiotic intramedullary nail. Temporary external fixation pins should not be placed close to the infected area or the area of subsequent definitive fixation. Staged reconstruction with the use of definitive fixation is performed after control of the infection has been achieved.

The definitive fixation method depends on the involved bone, the type of nonunion, the local soft tissues, and the health status of the host.[3-5] Patients with an infected nonunion require a more robust fixation construct because of the compromised local biology and the prolonged healing time. Similarly, type B hosts may benefit from more rigid fixation because healing is expected to be delayed. The condition of the soft-tissue envelope affects the type of fixation that can be used for nonunion stabilization. Better soft-tissue coverage is required for plate-and-screw fixation, even if placed percutaneously. Intramedullary nailing is less likely to injure the soft tissues but may not be possible depending on the location of the nonunion or the presence of bone deformity. Ring external fixation provides adequate stability for weight bearing with the least amount of surgical insult to the soft tissues but is associated with exposed hardware and increased cost.

Different techniques may be applicable for each anatomic location. Surgeons must analyze the reason initial fixation failed and modify fixation to maximize the likelihood of healing in the most straightforward and expedient manner without further complications. The goal of revised fixation is adequate stability at the fracture/nonunion site to allow early functional active range of motion and weight bearing. Mechanical strategies for internal and external fixation that promote compression forces and minimize shearing forces during weight bearing help promote union.[3,5]

Plate fixation is often used in fractures/nonunion located at periarticular areas or at the diaphysis of the humerus, radius, and ulna.[37,38] The fixation construct must be carefully planned based on whether the goal is relative or absolute stability. The weakest fixation block determines the stability of the entire construct; therefore, balanced fixation is essential in both relative and absolute stability constructs. Placement of locked screws in the plate provides additional stability and is particularly important in periarticular fractures/nonunion and osteoporotic bone. Unnecessary exposure and soft-tissue stripping should be avoided to maximally preserve local soft-tissue biology.

Intramedullary fixation is often used in diaphyseal fractures/nonunion of the femur and tibia but can also be used for the management of metaphyseal ones.[39,40] Intramedullary nails are biomechanically advantageous because of their load-sharing properties, and the larger the nail, the more likely translational stability will be attained and the less likely shearing forces will occur at the nonunion site. Nails can be placed without further disruption of the soft-tissue envelope and are best used for the management of diaphyseal fractures/nonunion if the medullary canal is patent and no angular correction is necessary.

The use of uniplanar external fixation for the definitive management of a fracture/nonunion is limited because monolateral external fixation frames are inherently unstable during weight bearing. However, provisional, uniplanar, non–weight-bearing external fixators provide temporary stability, allow for easy wound access, and are very useful during the first stage of management.

Ring external fixation constructs, specifically the hexapod external fixation frame, are very useful for the definitive nonunion fixation and management, especially in the lower extremity.[3,5,41] A stable ring external fixator promotes compression forces, which stimulate healing, and minimizes shearing forces, which delay healing, at the nonunion site during weight bearing. Ring external fixation provides enough stability for early weight bearing and does not reintroduce metal into the area of infection; therefore, it can be very useful for patients with an infected nonunion, especially of the lower extremity. An understanding of cross-sectional anatomy is necessary for the safe placement of wires and half-pins. Selection of ring external fixation rather than standard internal fixation techniques may be preferable in infected nonunion with segmental bone loss and/or a short extremity because ring external fixation allows for lengthening.

SOFT-TISSUE COVERAGE

Depending on the extent of the infection, delayed or primary closure may be performed in patients with an adequate soft-tissue envelope. In the presence of compromised soft tissues, soft-tissue reconstruction is necessary to improve the local biologic environment, which is very important for both bone healing and infection control. Soft-tissue coverage with healthy, well-vascularized tissue eliminates dead space, prevents secondary contamination, enhances vascularity at the defect site, improves local host defenses, and facilitates the healing process. Therefore, in extremities with local soft-tissue compromise, early consultation with a microvascular surgeon should be obtained.

Soft-tissue coverage may be accomplished by local or free muscle flaps depending on the location and size of the soft-tissue defect.[42-45] Local transfer of muscle that has been damaged because of previous injury or compartment syndrome should be avoided. Free fasciocutaneous flaps are a viable alternative and achieve comparable rates of limb salvage and functional recovery.[45] A multicenter retrospective review from 2018 of 518 lower extremity free flaps that were performed for acute traumatic injuries ($n = 238$) or chronic traumatic sequelae ($n = 280$) found that muscle ($n = 307$) and fasciocutaneous ($n = 211$) flaps achieved similar limb salvage rates in both the acute trauma (90% versus 94%) and the chronic trauma subgroups (90% versus 88%).[45] The reconstruction and functional outcomes were not influenced by the type of flap but by injury severity.[45]

Soft-tissue coverage, if needed, is usually performed at a second stage, preferably within 5 to 7 days after the initial débridement, once the infection has been controlled.[44] With staged coverage, the surgeon can treat organisms present from the first débridement with specific antibiotics based on deep cultures and can perform a repeat débridement before flap transfer, which will help eliminate residual organisms. In the meantime, nosocomial contamination of the wound should be avoided by sealing the wound with either an antibiotic bead pouch or a negative-pressure wound dressing.[34,35,46] Coverage at the initial débridement procedure is a viable option when the surgeon is confident that all infected tissue has been removed.[42,43,47] A 2020 retrospective study of 57 consecutive patients with chronic osteomyelitis or infected nonunion who underwent simultaneous débridement and reconstruction with Ilizarov fixation and free muscle flap transfer reported infection control in 55 of 57 patients (96%) at a mean follow-up of 36 months and bony union after the initial surgery in 52 of 57 patients (91%).[47] However, simultaneous reconstruction requires careful planning and it may be logistically challenging for most institutions.

PROMOTION OF HEALING AND BONE DEFECT RECONSTRUCTION

Bone Grafting

Bone grafting is indicated in patients in whom nonunion repair augmentation or skeletal defect reconstruction is required. The preferred method for bone grafting is autogenous cancellous bone grafting, which results in osteoconduction, osteoinduction, and osteogenesis at the nonunion site. Autogenous bone graft revascularizes relatively quickly and is replaced by creeping substitution. Weak structural mechanics are present for at least 6 months in patients who undergo autogenous bone grafting; however, normal structural mechanics have been reported 1 year postoperatively.

The timing of bone grafting is important. In patients with a nonunion in whom a poor soft-tissue envelope and infection is present, bone grafting should be postponed (usually 6 to 8 weeks) until adequate soft-tissue coverage is achieved and infection is controlled. Autogenous cancellous bone graft should be placed in a well-vascularized noninfected bed at the nonunion site and should be used only in patients with defects smaller than 6 cm because it lacks structural integrity. Larger defects are optimally reconstructed with the techniques of bone transport and free vascularized autografts, which are discussed later.

Common sources of autogenous bone graft include the anterior and posterior iliac crests and the femur.[48-50] An RCT of 113 patients with nonunion or posttraumatic segmental bone defects requiring surgical intervention compared iliac crest bone autograft (from the anterior or posterior crest) with femoral autograft harvested with the reamer-irrigator-aspirator (RIA) device.[49] Union rates and time to union were comparable between the iliac crest and the RIA autografts; 49 of 57 patients (86%) who received iliac crest bone autograft achieved union at a mean of 22.5 weeks, whereas 46 of 56 patients (82%) who received RIA autograft achieved union at a mean of 26 weeks. There was no difference in donor-site complications, persistent nonunion, or infection at the grafted site.[49] A retrospective review of 108 patients requiring bone grafting for nonunion or failed arthrodesis reported a higher volume of graft harvested with the RIA compared with the anterior iliac crest (53 versus 27 mL) but an increased need for blood transfusion with the RIA (44% versus 21%).[50]

The induced membrane technique for staged reconstruction of larger bone defects has been developed and popularized by Masquelet.[51,52] This technique can be particularly helpful when treating an FRI as it is imperative to avoid placing bone graft into an infected site. The first stage consists of débridement, soft-tissue coverage if needed, and insertion of an antibiotic-impregnated PMMA cement spacer into the bone defect. It is extremely important to control infection with a thorough débridement; in select cases, more than one débridement may be necessary. The placement of a PMMA spacer allows for the local release of antibiotics into the site of infection, maintains the space for the eventual bone graft by preventing fibrous tissue growth into the defect, and induces formation of a membrane around the spacer. The second stage is performed 6 to 8 weeks later. The spacer is removed, but the membrane that is induced by the cement is left in place and the cavity is filled with cancellous bone autograft. The induced membrane acts as a biologic chamber; it prevents resorption of the cancellous bone, promotes its vascularization and corticalization, and acts as an in situ delivery system for growth and osteoinductive factors.[51,52]

A retrospective study of 69 patients with a mean bone loss of 5 cm who underwent treatment with the induced membrane technique found that union was obtained in 83% of patients.[53] Significant risk factors for nonunion included infection before grafting, postoperative wound dehiscence, and postgrafting infection.[53] A 2019 retrospective study of 123 patients treated with the induced membrane technique reported that multiple grafting procedures were required in a significantly lower proportion of patients treated with intramedullary nail fixation (11%, 6 of 57 patients) compared with patients treated with plate fixation (28%, 18 of 64 patients).[54] Osteodecortication is another option to promote healing.[55] Osteodecortication involves the elevation of cortical chips that remain attached to the periosteum and the overlying soft tissue surrounding the fracture site. Osteodecortication increases the surface area for healing, exposes the vascular subcortical haversian system, and results in osteogenic stimulation.

Biologics

Bone morphogenetic proteins have been used for the management of nonunion and delayed union. Bone morphogenetic proteins provide a primordial signal that regulates the differentiation of mesenchymal cells to osteoblasts and are more effective if surrounded by pluripotent cells, such as those in autogenous bone graft.[56,57]

Recombinant human bone morphogenetic protein 7 and recombinant human bone morphogenetic protein 2 have been reported to be safe and effective for the management of nonunion.[58,59] In patients with an atrophic long bone nonunion who undergo open reduction and internal fixation, the use of bone morphogenetic protein alone has been reported to be as effective as the use of bone morphogenetic protein in combination with autogenous cancellous bone grafting, with union achieved in more than 80% of the patients.[60,61] Surgeons must understand that there is an increased risk for prolonged serous wound drainage in patients with a nonunion who undergo treatment with the use of biologics. However, biologics are not associated with an increased risk for wound infection or need for revision surgery.[62]

Bone Transport

Bone transport is a very useful reconstruction technique to address bone defects. Bone transport can be achieved with either a standard Ilizarov frame or a hexapod external fixation frame. Ring external fixation allows for bone lengthening, does not reintroduce metal into the area of infection, and allows for postoperative alignment adjustments without future surgery.[5,41,63,64]

The surgeon and the patient must understand that bone transport for the management of infected nonunion with a bone defect is a limb salvage technique, which is associated with complications and requires an external fixation frame to be used for many months.[5,64] In a study of 19 patients with a mean bone defect of 10 cm, the mean external fixation time was 16 months and there were 19 major complications; however, infection control and union were achieved in all patients.[64] Moreover, prolonged time may be required before potential maximum functional improvement is achieved. A retrospective study of 38 patients with infected nonunion of the tibia and defects of mean size of 5.1 cm treated with stacked hexapod bone transport reported that mean musculoskeletal functional outcome scores improved from 2 to 8 years after external fixator removal (26.5 versus 19.4, respectively), approaching a normal range.[41]

Free Vascularized Bone Grafting

Free vascularized corticocancellous grafts can successfully reconstruct large bone defects. They have beneficial biologic and mechanical properties and they result in osteoconduction, osteoinduction, and osteogenesis at the nonunion site while offering structural support in patients with defects larger than 6 cm.[65,66] The free vascularized fibular graft is a versatile flap that in addition to bone can include muscle, skin, and fascia. It is particularly useful in upper extremity defects, in combined bone and soft-tissue defects, and in patients opposed to having an external fixator.

SUMMARY

FRIs are challenging to treat and are associated with considerable morbidity and socioeconomic effect. FRI management should be undertaken by a multidisciplinary team with the goals of infection control, fracture healing, and restoration of function. However, patient comorbidities, associated injuries, and bone/soft-tissue loss from previous trauma or surgical débridement may make these goals challenging to achieve. The management principles of FRIs include host optimization, aggressive surgical débridement, appropriate systemic and local antibiotic administration, fracture stabilization, soft-tissue coverage, and promotion of healing and/or bone defect reconstruction.

KEY STUDY POINTS

- The patient with an FRI should be optimized and comorbidities corrected to the extent possible.
- Surgical débridement aims to remove all foreign material, nonviable tissue, and the biofilm that has formed on their surface.
- Systemic antibiotics are needed and can be administered orally instead of intravenously.
- Stability at the fracture/nonunion site should be achieved.
- A compromised soft-tissue envelope should be reconstructed with local or free flaps.

ANNOTATED REFERENCES

1. Iliaens J, Onsea J, Hoekstra H, Nijs S, Peetermans WE, Metsemakers WJ: Fracture-related infection in long bone fractures: A comprehensive analysis of the economic impact and influence on quality of life. *Injury* 2021;52(11):3344-3349.

   This matched-pair analysis of 15 patients each in the FRI and non-FRI groups found that direct hospital-related health care costs of FRI are eight times that of non-FRI long bone fractures. Level of evidence: III.

2. Patzakis MJ, Zalavras CG: Chronic posttraumatic osteomyelitis and infected nonunion of the tibia: Current management concepts. *J Am Acad Orthop Surg* 2005;13(6):417-427.

3. Zalavras CG, Marcus RE, Sontich JK: How can I get this bone to heal? *Instr Course Lect* 2018;67:511-528.

   This is a review on the assessment and treatment of patients with nonunion.

4. Metsemakers WJ, Morgenstern M, Senneville E, et al: General treatment principles for fracture-related infection: Recommendations from an international expert group. *Arch Orthop Trauma Surg* 2020;140(8):1013-1027.

   This article presents recommendations from an international expert group on the diagnosis and management of FRI.

5. Sontich JK, Zalavras CG, Marcus RE: Secrets of success in the management of lower extremity nonunions. *Instr Course Lect* 2021;70:163-180.

   This is a review on the assessment and treatment of patients with nonunion of the lower extremity.

6. Wittauer M, Burch MA, McNally M, et al: Definition of long-bone nonunion: A scoping review of prospective clinical trials to evaluate current practice. *Injury* 2021;52(11):3200-3205.

   This literature review reported a lack of consensus with regard to the definition of long bone nonunion.

7. Cierny G 3rd, Mader JT, Penninck JJ: A clinical staging system for adult osteomyelitis. *Clin Orthop Relat Res* 2003;10(414):17-24.

8. Macey LR, Kana SM, Jingushi S, Terek RM, Borretos J, Bolander ME: Defects of early fracture-healing in experimental diabetes. *J Bone Joint Surg Am* 1989;71(5):722-733.

9. Henderson S, Ibe I, Cahill S, Chung YH, Lee FY: Bone quality and fracture-healing in type-1 and type-2 diabetes mellitus. *J Bone Joint Surg Am* 2019;101(15):1399-1410.

   This review summarizes the effects of diabetes mellitus on fracture healing and perioperative complications.

10. Rothman RH, Klemek JS, Toton JJ: The effect of iron deficiency anemia on fracture healing. *Clin Orthop Relat Res* 1971;77:276-283.

11. Hughes MS, Kazmier P, Burd TA, et al: Enhanced fracture and soft-tissue healing by means of anabolic dietary supplementation. *J Bone Joint Surg Am* 2006;88(11):2386-2394.

12. Amling M: Calcium and vitamin D in bone metabolism: Clinical importance for fracture treatment. *Unfallchirurg* 2015;118(12):995-999.

13. Hood MA, Murtha YM, Della Rocca GJ, Stannard JP, Volgas DA, Crist BD: Prevalence of low vitamin D levels in patients with orthopedic trauma. *Am J Orthop (Belle Mead NJ)* 2016;45(7):E522-E526.

14. Brinker MR, O'Connor DP, Monla YT, Earthman TP: Metabolic and endocrine abnormalities in patients with nonunions. *J Orthop Trauma* 2007;21(8):557-570.

15. Patton CM, Powell AP, Patel AA: Vitamin D in orthopaedics. *J Am Acad Orthop Surg* 2012;20(3):123-129.

16. Castillo RC, Bosse MJ, MacKenzie EJ, Patterson BM, LEAP Study Group: Impact of smoking on fracture healing and risk of complications in limb-threatening open tibia fractures. *J Orthop Trauma* 2005;19(3):151-157.

17. Scolaro JA, Schenker ML, Yannascoli S, Baldwin K, Mehta S, Ahn J: Cigarette smoking increases complications following fracture: A systematic review. *J Bone Joint Surg Am* 2014;96(8):674-681.

18. Warner DO: Preoperative smoking cessation: How long is long enough. *Anesthesiology* 2005;102(5):883-884.

19. Egan TD, Wong KC: Perioperative smoking cessation and anesthesia: A review. *J Clin Anesth* 1992;4(1):63-72.

20. Kuri M, Nakagawa M, Tanaka H, Hasuo S, Kishi Y: Determination of the duration of preoperative smoking cessation to improve wound healing after head and neck surgery. *Anesthesiology* 2005;102(5):892-896.

21. Pountos I, Georgouli T, Blokhuis TJ, Pape HC, Giannoudis PV: Pharmacological agents and impairment of fracture healing: What is the evidence? *Injury* 2008;39(4):384-394.

22. Tetsworth K, Cierny G 3rd: Osteomyelitis debridement techniques. *Clin Orthop Relat Res* 1999;360:87-96.

23. Costerton JW: Biofilm theory can guide the treatment of device-related orthopaedic infections. *Clin Orthop Relat Res* 2005;437:7-11.

24. Zalavras CG, Costerton JW: Biofilm, biomaterials, and bacterial adherence, in Cierny G III, McLaren AC, Wongworawat MD, eds: *Orthopaedic Knowledge Update®: Musculoskeletal Infection*. American Academy of Orthopaedic Surgeons, 2009, pp 33-42.

25. Foster AL, Moriarty TF, Zalavras C, et al: The influence of biomechanical stability on bone healing and fracture-related infection: The legacy of Stephan Perren. *Injury* 2021;52(1):43-52.

    This review examines the role of biomechanical stability on fracture healing and provides a detailed analysis of the preclinical animal studies addressing this in the context of FRI.

26. Berkes M, Obremskey WT, Scannell B, et al: Maintenance of hardware after early postoperative infection following fracture internal fixation. *J Bone Joint Surg Am* 2010;92(4):823-828.

27. Morgenstern M, Kuehl R, Zalavras CG, et al: The influence of duration of infection on outcome of debridement and implant retention in fracture-related infection. *Bone Joint J* 2021;103-B(2):213-221.

    This systematic literature review analyzed the influence of the interval between fracture fixation and FRI revision surgery on infection control rates after DAIR. The limited available data suggest that chronic/late-onset FRI managed with DAIR may be associated with a higher rate of recurrence. Level of evidence: IV.

28. Zalavras CG, Singh A, Patzakis MJ: Novel technique for medullary canal débridement in tibia and femur osteomyelitis. *Clin Orthop Relat Res* 2007;461:31-34.

29. Zalavras CG, Sirkin M: Treatment of long bone intramedullary infection using the RIA for removal of infected tissue: Indications, method and clinical results. *Injury* 2010;41(suppl 2):S43-S47.

30. Scarborough M, Li HK, Rombach I, et al: Oral versus intravenous antibiotics for bone and joint infections: The OVIVA non-inferiority RCT. *Health Technol Assess* 2019;23(38):1-92.

This large randomized, open label, noninferiority trial showed that in adults with a clinical diagnosis of bone, joint, or orthopaedic implant–associated infection, there was no outcome difference between oral and intravenous therapy for 6 weeks. Level of evidence: I.

31. Bernard L, Dinh A, Ghout I, et al: Antibiotic treatment for 6 weeks versus 12 weeks in patients with pyogenic vertebral osteomyelitis: An open-label, non-inferiority, randomised, controlled trial. *Lancet* 2015;385(9971):875-882.

32. Tone A, Nguyen S, Devemy F, et al: Six-week versus twelve-week antibiotic therapy for nonsurgically treated diabetic foot osteomyelitis: A multicenter open-label controlled randomized study. *Diabetes Care* 2015;38(2):302-307.

33. Benkabouche M, Racloz G, Spechbach H, Lipsky BA, Gaspoz JM, Uçkay I: Four versus six weeks of antibiotic therapy for osteoarticular infections after implant removal: A randomized trial. *J Antimicrob Chemother* 2019;74(8):2394-2399.

   This trial found no statistically significant difference in the rates of clinical or microbiologic remission between 62 patients randomized to 4 weeks of systemic antibiotic therapy and 61 patients randomized to 6 weeks of therapy after removal of an infected osteoarticular implant. Level of evidence: I.

34. Zalavras CG, Patzakis MJ, Holtom P: Local antibiotic therapy in the treatment of open fractures and osteomyelitis. *Clin Orthop Relat Res* 2004;427:86-93.

35. Metsemakers WJ, Fragomen AT, Moriarty TF, et al: Evidence-based recommendations for local antimicrobial strategies and dead space management in fracture-related infection. *J Orthop Trauma* 2020;34(1):18-29.

   This article summarizes recommendations from an international expert group on the use of local antimicrobials and dead space management in FRIs.

36. Prasarn ML, Ahn J, Achor T, Matuszewski P, Lorich DG, Helfet DL: Management of infected femoral nonunions with a single-staged protocol utilizing internal fixation. *Injury* 2009;40(11):1220-1225.

37. Miller DL, Goswami T, Prayson MJ: Overview of the locking compression plate and its clinical applications in fracture healing. *J Surg Orthop Adv* 2008;17(4):271-281.

38. Wiss DA, Garlich JM: Healing the index humeral shaft nonunion: Risk factors for development of a recalcitrant nonunion in 125 patients. *J Bone Joint Surg Am* 2020;102(5):375-380.

   This retrospective study of 125 patients with humeral shaft nonunion reported that plate fixation with bone graft augmentation remains a successful treatment method. A history of deep infection and two or more prior surgical procedures is associated with the development of a recalcitrant nonunion. Level of evidence: IV.

39. Iqbal HJ, Pidikiti P: Treatment of distal tibia metaphyseal fractures; plating versus intramedullary nailing: A systematic review of recent evidence. *Foot Ankle Surg* 2013;19(3):143-147.

40. Makridis KG, Tosounidis T, Giannoudis PV: Management of infection after intramedullary nailing of long bone fractures: Treatment protocols and outcomes. *Open Orthop J* 2013;7:219-226.

41. Napora JK, Weinberg DS, Eagle BA, Kaufman BR, Sontich JK: Hexapod stacked transport for tibial infected nonunions with bone loss: Long-term functional outcomes. *J Orthop Trauma* 2018;32(1):e12-e18.

   This retrospective cohort study analyzed long-term functional outcomes in patients with posttraumatic infected tibial nonunion having undergone bone transport with hexapod external fixator. This is a reliable technique for infected nonunion of the tibia with bone loss. Improved short Musculoskeletal Functional Assessment scores can be expected from 2 to 8 years, suggesting that full recovery takes longer than previously anticipated. Level of evidence: IV.

42. Anthony JP, Mathes SJ, Alpert BS: The muscle flap in the treatment of chronic lower extremity osteomyelitis: Results in patients over 5 years after treatment. *Plast Reconstr Surg* 1991;88(2):311-318.

43. Swiontkowski MF, Hanel DP, Vedder NB, Schwappach JR: A comparison of short- and long-term intravenous antibiotic therapy in the postoperative management of adult osteomyelitis. *J Bone Joint Surg Br* 1999;81(6):1046-1050.

44. Patzakis MJ, Greene N, Holtom P, Shepherd L, Bravos P, Sherman R: Culture results in open wound treatment with muscle transfer for tibial osteomyelitis. *Clin Orthop Relat Res* 1999;360:66-70.

45. Cho EH, Shammas RL, Carney MJ, et al: Muscle versus fasciocutaneous free flaps in lower extremity traumatic reconstruction: A multicenter outcomes analysis. *Plast Reconstr Surg* 2018;141(1):191-199.

   This multicenter retrospective review found that muscle and fasciocutaneous free flaps achieved comparable rates of limb salvage and functional recovery in acute trauma and chronic traumatic sequelae. Level of evidence: III.

46. Haidari S, IJpma FFA, Metsemakers WJ, et al: The role of negative-pressure wound therapy in patients with fracture-related infection: A systematic review and critical appraisal. *Biomed Res Int* 2021;2021:7742227.

   This systematic review assessed the role of negative-pressure wound therapy in the management of soft-tissue defects in patients with FRI and found no clear scientific evidence to support the use of negative-pressure wound therapy as definitive treatment. Negative-pressure wound therapy may be safe for a few days as temporary soft-tissue coverage until definitive soft-tissue management can be achieved with a local or free flap. Level of evidence: IV.

47. Mifsud M, Ferguson JY, Stubbs DA, Ramsden AJ, McNally MA: Simultaneous debridement, Ilizarov reconstruction and free muscle flaps in the management of complex tibial infection. *J Bone Jt Infect* 2020;6(3):63-72.

   This is a retrospective study of 57 consecutive patients with chronic osteomyelitis or infected nonunion who underwent simultaneous débridement and reconstruction with an Ilizarov fixator and free muscle flap transfer. Simultaneous reconstruction is safe but requires careful planning and logistic considerations. Level of evidence: IV.

48. Ahlmann E, Patzakis M, Roidis N, Shepherd L, Holtom P: Comparison of anterior and posterior iliac crest bone grafts in terms of harvest-site morbidity and functional outcomes. *J Bone Joint Surg Am* 2002;84(5):716-720.

49. Dawson J, Kiner D, Gardner W 2nd, Swafford R, Nowotarski PJ: The reamer-irrigator-aspirator as a device for harvesting bone graft compared with iliac crest bone graft: Union rates and complications. *J Orthop Trauma* 2014;28(10):584-590.

50. Marchand LS, Rothberg DL, Kubiak EN, Higgins TF: Is this autograft worth it?: The blood loss and transfusion rates associated with reamer irrigator aspirator bone graft harvest. *J Orthop Trauma* 2017;31(4):205-209.

51. Masquelet AC, Begue T: The concept of induced membrane for reconstruction of long bone defects. *Orthop Clin North Am* 2010;41(1):27-37.

52. Mauffrey C, Hake ME, Chadayammuri V, Masquelet AC: Reconstruction of long bone infections using the induced membrane technique: Tips and tricks. *J Orthop Trauma* 2016;30(6):e188-e193.

53. Taylor BC, Hancock J, Zitzke R, Castaneda J: Treatment of bone loss with the induced membrane technique: Techniques and outcomes. *J Orthop Trauma* 2015;29(12):554-557.

54. Morwood MP, Streufert BD, Bauer A, et al: Intramedullary nails yield superior results compared with plate fixation when using the Masquelet technique in the femur and tibia. *J Orthop Trauma* 2019;33(11):547-552.

    This retrospective study of 123 patients treated with the induced membrane technique compared intramedullary nail with plate fixation and reported that multiple grafting procedures were required in a significantly lower proportion of patients treated with intramedullary nail fixation. Level of evidence: III.

55. Judet R, Judet J, Orlandini J, Patel A: Osteo-muscular decortication (osteo-periosteal pediculated grafts). *Rev Chir Orthop Reparatrice Appar Mot* 1967;53(1):43-63.

56. Urist MR: Bone: Formation by autoinduction. *Science* 1965;150(3698):893-899.

57. Cheng H, Jiang W, Phillips FM, et al: Osteogenic activity of the fourteen types of human bone morphogenetic proteins (BMPs). *J Bone Joint Surg Am* 2003;85(8):1544-1552.

58. Friedlaender GE, Perry CR, Cole JD, et al: Osteogenic protein-1 (bone morphogenetic protein-7) in the treatment of tibial nonunions. *J Bone Joint Surg Am* 2001;83-A(suppl 1, pt 2):S151-S158.

59. Tressler MA, Richards JE, Sofianos D, Comrie FK, Kregor PJ, Obremskey WT: Bone morphogenetic protein-2 compared to autologous iliac crest bone graft in the treatment of long bone nonunion. *Orthopedics* 2011;34(12):e877-e884.

60. Morison Z, Vicente M, Schemitsch EH, McKee MD: The treatment of atrophic, recalcitrant long-bone nonunion in the upper extremity with human recombinant bone morphogenetic protein-7 (rhBMP-7) and plate fixation: A retrospective review. *Injury* 2016;47(2):356-363.

61. Papanagiotou M, Dailiana ZH, Karachalios T, et al: RhBMP-7 for the treatment of nonunion of fractures of long bones. *Bone Joint J* 2015;97-B(7):997-1003.

62. Chan DS, Garland J, Infante A, Sanders RW, Sagi HC: Wound complications associated with bone morphogenetic protein-2 in orthopaedic trauma surgery. *J Orthop Trauma* 2014;28(10):599-604.

63. Lowenberg DW, Feibel RJ, Louie KW, Eshima I: Combined muscle flap and Ilizarov reconstruction for bone and soft tissue defects. *Clin Orthop Relat Res* 1996;332:37-51.

64. Paley D, Maar DC: Ilizarov bone transport treatment for tibial defects. *J Orthop Trauma* 2000;14(2):76-85.

65. Duffy GP, Wood MB, Rock MG, Sim FH: Vascularized free fibular transfer combined with autografting for the management of fracture nonunions associated with radiation therapy. *J Bone Joint Surg Am* 2000;82(4):544-554.

66. Malizos KN, Zalavras CG, Soucacos PN, Beris AE, Urbaniak JR: Free vascularized fibular grafts for reconstruction of skeletal defects. *J Am Acad Orthop Surg* 2004;12(5):360-369.

SECTION 6

Bone, Joint, and Soft-Tissue Infections

Section Editor:
Aaron J. Tande, MD, FIDSA

CHAPTER 22

Pediatric Musculoskeletal Infections

ISAAC P. THOMSEN, MD, MSCI • LAWSON A. COPLEY, MD, MBA, FAAOS

ABSTRACT

Musculoskeletal infection in children is different from that commonly occurring in adults. Musculoskeletal infection in adults predominantly occurs among populations at risk for acquiring infections through inoculation from surgical implants, intravenous drug use, and trauma (open fractures) or alteration of the ability of the host to respond to the infection (eg, diabetes and vasculopathy). Children are generally a healthy, immunocompetent population who acquire infection through the bloodstream. Given the circulatory pattern that distributes blood flow to the end of long bones with large joint capsules and open epiphyseal plates, a unique and important feature of pediatric bone, the pathophysiology of the disease in pediatrics favors hematogenous distribution to these regions, allowing a mechanism for initiation. Another unique feature of pediatric infection is the age-based distribution of causative pathogens, which leads to specific organism identification based on the maturation of the immune system and environmental exposure risks. Therefore, neonates are exposed to *Streptococcus agalactiae* and *Enterobacteriaceae* during the perinatal period, preschool-age children to *Kingella kingae* and *Streptococcus pneumoniae*, and school-age children to *Staphylococcus aureus* and *Streptococcus pyogenes*. It is important to summarize recent developments in the evaluation and treatment of children with bone and/or joint infections.

Dr. Thomsen or an immediate family member serves as a paid consultant to or is an employee of Horizon Therapeutics. Neither Dr. Copley nor any immediate family member has received anything of value from or has stock or stock options held in a commercial company or institution related directly or indirectly to the subject of this chapter.

Keywords: acute hematogenous osteomyelitis; infection; septic arthritis; *Staphylococcus aureus*

INTRODUCTION

Evidence-based evaluation and treatment of children with acute hematogenous osteomyelitis and septic arthritis are challenging because there have been relatively few randomized prospective investigations devoted to pediatric musculoskeletal infection. Important aspects of the pathogenesis, diagnosis, and treatment of these important invasive pediatric infections all should be considered.

ACUTE HEMATOGENOUS OSTEOMYELITIS

In 2021, the Pediatric Infectious Diseases Society and Infectious Diseases Society of America formed a study group that systematically reviewed the relevant literature to create a comprehensive clinical practice guideline for AHO using the Grading of Recommendations Assessment, Development, and Evaluation (GRADE) method.[1] This study group determined the need for separate guidelines for acute bacterial arthritis, given the substantial differences between children who have bone infections and those who have primary septic arthritis. Together, these guidelines will help to frame decision making during the evaluation and treatment of children with bone and/or joint infections as well as demonstrate gaps in existing evidence and identify opportunities for future research that may help close the gaps. **Figures 1** through **5** provide case illustrations of several principles involved with imaging, diagnosis, and surgical decision making for children with osteomyelitis and septic arthritis.

Given the high rate of culture positivity and moderate rate of initial bacteremia, the diagnosis of acute bone infection in children is typically straightforward. Common presenting symptoms include subjective fever, focal pain in the region of the infection, and limited use of the affected

Section 6: Bone, Joint, and Soft-Tissue Infections

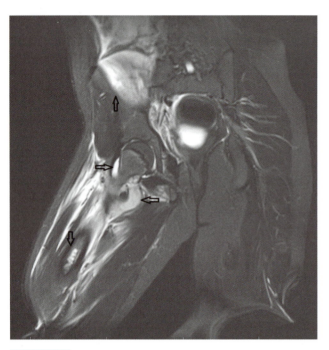

FIGURE 1 Coronal short tau inversion recovery (STIR) magnetic resonance image from a 13-year-old boy with fever, inability to bear weight, and methicillin-sensitive *Staphylococcus aureus* bacteremia. Magnetic resonance image was obtained to visualize surgically drainable infection for source control. Findings on this image include infectious myositis of the right iliacus muscle (up arrow); moderate hip joint effusion concerning for possible septic arthritis (right arrow); extensive fluid collection of the iliopsoas tendon sheath (left arrow); and marrow signal abnormality of the right femur shaft suggestive of osteomyelitis (down arrow). The coronal STIR sequence additionally showed osteomyelitis of the right proximal and distal femur.

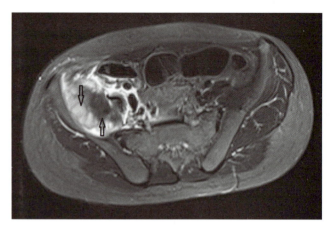

FIGURE 2 Axial short tau inversion recovery (STIR) magnetic resonance image of the pelvis showing a moderately large abscess (down arrow) under the displaced right iliacus muscle (up arrow). The axial STIR sequence additionally confirmed the iliopsoas tendon sheath abscess, right hip joint effusion, and right proximal femur osteomyelitis.

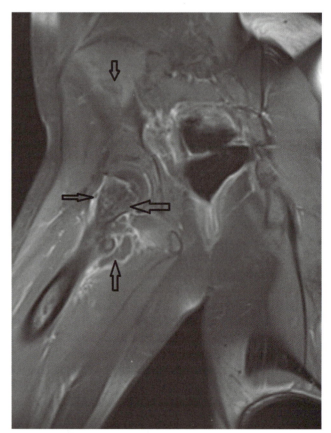

FIGURE 4 Postcontrast coronal fat-saturated T1-weighted magnetic resonance image of the pelvis and proximal femur showing the osteomyelitis (left arrow), septic arthritis (right arrow), iliopsoas tendon sheath abscess (up arrow), and iliacus infectious myositis with abscess (down arrow). The magnetic resonance image was interpreted as showing evidence of the iliopsoas tendon sheath abscess, but the other findings were not recognized by the radiologist or the orthopaedic surgeon. The child was therefore taken to surgery only to drain the iliopsoas tendon sheath abscess.

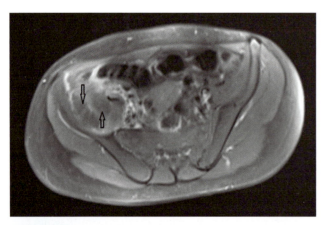

FIGURE 3 Postcontrast axial fat-saturated T1-weighted magnetic resonance image of the pelvis showing the iliac fossa abscess (down arrow) under the right iliacus muscle (up arrow).

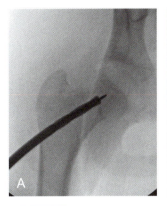
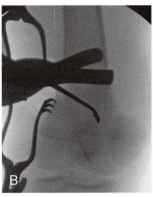

FIGURE 5 Three days after no appropriate clinical or laboratory improvement was demonstrated, the child described in Figure 4 was returned to the operating room, without additional imaging and underwent exploration with irrigation and drainage of the right iliac fossa abscess, irrigation and drainage of the right hip septic arthritis, drill decompression of the right proximal femur (**A**, AP intraoperative fluoroscopic view), and incision of bone cortex with irrigation and débridement of the right distal femur (**B**, AP intraoperative fluoroscopic view). All four intraoperative cultures were positive for methicillin-sensitive *Staphylococcus aureus*. The following day, the patient became afebrile, the bacteremia resolved, and his C-reactive protein level began to decrease.

region of the musculoskeletal system. Signs of osteomyelitis include measured fever (>38.0°C) and focal tenderness in the region of the metaphysis of long bones or equivalent sites (eg, posterior tuberosity of the calcaneus or inferior pubic ramus of the pelvis). Although osteomyelitis may occur in children of any age, the median age of children with osteomyelitis is approximately 8 years. Preverbal children are often unable to clearly communicate symptoms, but the physical findings are very similar across all age groups. Antibiotic treatment is the mainstay of therapy but, in some situations, surgical source control is a necessary supplement.[2] Antibiotic selection should be guided by culture acquisition and susceptibility testing of the causative organism whenever it is practical to obtain a specimen from the site of infection. In 2020, a multicenter pediatric orthopaedic study group investigated the rate and spectrum of culture-positive bone infections at 18 tertiary pediatric medical centers in the United States.[3] It was noted that *Staphylococcus aureus* remains the most frequently identified pathogen across the United States, but there is substantial regional variation in the relative prevalence of other causative pathogens, as well as local rates of methicillin and clindamycin susceptibility among *S aureus*.[3] Because antibiotic resistance evolves over time, attempting to identify the causative pathogen whenever possible remains best practice. At a minimum, an aerobic blood culture should be obtained for every child who is suspected to have a deep infection of bone, before the administration of antibiotics. This practice is helpful given the moderate rate of bacteremia among children with osteomyelitis.[4] In addition, in 2019, it was reported that if MRI with sedation is performed to evaluate a child suspected to have osteomyelitis, a biopsy and culture by trocar, with an 11-gauge needle, should be considered while the child is still under anesthesia for the MRI.[5] Given that *S aureus* is responsible for most childhood osteomyelitis, antibiotic selection is sometimes made empirically and tailored according to methicillin or clindamycin susceptibility rates within local communities or institutions.

Antibiotic Treatment

Antimicrobial therapy should be guided by culture results and susceptibility data whenever possible. Empiric antimicrobial therapy includes, at a minimum, an agent with activity against methicillin-susceptible *S aureus* (eg, clindamycin). Activity against methicillin-resistant *S aureus* (MRSA) is warranted in regions where local prevalence is high, and for preschool-age children, an agent with activity against *Kingella kingae* (eg, cephalexin) is typically warranted as well. Antibiotic treatment is commonly given in a sequential parenteral-to-oral manner, with intravenous administration continued until sufficient clinical and laboratory improvement has occurred to minimize concern regarding relapse or hospital readmission. This decision is often guided by temperature trending, resolution of bacteremia, and decline of inflammatory marker values over time.[6] Before discharge and transition to oral antibiotic therapy, the child should be afebrile and clinically improving with a reassuring C-reactive protein (CRP) trend.

According to a prospective randomized trial, uncomplicated cases of osteomyelitis may be treated with antibiotic therapy that lasts for as little as 3 weeks.[7] However, this study population did not include MRSA or other virulent *S aureus* strains commonly encountered in the United States. Consideration may be given to targeting approximately 3 to 4 weeks of total therapy in uncomplicated cases, provided there is clinical and laboratory resolution within that time frame. Two studies of pediatric AHO demonstrated that even in the setting of concomitant *S aureus* bacteremia, early transition to oral therapy (often 3 to 5 days) and a duration of 3 to 4 weeks for mild to moderate cases was not associated with treatment failure compared with prolonged courses of therapy.[8,9]

Surgical Treatment

As of 2022, surgical decision making has yet to be standardized for children with acute hematogenous osteomyelitis (AHO).[10] Some children undergo multiple surgeries in the effort to achieve source control, whereas others are treated with minimal or no surgery.[2] Indications for surgical intervention are often based on the presence and size of abscess identified on MRI and the existence of contiguous septic arthritis. Children with large abscesses or suspected contiguous septic arthritis routinely undergo surgery, with the occasional occurrence of multiple surgeries. Other findings that generally indicate that surgical evaluation may be warranted include prolonged fever, persistent bacteremia, and/or progressive increase of inflammatory markers despite appropriate antimicrobial therapy. However, the specific techniques of surgical source control may vary widely from surgeon to surgeon.[10] Because surgical source control is only a part of the management of osteomyelitis, the consideration of differences in outcomes for surgically treated children versus those for children treated solely with antibiotics is based simply on differences in severity of illness that might drive surgical treatment. Children treated with antibiotics with or without surgery tend to have similar resolution of infection. However, infected bone, which has been architecturally altered by surgical decompression, is vulnerable to pathologic fracture and other intermediate or long-term adverse outcomes that would not be anticipated among children who were treated with antibiotics alone. The treatment of these children is invariably less complicated than for those who required surgery to attain source control.

Complications and Outcomes

Children with osteomyelitis have an increased risk for deep vein thrombosis (DVT). In 2018, it was noted that recognizing the pattern of clinical presentation for this occurrence is important as there is a tendency for these children to have greater severity of illness with a high rate of bacteremia with MRSA as the clinical isolate.[11] Awareness of these characteristics may lead to earlier diagnosis of the DVT through liberal use of ultrasonography whenever children with osteomyelitis are admitted to the intensive care unit. One study found that surgery occurred at a higher rate among children with osteomyelitis and DVT compared with that of children without DVT (89.3% versus 21.2%) with more surgeries per child (2.1 versus 0.7).[11] Anticoagulation therapy is a necessary adjunct for these children due to the risk of pulmonary embolism. Because the anticoagulation must be managed for children who may have more than one trip to the operating room, it is prudent to use unfractionated heparin until the surgical source control has been established. Because postthrombotic syndrome is exceedingly rare among children with osteomyelitis and DVT, a prolonged anticoagulation course may not be necessary.[11]

Overall, children with osteomyelitis have good long-term clinical outcomes. A 2019 study of 195 children with acute osteomyelitis found a long-term adverse outcome rate of 7.9% that occurred disproportionately among children with the highest risk, based on a clinical severity of illness score that was determined during the first few days of their initial hospitalization.[12] At a mean follow-up of 2.5 years, 41% of children with osteomyelitis had normal radiographic findings and a normal physical examination and 51.1% had minor radiographic findings but were without clinical abnormalities.[12] The children who were found to have profound skeletal abnormalities required ongoing surveillance or surgical intervention given the effect on their skeletal anatomy and function. These adverse outcomes, including osteonecrosis, joint destruction, deformity, and limb length inequality, occurred in 32.0% of children with severe illness but only in 5.9% and 1.3% of children with moderate or mild illness, respectively.[12]

Understanding the risk for long-term complications among children with osteomyelitis is an important factor in consideration of follow-up duration and need for subspecialty evaluations at tertiary pediatric centers. Given the rarity of long-term adverse outcomes, prolonged subspecialty follow-up may be rarely needed, except among children with severe illness. In general, children with uncomplicated osteomyelitis do not require follow-up beyond the duration of antibiotic therapy. This benefits families of children with mild or moderate illness who would otherwise be obligated to travel long-distance and require days off work for these follow-up evaluations. Children who undergo multiple surgeries and who have high severity of illness are often treated with antibiotics for a longer duration, up to 2 to 3 months, to achieve clinical and laboratory normalization. It is appropriate for these children who are at higher risk of long-term adverse outcomes to be seen by a subspecialist to obtain radiographs of the region of infection. This will generally allow detection of problems that are evolving and that may need to be followed up for a longer period.

PRIMARY SEPTIC ARTHRITIS

The evaluation of children suspected to have primary septic arthritis is inherently uncertain because of a variety of inflammatory and reactive conditions that mimic infection. There is also a high rate of culture-negative septic arthritis, which is reported in up to 65% of patients, even when nucleated cell counts are higher than 50,000 cells/mL.[3,13,14] A 2022 study reported that among the conditions that mimic septic arthritis are viral processes, reactive arthritis, inflammatory arthritis, minor trauma, and hematologic disorders.[14] Clinical prediction algorithms have been developed to differentiate septic arthritis from noninfectious conditions with variable results. These algorithms offer limited guidance in cases that seemingly contradict the rules of prediction. A 2022 report advocates for a systematic approach that takes into consideration laboratory normalcy and the relative elevation of a variety of laboratory values of the affected child to establish a level of concern to guide judgment under uncertainty.[14] In general, a careful history and physical examination followed by systematic review of laboratory studies and basic imaging will help clinicians to distinguish between an evolving infection and other conditions. However, trending of inflammatory markers with close, early follow-up is a helpful and safe practice when one is considering inflammatory or reactive etiologies. This practice minimizes sedated imaging and procedural intervention in cases of transient synovitis or poststreptococcal reactive arthritis. Children with septic arthritis typically present with symptoms of subjective fever, limited use of the affected extremity, warmth, and swelling of the joint involved. On physical examination, an effusion is sometimes palpable in the joints, which are accessible (knee, ankle, elbow, and wrist). They also have tenderness when palpating the joint capsule and painful range of motion, even when minimal range of motion is passively attempted. Similar to that which occurs in adults, joint infections in children tend to involve larger joints with the hip, knee, and shoulder among the most commonly affected.

Spectrum of Primary Septic Arthritis

Septic arthritis is challenging because of the heterogeneity of pathogens that aggregate into age-specific groups.[14] Identifying the causative bacteria may be challenging in centers with limited access to polymerase chain reaction (PCR) testing, which greatly improves the pathogen detection rate compared with culture-based methods.[13] *K kingae* is the most common pathogen identified among children aged 6 to 48 months.[14,15] This pathogen often has a milder clinical presentation. In a 2021 study, children with *Kingella* septic arthritis had lower initial CRP levels (4.8 versus 9.3 mg/dL) than that of children with other confirmed pathogens.[15] A study of children in Israel with *Kingella* infections found that 22% had a normal CRP level, 31.8% had a normal erythrocyte sedimentation rate, and 25% were afebrile.[16] In another study, 70.4% of children with *Kingella* septic arthritis were afebrile and had lower inflammatory markers, a lower bacteremia rate (3.6% versus 61.9%), and a lower complication rate.[17] This mild clinical presentation in the 6- to 48-month age group raises concern regarding the use of clinical predictive algorithms to differentiate noninfectious conditions from *Kingella* septic arthritis because viral reactive arthritis or transient synovitis is occasionally incorrectly diagnosed in these children. Children with septic arthritis due to other pathogens tend to have a more traditional clinical presentation with fever and moderately elevated inflammatory markers.

Approach to Management

It is common to initiate treatment of primary septic arthritis with invasive procedures that have a twofold purpose. First, acquisition of material for cell count, culture, and PCR may be performed in a variety of settings including the emergency department, fluoroscopy suite, with or without ultrasonographic guidance, hospital bedside, or operating room. If a period of observation is available after aspiration, a small percentage of these children who have undergone aspiration and received antibiotics may improve to the extent that the treating clinicians may elect to forgo additional invasive treatment. In the United States, surgery is frequently elected as part of the treatment for primary septic arthritis. This may involve aspiration lavage, arthroscopy, or arthrotomy for irrigation and drainage. Surgeon preference and comfort with arthroscopy often determine the selection of method for surgery, as outcomes are sufficiently similar regardless of the selection.

Following surgical drainage, antibiotic therapy is the mainstay of management leading to resolution. Complicated cases may undergo more than one surgical drainage procedure and receive a longer antibiotic course, but most uncomplicated cases are amenable to a relatively brief hospitalization with sequential parenteral-to-oral antibiotic therapy. A study of short-duration antimicrobial therapy involved children randomized to receive either a short course (10 days) or long course (30 days) of antibiotics for primary septic arthritis, and short-duration therapy was found to be as effective as a longer course outside the neonatal age group.[18] However, one important caveat to these data was that MRSA was rare in this cohort, and although MRSA is not highly prevalent in many other countries, it continues to be a major concern in the United States. MRSA, by virtue of resistance to the highly effective and rapidly bactericidal beta-lactam class of antimicrobials, may require more prolonged therapy. Therefore, in the absence of clinical outcome data for a short-duration treatment of acute bacterial arthritis due to MRSA, there is not enough support for this in the United States. One study found no difference in outcomes when children were treated with a shorter course of parenteral therapy (7.4 days) when compared with a longer therapy (18.6 days) before transition to oral therapy for 4 weeks of total treatment.[19] It is current practice to transition children from intravenous to oral therapy as soon as they demonstrate clinical improvement with a sustained decline in inflammatory markers. Some groups advocate for the sole use of CRP to guide decision making while transitioning to oral therapy. It has been suggested that CRP is a better indicator for infection resolution than erythrocyte sedimentation rate, which tends to remain elevated after infection is resolved.[20] In one prospective randomized trial, no child relapsed when CRP level reached less than 2 mg/dL.[21] However, in a 2019 retrospective study evaluating the efficacy of using CRP level of less than 2 mg/dL for discharge of children with septic arthritis, this was found to be a poor predictor of readmission and relapse.[22]

CONTIGUOUS OSTEOMYELITIS AND SEPTIC ARTHRITIS

It is commonly thought that osteomyelitis and septic arthritis are different manifestations of a deep infection process along a continuum of disease. In 2021, this paradigm was challenged with evidence illuminating many marked differences between primary and secondary forms of septic arthritis.[23] In a study comparing 134 children with primary septic arthritis with 105 children who had contiguous osteomyelitis, children with primary septic arthritis were younger (2.4 versus 7.4 years), had lower initial CRP level (6.4 versus 15.7 mg/dL), and had lower bacteremia rate (20% versus 69.5%).[23] Children with contiguous osteomyelitis were more likely infected with *S aureus* (77.1% versus 32.1%).[23] Children with primary septic arthritis had shorter hospitalizations (4 versus 8 days), required less intensive care (1.5% versus 21%), had fewer readmissions (5.2% versus 17.2%), and had a lower complication rate (0.7% versus 38.1%).[23] Similarly, a 2021 study of 450 patients with pediatric musculoskeletal infections (including 218 AHO, 132 primary septic arthritis, and 103 with septic arthritis and contiguous osteomyelitis) found that patients with concurrent AHO/septic arthritis had longer hospital stays, required longer duration of antibiotic therapy, and were more likely to have prolonged bacteremia and require intensive care.[9] Therefore, distinguishing between primary and secondary septic arthritis provides a better framework by which to improve evaluation and treatment guidelines.

Initial Imaging

Imaging of children with contiguous bone and joint infections always starts with plain radiograph. The typical findings often include deep soft-tissue swelling overlying the metaphyseal bone in the area of the infection. In many cases, the plain radiographs may reveal a joint effusion of the adjacent joint. If this is not visible on a radiograph, ultrasonography may be used, particularly for the hip joint, to visualize the joint effusion and help consider the possibility that septic arthritis may be part of the clinical spectrum of the infection. Because concurrent osteomyelitis and septic arthritis may be best detected with MRI, some institutions have increasingly turned toward this modality for musculoskeletal infection evaluations.[4] This has potential for excessive resource utilization and greater anesthesia exposure for young children. It also risks delay of intervention for children with primary joint infections. To guide the decision for MRI, prediction algorithms have been developed to recognize children at greater risk of having contiguous osteomyelitis.[24-26] One study identified predictors of osteomyelitis including age older than 3.6 years, CRP level greater than 13.8 mg/L, symptoms longer than 3 days, and absolute neutrophil count greater than 8,600 cells/mL.[24] The presence of three or more of these criteria resulted in a sensitivity of 90% and specificity of 67% for adjacent osteomyelitis.[24] This model was later validated in 2018, which led to recommendations that children with three or more predictors should undergo MRI, whereas those with one or no risk factors should forgo MRI.[26]

Plain radiographs play an important role in the aftermath of treatment for osteomyelitis as this modality will help to identify the intermediate and long-term adverse outcomes that may emerge. Repeat MRI during disease resolution is not recommended as this form of imaging will often raise concern regarding the amount of residual inflammation and healing, which is part of the process of recovery. If a child is demonstrating appropriate clinical and laboratory improvement, the plain radiograph is a better imaging tool to see the big picture of bone and joint health. Because children with contiguous bone and joint infection are at higher risk of adverse long-term outcomes, this population often requires longer follow-up with subspecialists, particularly if they had high severity of illness or had a prolonged and complicated hospital-based course of treatment as a result of multiple surgeries.

Advanced Imaging and Use of Contrast Enhancement

Adoption of MRI has allowed more precise visualization of suspected musculoskeletal infection. This has reduced unplanned returns to the operating room via earlier detection of adjacent infections that may be addressed during the index surgical procedure. However, gadolinium-based contrast agents are increasingly scrutinized because of long-lasting retention in the brain. Because contrast use results in a longer imaging duration, adoption of protocols for imaging without contrast is potentially advantageous. It was reported in 2019 that T1- and T2-weighted fat saturation and short tau inversion recovery sequences have similar sensitivity and specificity as do contrast imaging.[27] An innovative approach for musculoskeletal infection MRI involves coordinated interdisciplinary communication between orthopaedic surgery, radiology, and anesthesiology services.[5] Compared with a fragmented workflow, the use of a coordinated MRI algorithm led to reduced scan duration (35 versus 73.6

minutes), fewer sequences (4.6 versus 7.5), shorter anesthesia time (53.2 versus 94.1 minutes), and more procedures performed under the same anesthesia session as the MRI (84.6% versus 70.2%).[5]

SUMMARY

The evaluation and treatment of children with osteomyelitis and septic arthritis have evolved over the past decade through better understanding of the age-specific microbiologic epidemiology of septic arthritis and the substantial differences between children with septic arthritis and those with associated osteomyelitis. Because of this, the osteoarticular infection continuum has been challenged with recognition of primary septic arthritis as a distinct clinical entity with a lower risk of complications compared with that of children with contiguous osteomyelitis. Osteomyelitis is predominantly a disease associated with *S aureus* with a severity-driven risk for DVT and adverse long-term outcomes. *K kingae* is now increasingly recognized for its role as a common pathogen affecting children aged 6 to 48 months. The use of MRI has greatly evolved over the past decade using carefully coordinated workflows. Concerns for long-term contrast material deposition in the brain as well as a desire to limit the duration of anesthesia for young children have led to refinement of imaging protocols without loss of fidelity. Although the optimal duration of antimicrobial treatment remains to be clearly defined, recent work has led to consideration of short-duration therapy for children with osteomyelitis and primary septic arthritis. However, caution should be given for children with osteomyelitis who may have greater severity of illness or for children with septic arthritis who may have contiguous osteomyelitis for whom a shorter course of treatment may lead to relapse from residual infection.

KEY STUDY POINTS

- A concerted effort has been made in the past decade to explore and publish evidence-based guidance on the topics of AHO and acute bacterial arthritis in children.
- AHO is predominantly due to *S aureus*, which causes illness ranging from mild to severe, which has implications for the risk of DVT and long-term adverse outcomes.
- Primary septic arthritis refers to acute bacterial arthritis in children, which is not associated with adjacent osteomyelitis and is due to a broad spectrum of pathogens that aggregate in age-specific groups.
- There are many marked differences between children with primary septic arthritis and those who have septic arthritis associated with contiguous osteomyelitis.
- Judicious use of MRI may help identify children with septic arthritis and contiguous osteomyelitis or recognize indications for surgical intervention that might otherwise be missed without this modality.

ANNOTATED REFERENCES

1. Woods CR, Bradley JS, Chatterjee A, et al: Clinical practice guideline by the Pediatric Infectious Diseases Society and the Infectious Diseases Society of America: 2021 guideline on diagnosis and management of acute hematogenous osteomyelitis in pediatrics. *J Pediatric Infect Dis Soc* 2021;10(8):801-844.

   This is the culmination of an 11-year endeavor using the Grading of Recommendations Assessment, Development, and Evaluation methodology following extensive literature review of the bone and joint infection guideline panel of Pediatric Infectious Diseases Society/Infectious Diseases Society of America. Representation from 19 tertiary pediatric centers in North America generated this clinical practice guideline to improve care for children with AHO and identify knowledge gaps for future research. Level of evidence: II.

2. Tuason D, Gheen T, Sun D, Huang R, Copley L: Clinical and laboratory parameters associated with multiple surgeries in children with acute hematogenous osteomyelitis. *J Pediatr Orthop* 2014;34(5):565-570.

3. Koehler RJ, Shore BJ, Hedequest D, et al: Defining the volume of consultations for musculoskeletal infection encountered by pediatric orthopaedic services in the United States. *PLoS One* 2020;15(6):e0234055.

   This work was accomplished by pediatric orthopaedic principal investigators at 18 tertiary pediatric centers. A retrospective database was gathered for all musculoskeletal infection consultations within these orthopaedic practices. This study recognized that 10% of all acute orthopaedic consultations in the emergency department and inpatient hospital are for the evaluation of musculoskeletal infection. The regional variation of causative pathogens and the rates of MRSA and methicillin-sensitive *S aureus* are reported. Level of evidence: III.

4. Section J, Gibbons SD, Barton T, Greenberg DE, Jo CH, Copley LA: Microbiological culture methods for pediatric musculoskeletal infection: A guideline for optimal use. *J Bone Joint Surg Am* 2015;97(6):441-449.

5. Ojeaga PO, Hammer MR, Lindsay EA, Tareen NG, Jo CH, Copley LA: Quality improvement of magnetic resonance imaging for musculoskeletal infection in children results in decreased scan duration and decreased contrast use. *J Bone Joint Surg Am* 2019;101(18):1679-1688.

   This study is a retrospective review of a 6-year process improvement initiative in which interdisciplinary coordination and communication among orthopaedic surgery, radiology, anesthesia, and the operating room nursing staff led to substantial, progressive improvement of MRI utilization and workflows. There was a decrease in MRI acquisition, imaging duration, sequences per image, anesthesia use, and anesthesia duration. There was an increase in the rate of surgery immediately following the MRI while under continued anesthesia while the child was transported from the imager to the operating room. Level of evidence: III.

6. Copley LA, Kinsler A, Gheen T, Shar A, Sun D, Browne R: The impact of evidence-based clinical practice guidelines applied by a multidisciplinary team for the care of children with osteomyelitis. *J Bone Joint Surg Am* 2013;95(8):686-693.

7. Peltola H, Pääkkönen M, Kallio P, Kallio MJ, Osteomyelitis-Septic Arthritis Study Group: Short- versus long-term antimicrobial treatment for acute hematogenous osteomyelitis of childhood: Prospective, randomized trial on 131 culture-positive cases. *Pediatr Infect Dis J* 2010;29(12):1123-1128.

8. Sanchez MJ, Patel K, Lindsay EA, et al: Early transition to oral antimicrobial therapy among children with *Staphylococcus aureus* bacteremia and acute hematogenous osteomyelitis. *Pediatr Infect Dis J* 2022;41(9):690-695.

   This study illustrates that a one-size-fits-all approach is not appropriate for the clinical occurrence of *S aureus* bacteremia and AHO. A severity-adjusted approach to the decision to transition to early oral therapy will avoid prolonged hospitalization and parenteral therapy for children with mild or moderate illness severity. However, children with severe illness will often need surgical source control and a prolonged inpatient course of antibiotic therapy to ensure resolution. Level of evidence: III.

9. Yi J, Wood JB, Creech CB, et al: Clinical epidemiology and outcomes of pediatric musculoskeletal infections. *J Pediatr* 2021;234:236-244.e2.

   This is a retrospective study of 453 children with osteomyelitis and/or septic arthritis. It confirms *S aureus* to be the most common pathogen for these conditions with a community rate of MRSA of 25%. The combination of osteomyelitis and septic arthritis was associated with longer hospitalization, longer duration of antibiotic therapy, prolonged bacteremia, and intensive care unit admissions. Level of evidence: IV.

10. Upasani VV, Burns JD, Bastrom TP, et al: Practice variation in the surgical management of children with acute hematogenous osteomyelitis. *J Pediatr Orthop* 2022;42(5):e520-e525.

    Data from 18 pediatric medical centers were aggregated to assess the surgical intervention practice variation in current use to manage osteomyelitis. More than 1,000 children were studied with a 62% rate of intervention. Some centers demonstrated a tendency toward greater frequency of surgical intervention, which ranged from 26% to 72%. Level of evidence: III.

11. Ligon JA, Journeycake JM, Josephs SC, Tareen NG, Lindsay EA, Copley LAB: Differentiation of deep venous thrombosis among children with or without osteomyelitis. *J Pediatr Orthop* 2018;38(10):e597-e603.

    This study evaluated DVT rates among children at a tertiary care pediatric center. Children who had underlying osteomyelitis were compared with those who did not. Children without osteomyelitis had many comorbidities and a high incidence of postthrombotic syndrome. The study also compared children with osteomyelitis with or without DVT and found that those with DVT had higher illness severity, intensive care admissions, and MRSA bacteremia levels. Level of evidence: III.

12. Vorhies JS, Lindsay EA, Tareen NG, Kellum RJ, Jo CH, Copley LA: Severity adjusted risk of long-term adverse sequelae among children with osteomyelitis. *Pediatr Infect Dis J* 2019;38(1):26-31.

    This is the first prospective long-term clinical outcomes study of 195 children with AHO over 3 years: 139 (71.3%) had clinical follow-up at a mean 2.4 years after their initial hospitalization. The study found a 7.9% rate of adverse outcomes including chondrolysis, osteonecrosis, deformity, and limb length inequality, which was disproportionately identified among children with high severity of illness scores during the hospitalization. Thirty-two percent of children in the severe cohort had complications compared with 5.9% and 1.3% of the moderate or mild cohorts, respectively. Level of evidence: III.

13. Carter K, Doern C, Jo CH, Copley LA: The clinical usefulness of polymerase chain reaction as a supplemental diagnostic tool in the evaluation and the treatment of children with septic arthritis. *J Pediatr Orthop* 2016;36(2):167-172.

14. Klosterman MM, Villani MC, Hamilton EC, Jo CH, Copley LA: Primary septic arthritis in children demonstrates presumed and confirmed varieties which require age-specific evaluation and treatment strategies. *J Pediatr Orthop* 2022;42(1):e27-e33.

    This study establishes the clinical epidemiology of primary septic arthritis within categories of confirmed and presumed varieties. A spectrum of clinical pathogens were identified by culture and/or PCR for children with confirmed primary septic arthritis. These pathogens tended to occur within age-specific groups of the affected children. The skewed age distribution and the relative rates of presumed cases (no identified pathogen) offer guidance for further analysis. The study acknowledges the moderate rate at which children who are initially thought to have presumed septic arthritis are subsequently found to have noninfectious conditions. Level of evidence: III.

15. Villani MC, Hamilton EC, Klosterman MM, Jo CH, Kang LH, Copley LAB: Primary septic arthritis among children 6 to 48 months of age: Implications for PCR acquisition and empiric antimicrobial selection. *J Pediatr Orthop* 2021;41(3):190-196.

    Children aged 6 to 48 months with primary septic arthritis were studied to determine the causative pathogens and the relative rates of presumed and confirmed varieties. *K kingae* was the most frequently identified pathogen followed by *S aureus* and *Streptococcus pneumoniae*. Children with presumed septic arthritis had similar clinical and laboratory presentations as those with *Kingella* infections. A lower rate of PCR acquisition among presumed cases (47.1%) compared with that of the *Kingella* cohort (95.0%) suggests that *Kingella* may be missed when PCR is not used. Level of evidence: III.

16. Dubnov-Raz G, Ephros M, Garty BZ, et al: Invasive pediatric *Kingella kingae* infections: A nationwide collaborative study. *Pediatr Infect Dis J* 2010;29(7):639-643.

17. Gouveia C, Duarte M, Norte S, et al: *Kingella kingae* displaced *S. aureus* as the most common cause of acute septic arthritis in children of all ages. *Pediatr Infect Dis J* 2021;40(7):623-627.

    This longitudinal observational study at a single center determined a high rate of *K kingae* infections, which were found in 51.9% of affected children with a median age of 2 years. The next most frequent pathogens were methicillin-sensitive *S aureus* (19.2%) and group A beta-hemolytic streptococci (9.6%). Level of evidence: IV.

18. Peltola H, Pääkkönen M, Kallio P, Kallio MJ, Osteomyelitis-Septic Arthritis OM-SA Study Group: Prospective, randomized trial of 10 days versus 30 days of antimicrobial treatment, including a short-term course of parenteral therapy, for childhood septic arthritis. *Clin Infect Dis* 2009;48(9):1201-1210.

19. Ballock RT, Newton PO, Evans SJ, Estabrook M, Farnsworth CL, Bradley JS: A comparison of early versus late conversion from intravenous to oral therapy in the treatment of septic arthritis. *J Pediatr Orthop* 2009;29(6):636-642.

20. Pääkkönen M, Kallio MJ, Kallio PE, Peltola H: Sensitivity of erythrocyte sedimentation rate and C-reactive protein in childhood bone and joint infections. *Clin Orthop Relat Res* 2010;468(3):861-866.

21. Pääkkönen M, Peltola H: Management of a child with suspected acute septic arthritis. *Arch Dis Child* 2012;97(3):287-292.

22. Bouchard M, Shefelbine L, Bompadre V: C-reactive protein level at time of discharge is not predictive of risk of reoperation or readmission in children with septic arthritis. *Front Surg* 2019;6:68.

    An 11-year retrospective review of children with septic arthritis determined that CRP levels are not reliable to prevent readmission or revision surgery. Clinical improvement and decreasing CRP levels were recommended as a better guide for discharge planning. Risk for readmission was more frequent for children with antibiotic-resistant strains and atypical bacteria. Level of evidence: III.

23. Hamilton EC, Villani MC, Klosterman MM, Jo CH, Liu J, Copley LAB: Children with primary septic arthritis have a markedly lower risk of adverse outcomes than those with contiguous osteomyelitis. *J Bone Joint Surg Am* 2021;103(13):1229-1237.

    This is a retrospective cohort comparison study of children with primary confirmed septic arthritis (n = 134) and children with septic arthritis associated with osteomyelitis (n = 105). The many marked differences between cohorts were most notable for the rate of adverse outcomes, which was much higher for children with osteomyelitis (38.1% versus 0.7%). Older children with *S aureus* bacteremia and markedly elevated inflammatory markers are more likely to have contiguous osteomyelitis. Level of evidence: III.

24. Rosenfeld S, Bernstein DT, Daram S, Dawson J, Zhang W: Predicting the presence of adjacent infections in septic arthritis in children. *J Pediatr Orthop* 2016;36(1):70-74.

25. Nguyen A, Kan JH, Bisset G, Rosenfeld S: Kocher criteria revisited in the era of MRI: How often does the Kocher criteria identify underlying osteomyelitis? *J Pediatr Orthop* 2017;37(2):e114-e119.

26. Welling BD, Haruno LS, Rosenfeld SB: Validating an algorithm to predict adjacent musculoskeletal infections in pediatric patients with septic arthritis. *Clin Orthop Relat Res* 2018;476(1):153-159.

    This 3-year review of surgically treated children with suspected septic arthritis (n = 109) validates the previously published prediction algorithm in which adjacent infection on MRI was identified by the presence of three or more of the risk factors including older age, longer duration of symptoms, higher CRP level, lower platelet count, and higher absolute neutrophil count. The sensitivity and positive predictive value (86% and 91%, respectively) were found when children satisfied at least three parameters and 100% when four or more were identified. Level of evidence: III.

27. Nguyen JC, Yi PH, Woo KM, Rosas HG: Detection of pediatric musculoskeletal pathology using the fluid-sensitive sequence. *Pediatr Radiol* 2019;49(1):114-121.

    This study compares MRI sequences of 99 studies from 96 children, performed with and without intravenous contrast enhancement. The fluid-sensitive sequences recommended for this purpose resulted in a high agreement between the two radiologists who reviewed the studies for detection of pathology (97% to 100%) and overall impression (93%). Level of evidence: IV.

CHAPTER 23

Septic Arthritis in Adults

DON BAMBINO GENO TAI, MD, MBA • OLIVIER BORENS, MD • PARHAM SENDI, MD

ABSTRACT

Septic arthritis is a serious joint infection that requires prompt recognition and treatment, with the incidence increasing in the past decade. The primary pathogenesis of septic arthritis is hematogenous seeding of the joint, with most caused by gram-positive bacteria. *Staphylococcus aureus* remains the top cause of septic arthritis. Synovial fluid cell count and cultures are the most widely used diagnostic tests. Management should focus on decreasing inflammation through joint lavage or decompression with arthrocentesis, establishing the microbiologic etiology through the timely collection of cultures, and proper antibiotic choice. Further research is needed on the role of molecular techniques in diagnosing septic arthritis. There is also a knowledge gap in the timing of joint lavage, duration, and route of antibiotics for treatment.

Keywords: arthritis; joint infection; septic arthritis; synovitis

---

Dr. Borens or an immediate family member is a member of a speakers' bureau or has made paid presentations on behalf of Lima and Medacta and serves as a board member, owner, officer, or committee member of Swiss Orthopaedic Society. Dr. Sendi or an immediate family member serves as an unpaid consultant to Medacta International SA and serves as a board member, owner, officer, or committee member of Member of the Expert Group on Infection of Swiss Orthopaedics. Neither Dr. Geno Tai nor any immediate family member has received anything of value from or has stock or stock options held in a commercial company or institution related directly or indirectly to the subject of this chapter.

INTRODUCTION

Septic arthritis is an inflammation of the joint space and the surrounding synovial membrane due to infection. Significant morbidity and mortality are associated with septic arthritis. Septic arthritis must be recognized early and requires prompt management by an interdisciplinary team (ie, infectious diseases physicians and orthopaedic surgeons). The delay in diagnosis and treatment leads to the destruction of the cartilage, impairment of joint function, and accelerated degenerative osteoarthritis. Clinicians caring for patients with septic arthritis must have a thorough understanding of the clinical presentations and management options in order to enhance patient outcomes.

INCIDENCE

A 2020 study reported that the in-hospital mortality rate of septic arthritis is estimated between 2% and 4%.[1] In concomitant *Staphylococcus aureus* bacteremia cases, a 2022 review reported that the bloodstream infection itself worsens prognosis with reported mortality rates higher than 50%.[2]

The incidence has been increasing throughout the past decade, possibly because of a growing elderly population alongside individuals with multiple comorbidities, and therefore, risk factors for infection.[3,4] A 2020 study reported an incidence rate of large joint septic arthritis of 13 per 100,000 person-years in New Zealand.[5]

PATHOGENESIS

Hematogenous seeding to the joint is the primary route of infection in septic arthritis. In these cases, bacteremia is either occult and transient or overt with metastatic infection elsewhere. Another route is through contiguous infection from a neighboring anatomic site (ie, necrotizing fasciitis or open fracture). An iatrogenic source (ie, steroid injections, postarthroscopy) is rare. The risk of procedure-related infections has been estimated at less than 1% for arthroscopy. Considering that these procedures are increasingly performed, a 2021 study reported that incidence is increasing.[6]

A 2022 case-control study reported that, the longer septic arthritis remains untreated, the more likely it accelerates osteoarthritis.[7] The biologic basis for this continuum of joint destruction is based on animal studies. The proteolytic and lysosomal enzymes produced from inflammation and bacterial invasion cause the destruction of the cartilage and the synovium[8] (**Figure 1**). Several authors have attempted to classify septic arthritis according to the severity of the synovial reaction and joint destruction. Inflamed synovium without cartilage destruction indicates the early stage of the infection, whereas osteomyelitis of the adjacent bone is a late stage of septic arthritis (continuum of disease progression from stage I to IV).[9] However, preexisting osteoarthritis, comorbidities, and the virulence of microorganisms may influence the dynamic from early to late stages. Although such a classification would be meaningful for several reasons (ie, compatibility of research questions, aiding in decision making for management), there is no uniformly accepted and well-validated classification.

MICROBIOLOGY

Most septic arthritis are monomicrobial infections; less than 10% of cases are polymicrobial.[4] Studies showed that most etiologic organisms are gram-positive bacteria, with more than one-half caused by *S aureus* followed by *Streptococcus* species in 10% to 20% of the cases.[5,10,11] Gram-negative bacteria cause up to 10% of cases. These proportions have been mainly stable throughout the years. However, a 2021 study from Western Australia reported increasing rates of septic arthritis caused by gram-negative bacilli.[12]

Certain organisms can be more common depending on specific patient characteristics or exposures. For example, in a 2020 study of people who inject drugs, there is proportionately more *S aureus*, including methicillin-resistant *S aureus* (MRSA), compared with the general population.[13] Gram-negative bacilli or atypical organisms may be more prevalent among people who are immunocompromised. *Mycoplasma* and *Ureaplasma* species should be considered among patients with hypogammaglobulinemia or a history of genitourinary tract manipulation. A 2022 case series reported that, in disseminated infections, these organisms can cause arthritis with or without genitourinary symptoms.[14] Molds and nontuberculous mycobacteria can cause septic arthritis in this population.[15-17]

Neisseria gonorrhoeae is a sexually transmitted infection that most commonly presents as urethritis or cervicitis. A disseminated infection develops in approximately 0.5% to 3% of patients, with an increasing incidence of gonococcal arthritis in some countries.[18,19] In endemic areas, arthritis can be a manifestation of Lyme disease. The estimated annual incidence of Lyme disease in the United States is 106 cases per 100,000.[20] Although there are high-incidence areas, such as the Northeast

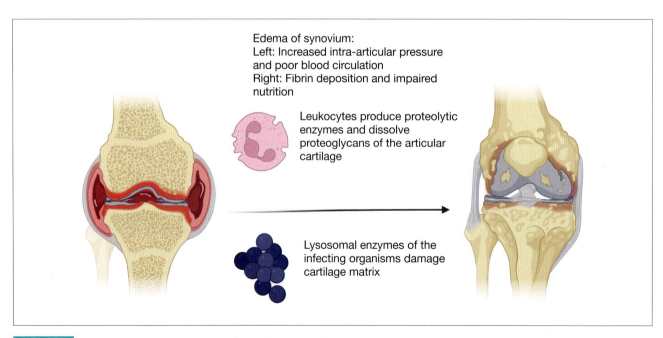

FIGURE 1 Schematic illustration showing the pathogenesis of joint destruction in septic arthritis.

and Upper Midwest regions of the United States, the geographic distribution is expanding into neighboring states.[21] The proportion of patients with Lyme disease who present with arthritis varies considerably between studies and ranges from 3% to 30%.[22,23] The association of clinical features and other uncommon pathogens are listed in **Table 1**.

CLINICAL PRESENTATION

Joint pain, erythema, and swelling are the cardinal manifestations of septic arthritis. Joint pain can be associated with systemic symptoms such as fever, chills, and malaise. However, only 30% to 40% present with fever.[24] Most patients (>90%) have involvement of a single large joint.[4] The most commonly affected joint is the knee, followed by the shoulder or hip. Elbow, wrist, foot, and ankle are less frequently affected (<10% of cases).[10] A 2023 case series reported that sternoclavicular, sacroiliac, and acromioclavicular septic arthritis are more common among persons who inject drugs.[25] A 2022 retrospective study reported that septic arthritis of the symphysis pubis is a rarer type that occurs among patients with a history of prostate or gynecologic cancer who underwent surgery and radiation therapy. These patients present with pelvic pain, particularly when sitting or standing.[26]

Involvement of multiple joints does not rule out the diagnosis, particularly in cases with prolonged *S aureus* bacteremia. Migratory polyarthritis (eg, knees, wrist, ankles) with weight loss, diarrhea, and abdominal pain is a frequent clinical feature in classic Whipple disease.[27] **Table 2** lists other possible differential diagnoses of septic arthritis.[28]

The examination should focus on determining if the findings are intra-articular or periarticular. The cardinal physical examination finding is difficulty moving the joint due to severe pain in conjunction with signs of inflammation, such as warmth, swelling, and tenderness. Some studies have demonstrated that pain with motion, warmth, and tenderness is the most sensitive sign with 92% to 100% sensitivity. No studies have extensively evaluated the accuracy of physical examination findings in septic arthritis. Thus, specificities and likelihood ratios are unknown.[29] Other physical examinations are necessary depending on the leading differential diagnoses. For example, a cardiovascular examination is essential if bacteremia is present. If a disseminated gonococcal infection is suspected, particular attention should be given to the presence of tenosynovitis and dermatitis.

DIAGNOSTIC TESTING

A 2021 review reported that among patients presenting with acute monoarticular arthritis, the diagnostic test strategy aims to differentiate between septic arthritis,

Table 1
Uncommon Pathogens Causing Septic Arthritis With Particular History

Microorganisms	Clinical Feature
Neisseria meningitidis, *Streptococcus pneumoniae*	Presence of meningitis
Listeria monocytogenes, *Brucella* spp.	Ingestion of nonpasteurized milk products
Mycobacterium tuberculosis	Indolent symptoms, presence of risk factors for tuberculosis
Pasteurella spp., *Capnocytophaga* spp., *Neisseria* spp.	Cat or dog bites
Streptobacillus moniliformis, *Spirillum minus*	Rat bites
Mycobacterium marinum, *Vibrio* spp., *Aeromonas hydrophila*	Aquatic injuries
Eikenella corrodens	Human bites
Tropheryma whipplei	Associated weight loss, abdominal pain

Table 2
Differential Diagnosis of Septic Arthritis

Acute Monoarthritis	Oligoarthritis
Bacterial septic arthritis	Multiple septic arthritis with bacteremia
Crystal arthropathy (gout, pseudogout)	Lyme arthritis
Fracture or tendon/ligament lesion due to trauma	Whipple disease
Hemarthrosis	Rheumatoid arthritis
Acute flare of inflammatory arthritis (eg, rheumatoid arthritis)	Behçet syndrome
Tenosynovitis or bursitis	Ankylosing spondylitis
Tumor: Metastasis, pigmented villonodular synovitis	Psoriatic arthritis
	Reactive arthritis
	Inflammatory bowel disease–related arthritis
	Sarcoidosis
	Systemic lupus erythematosus
	Still disease

Data from Alpay-Kanıtez N, Çelik S, Bes C: Polyarthritis and its differential diagnosis. *Eur J Rheumatol* 2019;6(4):167-173.

crystal arthropathy, and flare-ups of inflammatory diseases (eg, rheumatoid arthritis).[30] No single clinical finding or diagnostic test can reliably differentiate among these disease entities. At initial presentation (before the availability of microbiologic results), a combination of clinical and laboratory findings can provide clues to the likelihood of each diagnosis. Of note, concomitant septic and crystal monoarthritis occurs in approximately 5% of patients. Furthermore, those with gout are at a higher risk of septic arthritis.[31,32]

In 1976, Newman published criteria for the diagnosis of septic arthritis. These include (1) organisms isolated from the joint, (2) organisms isolated elsewhere, and (3) no organism isolated but (i) histologic or radiologic evidence of infection or (ii) turbid fluid aspirated from the joint.[33] Currently, isolating an organism from the joint or concurrent bacteremia remains the gold standard in diagnosing septic arthritis. In addition, the white blood cell (WBC) count in the synovial fluid is used as an adjunct to the diagnosis.

Microbiologic Testing

As most instances of septic arthritis are hematogenous, blood cultures are of paramount importance. Blood cultures are positive in approximately 40% to 60% of patients, with some studies showing that up to 78% of patients have positive blood cultures.[34] The presence of bacteremia may change the treatment duration and necessitate additional diagnostic testing for concomitant endovascular infection. Synovial fluid culture is the gold standard in the diagnosis of septic arthritis. A 2020 study reported that using blood culture bottles for synovial fluid cultures is more accurate and efficient than classic agars and broths. The sensitivity is higher at 50% versus 42% and the specificity is higher at 96% versus 93%, respectively.[35]

Molecular techniques such as 16S ribosomal RNA gene polymerase chain reaction (PCR), multiplex PCR, and metagenomic next-generation sequencing are under investigation for cases of culture-negative septic arthritis. Currently, investigations show that molecular techniques add little to the diagnosis of septic arthritis. In select cases, molecular technique helps in identifying microorganisms that did not grow in culture.[36,37]

Serologic testing with organism-specific PCR from biopsy samples is the best test for *Borrelia burgdorferi*, *Brucella* spp., and *Coxiella burnetii* (Q fever). Specific PCR is recommended for *N gonorrhoeae*, *Ureaplasma* spp., and *Mycoplasma* spp. The diagnosis of *Mycobacterium tuberculosis* arthritis is challenging because it requires specific media and culture time of at least 8 weeks. The suspicion of diagnosis relies on the epidemiology and other sites of infection (ie, lung, lymph nodes). A 2019 prospective study reported that the sensitivity of culture and PCR for *M tuberculosis* using joint samples is low, and investigations are based on low sample numbers.[38]

Synovial Fluid Analysis

Synovial fluid should also be analyzed for WBC count and differential. Synovial WBC counts confirm or rule out the diagnosis, mainly when the counts are incredibly high (>100,000/mm^3) or normal (<200/mm^3). The range between these numbers is less reliable in predicting the etiology of arthritis, either infectious or noninfectious. Traditionally, a WBC count of more than 50,000/mm^3 or polymorphonuclear cell percentage of greater than 90% has been set as diagnostic of septic arthritis. Although it has high specificity (>90%), the sensitivity is poor (approximately 50%); thus, a low cell count cannot rule out septic arthritis. A 2020 study reported that up to 29% of crystal arthropathies present with more than 50,000/mm^3. Even a higher count of 85,000/mm^3 would not exclude concomitant disease.[39] For this reason, crystal analysis should always be part of the synovial fluid analysis.

Another confounder of the interpretation of synovial cell counts is antibiotic exposure. A higher threshold level will miss many true cases of septic arthritis among patients who received antibiotics before the arthrocentesis. A 2021 study showed that 16,000/mm^3 should be the ideal threshold level.[40] Notably, most studies on synovial cell counts are based on lower extremity septic arthritis, and it is a gap in the knowledge of how applicable these are to upper extremity and other joints.

Imaging

Imaging has a limited role in diagnosing septic arthritis, especially because it rarely changes the approach to treatment. However, in cases of acute joint pain in which diagnosis is not sufficiently clear, a radiograph can help diagnose fractures, osteoarthritis, and chondrocalcinosis. In addition, repeat imaging at follow-up examinations can help estimate the dynamics and extent of cartilage destruction (ie, narrowing of the joint space) and the development of degenerative osteoarthritis (ie, destruction of the subchondral bone) over time. There is no evidence-based recommendation for this practice. Ultrasonography can guide arthrocentesis. A 2021 study reported that MRI alone cannot distinguish septic arthritis versus other inflammatory arthritis. However, if adjacent osteomyelitis is being considered, MRI is the imaging of choice.[41]

Other Tests

Traditionally used blood tests such as inflammatory markers (ie, C-reactive protein level and erythrocyte sedimentation rate) and serum WBC count are unreliable markers of septic arthritis due to their poor specificity. Other serum and synovial biomarkers, such as calprotectin, synovial lactate, glucose, apolipoprotein, and procalcitonin, have not been proven helpful in diagnosing septic arthritis.[42,43] If surgery is performed, histopathologic examination of samples may characterize the type and extent of the inflammation and offer clues into the causes of culture-negative septic arthritis, such as atypical bacteria, mycobacteria, and molds.

TREATMENT

Source Control

The following interventions have been described as a treatment modality for septic arthritis: (1) repeat arthrocentesis, (2) arthroscopy, and (3) arthrotomy. The primary goal of surgical therapy is to remove intra-articular pus, leukocytes, proteases, and cytokines responsible for joint destruction. A 2019 study showed that drainage also lowers the microbial burden, although antibiotics penetrate well into the synovial fluid.[44] There are wide variations in preference of procedure for acute septic arthritis globally.

The most common surgical treatment of septic arthritis is joint lavage, performed either open or arthroscopically. Arthroscopy is the favored approach due to less soft-tissue disruption, less bleeding, and quicker recovery of joint motion than open surgery. Arthroscopy also has a reduced risk of recurrence of infection and decreased length of stay, especially in knee and shoulder joints.[45-47] Late-stage septic arthritis associated with necrosis and osteomyelitis may require open arthrotomy. Recent data suggest similar outcomes when comparing nonsurgical management (ie, repeated arthrocentesis) with surgical management for early stages of septic arthritis in clinically stable patients. These studies are preliminary and more research is needed before widespread adoption.[48-50]

Traditionally, septic arthritis was considered to need emergent joint lavage because of the risk of joint destruction. However, these data are derived from animal experiments with high-dose bacterial inoculation.[51] There is little clinical evidence to support this practice. A 2018 retrospective review showed that, among hemodynamically stable patients, emergency joint lavage results did not demonstrate better outcomes than lavage within 24 or 48 hours.[52]

Antibiotic Therapy

Antibiotic therapy must be withheld before collecting synovial fluid cultures, except in hemodynamic instability or bacteremia cases. Previous antibiotic exposure reduces the sensitivity of cultures.[53] Therefore, it is good practice to perform arthrocentesis for synovial fluid cultures expeditiously at the first clinical presentation and start empiric antibiotics afterward. The best approach for patients exposed to antibiotics is unclear as no studies have explored this topic.

The initial choice of antibiotics should cover gram-positive bacteria because these are the most common causes of septic arthritis. Depending on local rates of MRSA, empiric treatment with vancomycin or daptomycin (in areas with a high prevalence of MRSA), cefazolin, or antistaphylococcal penicillin derivates (in areas with a low prevalence of MRSA) might be considered. The routine addition of coverage for gram-negative bacteria is not necessary. It is reasonable to add antimicrobial agents with activity against gram-negatives if there is the presence of sepsis, history of trauma, or postprocedural infection or among people with compromised immune systems. For gonococcal arthritis, medical treatment alone with ceftriaxone is recommended. Once the causative organism has been established, antibiotics should be tailored to complete therapy. Table 3 lists suggested antibiotic regimens for common organisms.

Table 3

Targeted Antibiotic Therapy Following Isolation of Causative Microorganism

	Intravenous Antibiotic	Oral Antibiotic
Methicillin-sensitive *Staphylococcus aureus*	Cefazolin Nafcillin/Oxacillin	Cefadroxil Cefalexin
Methicillin-resistant *S aureus*	Vancomycin Daptomycin	Doxycycline Trimethoprim/Sulfamethoxazole Linezolid
Streptococcus species	Penicillin Cefazolin Ceftriaxone	Penicillin Amoxicillin Cefadroxil
Enterobacterales	Cefepime Ceftriaxone Piperacillin-tazobactam	Fluoroquinolones Trimethoprim/Sulfamethoxazole Cefdinir
Neisseria gonorrhoeae	Ceftriaxone Gentamicin	None

There is limited evidence on the optimal duration of therapy for septic arthritis, and there are wide variations in practices worldwide. One randomized trial from 2019 showed that 2 weeks of treatment is noninferior to 4 weeks.[54] However, most trial participants had septic arthritis of the hand and wrist, limiting the generalizability to larger joints such as hips and knees. For larger joints, 3 to 6 weeks of treatment is standard practice. Currently, intravenous antibiotics are considered the gold standard in the United States in treating septic arthritis. This view is being challenged by more recent evidence showing that oral antibiotics are noninferior in other bone and joint infections.[55,56]

Several factors may influence the decision on the treatment duration. Clinicians can consider the causative microorganism, the disease stage of septic arthritis, the joint size, and host factors. If there is concomitant bacteremia and endovascular infection, treatment duration for these infectious syndromes should be followed. Monitoring clinical and laboratory responses may also guide decision-making on the switch from parenteral to oral antibiotics and the total duration of treatment. Infections such as gonococcal and Lyme arthritis are treated for 7 and 28 days, respectively.

Physical Therapy

A 2022 study reported that early rehabilitation and joint movement have been advocated in septic arthritis. Historically, passive movement has been postulated to improve functional outcomes and reduce inflammation and joint destruction.[57] It is a poorly studied topic in septic arthritis and needs more studies, and many institutions are not in favor of this practice.

SUMMARY

Septic arthritis is a serious disease that requires prompt diagnosis and treatment. Establishing the microbiologic etiology is essential to the management of septic arthritis, and arthrocentesis for culture collection must be performed before initiating antibiotic therapy in patients without sepsis. Once the microbiologic diagnosis is established, antibiotic therapy should be tailored. There is no evidence that emergent arthroscopy or open arthrotomy results in better outcomes. There is increasing evidence that an early switch to oral antibiotics and nonsurgical management with repeated arthrocentesis are viable options in the management of septic arthritis. However, these approaches are undergoing further investigations before becoming standard of care.

KEY STUDY POINTS

- Gram-positive bacteria, notably, *S aureus*, cause most instances of septic arthritis regardless of individual patient characteristics.
- Identification of causative organisms is critical in the management of septic arthritis. Every effort should be made to ensure cultures are performed before initiating antibiotic therapy.
- No single physical examination finding or laboratory test can distinguish septic arthritis from other differential diagnoses. Low synovial fluid white cell count does not rule out septic arthritis.
- Arthroscopy is the preferred approach for joint lavage compared with open arthrotomy in early-stage septic arthritis because of reduced risk of recurrence of infection and quicker patient recovery.
- The optimal duration of antibiotic therapy for septic arthritis is unknown, and current practice is 2 weeks for small joints and 3 to 6 weeks for large joints.

ANNOTATED REFERENCES

1. Huang YC, Ho CH, Lin YJ, et al: Site-specific mortality in native joint septic arthritis: A national population study. *Rheumatology (Oxford)* 2020;59(12):3826-3833.

   Risk factors for death associated with native joint septic arthritis are hip infection, shoulder infection, multiple-site infection, male sex, and age 65 years or older.

2. Bai AD, Lo CKL, Komorowski AS, et al: What is the optimal follow-up length for mortality in *Staphylococcus aureus* bacteremia? Observations from a systematic review of attributable mortality. *Open Forum Infect Dis* 2022;9(5):ofac096.

   The optimal follow-up duration of *S aureus* bacteremia is between 1 and 3 months.

3. Darbà J, Marsà A: Hospital care and medical costs of septic arthritis in Spain: A retrospective multicenter analysis. *J Med Econ* 2022;25(1):381-385.

   The median duration of hospitalization among patients with septic arthritis is 14 days, with an in-hospital mortality rate of 3.7%.

4. Kennedy N, Chambers ST, Nolan I, et al: Native joint septic arthritis: Epidemiology, clinical features, and microbiological causes in a New Zealand population. *J Rheumatol* 2015;42(12):2392-2397.

5. McBride S, Mowbray J, Caughey W, et al: Epidemiology, management, and outcomes of large and small native joint septic arthritis in adults. *Clin Infect Dis* 2020;70(2):271-279.

   The native joint septic arthritis incidence in New Zealand is 21 per 100,000 person-years. The risk factors are increasing age and lower socioeconomic status; *S aureus* is the most common causative organism.

6. Voss A, Pfeifer CG, Kerschbaum M, Rupp M, Angele P, Alt V: Post-operative septic arthritis after arthroscopy: Modern diagnostic and therapeutic concepts. *Knee Surg Sports Traumatol Arthrosc* 2021;29(10):3149-3158.

   Infection after arthroscopy is rare (<1%). The diagnostic and treatment approach is similar to other forms of septic arthritis.

7. Bettencourt JW, Wyles CC, Osmon DR, Hanssen AD, Berry DJ, Abdel MP: Outcomes of primary total hip arthroplasty following septic arthritis of the hip: A case-control study. *Bone Joint J* 2022;104-B(2):227-234.

   There is a 10-fold higher risk of periprosthetic joint infection for patients with a history of septic arthritis and who underwent total hip arthroplasty. The risk is higher if arthroplasty is performed less than 5 years from an episode of septic arthritis compared with longer than 5 years.

8. Ateschrang A, Albrecht D, Schroeter S, Weise K, Dolderer J: Current concepts review: Septic arthritis of the knee pathophysiology, diagnostics, and therapy. *Wien Klin Wochenschr* 2011;123(7-8):191-197.

9. Stutz G, Kuster MS, Kleinstück F, Gächter A: Arthroscopic management of septic arthritis: Stages of infection and results. *Knee Surg Sports Traumatol Arthrosc* 2000;8(5):270-274.

10. Letarouilly JG, Clowez A, Senneville E, Cortet B, Flipo RM: Épidémiologie et écologie des infections ostéo-articulaires bactériennes. *Revue du Rhumatisme Monographies* 2022;89(2):79-83.

    The incidence of septic arthritis is increasing in France. The predominant causative organisms are staphylococci and streptococci.

11. Dubost JJ, Couderc M, Tatar Z, et al: Three-decade trends in the distribution of organisms causing septic arthritis in native joints: Single-center study of 374 cases. *Joint Bone Spine* 2014;81(5):438-440.

12. Nossent J, Raymond W, Keen H, Preen DB, Inderjeeth CA: Non-gonococcal septic arthritis of native joints in Western Australia. A longitudinal population-based study of frequency, risk factors and outcome. *Int J Rheum Dis* 2021;24(11):1386-1393.

    The most frequently affected joint is the knees (33.6%). Approximately 37% of cases were caused by microorganisms other than gram-positive cocci, and complications were higher for cases of culture-positive septic arthritis.

13. Ross JJ, Ard KL, Carlile N: Septic arthritis and the opioid epidemic: 1465 cases of culture-positive native joint septic arthritis from 1990–2018. *Open Forum Infect Dis* 2020;7(3):ofaa089.

    There has been an increase in people who inject drugs in the latest decade. Most cases were caused by *S aureus*.

14. Moussiegt A, François C, Belmonte O, et al: Gonococcal arthritis: Case series of 58 hospital cases. *Clin Rheumatol* 2022;41(9):2855-2862.

    The most frequently infected joint in this case series was the knee, followed by the ankle, wrist, and fingers or carpal joints. Notably, only 16% of cases had genital symptoms.

15. Chen Y, Huang Z, Fang X, Li W, Yang B, Zhang W: Diagnosis and treatment of mycoplasmal septic arthritis: A systematic review. *Int Orthop* 2020;44(2):199-213.

    Mycoplasma septic arthritis is rare and limited to case reports. Most patients (70%) in this review are immunocompromised.

16. Saha B, Young K, Kahili-Heede M, Lim SY: Septic arthritis of native joints due to Mycobacterium avium complex: A systematic review of case reports. *Semin Arthritis Rheum* 2021;51(4):813-818.

    Mycobacterium avium complex septic arthritis most frequently presents as monoarthritis involving the knees and wrist. Septic arthritis may be in the setting of disseminated infection or primary septic arthritis.

17. Taj-Aldeen SJ, Rammaert B, Gamaletsou M, et al: Osteoarticular infections caused by non-aspergillus filamentous fungi in adult and pediatric patients: A systematic review. *Medicine (Baltimore)* 2015;94(50):e2078.

18. Belkacem A, Caumes E, Ouanich J, et al: Changing patterns of disseminated gonococcal infection in France: Cross-sectional data 2009-2011. *Sex Transm Infect* 2013;89(8):613-615.

19. Nossent J, Raymond W, Keen H, Preen DB, Inderjeeth CA: Septic arthritis due to Neisseria gonorrhoea in Western Australia. *Intern Med J* 2022;52(6):1029-1034.

    The annual incidence of gonococcal arthritis increased from 1.35 to 2.10 per 1 million between 1990 and 2014 in Western Australia.

20. Nelson CA, Saha S, Kugeler KJ, et al: Incidence of clinician-diagnosed lyme disease, United States, 2005-2010. *Emerg Infect Dis* 2015;21(9):1625-1631.

21. Schwartz AM, Hinckley AF, Mead PS, Hook SA, Kugeler KJ: Surveillance for Lyme Disease – United States, 2008-2015. *MMWR Surveill Summ* 2017;66(22):1-12.

22. Kwit NA, Nelson CA, Max R, Mead PS: Risk factors for clinician-diagnosed lyme arthritis, facial palsy, carditis, and meningitis in patients from high-incidence states. *Open Forum Infect Dis* 2018;5(1):ofx254.

    The most common manifestations of disseminated Lyme disease are arthritis, facial palsy, and carditis. Younger age and male sex are risk factors for disseminated disease.

23. Udziela S, Biesiada G, Osiewicz M, et al: Musculoskeletal manifestations of Lyme borreliosis – A review. *Arch Med Sci* 2020;18(3):726-731.

    Arthritis is a common manifestation of Lyme disease. The diagnosis is made clinically and by means of serology, and one course of antibiotic therapy is sufficient for treatment.

24. García-Arias M, Balsa A, Mola EM: Septic arthritis. *Best Pract Res Clin Rheumatol* 2011;25(3):407-421.

25. Orbay H, Seng S, Kim DW, Geller CM: Increasing incidence of sternoclavicular joint infections in intravenous drug users. *Thorac Cardiovasc Surg* 2023;71(1):73-75.

    This is a case series of four patients with sternoclavicular septic arthritis. The most common symptoms were pain and swelling; two patients were treated medically.

26. Hansen RL, Bue M, Borgognoni AB, Petersen KK: Septic arthritis and osteomyelitis of the pubic symphysis – A retrospective study of 26 patients. *J Bone Jt Infect* 2022;7(1):35-42.

    Most patients with septic arthritis of pubic symphysis had undergone pelvic surgery (81%). The most common symptoms were severe suprapubic/pubic pain, gait difficulties, and intermittent fever.

27. Puéchal X: Whipple's arthritis. *Joint Bone Spine* 2016;83(6):631-635.

28. Alpay-Kanıtez N, Çelik S, Bes C: Polyarthritis and its differential diagnosis. *Eur J Rheumatol* 2019;6(4):167-173.

    This is a comprehensive review on the approach to polyarthritis. A thorough history and physical examination are required, while the differential diagnosis is broad.

29. Carpenter CR, Schuur JD, Everett WW, Pines JM: Evidence-based diagnostics: Adult septic arthritis. *Acad Emerg Med* 2011;18(8):781-796.

30. Earwood JS, Walker TR, Sue GJC: Septic arthritis: Diagnosis and treatment. *Am Fam Physician* 2021;104(6):589-597.

    The authors outline some key concepts in this review. Empiric antibiotic therapy can be initiated if there is clinical concern for septic arthritis after obtaining synovial fluid. A treatment duration of 2 to 6 weeks was also recommended.

31. Lim SY, Lu N, Choi HK: Septic arthritis in gout patients: A population-based cohort study. *Rheumatology (Oxford)* 2015;54(11):2095-2099.

32. Papanicolas LE, Hakendorf P, Gordon DL: Concomitant septic arthritis in crystal monoarthritis. *J Rheumatol* 2012;39(1):157-160.

33. Newman JH: Review of septic arthritis throughout the antibiotic era. *Ann Rheum Dis* 1976;35(3):198-205.

34. Nolla JM, Lora-Tamayo J, Gómez Vaquero C, et al: Pyogenic arthritis of native joints in non-intravenous drug users: A detailed analysis of 268 cases attended in a tertiary hospital over a 22-year period. *Semin Arthritis Rheum* 2015;45(1):94-102.

35. Cohen D, Natshe A, Ben Chetrit E, Lebel E, Breuer GS: Synovial fluid culture: Agar plates vs. blood culture bottles for microbiological identification. *Clin Rheumatol* 2020;39(1):275-279.

    Using blood culture bottles for synovial fluid cultures improves the detection rates of causative organisms for septic arthritis (higher sensitivity, specificity, positive predictive value, negative predictive value, and a higher significant positive likelihood ratio).

36. Morgenstern C, Renz N, Cabric S, Perka C, Trampuz A: Multiplex polymerase chain reaction and microcalorimetry in synovial fluid: Can pathogen-based detection assays improve the diagnosis of septic arthritis? *J Rheumatol* 2018;45(11):1588-1593.

    Synovial fluid automated multiplex PCR performed poorly and missed important pathogens such as *S aureus* and *Streptococcus* species. There was no significant difference between PCR and cultures.

37. Fida M, Khalil S, Abu Saleh O, et al: Diagnostic value of 16S ribosomal RNA gene polymerase chain reaction/Sanger sequencing in clinical practice. *Clin Infect Dis* 2021;73(6):961-968.

    Bacterial cultures outperformed 16S RNA PCR for musculoskeletal specimens. Specimens with a gram-positive stain had 12 times greater odds of having a positive molecular result than those with a gram-negative stain.

38. Jacquier H, Fihman V, Amarsy R, et al: Benefits of polymerase chain reaction combined with culture for the diagnosis of bone and joint infections: A prospective test performance study. *Open Forum Infect Dis* 2019;6(12):ofz511.

    Bacterial 16S RNA PCR test sensitivity was only 55% compared with cultures at 81%. The sensitivity was also low when used for *M tuberculosis*. However, it increased to 88% when used together with mycobacterial culture.

39. Luo TD, Jarvis DL, Yancey HB, et al: Synovial cell count poorly predicts septic arthritis in the presence of crystalline arthropathy. *J Bone Jt Infect* 2020;5(3):118-124.

    Almost one-third of aseptic aspirates with crystal arthropathy had synovial WBC count of 50,000/mm^3 or greater; thus, the cutoff positive predictive value for septic arthritis is only 6%. Concomitant septic arthritis and crystal arthropathy cases had synovial WBC count of 85,000/mm^3 or greater in this cohort.

40. Massey PA, Clark MD, Walt JS, Feibel BM, Robichaux-Edwards LR, Barton RS: Optimal synovial fluid leukocyte count cutoff for diagnosing native joint septic arthritis after antibiotics: A receiver operating characteristic analysis of accuracy. *J Am Acad Orthop Surg* 2021;29(23):e1246-e1253.

    Among patients with septic arthritis who received antibiotics, the optimal cutoff is 16,000 cells. The sensitivity was 82% and specificity was 76%. Level of evidence: III.

41. Alaia EF, Chhabra A, Simpfendorfer CS, et al: MRI nomenclature for musculoskeletal infection. *Skeletal Radiol* 2021;50(12):2319-2347.

    Inflammatory arthritis, crystal arthropathies, and reactive arthritis present similarly to septic arthritis in MRI. MRI alone cannot distinguish one from another. Monoarthritis should be considered septic until proven otherwise.

42. Clapasson M, Trocmé C, Courtier A, Gaudin P, Epaulard O, Baillet A: Apolipoprotein C1 in synovial fluid discriminates septic arthritis from rheumatoid arthritis but not from pseudogout. *Clin Rheumatol* 2020;39(7):2239-2241.

    Mean synovial ApoC1 level was lower in septic arthritis compared with inflammatory arthritis. However, ApoC1 does not discriminate between patients with septic arthritis and pseudogout.

43. Baillet A, Trocmé C, Romand X, et al: Calprotectin discriminates septic arthritis from pseudogout and rheumatoid arthritis. *Rheumatology (Oxford)* 2019;58(9):1644-1648.

    Synovial calprotectin (>150 mg/L) has 76% sensitivity, 94% specificity, and a positive likelihood ratio of 12.2 for septic arthritis.

44. Thabit AK, Fatani DF, Bamakhrama MS, Barnawi OA, Basudan LO, Alhejaili SF: Antibiotic penetration into bone and joints: An updated review. *Int J Infect Dis* 2019;81:128-136.

    A review of more than 30 antibiotics showed that most antibiotics have good penetration into bone and joint tissues reaching concentrations exceeding the MIC90 and/or minimum inhibitory concentration breakpoints of common bone and joint infection pathogens.

45. Acosta-Olivo C, Vilchez-Cavazos F, Blázquez-Saldaña J, Villarreal-Villarreal G, Peña-Martínez V, Simental-Mendía M: Comparison of open arthrotomy versus arthroscopic surgery for the treatment of septic arthritis in adults: A systematic review and meta-analysis. *Int Orthop* 2021;45(8):1947-1959.

    Arthroscopy has significantly lower risk of reinfection, reduced hospital stay, and fewer complications compared with arthrotomy.

46. Dobek A, Cohen J, Ramamurti P, et al: Comparison of arthroscopy versus open arthrotomy for treatment of septic arthritis of the native knee: Analysis of 90-day postoperative complications. *J Knee Surg* 2023;36(9):949-956.

    Patients who underwent open arthrotomy had increased rates of readmission to the hospital, postoperative anemia, and blood transfusion compared with those who underwent arthroscopy.

47. Padaki AS, Ma GC, Truong NM, et al: Arthroscopic treatment yields lower reoperation rates than open treatment for native knee but not native shoulder septic arthritis. *Arthrosc Sports Med Rehabil* 2022;4(3):e1167-e1178.

    Reoperation rates are higher after open compared with arthroscopic treatment at 1 month, 1 year, and 2 years for knee septic arthritis. There were no significant differences for shoulder septic arthritis.

48. Harada K, McConnell I, DeRycke EC, Holleck JL, Gupta S: Native joint septic arthritis: Comparison of outcomes with medical and surgical management. *South Med J* 2019;112(4):238-243.

    There was no statistically significant difference in long-term outcomes between surgical treatment and needle aspirations. Patients treated medically had faster recovery at 3 months.

49. Mabille C, El Samad Y, Joseph C, et al: Medical versus surgical treatment in native hip and knee septic arthritis. *Infect Dis Now* 2021;51(2):164-169.

    The rate of treatment failure is higher among patients with septic arthritis of the knee who underwent medical treatment compared with surgery. The opposite is true for hip joints.

50. Flores-Robles BJ, Jiménez Palop M, Sanabria Sanchinel AA, et al: Medical versus surgical approach to initial treatment in septic arthritis: A single Spanish center's 8-year experience. *J Clin Rheumatol* 2019;25(1):4-8.

    Among patients treated nonsurgically with arthrocentesis, 30% eventually required surgery. Joint function at 1 year did not show significant differences.

51. Daniel D, Akeson W, Amiel D, Ryder M, Boyer J: Lavage of septic joints in rabbits: Effects of chondrolysis. *J Bone Joint Surg Am* 1976;58(3):393-395.

52. Lauper N, Davat M, Gjika E, et al: Native septic arthritis is not an immediate surgical emergency. *J Infect* 2018;77(1):47-53.

    Patients who underwent joint lavage within 6 hours of presentation had similar functional outcomes as those with lavage performed later up to longer than 24 hours.

53. Hindle P, Davidson E, Biant LC: Septic arthritis of the knee: The use and effect of antibiotics prior to diagnostic aspiration. *Ann R Coll Surg Engl* 2012;94(5):351-355.

54. Gjika E, Beaulieu JY, Vakalopoulos K, et al: Two weeks versus four weeks of antibiotic therapy after surgical drainage for native joint bacterial arthritis: A prospective, randomised, non-inferiority trial. *Ann Rheum Dis* 2019;78(8):1114-1121.

    Two weeks of antibiotic therapy is noninferior to 4 weeks regarding cure rates for septic arthritis. However, most patients had hand and wrist infection.

55. Li HK, Rombach I, Zambellas R, et al: Oral versus intravenous antibiotics for bone and joint infection. *N Engl J Med* 2019;380(5):425-436.

    Early switch to oral antibiotics is noninferior to completing the entire regimen with intravenous antibiotics. The cohort was diverse but did not include septic arthritis.

56. Uçkay I, Tovmirzaeva L, Garbino J, et al: Short parenteral antibiotic treatment for adult septic arthritis after successful drainage. *Int J Infect Dis* 2013;17(3):e199-e205.

57. Chabaud A, Tetard M, Descamps S, et al: Early rehabilitation management strategy for septic arthritis of the knee. *Infect Dis Now* 2022;52(3):170-174.

    A protocol for early-phase rehabilitation management of septic arthritis of the knee in a native joint was developed and validated. However, there is reluctance among health professionals in adopting the practice.

CHAPTER 24

Diabetic Foot Infections

BÜLENT M. ERTUĞRUL, MD • SERKAN AKÇAY, MD • İLKER UÇKAY, MD

ABSTRACT

Of all complications of diabetes mellitus, foot problems remain a common cause of hospital admissions. Among them, diabetic foot infections (DFIs) are one of the most significant life-threatening complications and usually represent the tip of the iceberg of other, underlying chronic problems in the foot. Overall, DFIs accompany 60% of all lower extremity amputations. Although soft-tissue infections can be treated rapidly with antibiotics alone (by sometimes requiring minor débridement), osteomyelitis remains difficult to manage and requires a multidisciplinary approach involving physicians, orthopaedic surgeons, other professionals, and the patients' compliance. A review of the management of DFI, with an emphasis on antibiotic therapy and the general surgical approach to DFI and osteomyelitis, is provided. Finally, patients with diabetes mellitus who have a history of DFIs need a lifelong close medical follow-up by podiatrists and nurses, controls, and iterative adjustments of the health, particularly of the feet. The coronavirus 2019 pandemic illustrates what happens if these control chains are interrupted.

Keywords: antibiotics; diabetic foot infection; management; osteomyelitis; surgical principles

None of the following authors or any immediate family member has received anything of value from or has stock or stock options held in a commercial company or institution related directly or indirectly to the subject of this chapter: Dr. Ertuğrul, Dr. Akçay, and Dr. Uçkay.

INTRODUCTION

Diabetic foot infections (DFIs), including osteomyelitis, are one of the most life-threatening local complications of diabetes and usually represent the tip of the iceberg of other underlying chronic problem in the ischemic and neuropathic diabetic foot. Although soft-tissue DFI can be managed rapidly, chronic osteomyelitis remains difficult to cure without amputation and requires a multidisciplinary approach involving medical, surgical, and other health care professionals and the patient. Patients with diabetes mellitus who have a history of DFI require lifelong, regular medical, podiatric, and surgical follow up, including with nurses. They need repetitive professional wound care as well as medical and surgical adjustments of their individual foot problems. The coronavirus 2019 (COVID-19) pandemic illustrates what happens if these control chains are interrupted. A narrative review of the literature on the management of DFI, with an emphasis on antibiotic therapy and general surgical approach to diabetic foot problems, is provided.

PATIENT CARE

Currently, experts estimate that at least 20 million people worldwide have a diabetic foot ulcer (DFU) and 130 million patients will have risk factors for the development of a DFU.[1] Patients with prior DFU or DFI are at even greater risk.[2,3]

The drastic containment and mitigation measures in the community and the ban of elective and semielective surgery during the first COVID-19 pandemic wave[4] left fragile patients without necessary services.[5] A 2020 study reported a 50% drop in the frequency of the foot clinic visits in Manchester, England, and approximately 70% drop in Los Angeles, California, during the first lockdown, leading to an increase in the number of complicated DFUs and DFIs and a higher amputation risk in many regions of the world.[6,7] Moreover, even in terms of antibiotic stewardship,[8] the relatively short lockdowns could also contribute to a rise in the proportion of multidrug-resistant pathogens in DFI because the patients received treatment too late or by less experienced physicians.[9] Multidrug-resistant organisms reduce the choice of available antibiotics overall, but not that of costly, parenteral-only agents.[10]

DIAGNOSIS OF SOFT-TISSUE INFECTION AND ASSESSMENT OF ITS SEVERITY

The clinical diagnosis of soft-tissue DFI is clear when there is pus or a rapidly spreading erysipelas. However, a 2021 review reported that proof of infection relies on several deep, microbiologically concordant (intraoperative) tissue samples.[11] However, in certain circumstances, soft-tissue infection is difficult to diagnose (eg, with concomitant acute ischemia, venous insufficiency, or intolerance to topical medication).[4,12-14] Moreover, the classic signs of acute inflammation—redness, heat, swelling, pain, and loss of function—may not always apply for the neuropathic foot. A 2020 review reported that systemic symptoms such as fever and chills or leukocytosis are uncommon with a localized DFI, but their presence might denote a more severe, potentially limb-threatening infection, such as necrotizing fasciitis or gas gangrene.[14] In these cases, the blood cultures may be positive. A possible clinical evaluation of disease severity derived from the International Working Group on the Diabetic Foot[3] is summarized in **Table 1**.

IMPORTANCE OF DIAGNOSING CHRONIC OSTEOMYELITIS

Chronic bone infections with advanced radiologic lesions (ie, beyond the cortical level, bone vanishing, shattering, or destruction) are difficult to cure by antimicrobial agents alone.[15] A randomized trial from 2022 reported that, typically, a recurrence of osteomyelitis is always a bone infection, whereas the recurrence of an initial soft-tissue DFI often impresses as a new osteomyelitis (transformation DFI to osteomyelitis),[16] highlighting the importance of identifying bone involvement from the start. In the best case, antibiotics may stop the progression of bone infection. Even if most bacteria are killed in the altered bone parts, these bone lesions can become infected again, as they represent a vulnerable point of that bone. The nonsurgical osteomyelitis therapy (defined by the authors as a minimal surgical débridement, if ever, without resection of the infected bone) can achieve midterm remissions in up to 70%.[11,14] This may occur in selected patients with rather superficial osteitis and without major alteration of the foot architecture.

Table 1
Clinical Characteristics Suggesting an Important Diabetic Foot Infection

Wound-Specific

Wound	Penetrates to subcutaneous tissues (eg, fascia, tendon, muscle, joint, bone)
Cellulitis	Extensive (greater than 2 cm), distant from ulceration or rapidly progressive
Local signs	Severe inflammation or induration, crepitus, bullae, discoloration, necrosis or gangrene, ecchymoses or petechiae, new anaesthesia

General

Presentation	Acute onset/worsening or rapidly progressive
Systemic signs	Fever, chills, hypotension, confusion, volume depletion
Laboratory tests	Leukocytosis, high C-reactive protein or erythrocyte sedimentation levels, severe/worsening hyperglycemia, acidosis, new/worsening azotemia
Complicating features	Presence of a foreign body, deep abscess, arterial or venous insufficiency, lymphedema, immunosuppressive illness or treatment
Current treatment	Progression while on appropriate antibiotic and supportive therapy

Adapted with permission from Lipsky BA, Senneville E, Abbas ZG, et al: Guidelines on the diagnosis and treatment of foot infection in persons with diabetes (IWGDF 2019 update). *Diabetes Metab Res Rev* 2020;36:3280. Copyright 2020, John Wiley & Sons Ltd.

Bone infection is suspected based on the patient's history and examination. Osteomyelitis is likely if there are prior DFUs and amputations or recurrent DFIs at the same localization.[17] The presence of a DFU larger than 2 cm, deeper than 3 mm, or greater than 4.5 cm^2 increases the osteomyelitis risk.[17,18] A sausage toe is a clinical surrogate for chronic osteomyelitis without accompanying DFU. The probe-to-bone is another method.[19,20] If the bone surface through the DFU is touched, there is a likelihood of contamination (at least of the cortical bone). Likewise, if the bone is clearly visible, or if it is weakened and easily shattered on light contact, the presence of relevant osteomyelitis, or of bacterial bone contamination, is suggested.[18,19] Serum inflammatory markers might serve as a surrogate for bone infection, but can also be false-negative, especially in chronic cases with spontaneous drainage from a chronic DFU.[11,14,18,19]

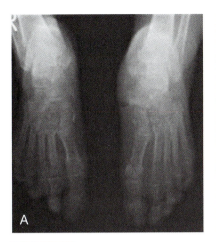 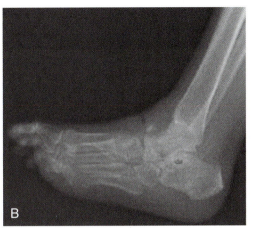 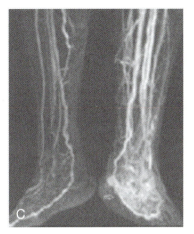

FIGURE 1 **A** and **B**, Radiographs and **C**, venogram of a diabetic Charcot foot without infection. Note the good vascularization (venous congestion) and the rocker-bottom aspect of the diabetic Charcot foot.

Imaging

Imaging studies alone do not ultimately prove the infectious nature of osteomyelitis, although it helps to strongly suggest it.[13] Similarly, MRI is frequently used as a gold standard for imaging to confirm the presence of osteomyelitis, although it can also be false-positive in up to 15% to 20% of the cases.[13,21] The standard radiograph is the initial radiologic study of choice.[13] Unless there is a clear acute DFI limited to the soft tissues, a radiograph is not recommended for every instance of DFI (especially in chronic DFI cases). The three classic findings suggestive for osteomyelitis are demineralization, periosteal reaction, and osteolysis. These signs usually become visible after 2 to 3 weeks of bone infection.[13] The more expensive MRI[21] as well as the newer scintigraphy techniques[22] might detect osteomyelitis much earlier, but they should be reserved for surgical decision making.[13,15,21,22] In retrospective evaluations, these sophisticated techniques ultimately lead to better outcomes and fewer recurrences after therapy for osteomyelitis.[21-23] Prospective trials using MRI for determining the presurgical amputation margin are under way, including one published in 2020.[24] Clinically, the diabetic Charcot foot is the most important differential diagnosis to bone infection. According to a 2019 illustrative radiologic review, the presence of joint destruction, cortical fractures, and joint dislocations is typical, and especially involving Lisfranc joints with a typically superior and lateral dislocation of the metatarsal bones and a collapse of the longitudinal arch[25] (**Figures 1** and **2**).

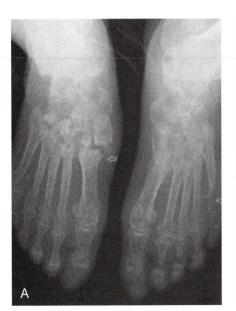 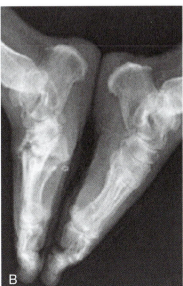 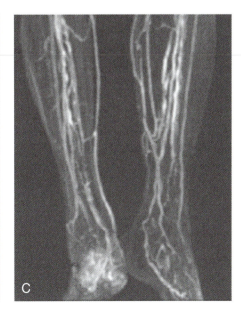

FIGURE 2 **A** and **B**, Radiographs demonstrating the diabetic Charcot foot. **C**, Venogram showing the substantial venous congestion unlikely with classic diabetic foot osteomyelitis.

Histology and Microbiology

The gold standard for proving osteomyelitis is still the growth of identical bacteria in several bone samples, together with a clinical history of osteomyelitis and/or histology.[26] Prospective studies are underway to demonstrate the bedside feasibility of bone biopsy performed by physicians. In many reports, the congruence of the retrieved pathogens between bone and soft-tissue culture results oscillated between 6% and 43%, whereas the proportion of polymicrobial infections was higher in soft-tissue DFIs compared with osteomyelitis.[27] However, the authors of this review do not think that all pathogens must be covered when treating soft-tissue DFIs.[8,11,14] In clinical practice, antimicrobial therapy often targets up to the three most important pathogens, leaving the others to be removed by débridement. In contrast, clinicians often treat every pathogen causing bone infection with systemic antibiotic agents.[8,11,14]

PATHOGENS AND BIOFILMS

The causative pathogens may depend on many factors, including the geographic location (eg, climate and socioeconomic issues), the chronicity of the wound, selection by current antibiotics, ischemia and maceration, exposures (eg, waterborne pathogens, nosocomial infections), or simply by chance.[11,14] In temperate geographic areas such as the United States and Europe, the most common pathogens are gram-positive cocci: *Staphylococcus aureus* and streptococci in acute soft-tissue DFI, and *S aureus* or coagulase-negative staphylococci in chronic osteomyelitis.[11] In contrast, almost all studies stemming from arid, tropical, and subtropical countries (eg, India), report a high proportion of gram-negative rods, for example, *Pseudomonas aeruginosa*, or mixed infections, for which the exact reasons remain unclear.[3,11] These reasons may be related to differences in the availability of over-the-counter antibiotic agents, foot sweating, or the type of (ritual) washing. It might also be that the microbiology of DFIs is evolving slowly toward more gram-negative organisms. Of note, bacteria with natural or acquired antibiotic resistances are becoming an important worldwide problem in DFIs.[10,14]

A 2019 study reported that molecular techniques and microbiome analyses might identify much more bacteria than traditional cultures, such as *Corynebacterium* spp., *Finegoldia* spp., *Porphyromonas* spp., *Anaerococcus* spp., and *Peptoniphilus* spp., especially in polymicrobial infections.[28] But these are expensive, and it is wise to apply them for a few restricted situations, in which the standard cultures cannot grow and are important:[28] for example, for patients already undergoing antibiotic therapy for nonsurgical treatment of osteomyelitis.[29]

Biofilms are another mechanical and chemical problem. The proportion of biofilm-forming bacteria in infected DFU may be as high as 60% to 80%.[28,30] Biofilms might explain why a systemic antibiotic treatment may often fail, because the sessile bacteria in biofilms display an increased resistance to blood-derived antibiotic drugs. The minimum inhibitory concentration for microorganisms embedded in the biofilms may be up to 100- to 1,000-fold higher compared with that for their free-floating planktonic bacteria, which makes mechanical removal by professional wound care or surgical débridement more powerful than a chemical action on the dormant bacterial cells.[30]

MANAGEMENT OF DFI

General Aspects

Provided that there is no emergency, the management of DFI should be preferably discussed and conducted using a multidisciplinary approach.[11,14] Patients needing surgery (eg, for gangrene, deep abscesses, or severe ischemia) with substantial comorbidities (eg, heart failure, renal failure) should be hospitalized. **Table 1** summarizes potential elements in favor of hospitalization. In contrast, clinicians should not always prescribe antibiotics based solely on the academic diagnosis of DFI or osteomyelitis.[11,29] In many chronic cases, the clinicians can withhold an (empirical) antibiotic treatment when they are not assured to cure infection, for example, in complete toe bone destruction with patients refusing surgery and having no symptoms. For such a patient, it may be appropriate to administer antibiotic therapy for relatively brief periods to suppress local worsening (soft-tissue flares) of a chronic osteomyelitis.[11,14]

Targeted Antibiotic Treatment

For all severe and rapid soft-tissue DFI, documented bacteremia, or clinical sepsis, an empirical broad-spectrum antibiotic therapy is initiated, preferably by the parenteral route. Recommendations[3] for treatment are provided in **Table 2**.[16,24,31-33] A 2019 study reported that, for moderate or mild DFIs, treatment can start either after the first microbiologic results are obtained and/or oral therapy is started immediately, including using oral beta-lactam drugs for osteomyelitis.[31] Finally, mild and superficial DFI can be treated by professional wound care, alone or only with topical antibiotics.[34] Reviews regarding the antibiotic choices for DFI and osteomyelitis[11,14] regularly fail to detect differences in the outcomes between various antimicrobial agents,[11,14] with one possible exception: rifampin.[11] Treatment with rifampin may yield a lower risk of amputation than that of the control group (odds ratio, 0.65).[11,35] Additional randomized trials should be performed to help resolve this clinical issue.

Table 2
Possible Empiric Antibiotic Regimens

Infection Severity	Additional Factors	Usual Pathogen(s)[a]	Potential Empirical Regimens[b]
Mild	Standard cases	GPC	S-S pen; first-generation cephalosporin
	Beta-lactam intolerance	GPC	Clindamycin; FQ; T/S; macrolide; doxycycline
	High risk for MRSA	MRSA	Linezolid; T/S; doxycycline; macrolide
Moderate/Severe	Standard cases	GPC ± GNR	ß-L-ase 1; second/third-generation cephalosporin
	Macerated ulcer or warm climate	GNR, including Pseudomonas	ß-L-ase 2; S-S pen + ceftazidime; S-S pen + antipseudomonal fluoroquinolone (ciprofloxacin); group 2 carbapenem
	Ischemic limb	GPC ± GNR ± Anaerobes	ß-L-ase 1 or 2; group 1 or 2 carbapenem; second/third-generation cephalosporin + clindamycin or metronidazole
	MRSA risk factors	MRSA	Consider adding glycopeptides; linezolid; daptomycin; fusidic acid; T/S (±rifamp[ic]in)[c]; doxycycline
	Risk factors for resistant GNR	ESBL	Carbapenems; piperacillin-tazobactam; FQ; aminoglycosides and/or colistin

ESBL = extended-spectrum ß-lactamase–producing organism, FQ = fluoroquinolone with good activity against aerobic gram-positive cocci (eg, levofloxacin or moxifloxacin), GNR = gram-negative rod, GPC = gram-positive cocci (staphylococci and streptococci), group 1 carbapenem = ertapenem, group 2 carbapenem = imipenem, meropenem, doripenem, MRSA = methicillin-resistant *Staphylococcus aureus*, S-S pen = semisynthetic penicillinase-resistant penicillin, T/S = trimethoprim/sulfamethoxazole, ß-L-ase = ß-lactam, ß-lactamase inhibitor, ß-L-ase 1 = amoxicillin/clavulanate, ampicillin/sulbactam, ß-L-ase 2 = ticarcillin/clavulanate, piperacillin/tazobactam

[a]Refers to isolates from an infected foot ulcer, not just colonization at another site.

[b]Given at usual recommended doses for serious infections. Where more than one agent is listed, only one of them should be prescribed, unless otherwise indicated. Consider modifying doses or agents selected for patients with comorbidities such as azotemia, liver dysfunction, and obesity.

[c]Rifamp(ic)in: because it is associated with higher risk of adverse events and its use is restricted in some countries, it may be most appropriately used for managing osteomyelitis or metal implant–related infections.

[d]Recommendations are based on theoretic considerations and results of available clinical trials.

[e]Oral antibiotic agents should generally not be used for severe infections, except as follow-on (switch) after initial parenteral therapy.

Adapted with permission from Lipsky BA, Senneville E, Abbas ZG, et al: Guidelines on the diagnosis and treatment of foot infection in persons with diabetes (IWGDF 2019 update). *Diabetes Metab Res Rev* 2020;36:3280. Copyright 2020, John Wiley & Sons Ltd.

Duration of Antibiotic Use

The minimal necessary duration of antibiotic treatment for a DFI (for which a surgery was performed) remains unclear[8,11,14] and should be individualized for each case. All retrospective studies with large databases failed to determine a minimum threshold for either the intravenous or the total duration of antibiotic use.[11,36] For mild to moderate tissue DFI, a 1- to 2-week duration is usually sufficient[3,11,16,24,37] (Table 3). For unresected osteomyelitis, 4 to 6 weeks are advocated.[11,14] The traditional approach of an initial parenteral antibiotic administration, often lasting weeks, can be replaced by oral regimens following only a brief intravenous duration, or even none.[11,14,36] All available literature suggests that a duration beyond 6 weeks is likely to be futile in terms of the prevention of recurrence. Within this long period, and provided that the patient complies with their medication, either the bone infection will be eradicated or it will require additional adjunct treatment. In some studies,[24] the treatment duration of investigation may be even shorter, especially if most of the infected bone has been resected. In a pilot randomized trial, remission and adverse events were compared in patients with osteomyelitis after surgical debridement, who were randomized to either 3 or 6 weeks of antibiotic therapy.[11,32] Among 93 enrolled patients, remission was noted in 84% of patients in the 3-week arm compared with 73% in the 6-week arm. The risk of antibiotic-related adverse events was similar and occurred within the first 2 to 3 weeks of therapy. Currently, a larger, confirmatory trial (with 436 cases planned) with soft-tissue DFI and osteomyelitis is conducted.[24]

Table 3

Suggested Administration Routes and Duration of Antibiotic Therapy

Site of Infection	Administration	Setting	Duration of Therapy
Soft Tissue Only			
Mild	Topical or oral	Outpatient	1-2 wk; may extend up to 4 wk if slow to resolve
Moderate	Oral (or initial parenteral)	Outpatient/inpatient	1-3 wk
Severe	Initial parenteral, switch to oral	Inpatient, then outpatient	2-4 wk
Bone/Joint Infection			
No residual infected tissue	Parenteral or oral	—	0-1 d
Residual infected soft tissue (but not bone)	Parenteral or oral	—	1-5 d
Residual osteomyelitis	Parenteral or oral	—	3-6 wk

Adapted with permission from Lipsky BA, Berendt AR, Cornia PB, et al: 2012 Infectious Diseases Society of America clinical practice guideline for the diagnosis and treatment of diabetic foot infections. *Clin Infect Dis* 2012;54(12):e132-e173, by permission of Oxford University Press.

ANTIBIOTIC THERAPY FOR RESIDUAL INFECTION AFTER AMPUTATION

Prolonging antibiotic administration after elective amputation for osteomyelitis is usually unnecessary if an experienced orthopaedic surgeon feels confident that all infection has been surgically removed.[11,38] However, frequently, the surgeon cannot be certain of this based only on the intraoperative appearance. There is no widely accepted standard for clinical practice in these doubts.[8,11,14] Various centers have developed strategies using an empirical continuation of antibiotics or case-by-case decision making.[11,38] A French study advocated that prescribing 1 to 3 weeks of additional therapy would be enough if all visibly infected bone has been resected.[11,33] One study found that, after a total excision of all infected bone, administering just 5 days of postsurgical antibiotic therapy was largely sufficient in terms of clinical failures.[10] Other studies routinely assessed the presence of residual bone infection (in the proximal residual bone) by bone biopsies for microbiology and/or histopathology and stop antibiotics if both return negative.[14,24] However, this practical attitude has not been clinically evaluated in large prospective trials and bone sampling of the residual bone through an infected site can also lead to erroneous false-positive result. This attitude is equally not recommended in the current International Working Group on the Diabetic Foot guidelines.[3] In the interim analysis of an ongoing prospective trial of patients with DFI and osteomyelitis in Zurich,[24] in which the therapy for residual osteomyelitis (in the proximal residual bone) is randomized to 1 versus 3 weeks, there are no apparent differences between the groups.[11,24] Residual soft-tissue infection is managed based on the visual evaluation of persistent infection, as it is advocated for all orthopaedic soft-tissue infections. Hence, the postamputation duration of antibiotics may range between 0 and 7 to 10 days, depending on the amount of infection.

ORTHOPAEDIC SURGERY FOR THE INFECTED DIABETIC FOOT

Major amputations were once common for osteomyelitis. However, improved and early nonsurgical surgery (ie, minimal débridement and no bone removal) is becoming commonplace, especially for the forefoot where a nonsurgical approach may be initially attempted.[11,14] Surgery may be required at the first line when bone protrudes through the DFU, when there is extensive bone destruction, lacking soft tissue, abscesses, phlegmons, or rapidly spreading soft-tissue DFI.[11] A 2021 narrative review, which included 14 studies that described seven types of nonsurgical surgeries, that is, nonamputation surgical procedures, concluded that all of them were safe, with clinical healing rates of 80% to 100%.[11,39]

Total amputation of all necrotic and infected tissue is probably the easiest way to achieve rapid cure, at least in the short term. However, this has consequences regarding mechanical sequelae, energy expenditure, postsurgical complications, costs, and quality of life.[11] Moreover, amputation, especially in the absence of reversing the reasons for the patient's initial DFI, does not protect against secondary, or new, infections.[11,14] Technically, surgeons often refer to the transcutaneous oxygen pressure measurements to select the amputation level in patients with ischemia. A 2019 study reported that 30 to 35 mm Hg is considered as an acceptable threshold for uneventful residuum healing, but this predictive role is bad.[40] The study included 303 amputations in 211 patients and found that a transcutaneous oxygen pressure threshold of 35 mm Hg did not discriminate between success and failure. Transcutaneous oxygen pressure values are highly depending on the local situations and the persons who measure. They may confirm a general clinical impression but do not replace it. Surgeons should avoid using them solely to select the amputation level.[40]

SUMMARY

Newer scientific studies have provided much useful new evidence on optimizing DFI and osteomyelitis treatment. On the surgical side, it appears that using surgical procedures that result in greater bone sparing is clinically effective and may also reduce postoperative problems. Regarding antibiotics, many DFIs can be treated with predominantly oral (rather than intravenous) therapy that have similar remission rates, fewer adverse effects, and lower financial costs. Treating for longer than 6 weeks is not necessary and might be even shortened, depending on the results of current and future prospective randomized trials.

KEY STUDY POINTS

- Most mild and moderate DFIs can be treated with oral antibiotics.
- The maximum duration of systemic antibiotic treatment for nonresected diabetic foot osteomyelitis is currently set at 6 weeks.
- The general management of DFI and osteomyelitis, or of any underlying foot problems, needs to be embedded in a multidisciplinary approach involving diabetologists, infectious disease specialist, off-loading, and eventual revascularization.

ANNOTATED REFERENCES

1. Lazzarini PA, Pacella RE, Armstrong DG, van Netten JJ: Diabetes-related lower-extremity complications are a leading cause of the global burden of disability. *Diabet Med* 2018; May 23 [Epub ahead of print].

   This is a relatively recent overview articles about the true and hidden burden and costs of diabetic foot infections, and non-infectious problems. The review is written by experts of resource-rich countries such as the US, but fairly resumes the global burden as well. Level of evidence: III.

2. Ertuğrul MB, Baktıroğlu S: Diyabetik ayak ve osteomyeliti. *Klimik Derg* 2005;18:8-13.

3. Lipsky BA, Senneville E, Abbas ZG, et al: Guidelines on the diagnosis and treatment of foot infection in persons with diabetes (IWGDF 2019 update). *Diabetes Metab Res Rev* 2020;36(suppl 1):3280.

   These are the most recent international guidelines (diagnosis, epidemiology, management, therapy) concerning the management of DFI. They are based on the PICO process. The PICO process (or framework) is a mnemonic used in evidence-based practice to frame and answer a clinical or healthcare-related question. The PICO acronym stands for P—patient, problem, or population; I—intervention; C—comparison, control, or comparator; O—outcome or outcomes (eg, pain, fatigue, nausea, infections, death). Level of evidence: III.

4. Laux CJ, Bauer DE, Kohler A, Uçkay I, Farshad M: Disproportionate case reduction after ban of elective surgeries during the SARS-CoV-2 pandemic. *Clin Spine Surg* 2020;33(6):244-246.

   This article on the experiences in Zürich, Switzerland, with the ban of elective orthopaedic surgery (and diabetic foot surgery) during the first lockdown for the COVID-19 pandemic in spring, 2020, targets the financial losses and the delays in providing necessary patient care. Level of evidence: III.

5. Najafi B: Post the pandemic: How will COVID-19 transform diabetic foot disease management? *J Diabetes Sci Technol* 2020;14(4):764-766.

   This is an article on the experience with COVID-19 lockdown and effects on the management and control of patients with DFI. This is also an opinion article predicting a new wave of innovations in the area of digital health, smart wearables, telehealth technologies, and hospital-at-home care delivery model for many patients with DFI. Level of evidence: III.

6. Shin L, Bowling FL, Armstrong DG, Boulton AJM: Saving the diabetic foot during the COVID-19 pandemic: A tale of two cities. *Diabetes Care* 2020;43(8):1704-1709.

   The advent of the COVID-19 pandemic has resulted not only in the closing of most outpatient clinics for face-to-face consultations but also in the inability to perform most laboratory and imaging investigations. This has resulted in a paradigm shift in the delivery of care for patients with DFUs, including virtual consultations using physician-to-patient and physician-to-home nurse telemedicine as well as home podiatry visits, as described in this review and illustrated by several case vignettes. Level of evidence: III.

7. Urbančič-Rovan V: Diabetic foot care before and during the COVID-19 epidemic: What really matters? *Diabetes Care* 2021;44(2):27-28.

   This opinion and experience article reported that the COVID-19 epidemic will lead to significant irreversible changes in diabetic foot care delivery. Level of evidence: IV.

8. Uçkay I, Berli M, Sendi P, Lipsky BA: Principles and practice of antibiotic stewardship in the management of diabetic foot infections. *Curr Opin Infect Dis* 2019;32(2):95-101.

This is a narrative review of the literature addressing the questions of whether antibiotic stewardship is possible in the community setting of DFI and how such a stewardship could be performed. Level of evidence: III.

9. Caruso P, Maiorino MI, Macera M, et al: Antibiotic resistance in diabetic foot infection: How it changed with COVID-19 pandemic in a tertiary care center. *Diabetes Res Clin Pract* 2021;175:108797.

   In a population of people with DFI admitted in a tertiary care center during the COVID-19 pandemic, the prevalence of antibiotic resistance was higher than the years before. Previous hospitalization and antibiotic self-administration/prescription by general practitioners were related to a higher risk of antibiotic-resistant infections. Level of evidence: IV.

10. Saltoğlu N, Ergönül Ö, Tülek N, et al: Influence of multidrug resistant organisms on the outcome of diabetic foot infection. *Int J Infect Dis* 2018;70:10-14.

    This is a multidisciplinary work of scientific experts and a nationwide evaluation of the Turkish Society for Diabetic Foot Infections (UDAIS). Turkey has long time been a country in between a predomination of gram-positive and gram-negative DFI pathogens. This epidemiology might change. The article clearly shows the relatively rent emergence of multi-drug-resistant gram-negative, including for community-acquired pseudomonas infections, and that successful management of these infections might become more and more difficult when facing multidrug-resistant pathogens, especially resistant *P aeruginosa*. Level of evidence: III.

11. Lipsky BA, Uçkay İ: Treating diabetic foot osteomyelitis: A practical state-of-the-art update. *Medicina (Kaunas)* 2021;57(4):339.

    This is an extensive recent review for internists on how to manage, diagnose, and treat DFI, based on the most recent scientific literature. Level of evidence: III.

12. Lipsky BA, Berendt AR, Deery HG, et al: Diagnosis and treatment of diabetic foot infections. *Plast Reconstr Surg* 2006;117:212-238.

13. Glaudemans AW, Uçkay I, Lipsky BA: Challenges in diagnosing infection in the diabetic foot. *Diabet Med* 2015;32(6):748-759.

14. Ertuğrul B, Uçkay I, Schöni M, Peter-Riesch B, Lipsky BA: Management of diabetic foot infections in the light of recent literature and new international guidelines. *Expert Rev Anti Infect Ther* 2020;18(4):293-305.

    This is an extensive, recent review on how to treat patients with diabetic foot osteomyelitis and their foot infections, especially in the community setting. Level of evidence: IV.

15. Lipsky BA: Osteomyelitis of the foot in diabetic patients. *Clin Infect Dis* 1997;25(6):1318-1326.

16. Pham TT, Gariani K, Richard JC, et al: Moderate to severe soft tissue diabetic foot infections: A randomized, controlled, pilot trial of post-debridement antibiotic treatment for 10 versus 20 days. *Ann Surg* 2022;276(2):233-238.

    This is a prospective randomized pilot trial investigating the optimal duration of postdébridement antibiotic therapy for soft-tissue DFI. Regardless of the severity of infection, a 10-day course of systemic antibiotics revealed the same outcomes as 20 days. Level of evidence: II.

17. Lipsky BA, Berendt AR, Deery HG, et al: Diagnosis and treatment of diabetic foot infections. *Clin Infect Dis* 2004;39(7):885-910.

18. Ertuğrul BM, Savk O, Öztürk B, Cobanoglu M, Öncü S, Sakarya S: The diagnosis of diabetic foot osteomyelitis: Examination findings and laboratory values. *Med Sci Monit* 2009;15(6):307-312.

19. Aragon-Sanchez J, Lipsky BA, Lazaro-Martinez JL: Diagnosing diabetic foot osteomyelitis: Is the combination of probe-to-bone test and plain radiography sufficient for high-risk inpatients? *Diabet Med* 2011;28(2):191-194.

20. Grayson ML, Gibbons GW, Balogh K, Levin E, Karchmer AW: Probing to bone in infected pedal ulcers. A clinical sign of underlying osteomyelitis in diabetic patients. *J Am Med Assoc* 1995;273(9):721-723.

21. Gariani K, Lebowitz D, Kressmann B, Gariani J, Uçkay I: X-ray versus magnetic resonance imaging in diabetic foot osteomyelitis: A clinical comparison. *Curr Diabetes Rev* 2021;17(3):373-377.

    This is a single-center retrospective evaluation concerning the clinical, and especially surgical, effect of an MRI on diabetic foot osteomyelitis. The authors show that diagnosing osteomyelitis with or without MRI does not change the management or the final outcomes significantly. Level of evidence: III.

22. Uçkay İ, Hüllner MW, Achermann Y, et al: The role of ^{99m}Tc-antigranulocyte SPECT/CT in community-acquired diabetic foot osteomyelitis: A clinical experience. *Curr Diabetes Rev* 2022;18(6):e030521193111.

    This is a single-center, clinical experience comparing MRI technique with a relatively new scintigraphic method in the diagnosis and management of diabetic foot osteomyelitis. This additional scintigraphy did not change the clinical approach. Level of evidence: III.

23. Eckman MH, Greenfield S, Mackey WC, et al: Foot infections in diabetic patients. Decision and cost-effectiveness analyses. *J Am Med Assoc* 1995;273(9):712-720.

24. Waibel F, Berli M, Catanzaro S, et al: Optimization of the antibiotic management of diabetic foot infections: Protocol for two randomized controlled trials. *Trials* 2020;21(1):54.

    This is the published protocol of several (in sum eight strata), ongoing, randomized controlled trials investigating the optimal duration of systemic antibiotic therapy in the nonsurgical and postamputation therapy of soft-tissue and osseous DFI. The primary outcome is remission of infection after a minimum follow-up of 2 months. The secondary outcomes are the incidence of adverse events and the overall treatment costs. The first randomized controlled trial will allocate the total therapeutic amputations in two arms of 50 patients each: 1 versus 3 weeks of antibiotic therapy for residual osteomyelitis (positive microbiologic samples of the residual bone) or 1 versus 4 days for remaining soft-tissue infection. The second randomized controlled trial will randomize the nonsurgical approach (only surgical débridement without in to amputation) in two arms with 50 patients each: 10 versus 20 days of antibiotic therapy for soft-tissue infections and 3 versus 6 weeks for osteomyelitis. All participants will have professional wound débridement, adequate off-loading, angiology evaluation, and a concomitant surgical, reeducational, podiatric, internist, and infectiology care. During the surgeries, tissues are collected for BioBanking and future laboratory studies.

25. Rosskopf AB, Loupatatzis C, Pfirrmann CWA, Böni T, Berli MC: The Charcot foot: A pictorial review. *Insights Imaging* 2019;10:77.

    This is a complete, pictorial, educational review on how to distinguish radiologically evident bone infection with non-infected Charcot deformities in the diabetic foot. Level of evidence: III.

26. Ertuğrul MB, Baktiroğlu S, Salman S, et al: The diagnosis of osteomyelitis of the foot in diabetes: Microbiological examination vs. magnetic resonance imaging and labelled leucocyte scanning. *Diabet Med* 2006;23(6):649-653.

27. Ertuğrul MB, Baktiroğlu S, Salman S, et al: Pathogens isolated from deep soft tissue and bone in patients with diabetic foot infections. *J Am Podiatr Med Assoc* 2008;98(4):290-295.

28. Johani K, Fritz BG, Bjarnsholt T, et al: Understanding the microbiome of diabetic foot osteomyelitis: Insights from molecular and microscopic approaches. *Clin Microbiol Infect* 2019;25(3):332-339.

    The microbiome of the infected diabetic foot, including osteomyelitis, is extremely complex. The presence of biofilms may explain why nonsurgical treatment, relying on systemic antibiotic therapy, may not resolve some chronic infections caused by biofilm-producing strains. Level of evidence: III.

29. Al-Mayahi M, Cian A, Lipsky BA, et al: Administration of antibiotic agents before intraoperative sampling in orthopedic infections alters culture results. *J Infect* 2015;71(5):518-525.

30. Malik A, Mohammad Z, Ahmad J: The diabetic foot infections: Biofilms and antimicrobial resistance. *Diabetes Metab Syndr* 2013;7(2):101-107.

31. Gariani K, Lebowitz D, Kressmann B, et al: Oral amoxicillin-clavulanate for treating diabetic foot infections. *Diabetes Obes Metab* 2019;21(6):1483-1486.

    For many experts, oral beta-lactam antibiotics should be avoided when treating DFI, especially osteomyelitis. In contrast, many general practitioners and other clinicians treat osteomyelitis with oral amoxicillin/clavulanic acid. In this single-center analysis with more than 700 cases of various foot infections, the combined or exclusive use of oral amoxicillin/clavulanic acid, at standard doses, did not change the incidence of clinical or microbiologic failures. Level of evidence: II.

32. Gariani K, Pham TT, Kressmann B, et al: Three weeks versus six weeks of antibiotic therapy for diabetic foot osteomyelitis: A prospective, randomized, noninferiority pilot trial. *Clin Infect Dis* 2021;73(7):1539-1545.

    In this prospective randomized noninferiority pilot trial, patients with osteomyelitis after surgical débridement were randomized (allocation 1:1) to either a 3- or a 6-week course of antibiotic therapy. The minimum duration of follow-up after the end of therapy was 2 months. Outcomes were compared using Cox regression and noninferiority analyses (25% margin). A postdébridement systemic antibiotic therapy course for osteomyelitis of 3 weeks resulted in similar incidences of remission and adverse events to a course of 6 weeks. Level of evidence: II.

33. Senneville E, Joulie D, Blondiaux N, Robineau O: Surgical techniques for bone biopsy in diabetic foot infection, and association between results and treatment duration. *J Bone Jt Infect* 2020;5(4):198-204.

    This is a review of bone biopsy performed at the margins of the resection, which permits the identification of residual osteomyelitis and the adjustment of the postsurgical antibiotic treatment. Some recent studies have reported the way to perform bone margin biopsies and have assessed the effect of the bone results on the patient's outcome. However, the effect of a residual osteomyelitis on the risk of recurrent osteomyelitis is still debated and questions regarding the interpretation of the results remain to be solved. Similarly, the consequences in terms of choice and duration of the antimicrobial treatment to use in case of positive bone margin are not established. Level of evidence: II.

34. Uçkay I, Kressmann B, Di Tommaso S, et al: A randomized-controlled trial of the safety and efficacy of a topical gentamicin-collagen sponge in diabetic patients with a mild foot ulcer infection. *SAGE Open Med* 2018;6:2050312118773950.

    This is a small pilot randomized-controlled trial in Geneva, Switzerland. It randomizes the treatment of mild and superficial ulcerated diabetic foot infections between the use of local gentamicin-sponges and professional wound care only. The diagnosis of mild infections is based on the latest IDSA criteria. In both arms, the clinicians avoid the use of systemic antibiotic agents. The professional wound care is as efficacious as the use of local gentamicin. This pilot trial shows that at least for mild superficial DFI, no systemic agents are probably necessary, which is in line with general principles of antibiotic stewardship in the diabetic foot. Whoever, confirmatory trials are necessary. Level of evidence: II.

35. Bessesen MT, Doros G, Henrie AM, et al: A multicenter randomized placebo-controlled trial of rifampin to reduce pedal amputations for osteomyelitis in veterans with diabetes (VA INTREPID). *BMC Infect Dis* 2020;20(1):23.

    This is a protocol of a prospective randomized double-blind investigation of the addition of rifampin 600 mg daily for 6 weeks versus matched placebo (riboflavin) to standard-of-care, backbone antimicrobial therapy for diabetic foot osteitis. Given that rifampin-adjunctive regimens are currently used for therapy for most osteomyelitis cases in Europe, and only in a small number of cases in the United States, the results may affect therapeutic decisions.

36. Gariani K, Lebowitz D, von Dach E, Kressmann B, Lipsky BA, Uçkay I: Remission in diabetic foot infections: Duration of antibiotic therapy and other possible associated factors. *Diabetes Obes Metab* 2019;21(2):244-251.

This large, single-center database with more than 1,000 cases of DFI found no threshold for the optimal duration or the route of administration (parenteral or oral) of antibiotic therapy to prevent recurrence. These limited data might support possibly shorter treatment duration for patients with DFI. Level of evidence: II.

37. Lipsky BA, Berendt AR, Cornia PB, et al: 2012 Infectious Diseases Society of America clinical practice guideline for the diagnosis and treatment of diabetic foot infections. *Clin Infect Dis* 2012;54:132-173.

38. Rossel A, Lebowitz D, Gariani K, et al: Stopping antibiotics after surgical amputation in diabetic foot and ankle infections – A daily practice cohort. *Endocrinol Diabetes Metab* 2019;2:e00059.

    This is a retrospective single-center analysis of a large database. When all bone and soft-tissue infection has been amputated, prolonging the prophylactic or therapeutic use of antibiotics does not change the outcome. Level of evidence: III.

39. Lázaro-Martínez JL, García-Madrid M, García-Álvarez Y, Álvaro-Afonso FJ, Sanz-Corbalán I, García-Morales E: Conservative surgery for chronic diabetic foot osteomyelitis: Procedures and recommendations. *J Clin Orthop Trauma* 2021;16:86-98.

    Seven types of nonsurgical surgical procedures for the management of osteomyelitis in the forefoot are described in this narrative review: (1) partial or total distal phalangectomy, (2) arthroplasty of the proximal or distal interphalangeal joint, (3) distal Syme amputation, (4) percutaneous flexor tenotomy, (5) sesamoidectomy, (6) arthroplasty of the metatarsophalangeal joint, and (7) metatarsal head resection. Because a lack of sufficient evidence supporting this procedure exists, future investigations should be focused on the randomized controlled trial design. Level of evidence: II.

40. Zingg M, Lacraz A, Robert-Ebadi H, Waibel F, Berli M, Uçkay I: Transcutaneous oxygen pressure values often fail to predict stump failures after foot or limb amputation in chronically ischemic patients. *Clin Surg* 2019;4:2366.

    Orthopaedic diabetic foot surgeons often overestimate the performance of preamputation transcutaneous oxygen pressure values in the prediction of wound healing after amputation for DFI. Low transcutaneous oxygen pressure values are certainly associated with more wound failures, but practically, they should not determine the amputation level alone. Level of evidence: III.

CHAPTER 25

Hand Infections

M. DANIEL WONGWORAWAT, MD, FAAOS • MILAN STEVANOVIC, MD, PhD

ABSTRACT

Acute infections of the hand often require urgent recognition and treatment. Delays in diagnosis and treatment and compromised patient health status are factors associated with poorer outcome. Although evaluation is performed primarily through physical examination, there are important roles for advanced imaging. Recent advances in diagnosis and treatment are highlighted. There also should be an awareness of other entities that may mimic infections.

Keywords: hand infections; human bites; microbiology; palmar space infections; tenosynovitis

INTRODUCTION

Infections of the hand can be a significant burden to health care. Sequelae of delayed treatment include pain, stiffness, and chronic infections. Treatment has become more challenging because of antibiotic resistance. Systemic illnesses such as diabetes and immunocompromised states and disparities in access to health care increase the risk of complications.

Dr. Wongworawat or an immediate family member serves as a board member, owner, officer, or committee member of American Orthopaedic Association, American Society for Surgery of the Hand, Association of Bone and Joint Surgeons, and Health Services International. Neither Dr. Stevanovic nor any immediate family member has received anything of value from or has stock or stock options held in a commercial company or institution related directly or indirectly to the subject of this chapter.

MICROBIOLOGY AND EPIDEMIOLOGY

Although most hand infections are caused by *Staphylococcus* species, the proportion of methicillin-resistant *Staphylococcus aureus* (MRSA) continues to increase. This poses an increasing burden on health care resources, where data suggest that patients with infection from community-acquired MRSA have a more severe clinical course.[1,2] Risk factors for community-acquired MRSA include intravenous drug use, living in close quarters, and previous hand infections.[3,4]

Certain systemic conditions and immunocompromised states increase the risk of developing hand infections and may complicate the course of treatment. In patients with HIV and decreased CD4 counts, aside from *S aureus*, other common organisms include alpha-hemolytic and beta-hemolytic streptococcus; these patients are also at increased risk of viral and fungal infections, such as herpes simplex virus, human papillomavirus, and opportunistic fungal infections. Patients with diabetes, particularly in the setting of neuropathy, may present with delayed infection, including late-stage osteomyelitis or septic arthritis. Diabetes is also a known risk factor for necrotizing fasciitis. Patients with diabetes are also more likely to have polymicrobial or fungal infections, including *Candida* species. Patients who underwent transplantation and are on immunosuppressive therapy face unique challenges, where infections were more likely to involve deeper anatomy and less likely to present with leukocytosis. Patients with autoimmune disorders often are placed on disease-modifying antirheumatic drugs. Although there are perioperative guidelines for holding medications before hip and knee arthroplasties, as of 2020, there is no consensus on applying these recommendations to hand surgery.[5]

EVALUATION

The mainstay of evaluation of hand infections is in the physical examination. Because of the variation in presentation, clinical diagnosis may not be straightforward. Laboratory workup and advanced imaging may be necessary. Erythrocyte sedimentation rate and C-reactive protein levels are usually elevated in the setting of infection; however, increased levels are not specific to hand infections, and in patients who are not able to mount a sufficient immune response, erythrocyte sedimentation rate and C-reactive protein levels may be normal. Commonly used advanced imaging modalities include ultrasonography, CT, and MRI. There has been increased interest in the use of ultrasonography as it offers some advantages over MRI and CT. A 2020 study reported that ultrasonography is sensitive in detecting fluid collections and in live point-of-care assessments; it is also useful for percutaneous aspirations. While being less costly than MRI and CT, one drawback is its operator dependence.[6]

BACTERIAL INFECTIONS

Felon

Infection of the fingertip pulp typically presents with erythema, swelling, and pain with associated congestion. Early cellulitis infections may be treated with antibiotics alone, with coverage of MRSA, if suspicion is reasonable. A 2020 study reported that surgical decompression is performed by incising over the area of maximum fluctuance, taking care to disrupt volar pulp septae that may harbor infective organisms; fish-mouth incisions may increase risk of soft-tissue necrosis and flap contracture and should be avoided.[7] After adequate drainage, antibiotics may not be needed.[8] However, the management of felons remains based on tradition and expert opinion.[9]

Paronychia

A 2022 study reported that infection of the proximal and lateral nail folds results from disruption of the protective barrier between the nail and the nail fold, most often caused by trauma.[10] Although *S aureus* is the most common organism, streptococci and pseudomonas may be seen in chronic infections. In a small study of pediatric patients from 2022, *S aureus* accounted for 58% of paronychia cases, other *Staphylococcus* species accounted for 40%, and streptococci were involved in 37%.[11] A study from 2021 reported that the differential diagnosis should include other organisms such as *Neisseria gonorrhea*, nontuberculous mycobacteria, and herpes simplex, which is often associated with paronychial vesicles.[12] In 2022, it was reported that acute bacterial infections of less than 6 weeks' duration are treated with abscess incision and decompression, and nail plate removal may be necessary if pus is present underneath the nail.[13] In a series of 26 patients with paronychia and 17 patients with combined paronychia and felon who were treated with surgical decompression alone with no antibiotics, only a single failure resulted, which was attributed to inadequate surgical excision. In uncomplicated paronychia treatment, antibiotics are not necessary after surgical treatment.[8]

Human Bites

Human bite injuries to the dorsal metacarpophalangeal joint result from a punch to the mouth, and the extensor tendon and joint capsule are often violated from tooth puncture. Most severe infections are caused by *S aureus*, and combined staphylococcal and streptococcal infections are common. *Eikenella corrodens* is characteristic of human bites and is associated with chronic abscess formation.[14] A cadaver study from 2023 reported that assessment of metacarpophalangeal joint integrity may be performed by a saline load test, where 0.3 mL may be sufficient in detecting joint arthrotomy.[15] In a 2020 retrospective study of 115 patients with a mean follow-up of 52 days, 62 patients were treated with antibiotics only; after adjusting for duration of follow-up and days to presentation, surgical treatment was not associated with lower complications, and time to presentation was the only variable associated with higher risk of complications.[16] When surgical débridement is necessary, a 2021 study of 210 patients treated with a bedside procedure under local anesthetic and field sterility found acceptable results; only 7% required repeat débridement.[17] A systematic review of 14 studies involving 756 patients found that complications were associated with delay in treatment, deeply penetrating injuries, proximal interphalangeal joint involvement, and *E corrodens* infections.[18]

Animal Bites

Dogs and cats account for most animal bites that present to the emergency department. Of dog bites, a 2020 systematic review found bites from German Shepherds and Pit Bulls to be the most common, with trends decreasing and increasing, respectively, from 1971 to 2018.[19]

A 2020 study reported that cat bites are twice as likely to become infected as dog bites, likely from deeper inoculation.[20] After irrigation, closure is acceptable only if débridement is adequate; wounds at high risk of infection (bites to the hand and deep puncture wounds) should be left to heal by secondary intention. Infected wounds often have multiple isolates, including *Pasteurella*, *Staphylococcus*, *Streptococcus*, *Moraxella*, and *Neisseria* species. Most characteristic is *Pasteurella*, an aerobic gram-negative bacillus, with *Pasteurella multocida* and *Pasteurella canis* found in cats and dogs, respectively. *Pasteurella* infection has a rapid onset, typically within the first day, with features of inflammation, cellulitis, and purulence in severe cases. These features may help distinguish *Pasteurella* infections from other organisms. Because multiple organisms may be implicated, polymicrobial antibiotic coverage is recommended in high-risk bite wounds; common oral therapy is with amoxicillin/clavulanic acid, and ampicillin/sulbactam is widely used for intravenous administration. There is controversy regarding prophylactic antibiotics in noninfected wounds; however, antibiotics are recommended for high-risk bite wounds. Characteristics of high risk include bites to the hand, deep or puncture wounds, wounds greater than 12 hours old, and immunocompromised states (such as diabetes and asplenia).

In addition to the aforementioned organisms, *Capnocytophaga canimorsus* is a rarer anaerobic gram-negative rod that is present in cat and dog oral flora. In immunocompromised patients, such as those with asplenia or cirrhosis, *C canimorsus* may cause severe sepsis and death, particularly when fever is present.[14] A low threshold for suspicion should be present for these patients.

Purulent Flexor Tenosynovitis

Suppurative flexor tenosynovitis is classically diagnosed based on cardinal signs of flexor sheath tenderness, flexed position of the digit, painful digital extension, and fusiform swelling. A study of 33 patients from 2022 showed increased diagnostic accuracy with the addition of A1 pulley tenderness to the four signs.[21] A 2022 study reported that infections of the index, long, and ring fingers are usually limited to the flexor sheath up to the A1 pulleys, and the thumb and small finger sheaths may communicate through the radial and ulnar bursae, forming a horseshoe abscess.[22] A 2022 case reported found that this communication occurs through the potential space of Parona, which is between the pronator quadratus fascia and the flexor digitorum profundus tendon sheath.[23]

Although diagnosis is made based on physical examination, a 2022 study comparing contrast-enhanced CT in patients with confirmed flexor tenosynovitis in the operating room demonstrated larger ratios, where coronal and sagittal ratios of 1.3 or greater (axial plane cut tendon sheath width divided by tendon width) had high sensitivity, specificity, and positive predictive value.[24] Other diagnostic imaging modalities include ultrasonography to visualize fluid within the flexor sheath and MRI; however, MRI is rarely used. Other processes such as nontuberculous mycobacterial infection or endemic mycoses may present as subacute flexor tenosynovitis. Advanced imaging may be helpful in identifying tendon sheath involvement.[22]

Early antibiotic treatment in the first few days may be successful, especially when there are fewer clinical signs present. There is little evidence for or against antibiotics alone for early cases, but there is consensus that this approach may be acceptable. A 2023 study reported that if symptomatic improvement is not seen within 2 days of antibiotic administration, or if symptoms worsen, surgical treatment is recommended.[25] A 2020 report found that the most commonly accepted method is the closed sheath technique with an incision at the A1 pulley (**Figure 1**) and another at the A5 pulley.[26] A 2023 report of six patients demonstrated effective irrigation under local anesthesia alone in the emergency department.[27] A larger study from 2023 compared 10 patients who underwent formal operating room drainage versus 24 patients who underwent emergency department drainage; time to intervention was approximately 5 hours sooner for an emergency department procedure, and there were no reported complications or need for additional surgical intervention.[28]

Palmar Space Infections

The midpalmar septum's attachment on the third metacarpal separates the thenar space from the midpalmar space, and the hypothenar space is ulnar to the hypothenar septum. The extensor tendons and fascia dorsally and metacarpals and interosseous muscles palmarly contain the dorsal subaponeurotic space. Interdigital subfascial web spaces can also develop infections, including the collar button abscess extending dorsally and palmarly (**Figure 2**). Multiple options exist for incision types. A 2020 study reported that, in general, incisions should be centered over fluctuance and not traverse flexion creases.[29]

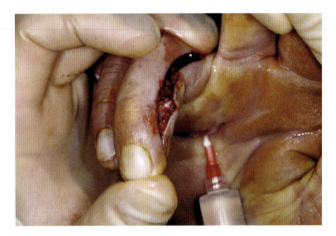

FIGURE 1 Clinical photograph showing how an A1 incision allows for drainage of purulence and insertion of irrigation catheter. Incision at the A5 pulley allows for outflow, and midlateral skin incision decompresses tight finger compartments, if present. (Courtesy of Milan Stevanovic, MD.)

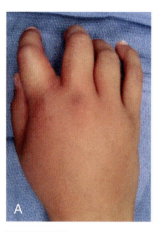
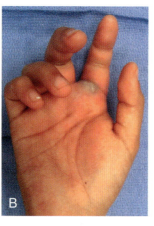

FIGURE 2 Clinical photographs showing a collar-button abscess presenting with (**A**) dorsal fluctuance, and (**B**) with extension into the palm. Because of the expanded space-occupying infection in the intermetacarpal space, the web space is widened with deviation of the digital rays. (Courtesy of Milan Stevanovic, MD.)

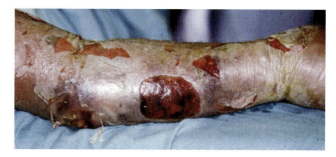

FIGURE 3 Clinical photograph shows rapidly progressing bullae, skin necrosis, and dishwater drainage, which should raise the clinical suspicion for necrotizing fasciitis. Emergency surgical treatment is required. (Courtesy of Milan Stevanovic, MD.)

Bone and Joint Infections

A 2020 study reported that osteomyelitis and septic joints are managed with timely débridement and irrigation followed by antibiotics, and recent evidence suggests that early transition to oral administration is noninferior to the intravenous route.[30] A 2021 study of 69 patients with hand osteomyelitis with a mean follow-up of 16 weeks found successful management using oral antibiotics, which resulted in substantial cost savings over intravenous administration.[31]

Surgical techniques are customized to the specific bone and joint. Although induced membrane technique is commonly used for large diaphyseal bone defects, a preliminary study from 2021 of seven patients undergoing staged surgeries, including an initial débridement of infected tissue and placement of cement spacer and second-stage bone grafting 4 weeks later, reported success in osteomyelitis control.[32]

Necrotizing Infections

Necrotizing soft-tissue infection progresses rapidly and requires early diagnosis. Physical examination findings include rapidly spreading edema, fever, tenderness, bullae, skin necrosis, and dishwater drainage (**Figure 3**). The Laboratory Risk Indicator for Necrotizing Fasciitis (LRINEC) score may assist in diagnosis (**Table 1**). Once diagnosed, emergency surgical management, often with serial débridement, combined with close monitoring is required. A 2020 study reported that, although group A *Streptococcus* is the most common organism, many cases involve multiple pathogens, and broad-spectrum coverage is critical.[33]

Even with the LRINEC score, differentiating necrotizing infection from severe cellulitis can be difficult. A 2021

Table 1

The Laboratory Risk Indicator for Necrotizing Fasciitis Score

Variable (Units)	Score
C-reactive protein level (mg/L)	
<150	0
≥150	4
Total white blood cell count (per mm^3)	
<15	0
15-25	0.5
>25	2.1
Hemoglobin level (g/dL)	
>13.5	0
11-13.5	0.6
<11	1.8
Sodium level (mmol/L)	
≥135	0
<135	1.8
Creatinine level (µmol/L)	
≤141	0
>141	1.8
Glucose level (mmol/L)	
≤10	0
>10	1.2
—	Total score
Clinical suspicion for necrotizing soft-tissue infection	≥6
Highly predictive of necrotizing soft-tissue infection	≥8

Data from Wong CH, Khin LW, Heng KS, et al: The LRINEC (Laboratory Risk Indicator for Necrotizing Fasciitis) score: A tool for distinguishing necrotizing fasciitis from other soft tissue infections. *Crit Care Med* 2004;32:1535-1541.

study compared 40 patients with necrotizing fasciitis and 40 patients with cellulitis and/or abscess with matched LRINEC scores and found additional factors that should increase the suspicion for necrotizing infections; these factors include elevated white cell count, high lactate levels, and homelessness.[34]

Complicating Factors

Diabetes and immunocompromised states are known factors that complicate the course of infection. An analysis of 39 patients with a septic wrist conducted in 2022 found that these factors increase the risk of *Pseudomonas* infection.[35] A 2022 study of 146 patients with hand osteomyelitis found that an increase in C-reactive protein level between diagnosis and follow-up was associated with an increase in amputation risk.[36] A 2019 study reported that delay in presentation of diagnosis, especially if greater than 6 months in cases of osteomyelitis, increases the risk of amputation.[37] A 2022 database study including 145 patients with diabetes found that osteomyelitis, ipsilateral upper extremity dialysis fistula, end-stage renal disease, and vascular disease were associated with amputation.[38]

Mimickers of Infection

Many clinical conditions may mimic hand infection. A 2021 case report determined that gouty tophi may present with erythema and drainage or as acute flexor tenosynovitis.[39] A 2018 case report showed that calcific tendinitis, such as involving the flexor carpi radialis or ulnaris, may present with erythema and mimic infection.[40] Pyogenic granuloma presents as a raised bed of friable tissue that may bleed easily, often associated with small papules and pustules with central necrosis (**Figure 4**). Biopsy shows heavy neutrophil infiltration, and treatment consists of

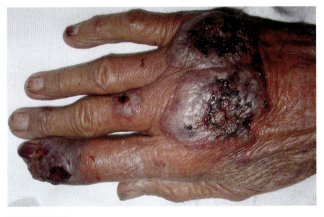

FIGURE 4 Photograph showing pyogenic granuloma, an inflammatory ulcerative dermatosis, presents as bullous lesions on the hand. Note surrounding erythema, tender nodules, and central ulceration. (Courtesy of Milan Stevanovic, MD.)

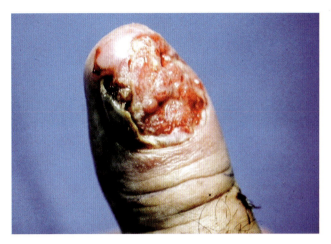

FIGURE 5 Photograph showing squamous cell carcinoma, presenting as red patches with crusting, scaling, and bleeding, which often arises in sun-exposed areas. (Courtesy of Milan Stevanovic, MD.)

local wound management; surgery is generally not indicated.[41] A 2021 study reported that squamous cell carcinoma often presents as chronic ulceration (**Figure 5**). Metastatic disease or systemic involvement, such as leukemic infiltrate, may mimic local inflammatory process.[42] Other considerations include deep penetrating injuries and foreign body reactions.[43,44]

SUMMARY

Hand infections are common. Infection with MRSA may complicate the clinical course. Immunosuppressed patients are at risk for prolonged course of infection. Although diagnosis and treatment plans are primarily made via physical diagnosis, inflammatory markers and advanced imaging may be helpful. Ultrasonography has the advantage of point-of-care application. The mainstay of treatment is incision and drainage. For localized uncomplicated infections, bedside irrigation may be sufficient. Early transition from intravenous to oral antibiotics is effective in many cases, allowing sooner discharge and lower hospital utilization. Gout, calcific tendinitis, pyogenic granuloma, squamous cell carcinoma, and other diseases may mimic hand infections.

KEY STUDY POINTS

- In acute hand infections, urgent diagnosis and treatment are necessary, and the focus of treatment should be appropriate incision and drainage.
- Surgical drainage that was traditionally performed in a formal operating room setting may be effectively performed at bedside under local anesthesia in select cases.

- Diabetes, immunocompromised states, and infection with resistant organisms complicate the clinical course.
- In uncomplicated bone and joint infections, oral antibiotics are noninferior to intravenous administration.
- Necrotizing infections require emergency treatment, including extensive débridement and close monitoring.

ANNOTATED REFERENCES

1. Gundlach BK, Sasor SE, Chung KC: Hand infections: Epidemiology and public health burden. *Hand Clin* 2020;36(3):275-283.

   Community-acquired MRSA is commonly isolated in upper extremity infections, and chronic health conditions and immunosuppression predispose patients to a complicated clinical course.

2. Flevas DA, Syngouna S, Fandridis E, Tsiodras S, Mavrogenis AF: Infections of the hand: An overview. *EFORT Open Rev* 2019;4(5):183-193.

   Clinical suspicion, medical history, and physical examination are mainstays of recognizing infections. Late diagnosis and delayed treatment are associated with morbidity of hand infections.

3. Luginbuhl J, Solarz MK: Complications of hand infections. *Hand Clin* 2020;36(3):361-367.

   Risk factors for complications from hand infections include diabetes mellitus, immunocompromised state, and delay in presentation. Complications include osteomyelitis, amputations, stiffness, and complex wound management needs.

4. Imahara SD, Friedrich JB: Community-acquired methicillin-resistant Staphylococcus aureus in surgically treated hand infections. *J Hand Surg Am* 2010;35(1):97-103.

5. Finley ZJ, Medvedev G: Hand infections associated with systemic conditions. *Hand Clin* 2020;36(3):345-353.

   Patients who have HIV, who have diabetes, or who are on immunosuppressive therapy are at risk for complicated hand infections, such as those from atypical organisms and necrotizing fasciitis.

6. Whitaker CM, Low S, Gorbachova T, Raphael JS, Williamson C: Imaging and laboratory workup for hand infections. *Hand Clin* 2020;36(3):285-299.

   Erythrocyte sedimentation rate and C-reactive protein levels are helpful for tracking disease progression and resolution. CT provides bony detail and is sensitive in detecting soft-tissue gas, MRI is useful for viewing soft-tissue and marrow detail, and ultrasonography can be applied for point-of-care evaluation.

7. Barger J, Garg R, Wang F, Chen N: Fingertip infections. *Hand Clin* 2020;36(3):313-321.

   Abscesses of the nail fold and infections of the fingertip pulp require adequate decompression.

8. Pierrart J, Delgrande D, Mamane W, Tordjman D, Masmejean EH: Acute felon and paronychia: Antibiotics not necessary after surgical treatment. Prospective study of 46 patients. *Hand Surg Rehabil* 2016;35(1):40-43.

9. Tannan SC, Deal DN: Diagnosis and management of the acute felon: Evidence-based review. *J Hand Surg Am* 2012;37(12):2603-2604.

10. Dulski A, Edwards CW: Paronychia, in *StatPearls*. StatPearls Publishing, 2022.

    Acute paronychia presenting within 6 weeks is most often caused by staphylococci. The mainstay of treatment is incision and drainage.

11. McKean AR, Williams GJ, Macneal P, Moore LS, Idowu A, Milroy C: Paediatric paronychia: A single centre retrospective, microbiological analysis and national survey. *J Plast Reconstr Aesthet Surg* 2022;75(7):2387-2440.

    A report of 84 children found that *S aureus* accounted for 58% of cases of pediatric paronychia, other *Staphylococcus* species accounted for 40%, whereas streptococci was involved in 37%.

12. Iorizzo M, Pasch MC: Bacterial and viral infections of the nail unit. *Dermatol Clin* 2021;39(2):245-253.

    Obtaining cultures is important in diagnosing and managing acute paronychia. Differential should include other organisms such as gonorrhea, atypical mycobacterium, and herpes simplex, which is often associated with paronychial vesicles.

13. Macneal P, Milroy C: Paronychia drainage, in *StatPearls*. StatPearls Publishing, 2022.

    Early paronychia may be treated with antibiotics alone, but many patients present with suppuration around the nail fold. In all cases with abscesses, surgical drainage is indicated.

14. Malahias M, Jordan D, Hughes O, Khan WS, Hindocha S: Bite injuries to the hand: Microbiology, virology and management. *Open Orthop J* 2014;8:157-161.

15. Chughtai M, Scollan JP, Emara AK, et al: The "Fight bite" saline joint loading test: Effectiveness in detecting simulated traumatic metacarpophalangeal arthrotomies. *Hand (N Y)* 2023;18(5):792-797.

    A cadaver study of sixteen hands found that injection volumes of 0.32 mL is 99% sensitive for identifying traumatic arthrotomy at the metacarpophalangeal joint.

16. Harper CM, Dowlatshahi AS, Rozental TD: Challenging dogma: Optimal treatment of the "Fight bite". *Hand (N Y)* 2020;15(5):647-650.

    This retrospective study of 115 patients found that irrigation in the emergency department and expectant wound may be sufficient in patients presenting within 24 hours in the absence of gross purulence. Level of evidence: IV.

17. Kay HF, Kang HP, Fisch R, Stevanovic M, Ghiassi A, Nicholson LT: The management of clenched fist injuries with local anaesthesia and field sterility. *J Hand Surg Eur Vol* 2021;46(4):411-415.

A study of 232 patients concluded that irrigation and débridement under local anesthesia with field stability, such as in the emergency department, is acceptable, with a low risk of complications or need for repeat débridement. Level of evidence: IV.

18. Smith HR, Hartman H, Loveridge J, Gunnarsson R: Predicting serious complications and high cost of treatment of tooth-knuckle injuries: A systematic literature review. *Eur J Trauma Emerg Surg* 2016;42(6):701-710.

19. Bailey CM, Hinchcliff KM, Moore Z, Pu LLQ: Dog bites in the United States from 1971 to 2018: A systematic review of the peer-reviewed literature. *Plast Reconstr Surg* 2020;146(5):1166-1176.

    This systematic review of 41 articles found that German Shepherd and Pit Bull breeds account for the largest subset of pure breeds implicated in severe dog bites.

20. Elcock KL, Reid J, Moncayo-Nieto OL, Rust PA: Biting the hand that feeds you: Management of human and animal bites. *Injury* 2022;53(2):227-236.

    Cat bites are more likely to become infected than dog bites because of deeper inoculation. Infected wounds often have multiple isolated organisms.

21. Siska RC, Davidson AL, Driscoll CR, et al: A1 pulley tenderness as a modification to tenderness along the flexor sheath in diagnosing pyogenic flexor tenosynovitis. *Plast Reconstr Surg Glob Open* 2022;10(3):e4165.

    A study of 33 patients found that while the classic Kanavel signs have reliable clinical utility, tenderness at the A1 pulley resulted in improved specificity. Level of evidence: IV.

22. Hermena S, Tiwari V: Pyogenic flexor tenosynovitis, in *StatPearls*. StatPearls Publishing, 2022.

    The flexor sheaths of the index, long, and ring fingers extend to the A1 pulleys, whereas those of the flexor pollicis longus communicate with the radial bursa proximally, and those of the small finger communicate with the ulna bursa. Interconnections may result in a horseshoe abscess.

23. Kuah T, Al Moslem FS, Banjar MA, Hallinan J: Parona space collection: A serious complication of hand infections. *Int J Infect Dis* 2022;120:121-124.

    This case report highlights the presence of the space of Parona, where interconnection in the distal forearm allows for potential abscess communication between the thumb and small finger.

24. Myers DM, Goubeaux C, Skura B, Warmoth PJ, Taylor BC: Contrast enhanced computed tomography in the diagnosis of acute pyogenic flexor tenosynovitis. *Hand (N Y)* 2022; May 24 [Epub ahead of print].

    This study of two adult cohorts with and without flexor tenosynovitis reports on the utility of CT ratios in the diagnosis of flexor sheath infections. Level of evidence: III.

25. Latario L, Abeler J, Clegg S, Thurber L, Igiesuorobo O, Jones M: Antibiotics versus surgery in treatment of early flexor tenosynovitis. *Hand (N Y)* 2023;18(5):804-810.

    A study of 40 patients, in which 20 were treated with surgical management and 20 were treated with antibiotics alone, found that shorter duration of symptoms and fewer Kanavel signs were associated with successful treatment with antibiotics alone. Level of evidence: III.

26. Goyal K, Speeckaert AL: Pyogenic flexor tenosynovitis: Evaluation and management. *Hand Clin* 2020;36(3):323-329.

    S aureus is the most common organism in pyogenic flexor tenosynovitis. Closed tendon sheath irrigation is usually successful.

27. Braza ME, Kelley JP, Kelpin JP, Fahrenkopf MP, Do VH: Treatment of pyogenic flexor tenosynovitis in the emergency department setting with WALANT technique. *Hand (N Y)* 2023;18(3):473-477.

    This report of six patients with pyogenic flexor tenosynovitis found that emergency department wide-awake surgery was effective and well-tolerated. Level of evidence: IV.

28. Rao V, Snapp WK, Crozier JW, Bhatt RA, Schmidt ST, Kalliainen LK: Limited flexor sheath incision and drainage in the emergency department in the management of early pyogenic flexor tenosynovitis. *Hand (N Y)* 2023;18(2):320-327.

    This retrospective study of 34 patients found that limited flexor sheath irrigation in the emergency department had shorter time to intervention, and there were no procedural complications or need for additional surgical intervention. Level of evidence: III.

29. Rekant MS, Tarr R: Hand abscesses: Volar and dorsal. *Hand Clin* 2020;36(3):307-312.

    Knowledge of hand anatomy is important in recognizing and treating hand abscesses. The mainstay of treatment is timely incision and drainage.

30. Chenoweth B: Septic joints: Finger and wrist. *Hand Clin* 2020;36(3):331-338.

    Finger and wrist septic joints often present with redness and swelling, sometimes associated with penetrating trauma. Prompt surgical débridement is required. Early transition to oral antibiotics is noninferior to prolonged intravenous administration.

31. Henry M, Lundy FH: Oral antibiotic management of acute osteomyelitis of the hand: Outcomes and cost comparison to standard intravenous regimen. *Hand (N Y)* 2021;16(4):535-541.

    This case series of 69 patients found that susceptibility-matched oral antibiotics after surgical débridement was associated with substantial direct and indirect cost savings when compared with central catheter administration. Level of evidence: IV.

32. Toyama T, Hamada Y, Horii E, Kinoshita R, Saito T: Finger rescue using the induced membrane technique for osteomyelitis of the hand. *J Hand Surg Asian Pac Vol* 2021;26(2):235-239.

    Induced membrane technique for osteomyelitis of the hand was shown to be successful in treating infection in seven patients. Level of evidence: IV.

33. Melillo A, Addagatla K, Jarrett NJ: Necrotizing soft tissue infections of the upper extremity. *Hand Clin* 2020;36(3):339-344.

Necrotizing soft-tissue infection of the upper extremity requires emergency surgical débridement. The risk of amputation and mortality is high.

34. Cohen LE, Kang H, Sochol K, et al: Differentiating upper extremity necrotizing soft tissue infection from serious cellulitis and abscess. *Cureus* 2021;13(9):e17806.

    This matched cohort study found additional factors that may differentiate necrotizing soft-tissue infections from cellulitis or abscess: elevated lactate, history of fever, male sex, and homelessness. Level of evidence: III.

35. Krauss S, Denzinger M, Rachunek K, Kolbenschlag J, Daigeler A, Illg C: Septic arthritis of the wrist: A retrospective review of 39 cases. *J Hand Surg Eur Vol* 2022;47(8):812-817.

    A retrospective series of 39 patients found that immunosuppression and diabetes were associated with *Pseudomonas* infection. Level of evidence: IV.

36. Wyman M, Dargan D, Kazzazi D, Caddick J, Giblin V: Serum inflammatory markers and amputations in hand osteomyelitis: A retrospective review of 146 cases. *Hand (N Y)* 2022; February 8 [Epub ahead of print].

    An analysis of 146 patients with hand osteomyelitis found that C-reactive protein level had higher sensitivity than white cell count, neutrophile-to-lymphocyte ratio, and platelet-to-lymphocyte ratio. White cell count and C-reactive protein level both within normal ranges were predictive against amputation. Level of evidence: III.

37. Koshy JC, Bell B: Hand infections. *J Hand Surg Am* 2019;44(1):46-54.

    Four main infectious conditions of the hand require emergent attention: necrotizing soft-tissue infections, flexor tenosynovitis, deep hand space infections, and septic arthritis. Treatment delay may increase the risk of amputation.

38. Gibson E, Bettlach CR, Payne E, et al: Predictors of digital amputation in diabetic patients with surgically treated finger infections. *Hand (N Y)* 2022; March 14 [Epub ahead of print].

    A study of 145 patients found that in patients with diabetes, four factors were associated with digital amputation: osteomyelitis, same arm dialysis fistula, end-stage renal disease, and vascular disease. Level of evidence: IV.

39. Cochrane E, Sandler RD, Dargan D, Hughes M, Caddick J: Gout presenting as acute flexor tenosynovitis mimicking infection. *J Clin Rheumatol* 2021;27(6):e236-e237.

    This case report highlights the importance of considering gout in the differential diagnosis of flexor tenosynovitis.

40. Shim MR: Unusual etiology of acute wrist pain: Acute calcific tendonitis of the flexor carpi ulnaris mimicking an infection. *Case Rep Orthop* 2018;2018:2520548.

    This case report illustrates the overlap of clinical presentation, where acute calcific tendonitis may mimic infection.

41. To D, Wong A, Montessori V: Atypical pyoderma gangrenosum mimicking an infectious process. *Case Rep Infect Dis* 2014;2014:589632.

42. Cruz D, Wild T, Glavynskyi I, et al: Unusual manifestation of chronic lymphocytic leukemia in the hand. *J Hand Surg Am* 2021;46(1):74.e1-74.e8.

    Pain on the dorsum of the hand from chronic lymphocytic leukemia may present as an infection.

43. Guss MS, Ruchelsman DE, Leibman MI: Deep penetrating kerosene exposure in the hand mimicking deep space infection. *J Hand Microsurg* 2020;12(2):125-127.

    Hydrocarbon penetration, such as that from kerosene, may present with midpalmar swelling and have an appearance similar to an infection.

44. Jacobs JWG, Schuurman AH: A prosthetic wrist joint complicated by metallosis and polyethylene synovitis, mimicking low-grade bacterial arthritis. *Clin Exp Rheumatol* 2021;39(2):438.

    Polyethylene synovitis and metallosis have the potential to mimic bacterial joint infections.

CHAPTER 26

Infections of the Spine

MAJA BABIC, MD • CLAUS S. SIMPFENDORFER, MD

ABSTRACT

Native spine infections are a heterogenous entity. Differences in clinical presentations are based on the affected anatomic structure of the spine. Except for cases of direct pathogen inoculation during instrumentation, native spine infections are caused by hematogenous seeding of the vertebral end plates, the disk space, and the facet joints. Undiagnosed and untreated, the infection can extend into the epidural space and form an epidural abscess, which can compress the spinal cord and result in significant morbidity and mortality. Diagnosis is based on advanced imaging. Better understanding of underlying anatomy and MRI has caused a shift toward more nonsurgical management of epidural abscesses. Clear-cut indications for early surgical intervention remain a major focus of research.

Keywords: diagnostic biopsy; epidural abscess; septic facet joint; Spondylodiscitis; surgical indications

INTRODUCTION

The incidence of spine infections involving both the native vertebral column and the instrumented spine is rising. The reasons are multifactorial. The population of older immunocompromised patients with significant comorbidities is growing. This population is subject to invasive medical procedures that carry a risk of transient bacteremia. Advanced, cross-sectional imaging is necessary to confirm the diagnosis and this type of imaging is widely available.

INCIDENCE

The annual incidence of spine infections of the native vertebral column is highly variable and ranges from 1 to 7 per 100,000 inhabitants.[1,2] In a 2018 retrospective review on spine infections in the United States, the mean annual incidence over a 15-year period from 1998 to 2013 was 4.7 in 100,000 admissions. A total of 228,044 patients were admitted with a diagnosis of vertebral osteomyelitis during this period, with an increasing annual trend, starting at 8,021 admissions per year in 1998 (an incidence of 2.9 of 100,000 and reaching 16,917 admissions per year in 2013 (5.4 of 100,000).[3] Prior studies on the epidemiology of spine infections that were conducted in Europe and showed a steady increase in incidence as the patient population aged, with a peak at age 70 years and older were compared with a US study that showed a shift to younger patients, with 49.5% of patients diagnosed in those younger than 59 years.[3] It is unclear what contributed to this marked difference, but factors could include heightened awareness, easier access to cross-sectional imaging, and the ongoing opioid crisis.

ANATOMY AND PHYSIOLOGY OF STRUCTURES RELEVANT IN SPINE INFECTIONS

Spine infections are a heterogeneous group of clinical syndromes. The basis for the variability is in the complex anatomic structure of the spinal column. The building blocks of the musculoskeletal spine include the vertebral bodies, the intervertebral disks (IVDs), the epidural space, the posterior elements, and the costovertebral joints (CVJs) in the thoracic spine. The IVDs connect adjacent vertebral bodies and function as a joint equivalent, providing the spine with flexibility. IVDs are

---

Neither of the following authors nor any immediate family member has received anything of value from or has stock or stock options held in a commercial company or institution related directly or indirectly to the subject of this chapter: Dr. Babic and Dr. Simpfendorfer.

composed of the inner gelatinous nucleus pulposus, the outer thick ringlike anulus fibrosus, and the hyaline end plates. In vertebrates, all spinal elements are mesodermal in origin, with the nucleus pulposus being the only derivative of the primordial notochord. All other structures are derived from sclerotomes.[4] The IVD in children is a vascularized structure, supplied by branches of interosseous arteries. These vessels involute in adults, making the IVD the largest avascular structure of the human body.[5] Vertebral bodies are the main weight-bearing elements of the spinal column, carrying 80% of its load in upright position. The bone-cartilage interface of the vertebral end plates is a physiologic equivalent of metaphyseal plates, which are supplied by terminal arteriolar loops.[6] Facet joints are synovial joints that can contain menisci. Together with the laminae and pedicles, they form the posterior elements. They interlock adjacent vertebral bodies posteriorly and are part of the weight-bearing tripod comprising vertebral bodies anteriorly and two symmetric facet joints in the back. Posterior elements bear approximately 20% of the load of a vertical spine. Their main function is to transfer load and constrain movement. With progressive degenerative disk disease and vertebral body loss of height, the weight balance shifts onto the posterior elements. The epidural space is located between the vertebral bone and the dura mater, the outer lining of the spinal cord. It is a potential space that contains fat, blood vessels, and traversing nerves. It is contiguous with the paraspinal space laterally and with the paravertebral space posteriorly.[7]

ETIOLOGY OF SPINE INFECTIONS

Infectious organisms can reach the spine hematogenously from a distant entry point or contiguously from an adjacent infected structure, or they can be introduced by instrumentation. In adults, the axial skeleton is the primary target for hematogenous osteomyelitis.[8] In contrast, young skeletons with open epiphyseal plates are at risk for hematogenous seeding of long bones, which does not occur in the adult population. The primary target is the metaphysis or its equivalent, where terminal blood vessels supply the bone-to-cartilage transition. Bacteria-laden clots of platelets lodge into end arteries, occlude them, and cause a septic bone infarct. In the adult spine, this happens at the vertebral end plates. The infection spreads to the adjacent IVD as it is an avascular structure that depends on the vertebral end plate supply for nutrients. Thus, osteomyelitis precedes the discitis and justifies the terms spondylitis and spondylodiscitis.[9,10] In children, the IVD is vascularized and can be the primary target of the infected clot, which leads to an isolated infection of the IVD or discitis. If left to progress unabated, the infection spreads locally from the disk and vertebral end plates into adjacent soft tissues. Anterior spread results in prevertebral collections in the retropharyngeal space of the cervical spine, the paravertebral space in the thorax, and the psoas muscles, which line the lumbar spine laterally.[11] Hematogenous seeding can affect synovial joints in the spine analogous to large joints such as the knee or hip during bacteremic episodes. Synovial joints are thought to be vulnerable to infection because the synovium lacks a protective basal membrane and is therefore porous and easily entered by infectious organisms.[12] Both the facet joint and the CVJ can be seeded hematogenously, although CVJs usually get infected because of direct extension from the adjacent vertebral body and IVD complex. Notable exceptions are the CVJ of the 1st, 11th, and 12th ribs as they join the lateral body of the vertebra and not the area of the IVD and two adjacent vertebra.[13,14] Extension of infection from both spondylodiscitis posteriorly and septic facet joint (SFJ) anteriorly expands the potential epidural space and causes and epidural abscess (EDA). Historically, EDA was labeled as primary and secondary. Primary EDA was thought to arise from the seeding of the potential space itself, which is unlikely. The widespread use of the term is attributed to limitations of the pre-MRI era, as the origin of infection cannot be delineated easily on a CT myelogram.[15] A secondary EDA results from spread of infection from either the vertebral body or disk posteriorly or from an SFJ spilling purulent material anteriorly. In a few cases, the spinal column is secondarily infected by spread from adjacent structures, namely esophageal leaks in patients with cancer who underwent head and neck irradiation, infected vascular grafts in the thorax or abdomen, fistulas from inflammatory bowel disease, or postoperative anastomotic bowel leaks. Direct inoculation of infection can happen following local steroid injections, pain pump implantations, instrumented fusion, or decompression procedures not involving hardware, such as diskectomies and laminectomies.[16]

MICROBIOLOGY

Hematogenous infections of the spine are monomicrobial; contiguous infections secondary to pelvic abscesses, dehisced surgical wounds, or decubitus ulcers can be polymicrobial.

Gram-positive bacteria account for most musculoskeletal infections, including the spine.[17] Staphylococci and streptococci are the leading cause of spondylodiscitis and comprise 60% to 90% of all infections in large case series of vertebral osteomyelitis.[18] This trend is confirmed in series of EDA with 90% of infections caused by gram-positive organisms.[19] *Staphylococcus aureus* remains the most frequent infectious agent isolated in infections of the native spine.[18-21] The nares are the main reservoir of *S aureus*, but as a commensal organism, it colonizes the skin, axillae, groin, pharynx, and vagina. Following a breach of skin or mucosal barrier, it gains access to the bloodstream and is well equipped to establish infections at distant sites.[22] *S aureus* has a unique ability to enter the osteoblast and survive intracellularly. Unlike the macrophage, the osteoblast is not an official phagocyte and cannot digest the bacterium in its lysosome.[23] *S aureus* remains protected inside a vesicle in the form of an indolent, resilient small colony variant that triggers the programmed death of the infected osteoblast. On disintegration of the infected cell, small colony variants are released and quickly revert to the aggressive wild type to infect adjacent osteoblasts. The loss of osteoblasts disrupts the equilibrium of bone formation as osteoclasts continue to degrade the mineralized matrix. An article from 2020 reported that this unabated activity of osteoclasts leads to net bone loss in infection.[24] Streptococci are gram-positive organisms that are the second most frequent bacterial pathogen causing spine infections. Streptococci are a heterogenous group of bacteria that range from highly virulent strains of *Streptococcus pyogenes*, *Streptococcus pneumoniae*, and *Streptococcus agalactiae/Streptococcus dysgalactiae* to indolent strains of *Streptococcus viridans*. Beta-hemolytic streptococci comprise most clinically overt spine infections, whereas the less virulent alpha-hemolytic *S viridans* tend to be associated with cases of dual infections of endocarditis and vertebral osteomyelitis.[25,26] *Staphylococcus epidermidis* is a coagulase-negative *Staphylococcus* that is a normal skin commensal with a low virulent potential. Prolonged bacteremia with *S epidermidis* requires the presence of infected artificial material, such as a hemodialysis catheter or an infected prosthetic valve. In cases of prolonged bacteremia, coagulase-negative staphylococci can cause spondylodiscitis.[27] In historical vertebral osteomyelitis series, gram-negative infections account for 15% to 30% of all cases.[18,28] The gastrointestinal and genitourinary systems harbor gram-negative commensals that gain access to the bloodstream during overt infection or following an invasive gastrointestinal/genitourinary procedure. Additional studies of vertebral osteomyelitis show a decreasing trend in gram-negative infections for unclear reasons.[19,29] A few infections are caused by fungi. A case series from 2019 reported that *Candida* and *Aspergillus* spp. affect high-risk patients with compromised immune systems or with injection drug use.[30] Tuberculosis, brucellosis, and parasitic spine infections are found in endemic areas. Gas-forming infections of the spine are exceedingly rare. Only 38 cases are described in literature and are a clinical curiosity. They include gas-containing EDA, emphysematous osteomyelitis, and necrotizing fasciitis of the spine and occur in elderly patients with diabetes who have rapid clinical deterioration and poor outcome. Most are monomicrobial gram-negative infections, such as *Escherichia coli* and *Klebsiella* spp., with only occasional clostridial and streptococcal cases documented. A literature review from 2021 reported on the distinct absence of *S aureus*.[31]

CLINICAL PRESENTATION AND DIAGNOSIS

Infections of the spine present as back pain in most cases (80%).[32,33] It is difficult to distinguish pain related to degenerative disease of the spine from that caused by a serious underlying disorder, namely infection, trauma, or cancer (**Table 1**). A delay in diagnosis is a hallmark of spine infections and has not been eliminated despite increased awareness of the condition and widespread availability of advanced imaging. Back pain in patients with the following risk factors should raise concern: susceptibility to episodes of bacteremia with chronic indwelling lines for hemodialysis access, chemotherapy or total parenteral nutrition, or injection drug use. Most studies also report diabetes, malignancy, alcoholism, and immunocompromised status as risk factors.[11,16,18] The back pain can be preceded by mechanical trauma; it is aggravated by movement and progresses to the point that it interferes with sleep. Patients describe it as throbbing or pulsating. Untreated, it evolves into unremitting pain at rest. Fever is an inconsistent symptom ranging from 16% to 97% in large case series.[1,18] Symptoms can be masked by use of anti-inflammatory agents or antibiotics administered for concomitant or preceding infection at a distant site. The onset, character of pain, and associated symptoms vary, depending on which of the different spinal elements are seeded. Spondylodiscitis presents gradually with midline pain that can radiate to either side. An SFJ presents acutely; frequently, patients recall the hour of pain onset. A study from 2020 reported that fever is more frequent in SFJ.[34]

CVJs are affected by lateral spread of infection from spondylodiscitis and can present as pleurisy. In the cervical spine, dysphagia or odynophagia can occur; in the thoracic spine, visceral symptoms related to the irritation of paravertebral ganglia can mask the clinical picture. Thoracic spondylodiscitis can present as chest or abdominal pain with associated sweating and palpitations mimicking a heart attack, cholecystitis, or pancreatitis. In the lumbar spine, extension into the psoas muscle can present as hip or leg pain. A serious and potentially life-threatening consequence of a spine infection is an EDA that compresses the spinal cord. Spinal cord compression causes neurologic deficits, loss of bladder or bowel control, or sudden weakness in extremities and is a surgical emergency. Because the spinal cord ends at the level of L2, serious neurologic deficits are mostly related to cervical and thoracic spine infections. Occasionally, an EDA

Table 1

Summary of Spine Infections: Clinical Presentation, Imaging, and Therapy

	Definition	Clinical Picture	CT	MRI	Therapy
Discitis	Isolated infection of vascularized disk in young child	Back pain in febrile toddler	Not helpful	Disk space enhances on T1-weighted postcontrast (**Figure 3**)	Antibiotic
Spondylodiscitis	Infection of vertebral end plates extending into disk	Indolent midline throbbing back pain, progresses to nocturnal pain	Eroded end plates (**Figure 5**) Paravertebral soft-tissue edema (**Figure 4, A** and **B**) Psoas muscle abscess (**Figure 6**) Useful for CT-guided biopsy	End plates and disk space enhance on postcontrast T1-weighted (**Figure 2**) Paravertebral soft-tissue edema on T2-weighted/STIR (**Figure 4, C**)	Antibiotic + surgery if epidural abscess with cord compression or loss of bone stock/mechanical instability
Septic facet joint	Pyogenic arthritis of synovial joint	Acute-onset unilateral back pain, often in febrile adult	Paraspinal soft-tissue edema with rim-enhancing collection (**Figure 7, A**) CT useful for aspiration	Fluid signal in facet joint and paraspinal tissue on T2-weighted/STIR (**Figure 7, B**) Smoking pipe sign (**Figure 8**)	Antibiotic + aspiration for prolonged bacteremia or pain relief
Epidural abscess	Extension of purulence into epidural space from spondylodiscitis or septic facet joint	Can compress spinal cord and cause weakness of extremities, loss of bladder/bowel control	Not helpful	Rim-enhancing collection on T1-weighted postcontrast originating from spondylodiscitis (**Figure 1, B**) or from septic facet joint (**Figure 9**)	Antibiotic + surgery only if cord compressed and neurologic deficits present

STIR = short tau inversion recovery

originating in the lumbar spine can ascend proximally to compress the cord. Neurologic symptoms occur in the setting of cord compression secondary to EDA or mechanical collapse of the vertebral column. Rarely, acute transverse myelitis can occur in the absence of mechanical compression and is attributed to an inflammatory response compromising the vascular supply of the spinal cord. The prognosis is poor in cases of acute transverse myelitis.[35]

As mentioned, the delay in diagnosis has not improved significantly over the past decades. Routine screening tools fail to alert the caretakers on initial presentation. The only laboratory marker that consistently points to a serious cause of back pain is C-reactive protein (CRP).[36] In patients with elevated CRP level, it behooves the clinician to exclude trauma, metastatic cancer, or infection. Imaging is the mainstay of establishing a diagnosis of spine infections. Plain radiographs are of little value in the early course of disease. End plate irregularities and loss of disk space can be seen with progression of untreated infection with a lag time of 2 weeks to 2 months.[9] The imaging modality of choice is MRI, preferably with administration of intravenous contrast material.[37] Following reports of a link between nephrogenic systemic fibrosis and the use of high-dose gadolinium preparations in patients undergoing dialysis, clinicians are hesitant to use contrast material in MRI. However, a study from 2020 reported that new generations of gadolinium have been developed and are safe to use in patients undergoing dialysis.[38] Although a diagnosis of infection can be established on a noncontrast MRI examination, the best information can be obtained if a fat-suppressed postcontrast sequence is included in the MRI protocols for infectious workup.[39] Contrast

Chapter 26: Infections of the Spine

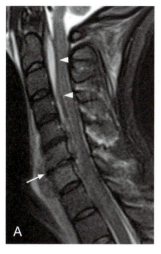
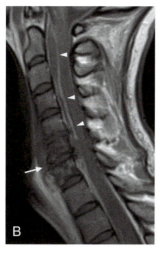

FIGURE 1 **A**, Fluid-sensitive T2-weighted magnetic resonance image of the cervical spine show C6-7 spondylodiscitis (arrow) and bright signal enhancement (arrowheads) in the epidural space: either a phlegmon or epidural abscess (EDA). **B**, Postcontrast T1-weighted image confirms that the rim-enhancing collection (arrowheads) is an EDA originating from C6-7 spondylodiscitis (arrow).

edema depicted in **Figure 4** is a specific finding that helps differentiate vertebral osteomyelitis from degenerative disease of the spine.[37] MRI is contraindicated in patients with certain cardiac implantable electronic devices, cochlear implants, and implantable neurostimulation systems.[42] If these patients cannot be urgently cleared for MRI, CT myelography is an alternative tool for EDA diagnosis and localization. It requires a lumbar puncture and injection of contrast material into the cerebrospinal fluid sac. A lack of free flow in contrast material outlines the EDA, though it cannot always trace its origin to the disk space, spondylodiscitis, or SFJ. In large series, CT myelograms were used to diagnose EDA; the term primary EDA was thus introduced for EDA of unknown origin.[15] If a spine infection is suspected in a neurologically intact patient, alternative imaging tools to MRI include contrast-enhanced CT, fluorodeoxyglucose positron emission tomography (FDG-PET), or combined gallium/^{99}Tc bone scanning.[43,44] CT is the modality of choice for evaluating bony structures and can diagnose

material is necessary to differentiate between EDA and phlegmon; EDA presents as a rim-enhancing collection on postcontrast T1-weighted images with a dark center and white rim. A phlegmon uniformly enhances and is not amenable to surgical drainage as it lacks the liquefied, purulent central part.[40] **Figure 1** demonstrates how addition of contrast material confirms an EDA diagnosis. Hallmarks of vertebral osteomyelitis on MRI include dark end plates on T1-weighted sequences that enhance with contrast material, narrowed disk space, enhancing disk space and fluid signal in surrounding soft tissue that enhances with contrast material (**Figures 2** and **3**). The earliest sign of acute vertebral osteomyelitis is enhancement of end plates.[41] Paravertebral soft-tissue

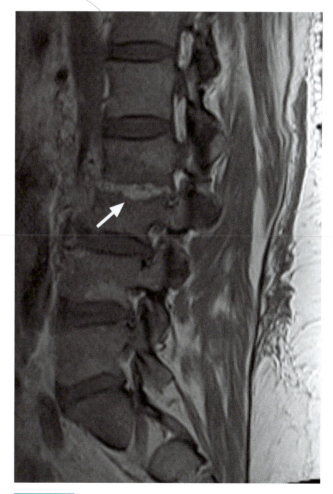

FIGURE 3 Postcontrast T1-weighted magnetic resonance image with uniformly enhancing disk space (arrow).

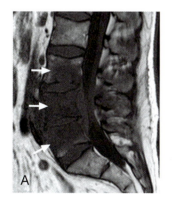
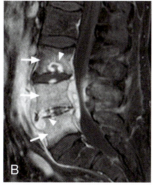

FIGURE 2 **A**, T1-weighted postcontrast magnetic resonance image of the lumbar spine with bright signal enhancement of L3-4 end plates marked by arrows. **B**, Postcontrast fat-suppressed T1-weighted image accentuates the bright signal intensity of the disk (arrowheads) and end plates (arrows).

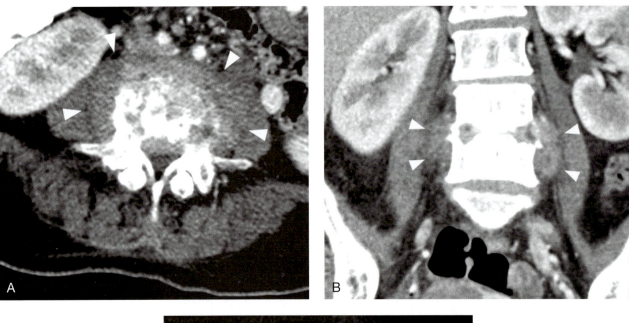

FIGURE 4 **A,** Axial CT scan shows soft-tissue edema (arrowheads) adjacent to the vertebral body. **B,** Coronal CT scan shows soft-tissue edema (arrowheads) adjacent to spondylodiscitis. **C,** T2-weighted magnetic resonance image shows soft-tissue edema (arrowheads) surrounding the vertebral body.

end plate erosions, narrowing of disk space, and bone loss of vertebral bodies (**Figure 5**). It shows edema and enhancement of the adjacent paravertebral and paraspinal soft tissues and reliably identifies psoas muscle abscesses secondary to lumbar spondylodiscitis (**Figure 6**). It is helpful in differentiating early changes of spondylodiscitis on MRI from degenerative disk disease as manifested by a vacuum disk phenomenon not seen on MRI.[45] FDG-PET scans are the best alternative to MRI for diagnosing spine infections and offer superior sensitivity to CT imaging, albeit at higher cost and limited availability. Neither contrast-enhanced CT nor can FDG-PET can be used to diagnose EDA.[46,47] SFJs are frequently overlooked and underreported. Plain radiographs only show degenerative changes of posterior elements and are not useful in screening for SFJ in the acute setting. CT imaging is not helpful, unless extensive inflammatory changes are present adjacent to the affected SFJ. Advanced SFJs show erosive cortical changes of the articular surfaces adjacent to rim-enhancing collections in the paraspinal soft tissues as shown in **Figure 7**. Occasionally, the infection extends from the SFJ into the ipsilateral psoas muscle and is visualized on CT contrast images as a psoas abscess. MRI is the most sensitive tool for diagnosing SFJ. Unilateral joint effusions of the facet joint with periarticular bone marrow edema are indicative of SFJ. They are associated

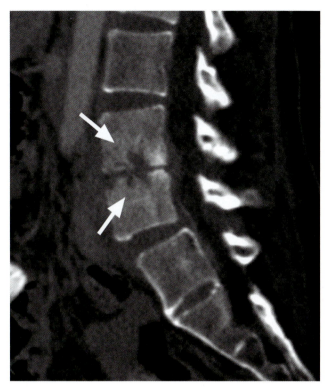

FIGURE 5 Sagittal CT scan shows erosive changes of end plates (arrows).

with inflammatory changes in the soft tissues, including collections in the paraspinal or psoas muscles (**Figure 7**). On sagittal views of fluid-sensitive sequences, SFJ resembles a smoking pipe, with the pipe represented by the distended joint effusion and the billowing smoke by

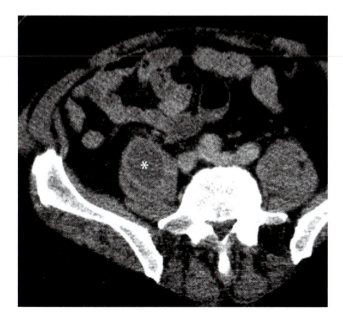

FIGURE 6 Contrast-enhanced axial CT scan shows rim-enhancing collection that represents a psoas abscess (*).

adjacent soft-tissue edema as demonstrated in **Figure 8**. Importantly, the origin of an EDA can be traced to an SFJ on MRI[34] (**Figure 9**).

If a diagnosis of spine infection is suspected on clinical basis and confirmed on imaging, every effort should be made to establish a microbiologic diagnosis. Blood cultures are routinely ordered for patients who present with fever and back pain or have suspicious imaging findings for spine infections. They are positive in approximately 60% of cases, ranging from 30% to 72%.[48] Cultures should preferably be obtained before the administration of empiric antibiotics. Most patients present with prolonged symptoms, and it is acceptable to withhold antibiotics in all but the critically ill patients with sepsis.[49] If blood cultures remain negative after 48 hours or yield a single set skin contaminant such as coagulase-negative staphylococci, a CT-guided or open biopsy is indicated. The reported yield of imaging-guided percutaneous biopsy ranges from 31% to 91% compared with open biopsy yield at 76% to 91%. Because the percutaneous route is less invasive and less costly, it should be performed first. A standard biopsy specimen should include a core sample of the affected end plates and a fluid aspirate of the disk space. Yield is improved if adjacent collections in paraspinal or paravertebral soft tissues are aspirated and if antibiotics are withheld up to 2 weeks. A study from 2021 reported that if an initial percutaneous biopsy is negative, it is acceptable to repeat it after 72 hours, given the importance of targeted antibiotic therapy.[50] Samples are sent for microbiology and histopathology. Standard bacterial and fungal stains and cultures are routinely performed. Mycobacterial stains for acid-fast bacilli and cultures are added in cases with significant exposure. Histopathology can show acute osteomyelitis with neutrophilic granulocytes infiltrating cancellous bone.[51] The absence of white blood cells in the biopsy sample is helpful in differentiating infection of the spine from its MRI mimickers such as degenerative Modic changes, neuropathic Charcot joints, ankylosing spondylitis, and hemodialysis-associated spondyloarthropathy.[52] If crystal deposits of uric acid or calcium pyrophosphate are seen on histopathology, a diagnosis of crystal arthropathy can be made, which is indistinguishable from infection on clinical and imaging grounds.[53] In culture-negative cases, granulomatous lesions can point toward mycobacterial etiology or brucellosis.[16] Broad-range PCR testing of biopsy samples is a novel methodology with a potential for better yield; it shows promise in culture-negative cases with prior antibiotic exposure or when fastidious organisms are suspected. The drawbacks of PCR are its high false-positive rate and the lack of antibiotic susceptibility reports to guide therapy.[54]

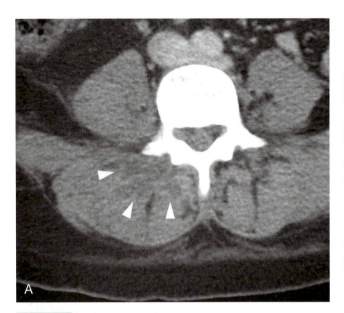
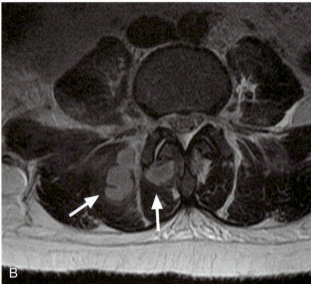

FIGURE 7 **A**, Contrast-enhanced axial CT scan of the spine shows rim-enhancing collection (arrowheads) in right-side paraspinal muscle image. **B**, Axial T2-weighted magnetic resonance image shows bright fluid signal in paraspinal muscle originating from a septic facet joint (arrows).

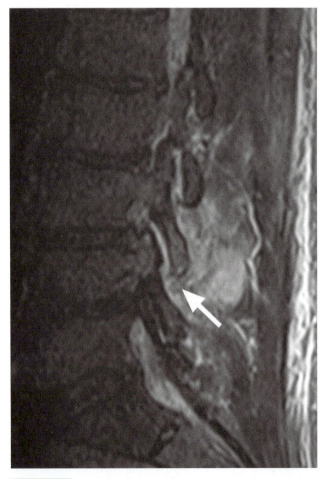

FIGURE 8 Sagittal short tau inversion recovery magnetic resonance image shows fluid signal in the facet joint (arrow) with adjacent billowing edema in paraspinal tissue demonstrating the smoking pipe sign of septic facet joint.

TREATMENT OF SPINE INFECTIONS

The treatment of spine infections has improved since 1936 when it was associated with a mortality rate of 70%.[55] The advent of effective antimicrobial therapy combined with surgical management provides optimal outcomes. The goals of treatment include control of infection and prevention or reversal of neurologic and mechanical deficits. The Infectious Diseases Society of America offers guidelines for antimicrobial management of spine infections.[49] Uncomplicated cases of spondylodiscitis, SFJ, and EDA without neurologic

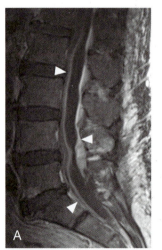
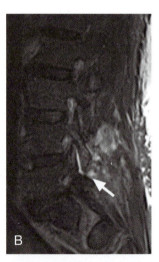

FIGURE 9 **A**, Postcontrast T1-weighted sagittal magnetic resonance image originating from shows rim-enhancing epidural abscess (EDA; arrowhead) in a septic facet joint (SFJ). **B**, Sagittal image shows fluid in a septic facet joint (arrows) as the origin of EDA in **A**.

deficits or significant loss of bone stock can be treated nonsurgically with targeted antibiotics for a duration of 6 weeks.[56] More extensive infections with significant paraspinal soft-tissue spread or significant spill into adjacent psoas muscles may benefit from longer courses of antibiotics of 8 to 12 weeks.[57] Therapeutic response is assessed by improvement of back pain and decrease in CRP, which is trended weekly. The initial administration of antibiotics intravenously can be switched to highly bioavailable oral agents once the CRP value has decreased by 50% and the patient reports significantly less back pain.[10] Success of treatment is determined by clinical response and normalization of inflammatory markers; end-of-treatment imaging is not recommended as findings on MRI can lag significantly and create unnecessary anxiety for the patient. Repeat cross-sectional imaging is warranted in cases of persistent, recurrent, or worsening pain or unexplained elevation of inflammatory markers.[58] Historically, all EDAs were treated surgically. Currently, it is acceptable to manage EDA with targeted antibiotics in patients who are neurologically intact. Treatment response is followed clinically and does not require repeat MRI. Neurologic deficits caused by cord compression, either from an EDA or mechanical instability of the spinal column, require surgical management. Because it is not known at which point in time neurologic deficits become irreversible, early decompression is imperative.[59] Minor neurologic deficits are treated nonsurgically and closely observed. The failure rate of nonsurgical management ranges from 30% to 40% and leads to delayed surgery. The outcome of delayed surgery is suboptimal, and it is therefore important to predict in which patients nonsurgical management is likely to fail. A 2018 review reported that multiple mathematical models based on a variety of risk factors have been suggested but have not been validated in subsequent cohorts and are of limited use in clinical practice.[60] The optimal approach to SFJ treatment is not established but most can be treated according to Infectious Diseases Society of America guidelines. Occasionally, prolonged bacteremia originating from the SFJ can be managed by percutaneous aspiration of the joint, which also provides symptomatic relief to the patient by decompressing the joint capsule.[34] The goal of surgery is to decompress a compromised spinal cord, remove all infected tissue, and maintain stability of the vertebral column. Instrumentation of the spine after radical débridement is safe and does not increase risk of recurrent infection.[61] Neither the addition of rifampin nor the use of chronic antimicrobial suppression is necessary following hardware placement. Treatment failures are infrequent and occur within the first year after surgery. The benefit of suppressive antimicrobial therapy beyond 1 year is minimal.[62]

SUMMARY

Infections of the native spine continue to rise as the population ages and is subject to more medical interventions. Because most spine infections are caused by hematogenous seeding, all conditions and procedures that predispose patients to transient episodes of bacteremia should be considered risk factors. The diagnostic delay remains unacceptably long because back pain as a presenting symptom is a common complaint. The complex structure of the spine accounts for the variability in presenting symptoms and reflects the underlying anatomic structure involved, specifically, discitis, spondylodiscitis, SFJ, and EDA. These categories are not mutually exclusive and represent a continuum of spread of infection in the spinal column. The diagnostic imaging of choice is contrast-enhanced MRI. Every effort should be made to establish a microbiologic diagnosis and withholding antibiotics for blood cultures, and subsequent biopsy is acceptable in patients who are not in septic shock. *S aureus* remains the most frequent organism isolated in spine infections. Therapy includes 6 weeks of antibiotics and surgery in select cases. Indications for surgery are twofold and include urgent decompression surgery for cord compression with neurologic deficits and delayed stabilization of the spinal column for residual mechanical pain due to loss of bone stock from infection. Placement of hardware in acute spine infection does not increase risk of recurrent infection and does not require long-term antibiotic suppression. End-of-treatment imaging is not indicated if inflammatory markers normalize and back pain improves.

KEY STUDY POINTS

- Infections of different anatomic structures of the spine present with different clinical symptoms.
- Imaging modalities are an essential tool in diagnosis but are fraught with limitations.
- Surgical indications have evolved in recent years and include decompression for a compromised cord in the acute setting and spine stabilization for mechanical pain.

ANNOTATED REFERENCES

1. Kehrer M, Pedersen C, Jensen TG, Lassen AT: Increasing incidence of pyogenic spondylodiscitis: A 14-year population-based study. *J Infect* 2014;68(4):313-320.
2. Lora-Tamayo J, Euba G, Narváez JA, et al: Changing trends in the epidemiology of pyogenic vertebral osteomyelitis: The impact of cases with no microbiologic diagnosis. *Semin Arthritis Rheum* 2011;41(2):247-255.

3. Issa K, Diebo BG, Faloon M, et al: The epidemiology of vertebral osteomyelitis in the United States from 1998 to 2013. *Clin Spine Surg* 2018;31(2):E102-E108.

   This study is an epidemiologic data analysis of vertebral osteomyelitis in the United States over a 15-year period showing an increasing burden of vertebral osteomyelitis in the United States.

4. Alkhatib B, Ban GI, Williams S, Serra R: IVD Development: Nucleus pulposus development and sclerotome specification. *Curr Mol Biol Rep* 2018;4(3):132-141.

   A review of basic research into embryologic development of the IVD is presented, which helps the understanding of its pathology.

5. Raj PP: Intervertebral disc: Anatomy-physiology-pathophysiology-treatment. *Pain Pract* 2008;8(1):18-44.

6. Nixon GW: Hematogenous osteomyelitis of metaphyseal-equivalent locations. *AJR Am J Roentgenol* 1978;130(1):123-129.

7. Newell RL: The spinal epidural space. *Clin Anat* 1999;12(5):375-379.

8. Friedman JA, Maher CO, Quast LM, McClelland RL, Ebersold MJ: Spontaneous disc space infections in adults. *Surg Neurol* 2002;57(2):81-86.

9. Govender S: Spinal infections. *J Bone Joint Surg Br* 2005;87(11):1454-1458.

10. Lam KS, Webb JK: Discitis. *Hosp Med* 2004;65(5):280-286.

11. Hadjipavlou AG, Mader JT, Necessary JT, Muffoletto AJ: Hematogenous pyogenic spinal infections and their surgical management. *Spine (Phila Pa 1976)* 2000;25(13):1668-1679.

12. Muffoletto AJ, Ketonen LM, Mader JT, Crow WN, Hadjipavlou AG: Hematogenous pyogenic facet joint infection. *Spine (Phila Pa 1976)* 2001;26(14):1570-1576.

13. Nathan H, Weinberg H, Robin GC, Aviad I: The costovertebral joints, anatomical-clinical observations in arthritis. *Arthritis Rheum* 1964;7:228-240.

14. Goldthwait JE: The rib joints. *New Engl J Med* 1940;223:568-573.

15. Reihsaus E, Waldbaur H, Seeling W: Spinal epidural abscess: A meta-analysis of 915 patients. *Neurosurg Rev* 2000;23(4):175-204.

16. Zimmerli W: Clinical practice. Vertebral osteomyelitis. *N Engl J Med* 2010;362(11):1022-1029.

17. Lew DP, Waldvogel FA: Osteomyelitis. *Lancet* 2004;364(9431):369-379.

18. McHenry MC, Easley KA, Locker GA: Vertebral osteomyelitis: Long-term outcome for 253 patients from 7 Cleveland-area hospitals. *Clin Infect Dis* 2002;34(10):1342-1350.

19. Artenstein AW, Friderici J, Holers A, Lewis D, Fitzgerald J, Visintainer P: Spinal epidural abscess in adults: A 10-year clinical experience at a Tertiary Care Academic Medical Center. *Open Forum Infect Dis* 2016;3(4):ofw191.

20. Arko L, Quach E, Nguyen V, Chang D, Sukul V, Kim BS: Medical and surgical management of spinal epidural abscess: A systematic review. *Neurosurg Focus* 2014;37(2):E4.

21. Gupta A, Kowalski TJ, Osmon DR, et al: Long-term outcome of pyogenic vertebral osteomyelitis: A cohort study of 260 patients. *Open Forum Infect Dis* 2014;1(3):ofu107.

22. Lowy FD: Staphylococcus aureus infections. *N Engl J Med* 1998;339(8):520-532.

23. Hamza T, Li B: Differential responses of osteoblasts and macrophages upon Staphylococcus aureus infection. *BMC Microbiol* 2014;14:207.

24. Wen Q, Gu F, Sui Z, Su Z, Yu T: The process of osteoblastic infection by Staphylococcus aureus. *Int J Med Sci* 2020;17(10):1327-1332.

   This article reviews basic science literature about the internalization of *S aureus* by osteoblasts and the basis of their failure to effectively kill the intracellular bacteria and eradicate infection.

25. Oppegaard O, Skrede S, Mylvaganam H, Kittang BR: Temporal trends of β-haemolytic streptococcal osteoarticular infections in western Norway. *BMC Infect Dis* 2016;16(1):535.

26. Murillo O, Grau I, Gomez-Junyent J, et al: Endocarditis associated with vertebral osteomyelitis and septic arthritis of the axial skeleton. *Infection* 2018;46(2):245-251.

   This study aims to understand the relationship between infective endocarditis and osteoarticular infections. It shows that patients with infective endocarditis mainly have axial skeleton involvement.

27. Bucher E, Trampuz A, Donati L, Zimmerli W: Spondylodiscitis associated with bacteraemia due to coagulase-negative staphylococci. *Eur J Clin Microbiol Infect Dis* 2000;19(2):118-120.

28. Nolla JM, Ariza J, Gómez-Vaquero C, et al: Spontaneous pyogenic vertebral osteomyelitis in nondrug users. *Semin Arthritis Rheum* 2002;31(4):271-278.

29. Loibl M, Stoyanov L, Doenitz C, et al: Outcome-related co-factors in 105 cases of vertebral osteomyelitis in a tertiary care hospital. *Infection* 2014;42(3):503-510.

30. Yang H, Shah AA, Nelson SB, Schwab JH: Fungal spinal epidural abscess: A case series of nine patients. *Spine J* 2019;19(3):516-522.

   This is a case series of nine cases of fungal spine infections outlining risk factors, clinical presentation, and management.

31. Beit Ner E, Chechik Y, Lambert LA, Anekstein Y, Mirovsky Y, Smorgick Y: Gas forming infection of the spine: A systematic and narrative review. *Eur Spine J* 2021;30(6):1708-1720.

   This is a literature review of published cases of gas-forming organisms causing spine infections. This is a clinical curiosity.

32. Chelsom J, Solberg CO: Vertebral osteomyelitis at a Norwegian university hospital 1987-97: Clinical features, laboratory findings and outcome. *Scand J Infect Dis* 1998;30(2):147-151.

33. Priest DH, Peacock JE Jr: Hematogenous vertebral osteomyelitis due to Staphylococcus aureus in the adult: Clinical features and therapeutic outcomes. *South Med J* 2005;98(9):854-862.

34. Babic M, Ilaslan H, Shrestha N, Simpfendorfer CS: Isolated septic facet joints: An underdiagnosed distinct clinical entity. *Skeletal Radiol* 2020;49(8):1295-1303.

    The authors present a review of 59 cases of isolated SFJs at a single institution. It describes the distinct clinical presentation and raise awareness of its increasing frequency.

35. Karakonstantis S, Galani D, Maragou S, Koulouridi A, Kalemaki D, Lydakis C: A rare case of acute transverse myelitis associated with Staphylococcusaureus bacteremia and osteomyelitis. *Spinal Cord Ser Cases* 2017;3:17029.

36. Siemionow K, Steinmetz M, Bell G, Ilaslan H, McLain RF: Identifying serious causes of back pain: Cancer, infection, fracture. *Cleve Clin J Med* 2008;75(8):557-566.

37. Diehn FE: Imaging of spine infection. *Radiol Clin North Am* 2012;50(4):777-798.

38. Soloff EV, Wang CL: Safety of gadolinium-based contrast agents in patients with stage 4 and 5 chronic kidney disease: A radiologist's perspective. *Kidney360* 2020;1(2):123-126.

    This review article summarizes the safety of newer gadolinium preparations used in MRI and compares it with the adverse effect profile of older generations of gadolinium.

39. Prodi E, Grassi R, Iacobellis F, Cianfoni A: Imaging in Spondylodiskitis. *Magn Reson Imaging Clin N Am* 2016;24(3):581-600.

40. Parkinson JF, Sekhon LH: Surgical management of spinal epidural abscess: Selection of approach based on MRI appearance. *J Clin Neurosci* 2004;11(2):130-133.

41. Dunbar JA, Sandoe JA, Rao AS, Crimmins DW, Baig W, Rankine JJ: The MRI appearances of early vertebral osteomyelitis and discitis. *Clin Radiol* 2010;65(12):974-981.

42. Korutz AW, Obajuluwa A, Lester MS, et al: Pacemakers in MRI for the Neuroradiologist. *AJNR Am J Neuroradiol* 2017;38(12):2222-2230.

43. Ohtori S, Suzuki M, Koshi T, et al: 18F-fluorodeoxyglucose-PET for patients with suspected spondylitis showing Modic change. *Spine (Phila Pa 1976)* 2010;35(26):E1599-E1603.

44. Love C, Patel M, Lonner BS, Tomas MB, Palestro CJ: Diagnosing spinal osteomyelitis: A comparison of bone and Ga-67 scintigraphy and magnetic resonance imaging. *Clin Nucl Med* 2000;25(12):963-977.

45. Resnick D, Niwayama G, Guerra J Jr, Vint V, Usselman J: Spinal vacuum phenomena: Anatomical study and review. *Radiology* 1981;139(2):341-348.

46. Prodromou ML, Ziakas PD, Poulou LS, Karsaliakos P, Thanos L, Mylonakis E: FDG PET is a robust tool for the diagnosis of spondylodiscitis: A meta-analysis of diagnostic data. *Clin Nucl Med* 2014;39(4):330-335.

47. Smids C, Kouijzer IJE, Vos FJ, et al: A comparison of the diagnostic value of MRI and (18)F-FDG-PET/CT in suspected spondylodiscitis. *Infection* 2017;45(1):41-49.

48. Mylona E, Samarkos M, Kakalou E, Fanourgiakis P, Skoutelis A: Pyogenic vertebral osteomyelitis: A systematic review of clinical characteristics. *Semin Arthritis Rheum* 2009;39(1):10-17.

49. Berbari EF, Kanj SS, Kowalski TJ, et al: 2015 Infectious Diseases Society of America (IDSA) clinical practice guidelines for the diagnosis and treatment of native vertebral osteomyelitis in adults. *Clin Infect Dis* 2015;61(6):e26-e46.

50. Husseini JS, Habibollahi S, Nelson SB, Rosenthal DI, Chang CY: Best practices: CT-guided percutaneous sampling of vertebral discitis-osteomyelitis and technical factors maximizing biopsy yield. *AJR Am J Roentgenol* 2021;217(5):1057-1068.

    This article offers a pragmatic guide for the use of CT-guided biopsy of the spine, including when to use it, what sample to obtain, and when it should be repeated.

51. Tiemann AH, Krenn V, Krukemeyer MG, et al: Infectious bone diseases [Article in German]. *Pathologe* 2011;32(3):200-209.

52. Hong SH, Choi JY, Lee JW, Kim NR, Choi JA, Kang HS: MR imaging assessment of the spine: Infection or an imitation? *Radiographics* 2009;29(2):599-612.

53. Bridges KJ, Bullis CL, Wanchu A, Than KD: Pseudogout of the cervical and thoracic spine mimicking infection after lumbar fusion: Case report. *J Neurosurg Spine* 2017;27(2):145-149.

54. Fuursted K, Arpi M, Lindblad BE, Pedersen LN: Broad-range PCR as a supplement to culture for detection of bacterial pathogens in patients with a clinically diagnosed spinal infection. *Scand J Infect Dis* 2008;40(10):772-777.

55. Kulowski J: Management of hematogenous pyogenic osteomyelitis. *Surgery* 1956;40(6):1094-1104.

56. Bernard L, Dinh A, Ghout I, et al: Antibiotic treatment for 6 weeks versus 12 weeks in patients with pyogenic vertebral osteomyelitis: An open-label, non-inferiority, randomised, controlled trial. *Lancet* 2015;385(9971):875-882.

57. Park KH, Cho OH, Lee JH, et al: Optimal duration of antibiotic therapy in patients with hematogenous vertebral osteomyelitis at low risk and high risk of recurrence. *Clin Infect Dis* 2016;62(10):1262-1269.

58. Kowalski TJ, Berbari EF, Huddleston PM, Steckelberg JM, Osmon DR: Do follow-up imaging examinations provide useful prognostic information in patients with spine infection? *Clin Infect Dis* 2006;43(2):172-179.

59. Tuchman A, Pham M, Hsieh PC: The indications and timing for operative management of spinal epidural abscess: Literature review and treatment algorithm. *Neurosurg Focus* 2014;37(2):E8.

60. Shah AA, Ogink PT, Nelson SB, Harris MB, Schwab JH: Nonoperative management of spinal epidural

abscess: Development of a predictive algorithm for failure. *J Bone Joint Surg Am* 2018;100(7):546-555.

This is a retrospective review of a large spinal epidural registry with a focus on outcome to develop a predictive algorithm for failure of nonsurgical management based on risk factors. This should help make the decision for surgical decompression more objective.

61. Rayes M, Colen CB, Bahgat DA, et al: Safety of instrumentation in patients with spinal infection. *J Neurosurg Spine* 2010;12(6):647-659.

62. Arnold R, Rock C, Croft L, Gilliam BL, Morgan DJ: Factors associated with treatment failure in vertebral osteomyelitis requiring spinal instrumentation. *Antimicrob Agents Chemother* 2014;58(2):880-884.

CHAPTER 27

Necrotizing Fasciitis and Other Complicated Skin and Soft-Tissue Infections

JOYA-RITA HINDY, MD • SARA F. HADDAD, MD
LARRY M. BADDOUR, MD, FIDSA, FAHA

ABSTRACT

Complicated skin and soft-tissue infections (SSTIs) characterize the more extreme zone of the SSTI spectrum and may involve any or all of the soft-tissue layers, namely epidermis, dermis, subcutaneous tissue, fascia, and skeletal muscle. Several complicated SSTIs have been defined and include necrotizing soft-tissue infections (NSTIs), surgical site infections, animal bite infections, and deep abscesses (such as pyomyositis). NSTIs, which include necrotizing cellulitis, necrotizing fasciitis, and necrotizing myositis, deserve special attention because they are life-threatening infections presenting acutely (within hours) and may lead to limb loss and in-hospital mortality with delays in surgical intervention. Early recognition and aggressive surgical débridement are fundamental in NSTIs management. In addition to antimicrobial therapy, complicated SSTIs usually require surgical management (typically serial interventions) including incision and drainage and débridement. Often, surgeons are involved in the treatment of patients with NSTIs and other complicated infections.

Keywords: complicated skin and soft-tissue infections; necrotizing fasciitis; outcomes; pyomyositis; surgical management

Dr. Baddour or an immediate family member has received royalties from UpToDate, Inc. Neither of the following authors nor any immediate family member has received anything of value from or has stock or stock options held in a commercial company or institution related directly or indirectly to the subject of this chapter: Dr. Hindy and Dr. Haddad.

INTRODUCTION

Microbial invasion of the skin and surrounding tissues leads to skin and soft-tissue infections (SSTIs). Surgery is often critical in the management of infectious syndromes addressed in this chapter, and a consultation may be needed on an immediate or emergent basis to ultimately save the affected limb and the patient's life. The limb perspective is of keen interest as most syndromes discussed herein involve an extremity. Without emergent surgical intervention for securing source control, and despite appropriate antimicrobial administration, important outcomes including the need for critical care support, hospital length of stay, readmission rates, ability to ambulate, multiple surgeries, and short-term and long-term mortality, worsen by the hour. This chapter focuses primarily on nonsurgical aspects of patient care, and reviews these complicated SSTIs: necrotizing soft-tissue infections (NSTIs) (such as cellulitis, fasciitis, myositis), animal bites in proximity to joints, and deep-seated abscesses (such as pyomyositis). The clinical variability and complexity of these complicated SSTIs, however, dictate that the diagnostic and management recommendations included herein be used to support and not supplant decisions regarding individual patient care.

CLASSIFICATION OF SSTIS

SSTIs are one of the most common types of infection encountered in an array of clinical settings.[1] These infections can involve any soft-tissue layer, including the epidermis, dermis, subcutaneous tissue, fascia, and skeletal muscle. Complicated SSTIs are usually deep soft-tissue infections and encompass an array of conditions that may be classified as necrotizing or nonnecrotizing. A proposed classification of SSTIs was created and divided by severity into three classes, of which classes 2B and 3 often require surgery.[2] A study from 2020 reported that certain noninfectious dermatologic diseases, including pyoderma gangrenosum and desomorphine-induced deep ulceration, can mimic infections and should be included in the differential diagnosis.[3] A 2022 nonsystematic review reported that in addition to a course of antimicrobial therapy, surgical management includes incision and drainage and débridement for source control.[4]

NECROTIZING SOFT-TISSUE INFECTIONS

Risk Factors

Although healthy individuals of any age without a clear portal of entry can be affected, there are several risk factors associated with NSTIs.[5-11] A 2022 study reported that patients presenting with SSTIs and any of these risk factors (**Table 1**) should be assessed to confirm or exclude NSTI. Diabetes mellitus, in particular, increases the risk of NSTIs, regardless of anatomic location.[12] A retrospective study from 2019 reported that necrotizing ulcers can be observed when people who inject drugs practice skin popping and use drugs and adulterants with irritant or toxic properties.[13]

Risk Factors Associated With Mortality in Patients With NSTIs

NSTIs may lead to limb loss and in-hospital mortality in up to 25% of patients.[11] Mortality in patients with NSTIs increases with age (especially those older than 60 years), having multiple comorbidities, chronic liver disease, coronary artery disease, chronic kidney disease, delayed surgery (longer than 24 hours), intensive care unit admission, transfer from an outside hospital, bacteremia at initial presentation, clostridial infection, monomicrobial NSTI (versus polymicrobial), streptococcal toxic shock syndrome, elevated peripheral white blood cell count (>30,000/μL), thrombocytopenia, lactic acidosis, and elevated serum creatinine (greater than 2.0 mg/dL).[14-17] Histopathologic findings in determining risk of mortality (the fewer the neutrophils and the more the bacteria, the higher the mortality) may be used to predict outcomes; however, cohort size used in this single-center study was relatively small.[18] Of note, during the COVID-19 pandemic, a significant increase in complicated dental infections and related mortality was described in patients presenting with NSTIs, possibly due to the hypercoagulable state associated with COVID-19 pandemic and delay in seeking medical care.[13,19]

Medicolegal Implications of NSTIs

NSTIs are implicated in an array of medical malpractice lawsuits, including six reported on in 2020, involving financial compensation and even homicide.[20] A 2020 report found

Table 1

Risk Factors Associated With Necrotizing Soft-Tissue Infections

Major penetrating trauma

Gunshot wounds[a], knife wounds[a], as a result of natural disasters (earthquake[a], hurricane[b], tsunami[b])

Blunt trauma

Compound fractures[a], crush injuries[a], muscle contusion, muscle sprain, muscle strain

Skin breach

Animal bite, insect bite, intramuscular injection[a], minor laceration (including in seawater[c] or freshwater settings[b]), varicella lesion

Genitointestinal mucosal breach

Episiotomy, hemorrhoids, rectal fissures

Recent surgery

Gastrointestinal tract (including biliary tract)[a], genitourinary tract, hip arthroplasty, liposuction[d], neonatal circumcision

Behavioral

Alcohol use disorder, heavy exercise, ingestion of contaminated oysters[c], injection drug use (especially use of black tar heroin and skin popping)[a], malnutrition, poor hygiene, tobacco use

Cardiovascular disease

Chronic kidney disease, diabetes mellitus, gout, hypertension, ischemic heart disease, obesity, peripheral vascular disease, stroke

Colonic diseases

Diverticulitis, inflammatory bowel disease, malignancy[e]

Immunocompromising conditions

Advanced HIV infection, chemotherapy, cirrhosis[c], leukemia, lymphoproliferative disorders, neutropenia (including cyclic neutropenia[e]), radiation therapy

Peripartum conditions

Childbirth, extremely low gestational age, gestational diabetes, pregnancy loss[a], preterm delivery, retained placenta[a], prolonged rupture of membranes[a], intrauterine fetal demise[a]

[a]These risk factors are associated with necrotizing soft-tissue infections (NSTIs) due to *Clostridium perfringens*. These can occur in victims of natural disasters (such as earthquakes) where there might be a delay in evacuation and treatment.
[b]This risk factor is associated with NSTIs due to *Aeromonas hydrophila*.
[c]These risk factors associated with NSTIs due to *Vibrio vulnificus*.
[d]Not limited to abdominal liposuction.
[e]These are risk factors associated with NSTIs due to *Clostridium septicum*.

that one of the major factors for concluding malpractice in court is the timely diagnosis and management of NSTIs.[21] In addition, although rare, cases of healthcare-associated NSTIs have been cited in malpractice claims.[22,23]

Microbiology of NSTIs

Almost all NSTIs are polymicrobial (type I) caused by various combinations of anaerobic and aerobic pathogens, with *Streptococcus* and *Bacteroides* spp. being the most common aerobic and anaerobic bacteria, respectively.[7,24] Other microbes involved in type I NSTIs include *Enterobacterales*, *Clostridium*, and *Peptostreptococcus* spp. NSTIs can also be monomicrobial (type II) caused by group A beta-hemolytic *Streptococcus* most commonly, other beta-hemolytic streptococci, or *Staphylococcus aureus*. Rarely, monomicrobial NSTI can be caused by *Vibrio vulnificus*, *Clostridium* spp., *Bacteroides* spp., *Escherichia* spp., or other organisms. Most clostridial infections are caused by *Clostridium perfringens*; other species causing clostridial infections include *Clostridium septicum*, *Clostridium novyi*, and *Clostridium histolyticum*. Less frequently, NSTIs can be caused by *Aeromonas hydrophila* and fungi such as *Candida* spp. and *Mucormycosis*.[25,26] A systematic review from 2022 reported that necrotizing myositis is usually caused by group A *Streptococcus* (and other beta-hemolytic streptococci), *C perfringens* (after penetrating trauma), or *C septicum* (after hematogenous seeding from the gastrointestinal tract).[27]

Clinical Findings in NSTIs

NSTIs can manifest with erythema, edema (sometimes extending beyond visible erythema), severe pain (out of proportion compared with physical examination findings), crepitus, and changes in skin color (such as bullae, necrosis, ecchymosis, and extensive tissue destruction) in the affected area (generally the extremities) (**Figures 1**

and **2**). In 2022, it was reported that nonspecific symptoms including diarrhea, malaise, and loss of appetite can precede the onset of skin manifestations. Fever and other systemic signs of toxicity (such as tachycardia or hemodynamic instability) can develop and then lead to shock and multiorgan failure.[28]

Necrotizing cellulitis only affects the skin and spares the fascia and skeletal muscles. Necrotizing fasciitis may be difficult to visualize because it involves the muscle fascia and overlying subcutaneous fat while initially the overlying tissue can look unaffected. One early clue to the presence of necrotizing fasciitis is the development of anesthesia due to destruction of superficial nerves in the subcutaneous tissue. Necrotizing myositis is a rare infection because of the generous blood supply of skeletal muscles; it has been called clostridial myonecrosis or gas gangrene when it is a clostridial infection. Although skin crepitus can be observed in necrotizing cellulitis, its presentation is less severe than gas gangrene.

Fournier gangrene is a form of polymicrobial (type I) necrotizing fasciitis affecting the perineum, the second most common site of NSTI after the extremities (lower more often than upper extremities).[7] It occurs more frequently in men, results from a breach of the urethral or gastrointestinal mucosa integrity, and may rapidly spread to the anterior abdominal wall and the gluteal muscles.

A 2018 systematic review of case reports found that NSTIs can affect the head and neck when there is rupture of the oropharynx mucous membrane following surgery or odontogenic infection.[29] A mixture of aerobic and anaerobic bacteria originating from dentition or the pharynx are usually identified. Although most NSTIs of the head and neck are polymicrobial, monomicrobial infection can be due to group A *Streptococcus*. Necrotizing fasciitis can spread to the lower neck, submandibular space (called Ludwig angina), jugular vein (Lemierre syndrome), and mediastinum. Factors increasing the risk of mediastinitis include prior corticosteroid use, infection due to gas-producing pathogens, and a pharyngeal source of infection.[30]

Diagnosis of NSTIs

The diagnosis of NSTIs is primarily clinical and suspected when there are symptoms of soft-tissue infection (such as erythema, edema, or warmth) and signs of systemic toxicity (such as fever, hemodynamic instability, organ dysfunction) with crepitus, rapid progression of symptoms, or extreme pain (sometimes out of proportion to skin findings). The definitive diagnosis of NSTIs is established by surgical exploration and direct examination of involved tissues including skin, subcutaneous tissue, fascia, and skeletal muscle. NSTIs are diagnosed when there is direct visualization of a swollen and dull-gray muscle fascia and easy separation of tissue planes by frank dissection (positive finger test).[31] Intraoperative

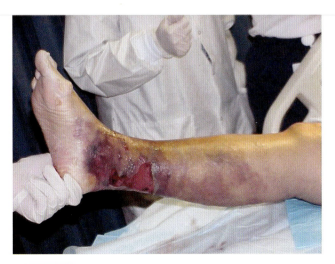

FIGURE 1 Photograph shows necrotizing fasciitis of the lower limb due to *Streptococcus agalactiae* in an elderly woman with obesity.

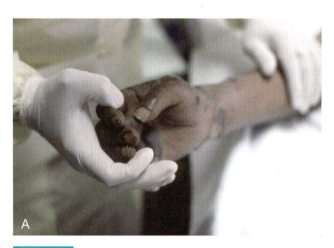 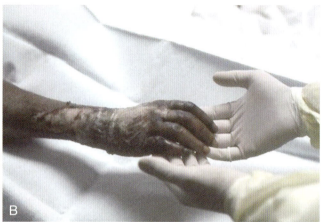

FIGURE 2 **A** and **B**, Necrotizing cellulitis of the upper limb due to *Streptococcus pyogenes* in an older man with a chronic underlying psychiatric disorder and severe malnutrition.

tissue should be sent for analysis by Gram stain, culture, and in vitro susceptibility screening. Although tissue biopsy is the most reliable for diagnosis, it is not required to establish a diagnosis of NSTIs.[18,32]

Laboratory Findings

The Laboratory Risk Indicator for Necrotizing Fasciitis (LRINEC) score is a tool based on laboratory parameters that has received considerable attention in its ability to discriminate between necrotizing and nonnecrotizing SSTIs,[33] especially those involving the head and neck.[34] The laboratory parameters included in the LRINEC score are C-reactive protein level, creatinine level, glucose level, hemoglobin level, sodium level, and white blood cell count. Because of its variable sensitivity, however, it is not recommended for ruling out NSTI.[34]

Before administering antibiotics, two sets of blood cultures (both aerobic and anaerobic bottles) should be drawn. Blood cultures are usually positive in patients with monomicrobial (type II) necrotizing fasciitis and necrotizing myositis, whereas it is not typically the case in patients with polymicrobial (type I) necrotizing fasciitis.

Imaging Findings

A retrospective study from 2022 reported that radiographic imaging should not delay surgical intervention, especially if there is crepitus on physical examination or rapid progression of symptoms.[35] A 2018 retrospective study showed that, compared with MRI and ultrasonography, CT is the best initial imaging modality.[36] It may show gas in soft tissues, prompting immediate surgical intervention as it is highly specific for NSTI and is most common in clostridial infection or polymicrobial (type I) necrotizing fasciitis. In addition, when a contrast-enhanced CT scan is negative, NSTI can be reliably ruled out in patients with initial suspicion.[36]

A 2019 systematic review and meta-analysis of 23 studies was conducted to compare the pooled sensitivity and specificity of physical examination, imaging, and LRINEC score in diagnosing NSTIs[37] (**Table 2**). It demonstrated that the lack of relevant findings on physical examination (eg, fever or hypotension) is not sufficient to rule out NSTI and that LRINEC should not be used to rule out NSTI because it had poor sensitivity. In addition, CT was superior to plain radiography. Thus, a high clinical suspicion justifies prompt surgical consultation for definitive diagnosis and management of NSTI.

Table 2

Accuracy of Some Parameters in Diagnosing Necrotizing Soft-Tissue Infections

Parameters	Pooled Sensitivity (%)	Pooled Specificity (%)
Fever	46.0	77.0
Hemorrhagic bullae	25.2	95.8
Hypotension	21.0	97.7
CT scan	88.5	93.3
LRINEC score ≥6	68.2	84.8
LRINEC score ≥8	40.8	94.9

LRINEC = Laboratory Risk Indicator for Necrotizing Fasciitis

Data obtained from Fernando SM, Tran A, Cheng W, et al: Necrotizing soft tissue infection: Diagnostic accuracy of physical examination, imaging, and LRINEC score – A systematic review and meta-analysis. *Ann Surg* 2019;269(1):58-65.

Management of NSTIs

Management of NSTIs entails early and thorough surgical exploration with débridement of necrotic tissue, along with broad-spectrum empiric antimicrobial therapy and hemodynamic support. Because patients with NSTIs may deteriorate within hours of their presentation, only a clinical suspicion of NSTI is warranted to incite surgical exploration, especially in patients who are immunocompromised, have diabetes mellitus, or have undergone surgery recently. A clear multidisciplinary approach among surgeons, microbiologists, infectious diseases specialists, pharmacists, and intensivists is fundamental in caring for these complex patients.[8]

Surgical Interventions

A 2023 review reported that aggressive débridement of all necrotic tissue should not be delayed for any reason as it is a surgical emergency.[38] A systematic review from 2018 reported that the goal of the surgical intervention is to reach healthy viable tissue that is bleeding[39] (**Figure 3**). A systematic review from 2020 reported that the initial débridement should be performed at the first center to which the patient presents with the suspected diagnosis; this way, control of infection source is achieved more promptly, ideally within 6 hours of presentation to reduce mortality.[40] A 2022 study showed that because prolonged surgical times may be associated with longer intensive care unit and hospital stays in patients with NSTIs, there should be a balance between adequate débridement and shorter surgical time.[41] In fact, débridement and reevaluation of tissue should be repeated every 1 to 2 days until all necrotic tissue is removed. This could be performed at a referral center that has a multidisciplinary team familiar with the management of complex wounds. Viable skin and subcutaneous tissue can be salvaged despite invasive débridement when it is focused only on necrosed tissue. Skin grafting and rehabilitation services are required to improve pain, joint mobility, and disfigurement after wide débridement.[42] A 2020 study reported that once necrotic tissue is resected, negative-pressure wound therapy may be helpful for physiologic wound healing.[43]

A surgical consult should occur early when patients have a prosthetic joint to help with the initial débridement and to direct decisions regarding implant removal.[10] In a 2020 review of cases of Fournier gangrene, urinary and fecal diversions may be warranted based on the extent of infection and débridement.[44] In addition, it was reported in 2018 that limb amputation may be needed in cases of severe NSTI, especially if the affected extremity is not viable or expected to be nonfunctional. Amputation performed in patients presenting with hemorrhagic bullae, peripheral vascular disease, bacteremia, or LRINEC score greater than 8 may reduce mortality risk.[45]

Antimicrobial Therapy

Initial empiric broad-spectrum antimicrobial agents with activity against gram-positive (including methicillin-resistant *S aureus* [MRSA]), gram-negative, and anaerobic pathogens should be administered after drawing blood cultures. An updated review from 2021 reported that adequate empiric antibiotic combinations include a carbapenem or piperacillin-tazobactam plus vancomycin or daptomycin (antibiotics with activity against MRSA) plus clindamycin (which is an antiribosomal agent active against organisms producing exotoxins as well as other beneficial aspects).[46] A 2023 review determined that deciding whether linezolid can be used instead of clindamycin in cases where group A *Streptococcus* is resistant

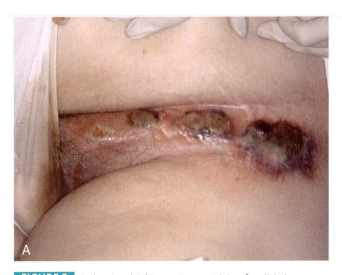
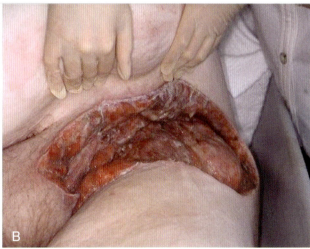

FIGURE 3 Polymicrobial (type I) necrotizing fasciitis in a woman with obesity and uncontrolled diabetes mellitus. Photographs were obtained on presentation (**A**) and after surgical exploration and débridement (**B**).

to clindamycin should be addressed by consulting an infectious diseases specialist.[47]

Antimicrobial agents should be tailored to results of Gram stain, culture, and sensitivity testing once available, and consultation from infectious disease specialists should be obtained[31] (Table 3). A retrospective study published in 2022 reported that the ideal duration of antimicrobial treatment is not well defined and could be shortened in select patients.[48] Continuation of antimicrobial agents is essential until the patient is hemodynamically stable and no further débridement is required.[43]

Additional Interventions

Guidelines published in 2021 emphasized that optimization of patient's physiologic state is crucial before surgery; aggressive supportive care with fluids and vasopressors may be required in hemodynamically unstable patients.[49] Intravenous immunoglobulin can be administered in patients with NSTI in the setting of streptococcal toxic shock syndrome.[50] Combining clindamycin with intravenous immunoglobulin is likely efficient by decreased circulating toxins produced by group A *Streptococcus* and by other mechanisms.[46,51] Although the role of hyperbaric oxygen therapy in wound healing has been debated because of the lack of strong research evidence, it could be considered if readily available. However, it should not delay standard care.[52] Patients with traumatic wounds should be vaccinated against tetanus if they have not been immunized in the past 5 years. In addition to standard precautions, patients with NSTIs due to group A *Streptococcus* require droplet and contact precautions, which may be stopped after 24 hours of initiating antimicrobial therapy.[53] A randomized double-blind placebo-controlled trial from 2020 showed that administering reltecimod (a molecule able to modulate the host immune response) within 6 hours of NSTI diagnosis lead to improvement of organ dysfunction and hospital discharge status.[54] However, further studies are warranted to establish recommendations in surgical and Infectious Diseases Society of America's guidelines.[31,43]

A patient who sustains close contact with an NSTI due to group A *Streptococcus* should imperatively be warned to promptly seek medical attention if signs and symptoms of NSTIs present within 30 days of diagnosing the index case. It was also suggested in 2019 that close contacts receive postexposure prophylaxis with penicillin, especially in highly susceptible individuals (recent surgery or immunocompromised), although the efficacy of this practice is undefined currently due to lack of clinical trial data.[55]

NONNECROTIZING COMPLICATED SSTIs

Pyomyositis is an acute skeletal muscle infection arising from hematogenous spread that can result in abscess formation. A review from 2021 reported that pyomyositis can also arise from direct injection in people who inject drugs.[56] A 2020 study determined that pyomyositis is most commonly caused by *S aureus*; *Streptococcus* spp. and other pathogens can also cause pyomyositis.[57] Risk factors associated with pyomyositis include trauma, vigorous exercise, injection drug use, concurrent infection with *Toxocara* spp, and malnutrition. A 2021 meta-analysis reported that immunocompromising conditions, including HIV infection, diabetes mellitus, malignancy, cirrhosis, chronic renal disease, organ transplant, rheumatologic conditions, and administration of immunosuppressive agents, can predispose to the development of pyomyositis.[58]

A retrospective study from 2021 reported that large muscles of the lower limbs (such as the quadriceps femoris and gluteal muscles) and the trunk muscles are most frequently involved.[59] The course of pyomyositis can vary and has been classified into three stages with most patients presenting at stage 2. Stage 1 is characterized by low-grade fever, swelling, induration, and crampy soreness of affected muscle. A frank fluctuating abscess may not be present and percutaneous aspiration of the muscle may

Table 3

Directed Antibiotic Therapy Based on Microbiologic Findings in Necrotizing Soft-Tissue Infection

Pathogens	Choice of Antibiotics
Polymicrobial[a]	Piperacillin-tazobactam[b]
Group A *Streptococcus*; *Clostridium* spp.	Penicillin G plus clindamycin
Aeromonas hydrophila	A fluoroquinolone plus ceftriaxone
Vibrio vulnificus	Doxycycline plus either cefotaxime or ceftriaxone
MRSA	Vancomycin or daptomycin plus linezolid or clindamycin
ESBL-producing Enterobacterales (*Escherichia coli*, *Klebsiella pneumoniae*)[a]	Meropenem

ESBL = extended-spectrum beta-lactamase, MRSA = methicillin-resistant *Staphylococcus aureus*, NSTI = necrotizing soft-tissue infection

[a]The treatment of aerobic gram-negative bacteria infection may vary depending on the prevalence of multidrug-resistant organisms with various mechanisms of resistance.

[a]In addition to piperacillin-tazobactam, antibiotic coverage for MRSA, Group A *Streptococcus*, and other beta-hemolytic streptococci should be added if culture results are positive. For MRSA, include the addition of vancomycin or daptomycin plus clindamycin or linezolid. For beta-hemolytic streptococci, this include clindamycin or linezolid.

not yield pus. When treatment is delayed, stage 2 occurs greater than 1 to 3 weeks after initial symptom onset and is suppurative. It is characterized by fever, muscle tenderness, and edema. A deep abscess may be present, and percutaneous aspiration of the affected muscle usually yields purulent material. A 2021 review determined that stage 3 is characterized by symptoms of systemic infection and toxicity with frank fluctuation in the affected muscle.[60] Another 2021 review reported that at this stage, various complications of *S aureus* bacteremia can occur, including osteomyelitis, septic arthritis, septic shock, infectious endocarditis, septic emboli, pneumonia, pericarditis, brain abscess, and acute kidney failure.[61]

A 2020 review reported that MRI is the most useful imaging technique for diagnosing pyomyositis, although other modalities could also be used for diagnosis such as ultrasonography or CT.[62] Because the pathogenesis of pyomyositis involves bacteremia, two sets of blood cultures should be obtained, especially in patients presenting with systemic symptoms or ectopic sites of complications. A 2020 review reported that ultrasonography and CT are also useful for percutaneous drainage or aspiration of purulent sites to identify a pathogen with antibiotic susceptibility screening, particularly in patients who have negative blood cultures.[63] Ideally, if the patient's condition permits, imaging with specimen collection will be performed before systemic antibiotics are initiated.

Stage 1 pyomyositis can be managed with parenteral antimicrobial agents alone and without percutaneous or open surgical drainage. The choice of initial empiric drug depends on the patient's immune status.[31,63] If the patient is immunocompetent, then gram-positive cocci (*S aureus* [including MRSA] and beta-hemolytic streptococci) should be covered, and the preferred therapy is vancomycin. If the patient is immunocompromised, broad coverage is needed against gram-positive, gram-negative, and anaerobic bacteria; the preferred therapy is a combination of vancomycin and a beta-lactam/beta-lactamase inhibitor (such as ampicillin-sulbactam, piperacillin-tazobactam, ticarcillin-clavulanate).[31,63] Duration of parenteral therapy is typically 3 to 4 weeks, and it should be adjusted based on clinical and radiographic improvement as well as microbiologic diagnosis. For example, if the patient has extensive, multifocal, or poorly drained infection, longer courses of therapy may be warranted. In addition, duration of therapy should be tailored if complicated bacteremia is present (eg, endocarditis or osteomyelitis).

In addition to a course of antibiotics, stages 2 and 3 of pyomyositis require image-guided percutaneous aspiration or surgical drainage and débridement depending on the abscess size, the depth of muscle involvement, and the presence of necrosis. An overview from 2020 determined that antimicrobial therapy should be administered in a timely manner, especially in patients with symptoms of systemic infections (stage 3).[64]

ANIMAL BITES

Infected animal bite wounds should be suspected with findings of fever, tenderness, erythema, swelling, warmth, purulent drainage, and lymphangitis 24 hours following dog bites and 12 hours following cat bites. In 2019, a retrospective study reported that younger patients typically have bites involving the head and neck as opposed to older patients whose upper extremities are usually affected.[65] A 2018 review reported that although cat bites are less common and have less damaging effect than dog bites, they can cause small puncture wounds that are often more difficult to manage with débridement.[66] It is important to note that cat bites can have a benign outward appearance and still put the patient at a greater risk for deep soft-tissue infections including abscesses, osteomyelitis, and septic arthritis/tenosynovitis.

Animal bite wound infections are usually polymicrobial caused by animal oral flora, human skin flora, and environmental organisms, with *Pasteurella* spp. being the most common organism isolated from both cat and dog bites.[66] Other pathogens, including aerobes (such as *Staphylococcus* spp. and *Streptococcus* spp.) and anaerobes (such as *Porphyromonas* spp., *Bacteroides* spp., and *Fusobacterium* spp.), are often identified and may lead to abscess formation. *Pasteurella multocida* tends to cause a more severe and rapidly spreading cellulitis that can lead to osteomyelitis. A 2021 report indicated that cat scratch fever caused by *Bartonella henselae* is another potential pathogen and is usually self-limited, but may rarely present with lymphadenitis, osteomyelitis, or prolonged fever.[67]

Prompt identification of the causative pathogen is essential, especially in a patient with immunocompromising conditions, asplenia, alcohol addiction, and cirrhosis and even sometimes in healthy individuals. Patients with infected animal bites should have aerobic and anaerobic bacterial wound cultures obtained and blood cultures drawn, especially in patients with immunocompromising conditions or signs of systemic infection. Because *Capnocytophaga canimorsus*, which is more common after dog bites, is difficult to isolate and identify on microbiologic media due to its slow growth, polymerase chain reaction is the gold standard for its bacteriologic diagnosis.[68] A retrospective study from 2020 determined that serologic assays should be obtained if *Bartonella* spp. are of concern. Radiography is recommended initially to detect debris or any residual teeth from the animal bite; however, MRI is the preferred modality for infection detection, especially osteomyelitis.[69]

Early treatment of animal bite injuries that are infected is associated with better outcome, shorter hospitalization, and reduced complications and the need for second-look surgeries.[69,70] Treatment of animal bites usually starts with thorough wound inspection to identify deep injuries and devitalized tissue; anesthesia is usually necessary for proper inspection and visualization of the bottom of the wound.[71] Copious irrigation with normal saline or antiseptic solutions is one of the most important means of infection prevention and the limb can be wrapped with a bandage for immobilization.[71,72] Although controversial, it is generally preferred to keep animal bite wounds open to reduce infection risk, except for facial wounds.[31,73] Tetanus and rabies prophylaxis should also be provided when indicated.[74]

The first-line empiric antibiotic for infected animal bite wounds is amoxicillin/clavulanic acid (or ampicillin/sulbactam if parenteral therapy is needed); then, antimicrobial therapy should be tailored to culture and susceptibility results if available. An effective antimicrobial treatment course is often 7 to 10 days. The total duration of therapy depends on the location and severity of the wound and the patient's clinical response; it should be extended for 4 to 6 weeks in the presence of bone and joint infections.[66] Surgeon consultation is warranted for deep wound infections that involve bone, tendons, joints, or other major structures and compromised neurovascular structures. Surgical débridement should be considered for dirty wounds notably for edges and nonviable tissue, as it has been shown to be effective in preventing infection.[71,72] Animal bite wounds are usually at greater risk of aesthetic sequelae because of their longer inflammatory phase that causes multiple edges, bruising, and laceration.[75] However, searching for deeper infections such as flexor tenosynovitis, necrotizing fasciitis, septic arthritis, and osteomyelitis is warranted in cases of persistent signs of infection despite adequate initial wound care and antibiotics administration.[66,70]

ABSCESS

S aureus is the most common cause of abscesses.[31] However, abscesses can be polymicrobial in up to 40% of cases in people who inject drugs because pathogens are inoculated into the skin layers and can originate from the individual's skin surface, contaminated drugs, or contaminated equipment.[76] In addition to *S aureus*, these include commensal organisms of the oral cavity (such as *Streptococcus anginosus*, other viridans group streptococci, and anaerobic organisms). In 2022, a retrospective study reported that in people who inject drugs, abscesses frequently occur at the antecubital fossa region, which is one of the most common injection sites and may use other injection sites throughout the body including the neck, groin, legs, or feet.[77] Early point-of-care ultrasonography can be used to rule out abscesses in uncertain cases.[78]

In some rare cases, these abscesses can contiguously spread to bone and joints and cause osteomyelitis and septic arthritis. Thus, incision and drainage, which is the primary therapeutic modality of abscess management, should be promptly performed. Pus directly drained from these lesions should be sent for Gram stain and culture testing. Blood cultures are not recommended by the Infectious Diseases Society of America in SSTIs because they have low yield, even in people who inject drugs who are febrile, and do not affect patient management significantly.[31] The authors of this chapter, however, disagree with this position and recommend obtaining blood cultures in this high-risk group for systemic complications of bacteremia; of note, a US population–based study from 2022 showed that 38% of *S aureus* bacteremia had SSTIs as a potential source.[79]

According to the IDSA, the administration of empiric antimicrobial agents covering *S aureus* (including MRSA), in addition to incision and drainage, depends on the presence or absence of signs of systemic infection, especially fever, hypotension, and sustained tachycardia.[31,80] Patients with immunocompromising conditions or inadequate improvement with incision and drainage should receive empiric coverage for MRSA.[31] In addition, antimicrobial agents with broad-spectrum covering gram-positive cocci are recommended in people who inject drugs as they represent most isolated organisms.[31,76] Patients at risk for infective endocarditis should receive antibiotic coverage 1 hour before incision and drainage with agents covering MRSA and beta-hemolytic streptococci. Other numerous conditions may warrant treatment with antimicrobial agents and these include size of single abscess (≥2 cm), multiple abscesses, surrounding cellulitis, major comorbidities, presence of an indwelling device (such as prosthetic joint, vascular graft, or permanent pacemaker), high risk for adverse outcomes with infective endocarditis (such as a history of infectious endocarditis, presence of prosthetic valve or prosthetic perivalvular material, unrepaired congenital heart defect, or valvular dysfunction in a transplanted heart), and high risk for community transmission of *S aureus* (such as military personnel and athletes).

SUMMARY

Complicated SSTIs encompass an array of conditions, such as necrotizing infections, pyomyositis, animal bites, and abscesses. In addition to a course of targeted antimicrobial therapy, these infections usually require substantial surgical management including incision and drainage or débridement, often on a recurrent basis. Without securing source control and despite appropriate antimicrobial administration, important outcomes, including need for critical care support, hospital length of stay, readmission rates, ability to ambulate, and short-term and long-term mortality, worsen by the hour in some cases without surgical intervention.

KEY STUDY POINTS

- NSTIs are limb and life threatening and are characterized by extensive and acute destruction of tissue associated with systemic signs of toxicity.
- Because NSTIs often result in increased morbidity (including limb loss) and mortality, they represent a surgical emergency where aggressive and prompt débridement, hemodynamic support, and antimicrobial therapy are required.
- Other types of complicated SSTIs also require surgical intervention as source control. Delays in diagnosis and surgical management have been associated with increased mortality rates.

ACKNOWLEDGMENTS

The authors are extremely grateful for the philanthropic support provided by a gift from Eva and Gene Lane (L.M.B.), which was paramount in the work to advance the science of cardiovascular infections, an ongoing focus of investigation at Mayo Clinic for more than 60 years.

ANNOTATED REFERENCES

1. Morgan E, Hohmann S, Ridgway JP, Daum RS, David MZ: Decreasing incidence of skin and soft-tissue infections in 86 US emergency departments, 2009-2014. *Clin Infect Dis* 2019;68(3):453-459.

   The rate of SSTIs decreased by 8% among all patients and by 14.6% among patients with HIV infection in the United States between 2009 and 2014. Level of evidence: II.

2. Lipsky BA, Silverman MH, Joseph WS: A proposed new classification of skin and soft tissue infections modeled on the subset of diabetic foot infection. *Open Forum Infect Dis* 2016;4(1):ofw255.

3. Saldana CS, Vyas DA, Wurcel AG: Soft tissue, bone, and joint infections in people who inject drugs. *Infect Dis Clin North Am* 2020;34(3):495-509.

   SSTIs have a wide variety of manifestations in people who inject drugs ranging from cellulitis to necrotizing fasciitis and are polymicrobial in up to 40%.

4. Sartelli M, Coccolini F, Kluger Y, et al: WSES/GAIS/WSIS/SIS-E/AAST global clinical pathways for patients with skin and soft tissue infections. *World J Emerg Surg* 2022;17(1):3.

   This extensive nonsystematic review conducted by several societies (including the World Society of Emergency Surgery/the Global Alliance for Infections in Surgery/the World Surgical Infection Society/the Surgical Infection Society Europe/the American Association for the Surgery of Trauma) drafted global clinical pathways for patients with SSTIs.

5. Gupta Y, Chhetry M, Pathak KR, et al: Risk factors for necrotizing fasciitis and its outcome at a tertiary care centre. *J Ayub Med Coll Abbottabad* 2016;28(4):680-682.

6. Liu TJ, Tai HC, Chien KL, Cheng NC: Predisposing factors of necrotizing fasciitis with comparison to cellulitis in Taiwan: A nationwide population-based case–control study. *J Formos Med Assoc* 2020;119(1 pt 1):18-25.

   Age and the presence of chronic diseases were major risk factors and prognostic factors of necrotizing fasciitis in Taiwan from 2002 to 2011. Level of evidence: III.

7. Pelletier J, Gottlieb M, Long B, Perkins JC: Necrotizing soft tissue infections (NSTI): Pearls and pitfalls for the emergency clinician. *J Emerg Med* 2022;62(4):480-491.

   This review assessed the current evidence regarding the presentation, evaluation, and management of NSTI from the emergency department perspective.

8. Peetermans M, de Prost N, Eckmann C, Norrby-Teglund A, Skrede S, De Waele JJ: Necrotizing skin and soft-tissue infections in the intensive care unit. *Clin Microbiol Infect* 2020;26(1):8-17.

   This review emphasizes the importance of multidisciplinary teams in the care of critically ill patients with NSTI.

9. Bruun T, Rath E, Madsen MB, et al: Risk factors and predictors of mortality in streptococcal necrotizing soft-tissue infections: A multicenter prospective study. *Clin Infect Dis* 2021;72(2):293-300.

   This prospective cohort identified risk factors associated with mortality in patients with group A *Streptococcus* NSTI, such as older age, septic shock, and lack of intravenous immunoglobulin administration. Level of evidence: II.

10. Eason TB, Cosgrove CT, Mihalko WM: Necrotizing soft-tissue infections after hip arthroplasty. *Orthop Clin North Am* 2022;53(1):33-41.

    This publication reviews two case reports of prosthetic joint infection presenting as NSTI in patients with hip implants. Level of evidence: IV.

11. Duane TM, Huston JM, Collom M, et al: Surgical Infection Society 2020 updated guidelines on the management of complicated skin and soft tissue infections. *Surg Infect (Larchmt)* 2021;22(4):383-399.

    The 2020 guidelines from the Surgical Infection Society on the management of complicated SSTI remain unchanged except for increased support for adjuvant antimicrobial therapy after drainage of complex abscess and updated findings regarding the use of alternative antimicrobial agents.

12. Lim SH, Tunku Ahmad TS, Devarajooh C, Gunasagaran J: Upper limb infections: A comparison between diabetic and non-diabetic patients. *J Orthop Surg (Hong Kong)* 2022;30(1):23094990221075376.

    Patients with diabetes were more likely to present with emergent scenarios, especially necrotizing fasciitis and infectious tenosynovitis, compared with patients without diabetes. Level of evidence: II.

13. Martin H, Bursztejn AC, Albuisson E, et al: Characteristics of chronic wounds in substance abuse: A retrospective study of 58 patients [Article in French]. *Ann Dermatol Venereol* 2019;146(12):793-800.

    Drug abuse–related chronic wounds were more likely to occur in young men with a history of injection drug abuse. Level of evidence: II.

14. Collins CM, McCarty A, Jalilvand A, et al: Outcomes of patients with necrotizing soft tissue infections: A propensity-matched analysis using the national inpatient sample. *Surg Infect (Larchmt)* 2022;23(3):304-312.

    This retrospective study from 2012 to 2018 identified older age and having two or more comorbidities as risk factors associated with mortality in NSTI. Level of evidence: II.

15. Al-Qurayshi Z, Nichols RL, Killackey MT, Kandil E: Mortality risk in necrotizing fasciitis: National prevalence, trend, and burden. *Surg Infect (Larchmt)* 2020;21(10):840-852.

    This retrospective cross-sectional study from 2010 to 2014 showed that NSTI with septicemia and lack of surgical intervention were associated with higher mortality. Level of evidence: II.

16. Naamany E, Shiber S, Duskin-Bitan H, et al: Polymicrobial and monomicrobial necrotizing soft tissue infections: Comparison of clinical, laboratory, radiological, and pathological hallmarks and prognosis. A retrospective analysis. *Trauma Surg Acute Care Open* 2021;6(1):e000745.

    This retrospective study from 2002 to 2019 showed that patients with monomicrobial NSTI had a significantly higher 90-day mortality rate in addition to higher rates of in-hospital mortality, intensive care unit admission, and vasopressor use than those with polymicrobial NSTI. Level of evidence: II.

17. Karnuta J, Featherall J, Lawrenz J, et al: What demographic and clinical factors are associated with in-hospital mortality in patients with necrotizing fasciitis? *Clin Orthop Relat Res* 2020;478(8):1770-1779.

    A retrospective study during a 10-year period identified risk factors associated with in-hospital mortality in necrotizing fasciitis, including older age, coronary artery disease, chronic kidney disease, and transfer from an outside hospital. Level of evidence: II.

18. Bakleh M, Wold LE, Mandrekar JN, Harmsen WS, Dimashkieh HH, Baddour LM: Correlation of histopathologic findings with clinical outcome in necrotizing fasciitis. *Clin Infect Dis* 2005;40(3):410-414.

19. Nguyen QD, Diab J, Khaicy D, et al: The impact of COVID-19 on delayed presentations of necrotising fasciitis. *J Surg Case Rep* 2022;2022(2):rjac015.

    This retrospective study from 2017 to 2020 showed that COVID-19 patients with necrotizing fasciitis had longer mean onset of symptoms until hospital presentation and were more likely to be admitted to the intensive care unit compared with non–COVID-19 patients with necrotizing fasciitis. Level of evidence: II.

20. Abder-Rahman H, Habash I, Alami R, Alnimer T, Al-Abdallat I: Medico-legal importance of necrotizing fasciitis. *J Forensic Leg Med* 2020;74:102019.

    Six cases in a forensic pathology practice where necrotizing fasciitis posed a unique medicolegal dilemma were examined in this article. Level of evidence: IV.

21. Kim MJ, Shin SH, Park JY: Medicolegal implications from litigations involving necrotizing fasciitis. *Ann Surg Treat Res* 2020;99(3):131-137.

    The outcome of 25 cases of medical malpractice litigation involving necrotizing fasciitis from 1998 to 2018 showed that physicians cannot be blamed for the failure to prevent necrotizing fasciitis. Level of evidence: IV.

22. Beaudoin AL, Torso L, Richards K, et al: Invasive group A Streptococcus infections associated with liposuction surgery at outpatient facilities not subject to state or federal regulation. *JAMA Intern Med* 2014;174(7):1136-1142.

23. Zhang JX, McSweeney CT, Bush KL: Nosocomial transmission of necrotising fasciitis organisms from prepartum patient to healthcare worker. *BMJ Case Rep* 2021;14(5):e240848.

    This is a case report of nosocomial transmission of necrotizing fasciitis from a prepartum patient to a health care worker. Level of evidence: IV.

24. Garcia NM, Cai J: Aggressive soft tissue infections. *Surg Clin North Am* 2018;98(5):1097-1108.

    This is a review on NSTI presentation, diagnosis, mortality, and surgical and antimicrobial treatment.

25. Geng C, Yu K, Li F: Necrotizing fasciitis caused by mucormycosis: A case report and literature review. *Int J Low Extrem Wounds* 2022; February 15 [Epub ahead of print].

    This is a case report of necrotizing fasciitis of the limb caused by mucormycosis managed with antifungal treatment and repeated débridement. Level of evidence: IV.

26. Horn DL, Roberts EA, Shen J, et al: Outcomes of β-hemolytic streptococcal necrotizing skin and soft-tissue infections and the impact of clindamycin resistance. *Clin Infect Dis* 2021;73(11):e4592-e4598.

    This retrospective study from 2015 and 2018 showed a high prevalence of beta-hemolytic streptococci (more specifically clindamycin resistant) in NSTI and a greater risk of amputation with this pathogen. Level of evidence: II.

27. Khanna A, Taylor MD: Necrotising myositis – Learnings for a plastic surgeon. *J Plast Reconstr Aesthet Surg* 2022;75(1):145-151.

    This is a systematic review on necrotizing myositis case reports showing that three-fourth of these cases were a result of group A *Streptococcus* infections.

28. Martin SJ, Stephen VS: Pitfalls in medicine: Pain out of proportion to examination findings. *Br J Hosp Med (Lond)* 2022;83(4):1-8.

    There is a raising awareness that NSTI can present with pain out of proportion to physical examination.

29. Gunaratne DA, Tseros EA, Hasan Z, et al: Cervical necrotizing fasciitis: Systematic review and analysis of 1235 reported cases from the literature. *Head Neck* 2018;40(9):2094-2102.

    This systematic review of case reports on cervical necrotizing fasciitis showed that most had odontogenic origin and required numerous débridement.

30. Petitpas F, Blancal JP, Mateo J, et al: Factors associated with the mediastinal spread of cervical necrotizing fasciitis. *Ann Thorac Surg* 2012;93(1):234-238.

31. Stevens DL, Bisno AL, Chambers HF, et al: Practice guidelines for the diagnosis and management of skin and soft tissue infections: 2014 update by the Infectious Diseases Society of America. *Clin Infect Dis* 2014;59(2):e10-e52.

32. Kazi FN, Sharma JV, Ghosh S, Prashanth D, Raja VOPK: Comparison of LRINEC scoring system with finger test and histopathological examination for necrotizing fasciitis. *Surg J (N Y)* 2022;8(1):e1-e7.

    This is a study showing that histopathology remained the gold standard for diagnosis of necrotizing fasciitis, whereas LRINEC score and finger test were good diagnostic tools for early diagnosis, with sensitivities of 83.33% and 86.11%, respectively.

33. Bechar J, Sepehripour S, Hardwicke J, Filobbos G: Laboratory risk indicator for necrotising fasciitis (LRINEC) score for the assessment of early necrotising fasciitis: A systematic review of the literature. *Ann R Coll Surg Engl* 2017;99(5):341-346.

34. Kim DH, Kim SW, Hwang SH: Application of the laboratory risk indicator for necrotizing fasciitis score to the head and neck: A systematic review and meta-analysis. *ANZ J Surg* 2022;92(7-8):1631-1637.

    This is a systematic review showing that LRINEC score is a useful adjunctive tool for predicting cervical necrotizing fasciitis in patients with a soft-tissue infection, with a more accurate diagnosis when using a cutoff value of 6. Level of evidence: III.

35. Tanaka S, Thy M, Khoury R, Tran-Dinh A, Khalil A, Montravers P: Severe necrotizing soft-tissue infection-associated mortality: Have a look at the computed tomography! *Crit Care* 2022;26:27.

    This retrospective study from 2009 to 2019 on patients with severe NSTI hospitalized in the intensive care unit showed that presence of inflammatory changes of the fascia parameter in the CT scan had a sensitivity of 60%, specificity of 92%, positive predictive value of 75%, and negative predictive value of 86%. Level of evidence: II.

36. Martinez M, Peponis T, Hage A, et al: The role of computed tomography in the diagnosis of necrotizing soft tissue infections. *World J Surg* 2018;42(1):82-87.

    This retrospective study from 2009 to 2006 showed that a negative intravenous contrast-enhanced CT scan can reliably rule out the need for surgical intervention in patients with initial suspicion of NSTI. Level of evidence: II.

37. Fernando SM, Tran A, Cheng W, et al: Necrotizing soft tissue infection: Diagnostic accuracy of physical examination, imaging, and LRINEC score – A systematic review and meta-analysis. *Ann Surg* 2019;269(1):58-65.

    A systematic review showed that LRINEC score had poor sensitivity and should not be used to rule out NSTI, reinforcing that high clinical suspicion warrants early surgical consultation for definitive diagnosis and management. Level of evidence: III.

38. Hua C, Urbina T, Bosc R, et al: Necrotising soft-tissue infections. *Lancet Infect Dis* 2023;23(3):e81-e94.

    This is a review focusing on practical approaches to management of NSTIs including prompt recognition, initiation of specific management, exploratory surgery, and care after treatment.

39. Gelbard RB, Ferrada P, Yeh DD, et al: Optimal timing of initial debridement for necrotizing soft tissue infection: A Practice Management Guideline from the Eastern Association for the Surgery of Trauma. *J Trauma Acute Care Surg* 2018;85(1):208-214.

    This is a systematic review showing that early surgical débridement within 12 hours of suspected diagnosis of NSTI is recommended. Level of evidence: III.

40. Nawijn F, Smeeing DPJ, Houwert RM, Leenen LPH, Hietbrink F: Time is of the essence when treating necrotizing soft tissue infections: A systematic review and meta-analysis. *World J Emerg Surg* 2020;15:4.

    This systematic review showed that early surgical débridement lowers the mortality rate for NSTI. Level of evidence: III.

41. Nawijn F, van Heijl M, Keizer J, van Koperen PJ, Hietbrink F: The impact of operative time on the outcomes of necrotizing soft tissue infections: A multicenter cohort study. *BMC Surg* 2022;22(1):3.

    This is a study showing that prolonged surgical time was associated with a prolonged intensive care unit and hospital stay. Level of evidence: II.

42. Tom LK, Maine RG, Wang CS, Parent BA, Bulger EM, Keys KA: Comparison of traditional and skin-sparing approaches for surgical treatment of necrotizing soft-tissue infections. *Surg Infect (Larchmt)* 2020;21(4):363-369.

    This is a study showing that skin-sparing débridement for source control of NSTI compared with traditional débridement resulted in significantly more wounds completely closed by delayed primary suture of existing skin flaps and a significantly lower overall wound percentage closed by skin graft, while demonstrating equivalent efficacy of source control and a similar low mortality rate. Level of evidence: II.

43. Sartelli M, Guirao X, Hardcastle TC, et al: 2018 WSES/SIS-E consensus conference: Recommendations for the management of skin and soft-tissue infections. *World J Emerg Surg* 2018;13:58.

    This task force created by the World Society of Emergency Surgery and the Surgical Infection Society Europe in 2018 emphasizes the need for multidisciplinary collaboration in treating patients with NSTI.

44. Tessier JM, Sanders J, Sartelli M, et al: Necrotizing soft tissue infections: A focused review of pathophysiology, diagnosis, operative management, antimicrobial therapy, and pediatrics. *Surg Infect* 2020;21(2):81-93.

    The Surgical Infection Society of North America and the World Society of Emergency Surgery emphasize on the importance of early diagnosis and surgical intervention in necrotizing fasciitis.

45. Chang CP, Hsiao CT, Lin CN, Fann WC: Risk factors for mortality in the late amputation of necrotizing fasciitis: A retrospective study. *World J Emerg Surg* 2018;13:45.

This retrospective cohort study from 2015 to 2018 in Taiwan identified significant risk factors for mortality in patients with NSTI who underwent late amputation: presence of hemorrhagic bullae, peripheral vascular disease, bacteremia, and LRINEC score greater than 8. Level of evidence: II.

46. Stevens DL, Bryant AE, Goldstein EJ: Necrotizing soft tissue infections. *Infect Dis Clin North Am* 2021;35(1):135-155.

    This is an updated review on risk factors, microbiology, diagnosis, and management of NSTI.

47. Cortés-Penfield N, Ryder JH: Should linezolid replace clindamycin as the adjunctive antimicrobial of choice in group A streptococcal necrotizing soft tissue infection and toxic shock syndrome? A focused debate. *Clin Infect Dis* 2023;76(2):346-350.

    This is a review comparing clindamycin and linezolid as adjunctive therapy to reduce mortality in invasive group A streptococcal infection.

48. Kenneally AM, Warriner Z, VanHoose JD, et al: Evaluation of antibiotic duration after surgical debridement of necrotizing soft tissue infection. *Surg Infect (Larchmt)* 2022;23(4):357-363.

    This retrospective study from 2010 to 2020 showed that shorter duration of antibiotic therapy after final surgical débridement of NSTI may be appropriate in patients without any other indications for antibiotic agents. Level of evidence: II.

49. Evans L, Rhodes A, Alhazzani W, et al: Surviving sepsis campaign: International guidelines for management of sepsis and septic shock 2021. *Intensive Care Med* 2021;47(11):1181-1247.

    The International Guidelines for Management of Sepsis and Septic Shock 2021 emphasized on appropriate source control as a key principle in the management of sepsis and septic shock including débridement of infected necrotic tissue.

50. Linnér A, Darenberg J, Sjölin J, Henriques-Normark B, Norrby-Teglund A: Clinical efficacy of polyspecific intravenous immunoglobulin therapy in patients with streptococcal toxic shock syndrome: A comparative observational study. *Clin Infect Dis* 2014;59(6):851-857.

51. Parks T, Wilson C, Curtis N, Norrby-Teglund A, Sriskandan S: Polyspecific intravenous immunoglobulin in clindamycin-treated patients with streptococcal toxic shock syndrome: A systematic review and meta-analysis. *Clin Infect Dis* 2018;67(9):1434-1436.

    This is a meta-analysis showing that the use of intravenous immunoglobulin in clindamycin-treated streptococcal toxic shock syndrome decreased mortality. Level of evidence: II.

52. Eskes A, Vermeulen H, Lucas C, Ubbink DT: Hyperbaric oxygen therapy for treating acute surgical and traumatic wounds. *Cochrane Database Syst Rev* 2013;12:CD008059.

53. Siegel JD, Rhinehart E, Jackson M, Chiarello L, Health Care Infection Control Practices Advisory Committee: 2007 guideline for isolation precautions: Preventing transmission of infectious agents in health care settings. *Am J Infect Control* 2007;35(10 suppl 2):S65-S164.

54. Bulger EM, May AK, Robinson BRH, et al: A novel immune modulator for patients with necrotizing soft tissue infections (NSTI): Results of a multicenter, phase 3 randomized controlled trial of reltecimod (AB 103). *Ann Surg* 2020;272(3):469-478.

    This randomized double-blind placebo-controlled trial showed that early administration of reltecimod in severe NSTI resulted in improved resolution of organ dysfunction and hospital discharge status. Level of evidence: I.

55. Moore DL, Allen UD, Mailman T: Invasive group A streptococcal disease: Management and chemoprophylaxis. *Paediatr Child Health* 2019;24(2):128-129.

    The Canadian guidelines emphasized on the importance of penicillin in the treatment of group A streptococcal disease.

56. Chambers HF: Skin and soft tissue infections in persons who inject drugs. *Infect Dis Clin North Am* 2021;35(1):169-181.

    This review on SSTI in people who inject drugs emphasized the importance of surgical incision, drainage, and débridement of devitalized tissue in management.

57. Maravelas R, Melgar TA, Vos D, Lima N, Sadarangani S: Pyomyositis in the United States 2002–2014. *J Infect* 2020;80(5):497-503.

    This US population–based study from 2002 to 2014 reported an increase in pyomyositis cases, with methicillin-susceptible *S aureus* being the most commonly identified organism. Level of evidence: II.

58. Ngor C, Hall L, Dean JA, Gilks CF: Factors associated with pyomyositis: A systematic review and meta-analysis. *Trop Med Int Health* 2021;26(10):1210-1219.

    This meta-analysis indicated a significant association between pyomyositis and HIV/AIDS. Level of evidence: II.

59. Radcliffe C, Gisriel S, Niu YS, Peaper D, Delgado S, Grant M: Pyomyositis and infectious myositis: A comprehensive, single-center retrospective study. *Open Forum Infect Dis* 2021;8(4):ofab098.

    This retrospective study from 2012 to 2020 on pyomyositis cases showed that *Staphylococcus* spp. accounted for 46% of all infections and that the most common symptom was muscle pain. Level of evidence: II.

60. Narayanappa G, Nandeesh BN: Infective myositis. *Brain Pathol* 2021;31(3):e12950.

    This is a review on the wide variety of pathogens causing infective myositis, including bacteria, fungi, viruses, and parasites.

61. Vij N, Ranade AS, Kang P, Belthur MV: Primary bacterial pyomyositis in children: A systematic review. *J Pediatr Orthop* 2021;41(9):e849-e854.

    This systematic review on tropical pyomyositis showed that the most commonly used imaging modality was MRI and that medical management alone can be successful, but surgical treatment was often needed. Level of evidence: II.

62. Altmayer S, Verma N, Dicks EA, Oliveira A: Imaging musculoskeletal soft tissue infections. *Semin Ultrasound CT MR* 2020;41(1):85-98.

    This review on radiologic findings of soft-tissue infections showed that the widespread use of cross-sectional imaging with MRI and CT has greatly increased the radiologic diagnosis in conditions where ultrasonography may be limited.

63. Shittu A, Deinhardt-Emmer S, Vas Nunes J, Niemann S, Grobusch MP, Schaumburg F: Tropical pyomyositis: An update. *Trop Med Int Health* 2020;25(6):660-665.

    This review on tropical pyomyositis suggested that there is strong evidence that Panton-Valentine leucocidin is the key toxin associated with disease.

64. Habeych ME, Trinh T, Crum-Cianflone NF: Purulent infectious myositis (formerly tropical pyomyositis). *J Neurol Sci* 2020;413:116767.

    This overview on purulent infectious myositis highlighted the need for combination of percutaneous or open surgical drainage along with antimicrobial therapy (including MRSA coverage).

65. Loder RT: The demographics of dog bites in the United States. *Heliyon* 2019;5(3):e01360.

    This US retrospective study from 2005 to 2013 reported a mean annual incidence of dog bites of 1.1 per 1,000 individuals with most located on the upper extremity. Level of evidence: II.

66. Bula-Rudas FJ, Olcott JL: Human and animal bites. *Pediatr Rev* 2018;39(10):490-500.

    This review on human and animal bites highlights the importance of amoxicillin-clavulanate as the antibiotic of choice for prophylaxis and empirical therapy in people nonallergic to penicillin.

67. Razafindrazaka H, Redl S, Aouchiche F, et al: Atteinte osseuse dans la maladie des griffes du chat. *La Revue de Médecine Interne* 2021;42(12):875-880.

    Approximately 30 cases of bartonellosis with bone involvement were reported. Level of evidence: IV.

68. Zajkowska J, Król M, Falkowski D, Syed N, Kamieńska A: Capnocytophaga canimorsus – An underestimated danger after dog or cat bite – Review of literature. *Przegl Epidemiol* 2016;70(2):289-295.

69. Seegmueller J, Arsalan-Werner A, Koehler S, Sauerbier M, Mehling I: Cat and dog bite injuries of the hand: Early versus late treatment. *Arch Orthop Trauma Surg* 2020;140(7):981-985.

    This retrospective study from 2010 to 2016 demonstrated that early management of cat and dog bite injuries results in less second-look surgeries and shorter hospitalization. Level of evidence: II.

70. Koshy JC, Bell B: Hand infections. *J Hand Surg Am* 2019;44(1):46-54.

    This is a review focusing on the importance of identifying serious hand infections requiring urgent or emergent treatment including necrotizing fasciitis.

71. Ellis R, Ellis C: Dog and cat bites. *Am Fam Physician* 2014;90(4):239-243.

72. Saul D, Dresing K: Surgical treatment of bites [Article in German]. *Oper Orthop Traumatol* 2018;30(5):321-341.

    This retrospective study examined bite injuries that were seen by healthcare professionals in Germany and found that 46% were caused by dogs and 32% by cats. Level of evidence: II.

73. Jaindl M, Oberleitner G, Endler G, Thallinger C, Kovar FM: Management of bite wounds in children and adults-an analysis of over 5000 cases at a level I trauma centre. *Wien Klin Wochenschr* 2016;128(9-10):367-375.

74. Fooks AR, Cliquet F, Finke S, et al: Rabies. *Nat Rev Dis Primers* 2017;3:17091.

75. Touzet-Roumazeille S, Jayyosi L, Plenier Y, Guyot E, Guillard T, François C: Surgical management of animal bites in children [Article in French]. *Ann Chir Plast Esthet* 2016;61(5):560-567.

76. Jenkins TC, Knepper BC, Jason Moore S, et al: Microbiology and initial antibiotic therapy for injection drug users and non-injection drug users with cutaneous abscesses in the era of community-associated methicillin-resistant Staphylococcus aureus. *Acad Emerg Med* 2015;22(8):993-997.

77. Lim J, Pavalagantharajah S, Verschoor CP, et al: Infectious diseases, comorbidities and outcomes in hospitalized people who inject drugs (PWID) infections in persons who inject drugs. *PLoS One* 2022;17(4):e0266663.

    This retrospective study from 2013 to 2018 showed that most abscesses in people who inject drugs were located on the upper extremities. Level of evidence: II.

78. Subramaniam S, Bober J, Chao J, Zehtabchi S: Point-of-care ultrasound for diagnosis of abscess in skin and soft tissue infections. *Acad Emerg Med* 2016;23(11):1298-1306.

79. Hindy JR, Quintero-Martinez JA, Lahr BD, et al: Incidence of monomicrobial *Staphylococcus aureus* bacteremia: A population-based study in Olmsted County, Minnesota – 2006 to 2020. *Open Forum Infect Dis* 2022;9(7):ofac190.

    This retrospective US population–based study from 2006 to 2020 showed that 38% of patients with *S aureus* bacteremia had SSTIs as a potential source. Level of evidence: II.

80. Hindy JR, Haddad SF, Kanj SS: New drugs for methicillin-resistant Staphylococcus aureus skin and soft tissue infections. *Curr Opin Infect Dis* 2022;35(2):112-119.

    This review highlights that several antibiotics received a fast-track approval by the FDA for the management of SSTI caused by MRSA but that the current Infectious Diseases Society of America guidelines and the recently published UK guidelines only consider them as alternative choices.

Index

Note: Page numbers followed by "*f*" indicate figures and "*t*" indicate tables.

A

Abscesses, 300
   epidural, 282, 285*f*
   subcutaneous, 64
   subperiosteal, 65
Acetic acid, 92–93, 95, 98
Acute hematogenous osteomyelitis (AHO), 243, 244*f*–245*f*
   antibiotic treatment, 245
   clinical outcomes, 246
   complications, 246
   surgical treatment, 245–246
Aerobic gram-negative bacteria, 72
Aerobic gram-positive bacteria
   coagulase-negative staphylococci, 72
   enterococci, 72
   Staphylococcus aureus, 71–72
   streptococci, 72
Airborne organism load
   air quality monitoring, 32
   organism profile, 32
   particles, as contamination, 32
   reducing air contamination, 32
Alcohol abuse, 22–23
Amputations, 268
   antibiotics, duration of, 200
   diabetic foot ulcer and, 264
   transfemoral, 174
Anaerobic bacteria, 4, 72–73
Anemia, 22, 230
   epidemiology, 50
   optimization strategy, 50
Animal bites. *See* Bite wounds
Antibiotics, 92, 106*t*, 132*t*–135*t*
   acute hematogenous osteomyelitis, 245
   allergy, 110
   antimicrobial selection, 107–108
   beads, 223
   biofilms, 107–108
   bone penetration, 108, 109*t*–110*t*
   diabetic foot infections, 267, 268*t*
   open fractures
      local delivery, 223
      systemic administration, 222–223
   oral, 200
   powder, 117
   prosthetic joint infection, 195–201
      culture negative, 196
      duration of, 199–200
      empiric treatment regimens, 196
      monitoring during, 200–201
      oral antimicrobial therapy for, 196–198
      postoperative, 187–188
      preoperative, 195
      rifampin combination therapy, 198–199
      targeted regimens, 196
   selection, 117, 118*t*
   septic arthritis, 257–258, 257*t*
   spacers, 168–171
   spectrum, 107
   suppressive, 200
Antimicrobial agents, 83, 149, 297–298
   choice of, 232, 233*t*–234*t*
   laboratory testing, 200
   pyomyositis, stage 1, 299
   rifampin, 198
Antimicrobial therapy
   bactericidal *vs.* bacteriostatic, 110
   local, 234
   necrotizing soft-tissue infections, 297–298, 298*t*
   outpatient parenteral antimicrobial therapy, 110–111
   suppressive, 148
   systemic
      choice of, 232, 233*t*–234*t*
      duration of therapy, 233–234
      route of administration, 232–233
Antiseptics
   acetic acid, 92–93
   chlorhexidine gluconate, 94–95
   commercial, 96–97
   hydrogen peroxide, 95
   hypochlorous acid, 96
   povidone-iodine, 93–94
   sodium hypochlorite, 95
Arthrocentesis, 156
Arthrodesis, 200
Arthroplasty
   single-stage revision
      clinical outcomes, 173
      indications, 173
      technique, 172–173
   two-stage revision, 167
      antibiotic spacers and, 168–171, 168*f*–170*f*
      outcomes following, 171–172
Autogenous bone graft, 236

B

Bacterial contamination, 81
Bacterial/fungal skin burden, 12
Bacterial infections
   animal bites, 274–275
   bone, 276
   complicating factors, 277
   felon, 274
   human bites, 274
   joint, 276
   mimickers of, 277, 277*f*
   necrotizing, 276–277, 276*f*, 276*t*
   palmar space infections, 275, 276*f*
   paronychia, 274
   purulent flexor tenosynovitis, 275, 275*f*
Benzoyl peroxide, 182
Beta-lactam antibiotics, 136–137
Biofilms, 70–71
   antibiotics in, 107–108
   bacterial contamination, 81
   biomaterial surface modifications, 86
   diabetic foot infections, 266
   diagnostic challenges, 84–85, 85*t*
   formation of, 85–86
   fracture-related infection, 231
   host immunity, 86, 86*t*
   life cycle, 82–83, 82*f*–83*f*
   musculoskeletal infections, 70–71
   physiologic fluid, 83
   proteinaceous transition, 83
   treatment, 83–84
      antibiotic susceptibility testing, 84
      dormant phenotypes, 84
      penetration, 84
      physiology, moving fluids on, 84
      slow-growing, 84
Biomarkers
   blood, 62–63
   orthopaedic infection, 62, 63*f*
   synovial fluid, 63–64
Biomaterial surface modifications, 86
Bite wounds
   animal, 274–275
   human, 274
   infections related to, 299–300
Blood biomarkers, 62–63
Bone
   biopsy, 266, 268
   destruction, 266
   healing, 230
   infections, 264, 276
   morphogenetic proteins, 237
   necrotic, 215
   transport, 237
Bone grafting
   autogenous, 236
   free vascularized, 237
   timing of, 236

C

Calcium, for fracture healing, 231
Calcium sulfate, 116–117, 122
Capnocytophaga canimorsus, 275, 299
Cefazolin, 42, 182, 196
Cefepime, 136–137

Ceftaroline, 136
Ceftriaxone, 196, 257
Cellulitis, necrotizing, 295, 296f
Cephalosporin, open fractures, 222
Charcot foot, 265f
Charlson Comorbidity Index, 166
Chitosans, 117, 122
Chlorhexidine, 182
Chlorhexidine gluconate (CHG), 94–95
Chronic renal disease, 25
Ciprofloxacin, bone formation, 231
Clindamycin, 138
Coagulase-negative staphylococci (CoNS), 72, 196
Compartment syndrome, 221
Computed tomography (CT), 65
    fracture-related infection, 214
    necrotizing soft-tissue infections, 296
    nonnecrotizing soft-tissue infections, 299
    prosthetic joint infection, 156, 184
    spine infections, 285–286, 286f–288f
Contiguous osteomyelitis, 248–249
Contraindications, 121–122
Coronavirus 2019 (COVID-19) pandemic, 263, 294
Corticosteroids, 231
Costovertebral joints (CVJs), 282
C-reactive protein (CRP)
    acute hematogenous osteomyelitis, 245
    fracture-related infection, 213
    primary septic arthritis, 247
    prosthetic joint infection, 156–157, 183, 200
    spine infections, 284, 289
CRIME80 score, 166, 167t
Culture-based methods, 69–70
Culture-negative prosthetic joint infection, 196
Cutibacterium acnes, 12, 181–182, 182f, 196
Cutibacterium avidum, 196
Cutibacterium granulosum, 196

D

Daptomycin, 137
D-dimer test, 63, 157
Débridement
    anemia, 22
    open fractures, 223–224
    prosthetic joint infections, 92
    surgical, 231–232
Débridement, antibiotics, and implant retention (DAIR) procedure
    clinical outcomes, 166–167, 167t
    indications, 165–166
    surgical technique, 166
Deep vein thrombosis (DVT), 246
Depression, 21, 22t
Device-related infections, 31
    infection after fracture fixation, 76
    prosthetic joint infections, 76
    spinal hardware, 76
Diabetes mellitus, 24, 230, 297, 297f
    epidemiology, 49
    optimization strategy, 49

Diabetic foot infections (DFI), 263
    antibiotic treatment, 266, 267t
    antibiotic use, duration of, 267, 268t
    biofilms, 266
    chronic osteomyelitis, 264–266
    clinical characteristics, 264, 264t
    orthopaedic surgery for, 268–269
    pathogens, 266
    patient care, 263–264
    residual infection, 268
    soft-tissue infection, 264
Diabetic foot ulcer (DFU), 263–264
Diphosphonates, 156
Duration of Antibiotic Treatment in Prosthetic Joint Infection (DATIPO) trial, 199

E

Eikenella corrodens, 274
Elution studies, antimicrobial delivery, 223
End-stage renal disease (ESRD), 25
Epidural abscess (EDA), 282, 285f
Erythrocyte sedimentation rate (ESR)
    fracture-related infection, 213
    prosthetic joint infection, 156–157, 200
Escherichia coli, 196
European Bone and Joint Infection Society, prosthetic joint infection, 161, 160f

F

Fasciitis, necrotizing, 295
Felon, 274
Fluorodeoxyglucose-positron emission tomography (FDG-PET), 65
    fracture-related infection, 214
    spine infections, 285–286
Fluoroquinolones, 136
Fournier gangrene, 295
Fracture-related infection (FRI), 4, 5f, 209
    biologics, 237
    bone grafting, 236
    bone transport, 237
    clinical assessment, 230
    clinical management, 229
    diagnostic criteria, 210t
        histopathology, 215
        medical imaging, 214
        microbiology, 213–214
        molecular diagnostics, 214–215
        monomicrobial, 211, 211f
        polymicrobial, 211, 212f–213f
    fracture stabilization, 234–236
    free vascularized bone grafting, 237
    host optimization, 230–231
    incidence of, 209–210
    local antimicrobial therapy, 234
    socioeconomic effect, 215–216
    surgical débridement, 231–232
    systemic antimicrobial therapy
        choice of, 232, 233t–234t
        duration of therapy, 233–234
        route of administration, 232–233

    treatment of, 229
Fractures
    fixation, 224
    open, 221, 223
        antibiotics, 222–223
        débridement, 223–224
        external fixation, 224
        Gustilo-Anderson classification system of, 222, 222t
        initial management of, 222
        injury evaluation, 221–222
        intramedullary nailing, 224
        irrigation, 223–224
        patient evaluation, 221–222
        plate-and-screw fixation, 224
        soft-tissue reconstruction, 225
        stabilization of, 224
        wound closure, 224–225
    stabilization
        external fixation, 234–235
        internal fixation, 234–235
        intramedullary fixation, 235
        plate fixation, 235
        soft-tissue coverage, 235–236
FRI. *See* Fracture-related infection (FRI)

G

Gentamycin, 169
Gram-negative bacilli infection, 196, 197t
Gunshot trauma, 15
Gunshot wounds (GSWs), 15
Gustilo-Anderson fracture classification system, 222, 222t

H

Hand infections, 273–277
    animal bites, 274–275
    bacterial, 274–277
    bone, 276
    complicating factors, 277
    epidemiology, 273
    evaluation, 273–274
    felon, 274
    human bites, 274
    joint, 276
    microbiology, 273
    mimickers of, 277, 277f
    necrotizing, 276–277, 276f, 276t
    palmar space, 275, 276f
    paronychia, 274
    purulent flexor tenosynovitis, 275, 275f
HEPA air filter, 33
Hepatitis disease, 25
Hip
    arthroscopy, 14
    prosthetic joint infection, clinical presentation in, 156
    two-stage revision arthroplasty, 168–171, 170f
Histopathologic assessment, of fracture-related infection, 214
Hydrogen peroxide, 95, 182

Index

Hyperglycemia
  epidemiology, 49
  optimization strategy, 49
Hypochlorous acid, 96

I

Immunosuppression, 24–25
Instrument trays, 35
Interleukin 6 (IL-6), 157
International Consensus Meeting (ICM), 62, 157, 159–161, 159f
Intervertebral disks, in children, 280–281
Intramedullary nailing, open fractures, 224
Irrigation agents
  antibiotics, 92
  antiseptics
    acetic acid, 92–93
    chlorhexidine gluconate, 94–95
    commercial, 96–97
    hydrogen peroxide, 95
    hypochlorous acid, 96
    povidone-iodine, 93–94
    sodium hypochlorite, 95
  delivery method, 97–98, 97t
  duration, 98
  open fractures, 223–224
  surfactants, 91–92
  volume, 98

J

Joint, prior surgery in, 12–14, 14f

K

Kingella kingae, 245
Knee
  arthrodesis, 173, 173f–174f
  prosthetic joint infection, 156
  two-stage revision arthroplasty, 168, 168f–170f

L

Laboratory Risk Indicator for Necrotizing Fasciitis (LRINEC) score, 276, 276t, 296
Laminar airflow (LAF), 33
Leukocyte esterase strip test, prosthetic joint infection, 157
Lipoglycopeptides, 137
Liver disease, 25
Local antibiotic delivery methods
  antibiotic powder, 117
  antibiotic selection, 117, 118t
  calcium sulfate, 116–117
  chitosans, 117
  clinical applications, 119t
  complications
    beads, 122
    calcium sulfate, 122
    chitosans, 122
    spacers, 122
  contraindications, 121–122
  future directions, 122–123, 123t
  history, 115–116
  orthopaedic infections, 115
  orthopaedic trauma, 118–119
  osteomyelitis, 119, 120t–121t
  polymethyl methacrylate, 116
  prosthetic joint infections, 119–121
Local patient risk factors
  bacterial/fungal skin burden, 12
  boils, 12
  gunshot trauma, 15
  hair management, 15
  joint/area, prior surgery in, 12–14, 14f
  prior local infection, 15
  skin breakdowns, 12
  skin lesions, 12
  skin preparation, 15
  Staphylococcus species, colonization with, 11
  ulcerations, 12
Low-friction articulating knee spacer, 168, 170f
Lyme disease, 254

M

Magnetic resonance imaging (MRI), 65
  acute hematogenous osteomyelitis, 245
  animal bites, 299
  diabetic foot infections, 265, 265f
  fracture-related infection, 214
  musculoskeletal infection, 248
  necrotizing soft-tissue infections, 296
  nonnecrotizing soft-tissue infections, 299
  prosthetic joint infection, 156–161, 184
  septic arthritis, 256
  spine infections, 284–285, 285f, 288f, 289
Malnutrition, 22
  epidemiology, 51
  optimization strategy, 51
Mass spectrometry analysis, prosthetic joint infection, 158
Methicillin-resistant *Staphylococcus aureus* (MRSA), 11
  acute hematogenous osteomyelitis, 245
  open fractures, 223
  primary septic arthritis, 247
  septic arthritis, 254, 257
Microbiologic diagnosis, 73–76, 74t–75t
Modifiable risk factors
  alcohol abuse, 22–23
  anemia, 22
  depression, 21, 22t
  malnutrition, 22
  obesity, 23
  smoking, 22
Monomicrobial fracture-related infection, 211, 211f
Musculoskeletal infections
  diagnostic radiology of
    computed tomography, 65
    fluorodeoxyglucose-positron emission tomography, 65
    magnetic resonance imaging, 65
    plain radiography, 64
    scintigraphy, 65
    single-photon emission computed tomography, 65
    ultrasonography, 64–65
  microbiology of, 69–76
  pediatric, 243
    acute hematogenous osteomyelitis, 243–246, 244f–245t
    contiguous osteomyelitis, 248–249
    primary septic arthritis, 246–248
    septic arthritis, 248–249
  in vitro studies, 66
  in vivo studies, 66
Musculoskeletal Infection Society (MSIS), 158–159
Mycobacteria, 73
Mycobacterium tuberculosis, 256
Myositis, necrotizing, 295

N

Nasal decolonization, 42
Native infections
  osteomyelitis, 73–75
  other orthopaedic infectious syndromes, 75–76
  septic arthritis, 75
Necrotizing cellulitis, 295, 296f
Necrotizing fasciitis, 295
Necrotizing infections, 276–277, 276f, 276t
Necrotizing myositis, 295
Necrotizing soft-tissue infections (NSTIs)
  antimicrobial therapy, 297–298, 298f
  clinical findings in, 295, 295f
  clinical management, 297–298
  diagnosis of, 295–296, 296t
  imaging findings, 296
  laboratory findings, 296
  medicolegal implications of, 294–295
  microbiology of, 295
  mortality, 294
  risk factors, 294, 294t
  surgical interventions, 297, 297f
Negative pressure wound therapy (NPWT), 225
Neisseria gonorrhoeae, 254
Next-generation sequencing (NGS)
  fracture-related infection, 214–215
  prosthetic joint infection, 158
Nicotine, 231
Nonarticulating (Girdlestone) spacers, 168, 170f
Nonmodifiable risk factors
  chronic renal disease, 25
  diabetes mellitus, 24
  dialysis, 25
  end-stage renal disease, 25
  gender, 23
  hepatitis and liver disease, 25
  immunosuppression, 24–25

Index

NSTIs. *See* Necrotizing soft-tissue infections (NSTIs)
Nuclear imaging
    fracture-related infection, 214
    prosthetic joint infection, 156, 184

O

Obesity, 23, 295*f*
    epidemiology, 47–48
    optimization strategy, 48, 48*f*
Open fractures, 221
    antibiotics
        local delivery, 223
        systemic administration, 222–223
    débridement, 223–224
    external fixation, 224
    Gustilo-Anderson classification system of, 222, 222*t*
    initial management of, 222
    injury evaluation, 221–222
    intramedullary nailing, 224
    irrigation, 223–224
    patient evaluation, 221–222
    plate-and-screw fixation, 224
    soft-tissue reconstruction, 225
    stabilization of, 224
    wound closure
        delayed, 225
        primary, 224–225
Open reduction and internal fixation (ORIF), 3, 5, 7, 13–14, 23–25
Operating room environmental risk factors
    airborne organism load
        air quality monitoring, 32
        organism profile, 32
        particles, as contamination, 32
        reducing air contamination, 32
    back table, 35
    device-related infection, 31
    HEPA air filter, 33
    instrument trays, 35
    laminar airflow, 33
    light handles, 34–35
    patient normothermia, 34
    personal protection suits, 34
    reducing operating room traffic, 32–33
    splash basins, 35
    temperature, 34
    ultraclean ventilation systems, 33
    ultraviolet light decontamination, 33–34
Oral antimicrobial therapy, for prosthetic joint infection, 196–198
Oral versus Intravenous Antibiotics for Bone and Joint Infection (OVIVA) trial, 196, 198
Orthopaedic infections, 115
    bacteria, 71–73
    biofilms, 70–71
    biomarkers, 62
    culture-based methods, 69–70
    fungi, 73
    microbiologic diagnosis, 73–76, 74*t*–75*t*
    microbiology laboratory, 70–71

    molecular pathogen detection in, 71
    mycobacteria, 73
    pathogenesis, 73–76, 74*t*–75*t*
Orthopaedic trauma, 118–119
Osteomyelitis, 73–75, 119, 120*t*–121*t*, 299. *See also* Acute hematogenous osteomyelitis (AHO)
    chronic, 264–266
    complications, 246
    contiguous, 248–249
    deep vein thrombosis, 246
    diabetic foot ulcer, 264
Outpatient parenteral antimicrobial therapy (OPAT), 110–111
Oxazolidinones, 138

P

Palmar space infections, 275, 276*f*
Paronychia, 274
Patient optimization, infection prevention
    anemia, 50
    diabetes mellitus, 49
    hyperglycemia, 49
    malnutrition, 51
    obesity, 47–48
    smoking, 49–50
    tobacco use, 49–50
Physical therapy, septic arthritis, 258
PJI. *See* Prosthetic joint infection (PJI)
Polymerase chain reaction (PCR)
    fracture-related infection, 214–215
    primary septic arthritis, 247
    prosthetic joint infection, 158
    septic arthritis, 256
    spine infections, 287
Polymethyl methacrylate (PMMA), 116, 223, 234
Polymicrobial fracture-related infection, 211, 212*f*–213*f*
Polymicrobial (type I) necrotizing fasciitis, 297, 297*f*
Polymorphonuclear leukocyte percentage, prosthetic joint infection, 157
Povidone-iodine, 93–94
Primary septic arthritis, 246
    management, approach to, 247–248
    spectrum of, 247
Procalcitonin, 157
Propionibacterium acnes, 181
Prosthetic joint infection (PJI), 76, 119–121
    antibiotic treatment of, 195–201
        culture-negative, 196
        duration of, 199–200
        empiric treatment regimens, 196
        monitoring during, 200–201
        oral antimicrobial therapy for, 196–198
        preoperative, 195
        rifampin combination therapy, 198–199
        targeted regimens, 196
    computed tomography, 156
    débridement, antibiotics, and implant retention procedure
        clinical outcomes, 166–167, 167*t*

        indications, 165–166
        surgical technique, 166
    diagnosis of, 156–161
    European Bone and Joint Infection Society criteria, 161, 160*f*
    hip
        clinical presentation in, 156
        surgical treatment of, 165–175
    International Consensus Meeting criteria, 159–161, 159*f*
    knee
        clinical presentation in, 156
        surgical treatment of, 165–175
    magnetic resonance imaging, 156–161
    Musculoskeletal Infection Society criteria, 158–159
    nuclear imaging, 156
    plain radiographs, 156
    preoperative and intraoperative testing
        microbial identification, 157–158
        pathology, 157
        serologic markers, 156–157
        synovial fluid analysis, 157
    salvage procedures, 173–174, 173*f*–174*f*
    shoulder, 181
        clinical outcomes, 188–189
        clinical presentation, 156, 182–183, 183*f*, 184*t*
        diagnostic criteria, 186, 186*t*
        epidemiology of, 181–182
        incidence of, 181–182
        postoperative antibiotics, 187–188
        surgical management of, 186–187, 187*f*–188*f*
        surgical prophylaxis, 182
        workup, 183–186, 185*f*
    single-stage revision arthroplasty, 172–173
    in total joint arthroplasty, 155–156
    two-stage revision arthroplasty, 167–172
    ultrasonography, 156
Pseudomonas aeruginosa, 196, 266
Purulent flexor tenosynovitis, 275, 275*f*
Pyomyositis, 298

Q

Quality of life (QoL), 6–7

R

Radiography, 170*f*
    animal bites, 299
    diabetic Charcot foot, 265*f*
    fracture-related infection, 214
    musculoskeletal infection, 64
    osteomyelitis, 248
    prosthetic joint infection, 156
Randomized controlled trials (RCTs)
    antibiotic spacers, 169
    prosthetic joint infection, 156
    rifampin, in staphylococcal prosthetic joint, 198, 198*t*
    systemic antimicrobial therapy, 232–233
Resistance, surgical site infections, 5–6

Index

Revision arthroplasty, prosthetic joint infection
  1.5-stage, 172
  single-stage
    clinical outcomes, 173
    indications, 173
    technique, 172–173
  two-stage, 167
    antibiotic spacers and, 168–171, 168f–170f
    outcomes following, 171–172
Rifampin
  for *Cutibacterium* species, 198–199
  for *Staphylococcus* species, 198, 198t
  for *Streptococcus* species, 198
Rifamycins, 131–136

S

SAT. *See* Suppressive antibiotic therapy (SAT)
Scintigraphy, 65
Septic arthritis, 75, 253
  blood tests, 256–257
  clinical presentation, 255
  contiguous osteomyelitis and, 248–249, 244f–245f
  diagnostic testing, 255–257
  differential diagnosis of, 255, 255t
  incidence of, 253
  joint destruction in, 254, 254f
  magnetic resonance imaging, 256
  microbiology, 254–255, 255t
    testing, 256
  pathogenesis of, 253–254
  primary, 246
    management, approach to, 247–248
    spectrum of, 247
  synovial fluid analysis, 256
  treatment
    antibiotic therapy, 257–258, 257t
    physical therapy, 258
    source control, 257
  ultrasonography, 256
Septic facet joints (SFJs), 286–287, 288f
Shoulder, prosthetic joint infection, 181
  clinical outcomes, 188–189
  clinical presentation, 156, 182–183, 183f, 184t
  diagnostic criteria, 186, 186t
  epidemiology of, 181–182
  incidence of, 181–182
  postoperative antibiotics, 187–188
  surgical management of, 186–187, 187f–188f
  surgical prophylaxis, 182
  workup, 183–186, 185f
Single-photon emission computed tomography (SPECT), 65
Single-purpose diagnostic tests, 62
Single-stage revision arthroplasty
  clinical outcomes, 173
  indications, 173
  technique, 172–173
Skin and soft-tissue infections (SSTIs), 293–300

abscess, 300
animal bites, 299–300
classification of, 293–294
necrotizing soft-tissue infections
  antimicrobial therapy, 297–298, 298t
  clinical findings in, 295, 295f
  clinical management, 297–298
  diagnosis of, 295–296, 296t
  imaging findings, 296
  laboratory findings, 296
  medicolegal implications of, 294–295
  microbiology of, 295
  mortality, 294
  risk factors, 294, 294t
  surgical interventions, 297, 297f
nonnecrotizing, 298–299
Skin hair management, 15
Skin integrity, 42
Skin preparation/decolonization, 15, 42
Smoking, 22, 231
  epidemiology, 49
  optimization strategy, 49–50
Sodium hypochlorite, 95
Soft-tissue coverage, 235–236
Spinal hardware, 76
Spine infections, 281–289
  anatomy, 281–282
  clinical presentation, 283–287, 284t
  diagnosis, 283–287
  etiology of, 282
  imaging, 284t
  incidence of, 281
  microbiology, 282–283
  physiology of, 281–282
  therapy, 284t
  treatment of, 288–289
Splash basins, 35
SSTIs. *See* Skin and soft-tissue infections (SSTIs)
Staphylococcus aureus, 71–72, 196, 266
  abscess, 300
  acute hematogenous osteomyelitis, 245
  prosthetic joint infection, 166
  pyomyositis, 298
  septic arthritis, 254
  spine infections, 282–283
Staphylococcus epidermidis, 12, 283
  coagulase-negative staphylococci infection, 196
  prosthetic joint infection, 166
Stealth infections, 183
Streptococcus agalactiae, 196, 283
Streptococcus dysgalactiae, 283
Streptococcus pneumoniae, 283
Streptococcus pyogenes, 283
Streptococcus viridans, 283
Suppressive antibiotic therapy (SAT), 200
  adverse events, 149
  antibiotic selection, 144–145, 145f
  efficacy, 145–148
  medical and surgical factors, 144t
  suppression, duration of, 148–149
Surgical site infections (SSIs)
  economics of, 6
  intraoperative strategies, 43t

  surgical techniques, 43
  wound closure, 43
local patient risk factors
  bacterial/fungal skin burden, 12
  boils, 12
  gunshot trauma, 15
  hair management, 15
  joint/area, prior surgery in, 12–14, 14f
  prior local infection, 15
  skin breakdowns, 12
  skin lesions, 12
  skin preparation, 15
  Staphylococcus species, colonization with, 11
  ulcerations, 12
organism profile, 4–5
preoperative strategies
  nasal decolonization, 42
  skin hair removal, 42
  skin integrity, 42
  skin preparation and decolonization, 42
prevalence, 3–4
quality of life, 6–7
resistance, 5–6
systemic patient risk factors
  modifiable, 21–23
  nonmodifiable, 23–25
Synovial alpha-defensin, 184
Synovial biomarker test, prosthetic joint infection, 157
Synovial fluid analysis, prosthetic joint infection, 157
Synovial fluid biomarkers, 63–64
Synovial leukocyte esterase testing, 184
Systemic antibiotic therapy
  antimicrobials, 132t–135t
  beta-lactam antibiotics, 136–137
  clindamycin, 138
  daptomycin, 137
  fluoroquinolones, 136
  lipoglycopeptides, 137
  oral *vs.* intravenous therapy, 130–131
  oxazolidinones, 138
  rifamycins, 131–136
  tetracyclines, 138
  trimethoprim/sulfamethoxazole, 138–139
  vancomycin, 137
Systemic patient risk factors
  modifiable
    alcohol abuse, 22–23
    anemia, 22
    depression, 21
    malnutrition, 22
    obesity, 23
    smoking, 22
  nonmodifiable
    chronic renal disease, 25
    diabetes mellitus, 24
    dialysis, 25
    end-stage renal disease, 25
    gender, 23
    hepatitis and liver disease, 25
    immunosuppression, 24–25

Index

T

Tetracyclines, 138
Tobacco use
    epidemiology, 49
    optimization strategy, 49–50
Tobramycin, 169
Total joint arthroplasty, prosthetic joint infection in, 155–156
Total knee arthroplasty (TKA)
    low-friction articulating knee spacer, 168, 170f
    prosthetic knee infection, 168, 169f
Trimethoprim/sulfamethoxazole (TMP-SMX), 138–139
Two-stage revision arthroplasty, 167
    antibiotic spacers and, 168–171, 168f–170f
    outcomes following, 171–172

U

Ulcerations, 12
Ultraclean ventilation systems, 33
Ultrasonography, 64–65
    necrotizing soft-tissue infections, 296
    nonnecrotizing soft-tissue infections, 299
    prosthetic joint infection, 156
    septic arthritis, 256
Ultraviolet light decontamination, 33–34

V

Vancomycin, 137, 169
    coagulase-negative staphylococci infection, 196
    open fractures, 223
Vitamin D homeostasis, for fracture healing, 231

W

Whipple disease, 255
Wounds
    closure, 43
        delayed, 225
        primary, 224–225
    contamination, 35
    cultures, 92
    dressing, 236
    environment, 223
    healing, 24, 92, 298
    serous drainage, 237